Cell Pathology

Cell Pathology

Edited by **Hans Affleck**

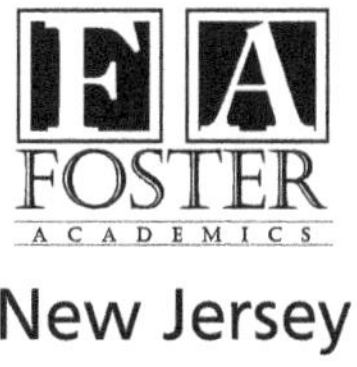

New Jersey

Published by Foster Academics,
61 Van Reypen Street,
Jersey City, NJ 07306, USA
www.fosteracademics.com

Cell Pathology
Edited by Hans Affleck

International Standard Book Number: 978-1-63242-455-6 (Hardback)

Printed in the United States of America.

Contents

Preface

This book unravels the recent studies in the field of cell pathology. It deals with the diagnosis of diseases at cellular level, and also determines how the cellular and molecular mechanisms work in these conditions. It is commonly used to detect thyroid lesions, sterile body cavities, infectious diseases, and some other inflammatory conditions. But one of the most important applications of cytopathology is to diagnose cancerous cells. This book strives to provide a fair idea about this discipline and to help develop a better understanding of the latest advances within this area. Students, researchers, pathologists, experts and all associated with cell pathology will benefit alike from this book.

This book is a result of research of several months to collate the most relevant data in the field.

When I was approached with the idea of this book and the proposal to edit it, I was overwhelmed. It gave me an opportunity to reach out to all those who share a common interest with me in this field. I had 3 main parameters for editing this text:

1. Accuracy – The data and information provided in this book should be up-to-date and valuable to the readers.
2. Structure – The data must be presented in a structured format for easy understanding and better grasping of the readers.
3. Universal Approach – This book not only targets students but also experts and innovators in the field, thus my aim was to present topics which are of use to all.

Thus, it took me a couple of months to finish the editing of this book.

I would like to make a special mention of my publisher who considered me worthy of this opportunity and also supported me throughout the editing process. I would also like to thank the editing team at the back-end who extended their help whenever required.

Editor

1

An Efficient Protocol for Deriving Liver Stem Cells from Neonatal Mice: Validating Its Differentiation Potential

Sugapriya Dhanasekaran,[1,2] Devilakshmi Sithambaram,[1] Kavitha Govarthanan,[1] Bijesh Kumar Biswal,[1] and Rama S. Verma[1]

[1] *Stem Cell and Molecular Biology Lab, Department of Biotechnology, Bhupat and Jyoti Mehta School of Biosciences, Indian Institute of Technology Madras, Chennai, Tamil Nadu 600036, India*
[2] *Department of Medical Laboratory Sciences (Haematology), College of Applied Medical Sciences, Prince Sattam Bin Abdul-Aziz University, Wadi Ad Dawaser Campus, P.O. Box 54, Riyadh, Saudi Arabia*

Correspondence should be addressed to Rama S. Verma; vermars@iitm.ac.in

Academic Editor: Alfredo Procino

The success of liver regeneration depends on the availability of suitable cell types and their potential to differentiate into functional hepatocytes. To identify the stem cells which have the ability to differentiate into hepatocytes, we used neonatal liver as source. However, the current protocol for isolating stem cells from liver involves enzymes like collagenase, hyaluronidase exposed for longer duration which limits the success. This results in the keen interest to develop an easy single step enzyme digestion protocol for isolating stem cells from liver for tissue engineering approaches. Thus, the unlimited availability of cell type favors setting up the functional recovery of the damaged liver, ensuring ahead success towards treating liver diseases. We attempted to isolate liver stem derived cells (LDSCs) from mouse neonatal liver using single step minimal exposure to enzyme followed by *in vitro* culturing. The cells isolated were characterized for stem cell markers and subjected to lineage differentiation. Further, LDSCs were induced to hepatocyte differentiation and validated with hepatocyte markers. Finally, we developed a reproducible, efficient protocol for isolation of LDSCs with functional hepatocytes differentiation potential, which further can be used as *in vitro* model system for assessing drug toxicity assays in various preclinical trials.

1. Introduction

The ability to isolate and expand liver-derived stem cells (LDSCs) is a crucial step towards the success of tissue engineering approaches for liver repair, regeneration for therapeutic purpose, and developing suitable scaffold for liver tissue engineering. Stem cells from the liver tissue can be good candidate cell types of interest in various approaches for regeneration therapy. Liver stem cells having potential to maintain liver homeostasis have considerable therapeutic potential. Hepatic progenitor cells are multipotent stem cells, which exhibit unlimited proliferation giving rise to hepatocytes and bile-duct epithelial cells, residing in the canals of Hering in human and animal livers [1, 2], and *in vivo* terminally differentiated hepatocytes lack the proliferative potential in response to liver injury [3–5]; hence, hepatic progenitor cells may serve as an ideal source for hepatocyte that can be used for transplantation approaches [6–12]. Human fetal liver progenitor cells maintain multipotent capability to differentiate into liver, mesenchymal lineages, and cartilage cells and also have repopulation capacity in a mouse model of liver injury [9].

These hepatocyte progenitor cells are capable of multiple cell divisions and have been identified without a preceding injury to the liver [13]. Earlier reports showed that bipotential clonal cell lines were isolated from adult murine liver [14], and also a report stated that α-fetoprotein (AFP) positive cells from adult liver with immature endodermal characteristics were capable of differentiating into both hepatic and biliary cell lineages [15]. Many studies have reported the isolation and purification of liver stem cells directly from the bone marrow using two-step magnetic bead cell sorting procedure [16]. Another report followed the isolation and purification of hepatic stem cell by two-step collagenase perfusion technique, simple gravity enrichment, and immunomagnetic cell sorting methods followed by flow cytometry cell sorting [17]. Earlier study showed that short repetitive trypsinization of heart tissue helps in obtaining a higher yield of viable cardiomyocytes rather than a single digestion for longer period [18].

Various current protocols used enzymes like collagenase, hyaluronidase, or both in combination exposed for a longer duration followed by high speed differential centrifugation using Ficoll density gradient method. Enzyme digestion and LDSCs enrichment are the two crucial steps which determine the success of isolation and culturing of the neonatal liver-derived stem cell *in vitro*. Several techniques, including slow speed centrifugation steps followed after partial collagenase digestion, and Ficoll fractionation, sorted based on the markers expression, have been used to culture neonatal murine LDSCs [11, 14, 19–21]. The enzyme digestion step for dissociating cells from liver tissue is too critical which determines the success of isolating viable neonatal liver stem cells [22]. Although the repetitive digestion with various enzyme combinations gives good yield, long-term enzyme digestion leads to toxicity which limits the success of higher yield in isolating viable cell [23].

In this study, we devised a simple and reproducible protocol for the isolation and culture of LDSCs from neonatal liver and their maintenance in primary cultures that consistently yield long-term liver-derived stem cell cultures. The protocol followed has advantages over the current available protocols, which circumvents the use of any growth supplements, without any collagenase digestion followed by single step enrichment for removing fibroblast contamination.

2. Materials and Methods

2.1. Animals. Commonly used mouse strains, BALB/c, were used in this protocol. The normal inbred 1- to 2-day-old neonatal mice (male and female) were procured from the King's Institute, Chennai, India. All experiments in this protocol were performed in accordance with the Institutional Animal Ethics Committee (IIT Madras, India, the Committee for the Purpose of Control and Supervision of Experiments on Animals, Government of India). It is preferred to use the neonatal mice (1-2 days old), as our previous observations for cardiomyocytes have shown that younger animals (newborn up to 1-2 days) produce more proliferative cell cultures enrichment [18].

2.2. Cell Preparation and Culture. Neonatal mice 1-2-day-old Balb/c pups were euthanized by cervical dislocation. The euthanized pups were rinsed completely in a beaker with 50 mL of 70% (vol/vol) ethanol for 2 min. Then, it was placed in a 100 mm sterile glass dish and incisions were made in the skin of the inguinal region; the muscles were disassociated and the liver was removed aseptically and immediately transferred into ice-cold phosphate-buffered saline (PBS; Ca^{2+} and Mg^{2+} free and 0.1% (vol/vol) penicillin/streptomycin) for 2-3 min. The excised livers were washed again with chilled PBS followed by another wash with sterile ice-cold balanced salt solution (20 mM hydroxyethyl piperazine ethanesulfonic acid, NaOH [pH 7.6], 130 mM NaCl, 1 mM NaH_2PO_4, 4 mM glucose, and 3 mM KCl), in which the tissue was kept for 10 min. The livers were then minced with a sterile scalpel blade into small pieces less than or equal to 1 mm^3 in 2 mL of 0.05% trypsin ethylenediamine tetraacetic acid (EDTA; Invitrogen, Carlsbad, CA; 0.1 mL per liver) and transferred into sterile 15 mL falcon tubes. The hepatic cells were digested by incubating with 0.25% (wt/vol) trypsin 0.02% (wt/vol) EDTA (~1 mL of 0.25% trypsin for every 100 mg of tissue), which was then mixed by intermittent pipetting along with stirring at 37°C in a water bath for 4 min. The cell suspension was allowed to stand for 1 min.

The supernatant containing single cells suspension was collected into a fresh 15 mL falcon tube kept on ice, to which 2 mL Dulbecco's modified Eagle's medium (DMEM)/F12 (1 : 1) medium (Gibco, Carlsbad, CA) supplemented with 20% fetal calf serum (Gibco) was added, and the digestion step was repeated three times. The cell suspension from each digestion was pooled and centrifuged at 3,500 rpm for 10 min at 4°C. The trypsin digestion was then neutralized with complete medium containing FCS. The cell pellet was washed twice in DMEM/F12 (1 : 1) medium supplemented with fetal calf serum (10%) and we finally seeded the enzyme-neutralized cell suspension into a 25 cm^2 plastic culture flask in the presence of 6 mL of growth medium containing DMEM/F12 (1 : 1) medium supplemented with fetal calf serum (20%), horse serum (Gibco) (5%), penicillin (100 U/mL), amphotericin B (25 μg/mL) and streptomycin (100 mg/mL; Cambrex, Verviers, Belgium), 2 mM L-glutamine (Cambrex), 0.1 mM nonessential amino acids (Gibco), 3 mM sodium pyruvate (Gibco), and bovine insulin (1 μg/mL; USV, India). The cells were plated on plates precoated with 1% gelatin and incubated in 95% air and 5% CO_2 at 37°C for ~2-3 h, to allow the differential attachment of fibroblast cells. The nonadhesive cells (LDSCs) were transferred into a sterile tube. Trypsin toxicity and cell viability of liver cells were assessed by trypan blue exclusion test as 85–90%. After counting, the LDSCs-enriched suspension was plated onto culture dishes at a density of 2×10^4 cells per cm^2. The cells were incubated in a humid 5% CO_2 incubator at 37°C.

Selective removal of nonadherent population ensures the success of getting homogenous population and minimizes the contamination with cells of hematopoietic origin. The medium was replenished after 3 d which removes nonadherent cells and tissue debris and replaced with 5 mL of the maintenance medium. The maintenance medium was changed after every 48 h. When it reached confluent, the adherent cells were harvested by removing the medium and adding 2 mL of 0.25% trypsin/EDTA and passaged with a split ratio of 1 : 3. The culture medium was changed every 48 h and passaged twice per week at a split ratio of 1 : 4 or 1 : 3. The cells at passages 3–8 were used for *in vitro* experiments.

2.3. LDSCs Characterizations

2.3.1. Immunophenotyping. Passage 4 LDSCs were harvested by trypsin digestion and the cells were centrifuged twice for 8 min, 300 ×g, at 4°C with 1 mL of cold PBS (range from 4 to 8°C). Then, resuspended 1×10^6 cells were mixed with 100 μL

Table 1: List of primers used in gene expression profiling.

Genes	Primer sequence (5′-3′)	Tm	Length
HNF-1α	FP: 5′-CGAAGATGGTCAAGTCGTAC-3′ RP: 5′-GGCAAACCAGTTGTAGACAC-3′	55°C	500 bp
HNF-1β	FP: 5′-TTCAGTCAACAGAACCAGGG-3′ RP: 5′-CTCTGTGCAATGGCCATGAC-3′	57.2°C	721 bp
HNF-3α	FP: 5′-CATGAGAGCAACGACTGGAA-3′ RP: 5′-TTGGCGTAGGACATGTTGAA-3′	55.2°C	182 bp
HNF-3β	FP: 5′-AGAGGACTGAGGTAACTGAC-3′ RP: 5′-GACTCGGACTCAGGTGAGGT-3′	60.2°C	415 bp
HNF-6	FP: 5′-CAGCGTATCACCACCGAGCT-5′ RP: 5′-CTCTGTCCTTCCCATGTTCT-3′	55°C	250 bp
C/EBP-α	FP: 5′-TGGACAAGAACAGCAACGAG-3′ RP: 5′-TCACTGGTCAACTCCAGCAC-3′	56°C	126 bp
C/EBP-β	FP: 5′-GAGCGACGAGTACAAGATGCG-3′ RP: 5′-TTGTGCTGCGTCTCCAGGTTG-3′	61°C	95 bp
GATA-4	FP: 5′-CTGTCATCTCACTATGGGCA-3′ RP: 5′-CAAGTCCGAGCAGGAATTTG-3′	59°C	257 bp
CK8	FP: 5′-ATCGAGATCACCACCTACCG-3′ RP: 5′-TGAAGCCAGGGCTAGTGAGT-3′	55°C	127 bp
CK18	FP: 5′-CGAGGCACTCAAGGAAGAAC-3′ RP: 5′-GCTGAGGTCCTGAGATTTGG-3′	57°C	130 bp
CK19	FP: 5′-ACCCTCCCGAGATTACAACC-3′ RP: 5′-CAAGGCGTGTTCTGTCTCAA-3′	58°C	160 bp
p450 Cyp3a11	FP: 5′-TGAGGCAGAAGGCAAAGAAA-3′ RP: 5′-GGTATTCCATCTCCATCACA-3′	55°C	590 bp
PXMP1-L	FP: 5′-CTTCAGACCCAGAGAGAGCTG-3′ RP: 5′-CCCGTGTTGCCTGTGATGAGC-3′	62°C	475 bp
Albumin	FP: 5′-TGAACTGGCTGACTGCTGTG-3′ RP: 5′-CATCCTTGGCCTCAGCATAG-3′	57°C	718 bp
Transthyretin	FP: 5′-AGTCCTGGATGCTGTCCGAG-3′ RP: 5′-TTCCTGAGCTGCTAACACGG-3′	62°C	440 bp
AFP	FP: 5′-TCGTATTCCAACAGGAGG-3′ RP: 5′-AGGCTTTTGCTTCACCAG-3′	55°C	174 bp
AAT	FP: 5′-AATGGAAGAAGCCATTCGAT-3′ RP: 5′-AAGACTGTAACTGCTGCAGC-3′	57.2°C	484 bp
β-actin (internal control)	FP: 5′-TTCCTTCTTGGGTATGGAAT-3′ RP: 5′-GAGCAATGATCTTGATCTTC-3′	55°C	206 bp

of cold PBS per Eppendorf tube and stain with anti-mouse or anti-goat EpCAM, Sca-1, CD29, CD44, CD105, GATA-4, CD34, CD45, and CD 90 for 1 h at 25°C and washed with cold PBS. The FITC-conjugated specific Ig antibodies and isotype antibodies were added, respectively, for 1 h at 25°C and washed with cold PBS. The concentrations of all primary antibodies were used in 1/200 dilution and 1/500 dilution of secondary antibodies was used for immunophenotype assays. The unstained cells were used as a control for all antibodies. The cells were washed again twice for 8 min, 300 ×g, at 4°C with 1 mL of cold PBS. Then paraformaldehyde (0.4%) was added to 200 μL of cold PBS and analyzed by FACS analysis, after excluding the dead cells by forward/side scatter gating (2,00,000 events per sample by FACS Calibur).

2.4. Multilineage Differentiation and Assessment

2.4.1. Differentiation of LDSCs to Osteogenic Lineage. Passage 4 LDSCs were harvested by trypsin digestion and the cells were seeded at a density of $5 \times 10^3/cm^2$ (or 1×10^4 per well) in a 24-well plate with α-MEM supplemented with 10% (vol/vol) FBS, 10^{-7} M dexamethasone, 10 mM β-glycerol phosphate, and 50 μM ascorbate-2-phosphate in a total volume of 500 μL. Cells cultured in α-MEM supplemented with 10% (vol/vol) FBS were used as a negative control. The medium was replenished twice per week and the culture was maintained for 4 weeks. During culture maintenance, the cells were not passaged. After 4 weeks, mineralization was confirmed by alizarin red S staining.

2.4.2. Assessment of Mineralization. Ca^{2+} mineralization of LDSCs induced to osteoblasts was assessed by Alizarin red biochemical staining, after 4 weeks of induction (with and without treatment for osteoblast for 4 weeks) [24]. The cells were rinsed with PBS and fixed with ice-cold 70% ethanol (Merck) for 1 h. The cells were washed twice with MQ H_2O and stained with 50 mM AR-S (pH 4.2) at RT for 10 min.

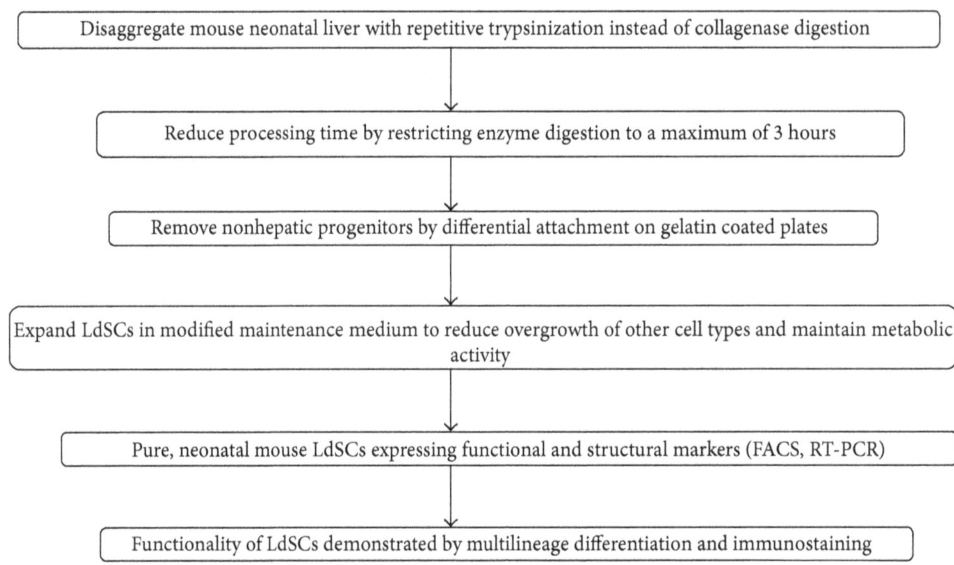

FIGURE 1: A schematic overview of the major steps followed in the isolation of LDSCs protocol.

The cells were rinsed five times with MQ H_2O succeeded by a 15 min wash with PBS with rotation to reduce nonspecific staining and the stained cells were photographed.

2.4.3. Differentiation of LDSCs to Adipogenic Lineage. Passage 4 LDSCs were seeded into a 24-well culture plate at a density of $1 \times 10^4/cm^2$ (or 2×10^4 per well) and incubated in α-MEM supplemented with 10% (vol/vol) FBS, 10^{-6} M dexamethasone, 0.5 μM IBMX, and 10 ng/mL (wt/vol) insulin in a total volume of 500 μL for 2 weeks. The cells were cultured in α-MEM supplemented with 10% (vol/vol) FBS as a negative control. Medium was changed twice per week and the culture was maintained for 2 weeks. Lipid accumulation was assessed biochemically by Oil Red O staining.

2.4.4. Assessment of Lipid Accumulation. To detect adipogenic differentiation following induction, Oil Red O (ORO) staining was performed as previously reported by [25] to monitor lipid accumulation with slight modifications. The cells were rinsed with PBS and fixed in 4% paraformaldehyde for 1 hr at RT. Cells were washed once with DPBS and twice with MQ H_2O. The cells were stained with 0.1% Oil Red O for 10 min at RT. The plates were washed with 60% of isopropanol to eliminate nonspecific staining and washed thrice with MQ H_2O and the cells were photographed.

2.4.5. Differentiation of LDSCs to Hepatocytes. Passage 4 LDSCs were seeded into a 24-well culture plate at a density of $1 \times 10^4/cm^2$ (2×10^4 per well) in serum deprived condition for two days in DMEM supplemented with 20 ng/mL epidermal growth factor (EGF) and 10 ng/mL basic fibroblast growth factor (bFGF), prior to differentiation. The medium was replenished after 2 d with differentiation medium that consisted of DMEM supplemented with 20 ng/mL hepatocyte growth factor (HGF), 10 ng/mL bFGF, and 0.61 g/L nicotinamide for six days (medium change was done every 3 days). The differentiation medium was replaced with maturation medium which consisted of DMEM supplemented with 20 ng/mL oncostatin M, 1 μmol/L dexamethasone (all from Sigma-Aldrich), and 50 mg/mL insulin. The medium was replenished twice per week and the culture was maintained for 3 weeks [26]. During cultural maintenance, the cells do not need to be passaged. Glycogen storage and albumin secretion were analyzed by periodic Acid-Schiff (PAS) staining and immunostaining, respectively.

2.4.6. Assessment of Glycogen Storage. Glycogen storage of LDSCs culture was evaluated using PAS staining. The cells were fixed with 4% paraformaldehyde, then oxidized in 1% periodic acid for 5 min, and rinsed in dH_2O. The cells were treated with Schiff's reagent for 15 min, and then color was developed in lukewarm dH_2O for 5–10 min and assessed under a light microscope.

2.5. Immunocytochemistry. Cells were fixed with 4% paraformaldehyde and for 30 min. Permeabilization was done with 0.5% Triton X-100 in PBS for 15 min. After the washing steps (3×5 min) with PBS, cells were kept in blocking buffer 3% BSA for 1 h. The samples were then incubated with primary antibody Anti-BSA rabbit polyclonal IgG (07-248 Upstate Biotechnology) at a 1:200 dilution for overnight at 4°C. The cells were washed twice with PBS and incubated with secondary antibody mouse anti-rabbit IgG-FITC for 1 h at 1:200 at 37°C. Nuclei staining was performed using Hoechst 33258. Cells were examined by fluorescence microscope.

2.6. Gene Expression Analysis by RT-PCR. Furthermore, expression profile of hepatic stem cell-specific transcription factors, structural and functional proteins were analyzed by reverse transcriptase-polymerase chain reaction (RT-PCR). Total RNAs from liver-derived stem cell, neonatal liver (NL), and adult liver (AL) were isolated on primary culture by using Trizol method. RNA was converted to cDNA by using M-MLV Reverse Transcriptase (New England Biologicals,

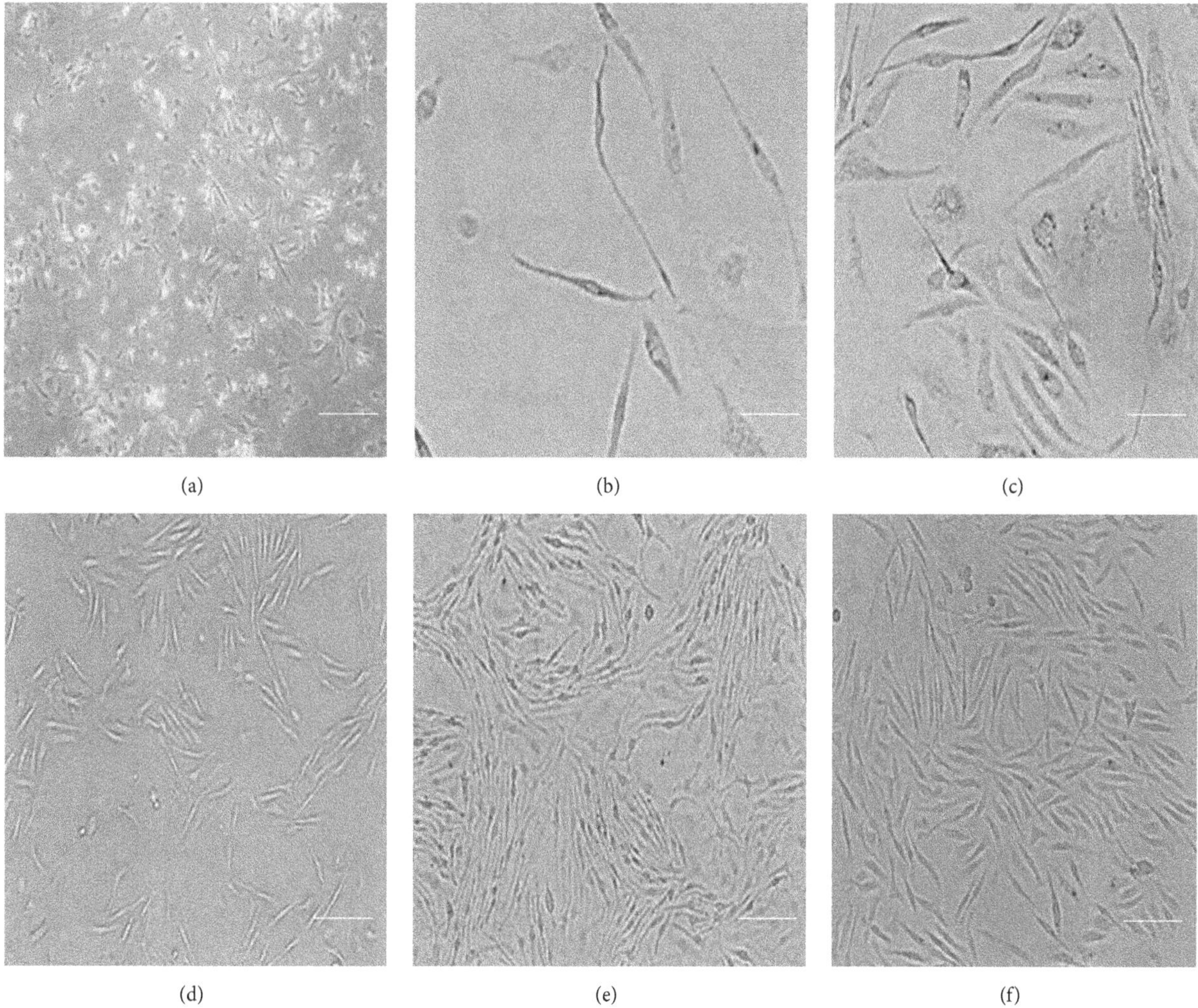

FIGURE 2: Morphological observation of liver-derived mouse stem cells. (a) LDSCs of different morphology were observed on 2nd day of culture (b, c) and after 3rd day elongated spindle shaped LDSCs were predominately observed from the initial culture. (d) LDSCs at their 60% confluency. (e) LDSCs at more than 90% confluent on day 6 of initial culture. (f) Passaged (P1) LDSCs at their 60% confluency. Scale bars represent 100 μm (a, d, e, and f) and 50 μm (a and b).

Beverly, MA) and was used as template for RT-PCR. The related PCR primers listed in Table 1 were used to produce the respective correlated products.

3. Results

3.1. Isolation of LDSCs. The aim of the current study is to derive stem cell populations from mouse neonatal liver using a simple and efficient protocol. LDSCs culture was isolated by digesting mouse neonatal liver with trypsin/EDTA for four minutes (Figure 1). The enzyme digested mixture was then seeded onto the flask already coated with 1% gelatin. Immediately after two to three hours, the culture medium along with the floating population of cells was transferred to another culture flask. Since most of all fibroblast-like cells adhere quickly to the gelatin coated culture flask, by changing to new culture flask it ensures the selective removal of fibroblasts. The reseeded suspension is mainly enriched with population of our interest, which adhered to the flask in 48 hours (Figure 2(a)). Further replenishing the adhered population with fresh media accelerated the growth and proliferation of the LDSC (Figures 2(b) and 2(c)) which was observed as increase in cell number inverted microscope (Nikon Eclipse TS100, Melville, NY).

An adherent population of spindle-shaped or vortex-shaped cells was observed after five days of culture (Figures 2(d) and 2(e)). The initial population of LDSC obtained after digestion was $0.3 \times 10^6/\text{mm}^2$ from every 100 mg of fetal liver tissue. Upon culture enrichment, the cell number of LDSC increased and reached confluency up to $0.2 \times 10^6/\text{mm}^2$ after 8 days (Figure 2(f)). After reaching confluency, the majority of the population morphologically appeared to be spindle-like cells. Briefly, after reaching confluency the cells were trypsinized, passaged, and maintained up to 4 weeks for further study.

3.2. Immunophenotyping of LDSCs. The cells were further characterized for their surface antigen by immunophenotyping. FACS analyses showed that majority of the populations were expressing markers like EpCAM, GATA-4, CD44,

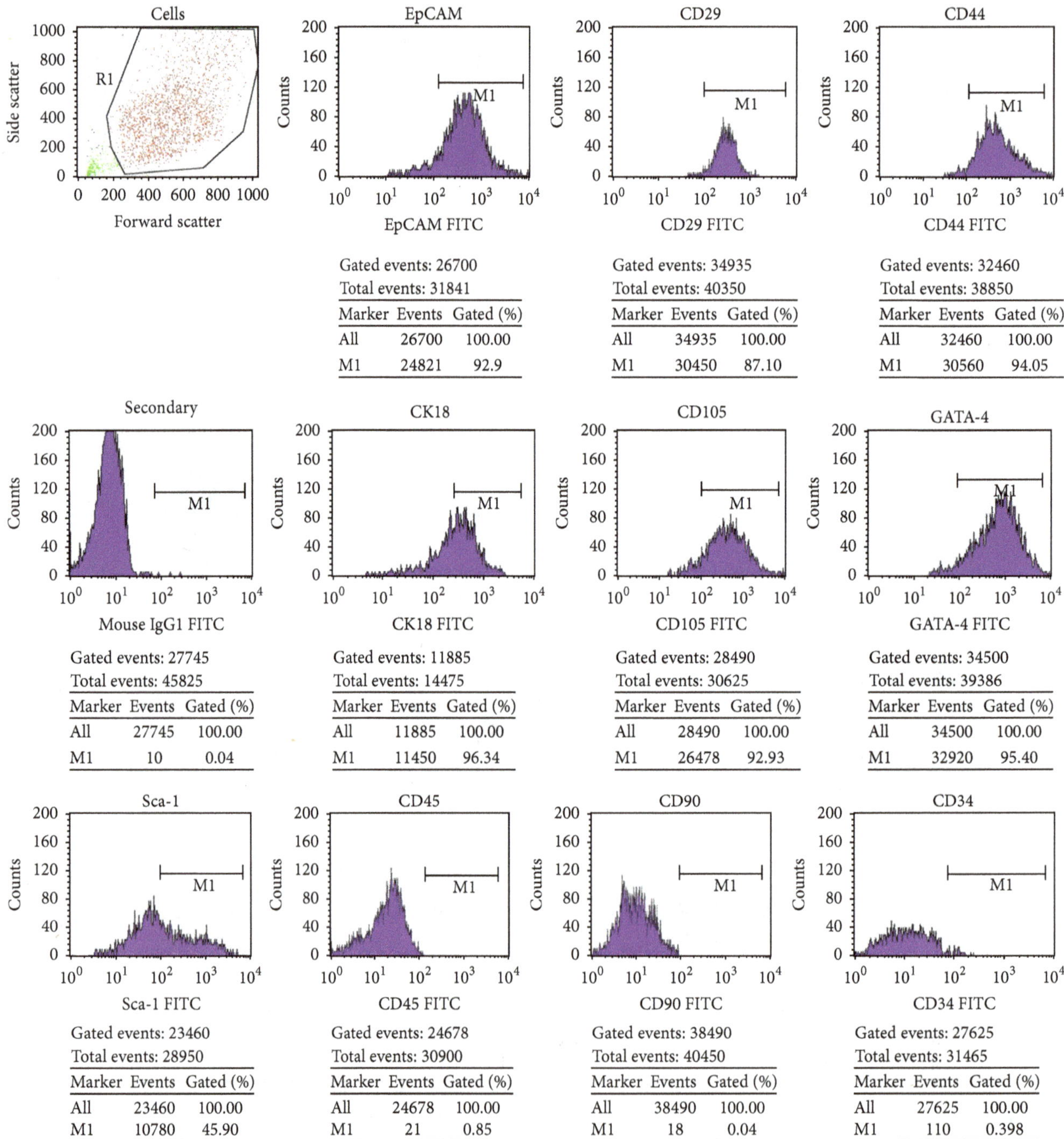

FIGURE 3: Immunophenotyping of LDSCs. Passaged 2 LDSCs were stained with fluorescein isothiocyanate (FITC) conjugated anti-mouse EpCAM, CD44, GATA-4, CD105, CD90, CD34, CK18 (Cytokeratin 18 (CK)), CD29, Sca-1, and CD45 along with its corresponding isotype control IgG1. FACS results showed that these cells were strong positive for liver stem cell markers EpCAM, GATA-4, CD44, CD105, CK18, and CD29 (β_1 integrin) in addition to weak positive for Sca-1 and negative for hematopoietic markers CD45, CD34, and CD 90.

CD105, and CD29 (β_1 integrin) more than 90% are suggesting strong positivity. In addition, LDSCs were found weak positive for Sca-1 and also negative for hematopoietic markers CD34, CD45, and CD 90 (Figure 3).

3.3. Multilineage Differentiation of LDSCs. LDSCs were induced to differentiate into lineages like osteoblasts, adipocytes, and hepatocytes. Passages 3–6 of LDSCs were used in the differentiation studies. Three weeks under the induction of osteogenic medium, LDSCs were differentiated into osteoblasts and was confirmed with alizarin red staining (Figures 4(c) and 4(d)) showed positive for the deposition of Ca^{2+} mineralization. Under adipogenic induction conditions for 3 weeks, the formation of intracellular microdroplets (accumulation of intracellular lipid droplets) was observed

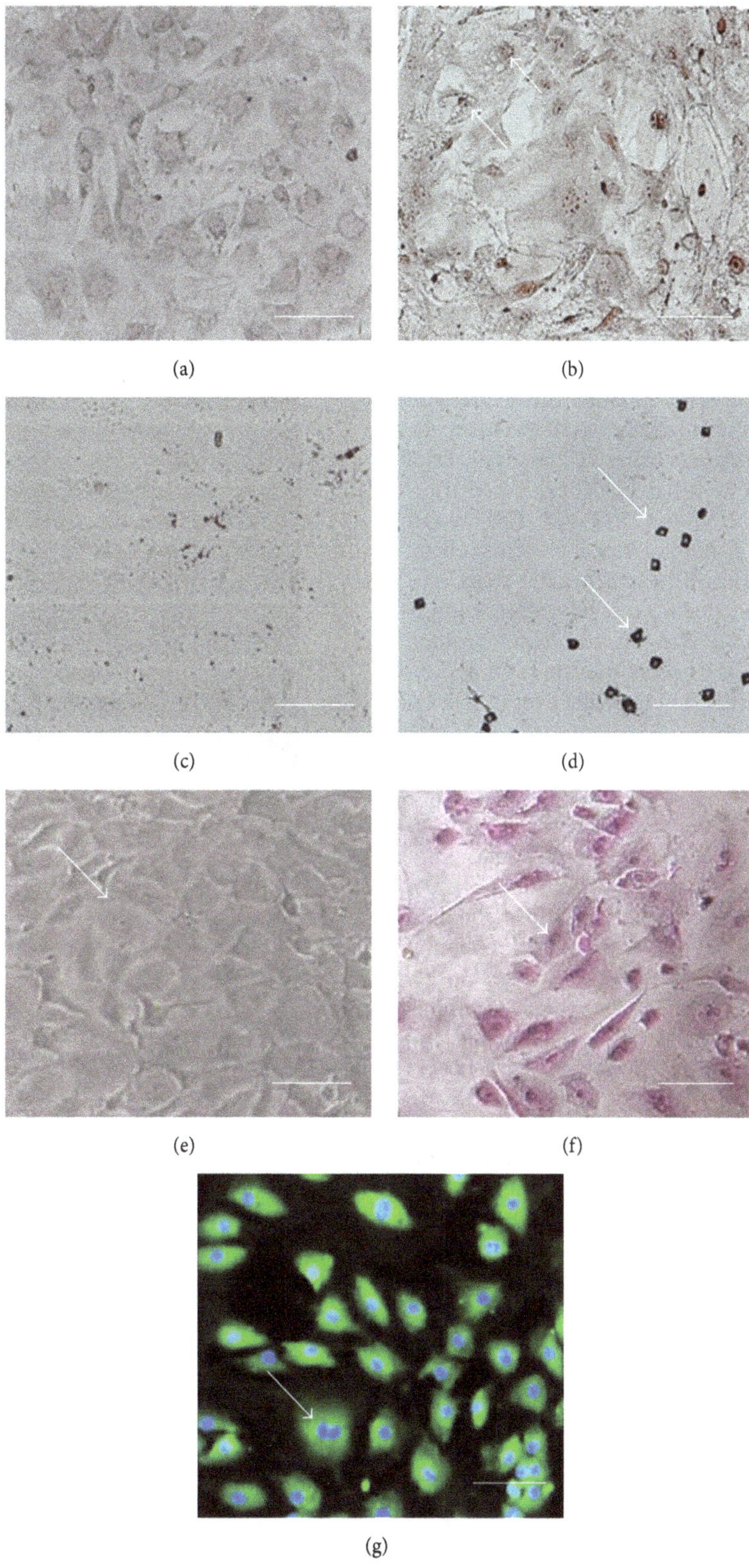

FIGURE 4: Differentiation potential of mouse liver-derived stem cells. (a, c) Uninduced LDSCs with their normal morphology stained negative for Oil Red O stain (a) and alizarin red (c). (b) Adipogenesis induced LDSCs were stained with Oil Red O stain showing positive for oil droplets after 4 weeks of induction. (d) Osteogenesis induced LDSCs were stained with alizarin red showing mineralized nodule after 4 weeks of induction. (e) Phase contrast image of hepatogenesis induced LDSCs showing typical polygonal shape from fibroblast shape. (f) Hepatogenesis was shown positive for PAS staining (glycogen storage). (g) Albumin expression in hepatocyte induced LdSCs showed by ICC. Scale bars represent 100 μm (a)–(g).

under microscope (Figure 4(b)) and it stained positive for Oil Red O (Figure 4(a)).

LDSCs showed hepatic differentiation by their phenotype from a spindle to a rather polygonal shape over a period of 36 days of culture, as observed by phase contrast microscope (Figure 4(g)). The presence of glycogen storage was also observed in differentiated hepatocyte by sensitive PAS staining (Figures 4(e) and 4(f)). Further, the functional potential of LDSC differentiated into hepatocytes was assessed by the liver specific marker of albumin secretion by immunocytochemistry and found to secrete albumin observed under phase fluorescent phase contrast microscope.

3.4. Gene Expression Profiling of LDSCs. The expression profile of liver-derived stem cell markers was screened for the presence of liver stem cell markers using PCR analysis. Data from the PCR analysis showed that LDSC expressed transcription factors (HNF-3β, HNF-6, C/EBP-β, C/EBP-α, and GATA-4) and also structural and functional proteins (CK18, CK19, p450 Cyp3a11, and PXMP1-L) of hepatic stem cells (Figure 5). Notably, the functional proteins mRNA expressions were negative (albumin, transthyretin, α-fetoprotein, and AAT) in case of LdSCs, whereas transthyretin and α-fetoprotein were found expressed in neonatal liver (Table 2).

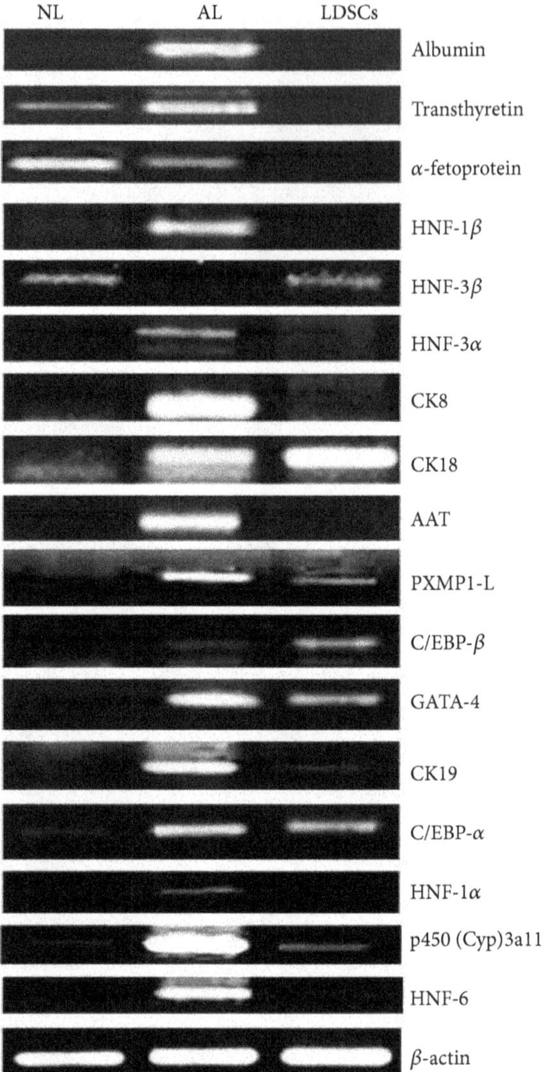

Figure 5: Hepatic markers and their transcription factor mRNA expression by RT-PCR. The RNA was isolated from LDSCs and the mRNA expressions were compared with neonatal liver (NL) and adult liver (AL) for albumin, transthyretin, AAT, AFP, CK8, CK18, CK19, p450 (Cyp)3a11, PXMP1-L HNF-1α, HNF-1β, HNF-3α, HNF-3β, HNF-4α, HNF-6, GATA-4, C/EBP-α, and C/EBP-β. LDSCs show the mRNA expression for HNF-3β, CK18, PXMP1-L, C/EBP-α, C/EBP-β GATA-4, CK18, p450 (Cyp)3a11, and HNF-6, negative for hepatic markers.

4. Discussion

The current study involved in the derivation of LDSCs from neonatal mice liver suggested that, when compared to adult mice liver, the neonatal mouse has a higher number of stem cells with high proliferation and differentiation potential [27]. LDSCs from neonatal liver possess features including spindle shape-like morphology, adherent to the plastic surface, devoid of hematopoietic markers, and possess multilineage differentiation potential into osteoblasts, adipocyte, and hepatocytes similar to MSCs [28]. Flow cytometric analysis showed that the cells were positive for EpCAM (CD326), GATA-4, CD105 (endoglin), and mesenchymal cells markers including CD29 (β_1 integrin) and CD44 (receptor for hyaluronate and osteopontin), in addition to being weak positive for Sca-1 (a murine hematopoietic stem cell and MSC marker). LDSCs were negative for hematopoietic markers such as CD34, CD45 (primitive hematopoietic progenitor and endothelial cell marker), and CD90 (GPI-anchored glycoprotein), which are congruent with their counterparts from human and murine. The cell surface antigen profile showed that the cultured LDSCs belong to a population of nonhematopoietic, nonendothelial, slightly mesenchyme origin, and it behaves similar to adult mouse hepatic stem cells under *in vitro* culture conditions. LDSCs are capable of self-renewal and are multipotent, able to give rise to committed biliary progenitors and hepatocyte lineages. Hepatic lineages were identified by morphological changes and stained with periodic Acid-Schiff (PAS) for glycogen storage and assessment of albumin secretion [29] by ICC as well as by another multilineage differentiation to osteoblasts and adipocytes (Figure 4).

The expression profiling showed the specific markers for transcriptional and structural proteins of LDSCs, with no expression of mature liver functional markers [10]. These findings suggested that the isolated cells resembled liver progenitors cells; however, they lack the mature hepatocyte marker like albumin and so forth. The reason for expressing the mesenchymal counter parts may be due to interaction of committed endodermal cells with mesenchymal components of the primitive liver during embryogenesis.

In the current study, LDSCs were efficiently isolated by a shortened protocol that limited the usage of enzyme cocktails like collagenase and hyaluronidase and also with minimal exposure to enzyme digestion time. This study followed a modified protocol as reported earlier by [30, 31] where 1%

Table 2: Summary of the phenotype and genotype of isolated LDSCs.

FACS	
Liver marker	Expression
EpCAM	+++
GATA-4	+++
CK18	+++
Mesenchyme marker	
CD105	+++
CD29	+++
CD44	+++
Sca-1	++
Hematopoietic marker	
CD34	−
CD45	−
CD90	−
RT-PCR	
Transcriptional markers	Expression
HNF-3β	++
HNF-6	+
C/EBP-α	++
C/EBP-β	++
HNF-1α	−
HNF-1β	−
HNF-3α	−
GATA-4	++
Structural markers	
CK8	−
CK18	++++
CK19	+
Functional markers	
Albumin	−
Transthyretin	−
α-fetoprotein	−
AAT	−
p450 Cyp3a11	++
PXMP1-L	+

Percentage of expression: ++++: 95–100%, +++: 75–95%, ++: 40–75%, +: 10–35%, and −: 0-1%.

gelatin has been used to coat culture dishes, which aids in selective removal of fibroblasts due to its higher affinity to a collagenous extracellular matrix like gelatin [32]. In our study we used one-step enrichment procedure followed by enzyme digestion that effectively removes fibroblasts and improves culture homogeneity. The culture conditions were optimized for DMEM/F12 which includes supplementation of insulin, sodium pyruvate, glutamine, nonessential amino acids, and horse serum were supported the LDSCs in stimulating the glycolysis, and preventing accumulation of metabolic end products like lactate, and reduces the overgrowth of epithelial and fibroblasts like-cells [16, 33] as compared to the maintenance medium M199, which was used by earlier workers [30, 34–36].

5. Conclusion

Current study describes a rapid, reproducible, and efficient protocol for isolation of homogenous population of LDSCs. These cells have potential to become functional hepatocytes. Further, LDSCs can be used as *in vitro* model system for assessing various drug toxicity assays and preclinical trials in pharmacokinetic studies and in various liver based tissue engineering approaches.

Conflict of Interests

The authors confirm that there is no conflict of interests.

Acknowledgment

The authors acknowledge grant and fellowship support from Department of Science and Technology, India (DST) (Grant no. SR/WOS-A/LS-205/2009).

References

[1] D. C. Hixson, R. A. Faris, L. Yang, and P. Novikoff, "Antigenic clues to liver development, renewal, and carcinogenesis: an integrated model," in *The Role of Cell Types in Hepatocarcinogenesis*, A. E. Sirica, Ed., pp. 151–182, CRC Press, Boca Raton, Fla, USA, 1992.

[2] R. Saxena, N. D. Theise, and J. M. Crawford, "Microanatomy of the human liver—exploring the hidden interfaces," *Hepatology*, vol. 30, no. 6, pp. 1339–1346, 1999.

[3] D. B. Solt, A. Medline, and E. Farber, "Rapid emergence of carcinogen-induced hyperplastic lesions in a new model for the sequential analysis of liver carcinogenesis," *The American Journal of Pathology*, vol. 88, no. 3, pp. 595–618, 1977.

[4] R. P. Evarts, Z. Hu, N. Omori, M. Omori, E. R. Marsden, and S. S. Thorgeirsson, "Precursor-product relationship between oval cells and hepatocytes: comparison between tritiated thymidine and bromodeoxyuridine as tracers," *Carcinogenesis*, vol. 17, no. 10, pp. 2143–2151, 1996.

[5] C. A. Lázaro, J. A. Rhim, Y. Yamada, and N. Fausto, "Generation of hepatocytes from oval cell precursors in culture," *Cancer Research*, vol. 58, no. 23, pp. 5514–5522, 1998.

[6] H. Kubota and L. M. Reid, "Clonogenic hepatoblasts, common precursors for hepatocytic and biliary lineages, are lacking classical major histocompatibility complex class I antigen," *Proceedings of the National Academy of Sciences of the United States of America*, vol. 97, no. 22, pp. 12132–12137, 2000.

[7] D. Mahieu-Caputo, J.-E. Allain, J. Branger et al., "Repopulation of athymic mouse liver by cryopreserved early human fetal hepatoblasts," *Human Gene Therapy*, vol. 15, no. 12, pp. 1219–1228, 2004.

[8] C. A. Lázaro, E. J. Croager, C. Mitchell et al., "Establishment; characterization; and long-term maintenance of cultures of human fetal hepatocytes," *Hepatology*, vol. 38, no. 5, pp. 1095–1106, 2003.

[9] Y. Y. Dan, K. J. Riehle, C. Lazaro et al., "Isolation of multipotent progenitor cells from human fetal liver capable of differentiating into liver and mesenchymal lineages," *Proceedings of the National Academy of Sciences of the United States of America*, vol. 103, no. 26, pp. 9912–9917, 2006.

[10] E. Schmelzer, E. Wauthier, and L. M. Reid, "The phenotypes of pluripotent human hepatic progenitors," *Stem Cells*, vol. 24, no. 8, pp. 1852–1858, 2006.

[11] E. Schmelzer, L. Zhang, A. Bruce et al., "Human hepatic stem cells from fetal and postnatal donors," *Journal of Experimental Medicine*, vol. 204, no. 8, pp. 1973–1987, 2007.

[12] W. S. Turner, E. Schmelzer, R. McClelland, E. Wauthier, W. Chen, and L. M. Reid, "Human hepatoblast phenotype maintained by hyaluronan hydrogels," *Journal of Biomedical Materials Research—Part B Applied Biomaterials*, vol. 82, no. 1, pp. 156–168, 2007.

[13] J. Wang, J. B. Clark, G.-S. Rhee, J. H. Fair, L. M. Reid, and D. A. Gerber, "Proliferation and hepatic differentiation of adult-derived progenitor cells," *Cells Tissues Organs*, vol. 173, no. 4, pp. 193–203, 2003.

[14] C. Fougère-Deschatrette, T. Imaizumi-Scherrer, H. Strick-Marchand et al., "Plasticity of hepatic cell differentiation: bipotential adult mouse liver clonal cell lines competent to differentiate in vitro and in vivo," *Stem Cells*, vol. 24, no. 9, pp. 2098–2109, 2006.

[15] T. Fujikawa, T. Hirose, H. Fujii et al., "Purification of adult hepatic progenitor cells using green fluorescent protein GFP-transgenic mice and fluorescence-activated cell sorting," *Journal of Hepatology*, vol. 39, no. 2, pp. 162–170, 2003.

[16] I. Avital, D. Inderbitzin, T. Aoki et al., "Isolation, characterization, and transplantation of bone marrow-derived hepatocyte stem cells," *Biochemical and Biophysical Research Communications*, vol. 288, no. 1, pp. 156–164, 2001.

[17] T. D. Shupe, A. C. Piscaglia, S.-H. Oh, A. Gasbarrini, and B. E. Petersen, "Isolation and characterization of hepatic stem cells, or 'oval cells,' from rat livers," *Methods in Molecular Biology*, vol. 482, pp. 387–405, 2009.

[18] P. Sreejit, S. Kumar, and R. S. Verma, "An improved protocol for primary culture of cardiomyocyte from neonatal mice," *In Vitro Cellular and Developmental Biology: Animal*, vol. 44, no. 3-4, pp. 45–50, 2008.

[19] H. Lilja, N. Arkadopoulos, P. Blanc et al., "Fetal rat hepatocytes: isolation, characterization, and transplantation in the nagase analbuminemic rats," *Transplantation*, vol. 64, no. 9, pp. 1240–1248, 1997.

[20] H. P. Lilja, P. Blanc, A. A. Demetriou, and J. Rozga, "Response of cultured fetal and adult rat hepatocytes to growth factors and cyclosporine," *Cell Transplantation*, vol. 7, no. 3, pp. 257–266, 1998.

[21] N. Tanimizu, M. Nishikawa, H. Saito, T. Tsujimura, and A. Miyajima, "Isolation of hepatoblasts based on the expression of Dlk/Pref-1," *Journal of Cell Science*, vol. 116, no. 9, pp. 1775–1786, 2003.

[22] D. Lee and K. Lee, "Hepatocyte isolation, culture and its clinical applications," *Hanyang Medical Reviews*, vol. 34, no. 4, pp. 165–172, 2014.

[23] R. B. Howard, A. K. Christensen, F. A. Gibbs, and L. A. Pesch, "The enzymatic preparation of isolated intact parenchymal cells from rat liver," *Journal of Cell Biology*, vol. 35, no. 3, pp. 675–684, 1967.

[24] C. M. Stanford, P. A. Jacobson, E. D. Eanes, L. A. Lembke, and R. J. Midura, "Rapidly forming apatitic mineral in an osteoblastic cell line (UMR 106-01 BSP)," *The Journal of Biological Chemistry*, vol. 270, no. 16, pp. 9420–9428, 1995.

[25] J. L. Ramírez-Zacarías, F. Castro-Muñozledo, and W. Kuri-Harcuch, "Quantitation of adipose conversion and triglycerides by staining intracytoplasmic lipids with oil red O," *Histochemistry*, vol. 97, no. 6, pp. 493–497, 1992.

[26] K.-D. Lee, T. K.-C. Kuo, J. Whang-Peng et al., "In vitro hepatic differentiation of human mesenchymal stem cells," *Hepatology*, vol. 40, no. 6, pp. 1275–1284, 2004.

[27] H. C. Fiegel, C. Lange, U. Kneser et al., "Fetal and adult liver stem cells for liver regeneration and tissue engineering," *Journal of Cellular and Molecular Medicine*, vol. 10, no. 3, pp. 577–587, 2006.

[28] M. Dominici, K. Le Blanc, I. Mueller et al., "Minimal criteria for defining multipotent mesenchymal stromal cells. The International Society for Cellular Therapy position statement," *Cytotherapy*, vol. 8, no. 4, pp. 315–317, 2006.

[29] C. Schudt, "Regulation of glycogen synthesis in rat-hepatocyte cultures by glucose, insulin and glucocorticoids," *European Journal of Biochemistry*, vol. 97, no. 1, pp. 155–160, 1979.

[30] W. Song, X. Lu, and Q. Feng, "Tumor necrosis factor-α induces apoptosis via inducible nitric oxide synthase in neonatal mouse cardiomyocytes," *Cardiovascular Research*, vol. 45, no. 3, pp. 595–602, 2000.

[31] K. Matsuura, H. Wada, T. Nagai et al., "Cardiomyocytes fuse with surrounding noncardiomyocytes and reenter the cell cycle," *Journal of Cell Biology*, vol. 167, no. 2, pp. 351–363, 2004.

[32] R. Haas, S. S. Banerji, and L. A. Culp, "Adhesion site composition of murine fibroblasts cultured on gelatin-coated substrata," *Journal of Cellular Physiology*, vol. 120, no. 2, pp. 117–125, 1984.

[33] M. C. Fioramonti, J. C. Bryant, W. T. Mcquilkin, V. J. Evans, K. K. Sanford, and W. R. Earle, "The effect of horse serum residue and chemically defined supplements on proliferation of strain L clone 929 cells from the mouse," *Cancer Research*, vol. 15, no. 11, pp. 763–766, 1955.

[34] P. Simpson and S. Savion, "Differentiation of myocytes in single cell cultures with and without proliferating nonmyocardial cells," *Circulation Research*, vol. 50, pp. 101–116, 1982.

[35] P. Nickson, A. Toth, and P. Erhardt, "PUMA is critical for neonatal cardiomyocyte apoptosis induced by endoplasmic reticulum stress," *Cardiovascular Research*, vol. 73, no. 1, pp. 48–56, 2007.

[36] V. Bryja, S. Bonilla, L. Čajánek et al., "An efficient method for the derivation of mouse embryonic stem cells," *Stem Cells*, vol. 24, no. 4, pp. 844–849, 2006.

2

Immunosuppressive Drugs Affect High-Mannose/Hybrid N-Glycans on Human Allostimulated Leukocytes

Ewa Pocheć,[1] Katarzyna Bocian,[2] Marta Ząbczyńska,[1] Grażyna Korczak-Kowalska,[2,3] and Anna Lityńska[1]

[1]*Department of Glycoconjugate Biochemistry, Institute of Zoology, Faculty of Biology and Earth Science, Jagiellonian University, Gronostajowa 9, 30-387 Krakow, Poland*
[2]*Department of Immunology, Institute of Zoology, Faculty of Biology, University of Warsaw, Miecznikowa 1, 02-096 Warsaw, Poland*
[3]*Department of Clinical Immunology, Transplantation Institute, Medical University of Warsaw, Nowogrodzka 59, 02-006 Warsaw, Poland*

Correspondence should be addressed to Ewa Pocheć; ewa.pochec@uj.edu.pl

Academic Editor: Consuelo Amantini

N-glycosylation plays an important role in the majority of physiological and pathological processes occurring in the immune system. Alteration of the type and abundance of glycans is an element of lymphocyte differentiation; it is also common in the development of immune-mediated inflammatory diseases. The N-glycosylation process is very sensitive to different environmental agents, among them the pharmacological environment of immunosuppressive drugs. Some results show that high-mannose oligosaccharides have the ability to suppress different stages of the immune response. We evaluated the effects of cyclosporin A (CsA) and rapamycin (Rapa) on high-mannose/hybrid-type glycosylation in human leukocytes activated in a two-way mixed leukocyte reaction (MLR). CsA significantly reduced the number of leukocytes covered by high-mannose/hybrid N-glycans, and the synergistic action of CsA and Rapa led to an increase of these structures on the remaining leukocytes. This is the first study indicating that β1 and β3 integrins bearing high-mannose/hybrid structures are affected by Rapa and CsA. Rapa taken separately and together with CsA changed the expression of β1 and β3 integrins and, by regulating the protein amount, increased the oligomannose/hybrid-type N-glycosylation on the leukocyte surface. We suggest that the changes in the glycosylation profile of leukocytes may promote the development of tolerance in transplantation.

1. Introduction

Most cell surface and secreted proteins in the immune system are N-glycosylated [1–4]. N-glycans added to the special protein sequence (Asn-X-Ser/Thr) during the posttranslational process form a large and important part of glycoprotein molecules; the oligosaccharide component reaches up to even 50% of glycoprotein molecular mass [5]. N-glycoproteins contain three different oligosaccharide structures: high-mannose, hybrid, and complex-type [6]. High-mannose glycans have been considered to be incomplete products of the N-glycosylation synthesis pathway, evolutionarily older than complex-type structures. They are thought to be typical for simpler organisms like yeast or fungi [5, 7, 8], but some studies have shown that these oligosaccharide structures are also abundant in mammalian cells and are no less important than completely processed complex-type sugar chains [9, 10]. Recognition of high-mannose structures by mannose receptors in macrophages and dendritic cells is critical to the innate immune response responsible for elimination of bacteria and viruses and for initiation of organ-specific autoimmunity [11, 12]. Other work established that mannose-rich oligosaccharides can suppress the immune response [13], ligand binding [14], and intracellular signal transduction [15].

Integrins are transmembrane receptors which mediate adhesive events critical to an effective immune response [16–19]. Leukocytes express a broad range of $\alpha\beta$ integrin heterodimers (at least 12) [17, 19]. The integrin repertoire on the leukocyte surface depends on the stage of leukocyte activation and is regulated by cytokines, chemokines, and other adhesion receptors [20]. The functions of leukocytes rely mostly on integrins belonging to the $\beta 2$ family but also to the $\beta 1$ family [16], and $\beta 3$ integrins are important to leukocyte biology as well [19, 20]. They are also called very late antigens (VLA), because some integrins appear on the cell surface days or even weeks after leukocyte activation [21]. Integrins take part in the formation of immunological synapses [21, 22], which serve immune cell communication [23]. These adhesion proteins are needed for leukocytes to move from the blood into peripheral tissues [20, 24] and they mediate leukocyte interactions with endothelial cells and extracellular matrix proteins (ECM) [20]. The most important integrins for leukocyte activation and migration are LFA-1 ($\alpha L\beta 2$), $\alpha 4\beta 1$ (VLA-4), and $\alpha 4\beta 7$ [25–27]. N-glycosylation of integrins, which are the highly N-glycosylated proteins, plays a crucial role in their functioning [28].

The proper functioning of immune cells in the response to alloantigens depends strongly on glycosylation of surface receptors [4]. Leukocytes modify cell interactions during each stage of the immune response by regulating the type and abundance of glycans; differentiation of leukocytes is also dependent on their glycosylation [8, 29–31]. The N-glycosylation process is very sensitive to different environmental agents and to the pathological conditions of immune diseases [29, 32, 33]. In transplantation, strong inflammatory signals are induced in the recipient, which need to be controlled through administration of immunosuppressive drugs [34, 35].

We posited that the pharmacological environment of immunosuppressive drugs may modulate leukocyte glycosylation. To the best of our knowledge there are no published studies evaluating the effects of cyclosporin A (CsA; inhibitor of calcineurin) and rapamycin (Rapa; inhibitor of mammalian target of rapamycin mTOR) on human immune cell glycosylation. In this study we assessed effects of these drugs on leukocyte glycosylation. These are immunosuppressive agents commonly used to inhibit leukocyte activation during a rapid immune response. We found that CsA significantly reduces the number of leukocytes covered with high-mannose/hybrid N-glycans, while the synergistic action of CsA and Rapa leads to an increase of these structures on the remaining leukocytes. We demonstrated, for the first time, that $\beta 1$ and $\beta 3$ integrins bearing high-mannose/hybrid structures are influenced by Rapa and CsA. Rapa taken separately and together with CsA significantly altered the expression of $\beta 1$ and $\beta 3$ integrins, and this caused an increase in the amount of oligomannose/hybrid N-glycans on leukocyte surfaces.

2. Materials and Methods

2.1. Materials. Peripheral blood samples were obtained from healthy volunteers aged 18–60 years. Gradisol L was provided by Aqua Medica (Łódź, Poland). RPMI1640 medium was purchased from Biomed, fetal calf serum (FCS), L-glutamine, and N-2-hydroxyethyl-piperazine-N′-2-ethanesulphonic acid (HEPES) from Gibco, and gentamicin from Biochemie. Rapamycin and cyclosporin A were obtained from Wyeth-Lederle and Novartis Pharma, respectively. Laemmli sample buffer (LSB, 161-0737) and β-mercaptoethanol (β-ME) were from Bio-Rad and RIPA buffer (89900) and PageRuler Prestained Protein Ladder (26616) from Thermo Scientific. Biotinylated *Galanthus nivalis* agglutinin (GNA, B-1246), agarose-bound GNA (AL-1243), agarose-bound streptavidin (SA-5010), and Carbo-Free Blocking Solution were obtained from Vector Lab. Mouse antibody against $\beta 1$ integrin subunit (MAB2251, clone B3B11), rabbit against $\beta 3$ subunit (AB1932), and alkaline phosphatase- (AP-) conjugated sheep anti-rabbit (AP322A) were obtained from Millipore. Rabbit polyclonal anti-GAPDH (G9545), AP-conjugated goat anti-mouse (084K4861) antibody, AP-conjugated ExtrAvidin (E2636), FITC-conjugated ExtrAvidin (E2761), Coomassie Brilliant Blue G (B2025), protease inhibitor cocktail (P2714), and trypan blue (T8154) were purchased from Sigma-Aldrich. Horseradish peroxidase- (HRP-) conjugated horse anti-mouse (7076S) and sheep anti-rabbit (70742) antibody were obtained from Cell Signaling Technology. Substrate for AP, nitro blue tetrazolium chloride (NBT) and 5-bromo-4-chloro-3-indolyl-phosphate (BCIP), and recombinant endo-β-N-acetylglucosaminidase H (Endo H) from *Streptomyces plicatus* (11088726001) were purchased from Roche. Western Bright Sirius chemiluminescent HRP substrate (K-12043-D10) was obtained from Advansta.

2.2. Mixed Leukocyte Reaction. Peripheral blood mononuclear cells (PBMCs) were isolated from heparinized venous blood by density-gradient centrifugation over Gradisol L. PBMCs were resuspended in RPMI1640 medium supplemented with 10% FCS, 20 mM L-glutamine, 10 μg/mL gentamicin, and 1 M HEPES and counted in a hemocytometer chamber using trypan blue dye. Cells from two healthy donors (1×10^6 per 1 mL medium) were mixed 1 : 1 for the two-way mixed leukocyte reaction (MLR). The cells were cultured in 24-well plates at 37°C for 6 days in a CO_2 incubator (Lab Line Instruments) in the presence of CsA (200 ng per 1 mL medium), Rapa (20 ng per 1 mL medium), and both drugs given together (150 ng CsA and 12 ng Rapa per 1 mL medium). The choice of immunosuppressive drug doses was based on earlier studies [36, 37].

2.3. Flow Cytometric Analysis. The cells were harvested from MLR cell culture and washed twice in cold PBS. All the steps were performed on ice. Cells were incubated with biotinylated GNA (1 : 100) for 30 min at RT, centrifuged (1800 rpm, 5 min, 4°C), and washed in PBS. Then the cells were incubated with FITC-conjugated ExtrAvidin (1 : 100) for 30 min at RT and centrifuged under the same conditions as previously. After washing in PBS, fluorescence was measured by flow cytometry in a FACSCalibur (BD Biosciences) using Cell Quest software (BD Biosciences).

2.4. GNA Precipitation. Cell lysate proteins (500 μg) were incubated with 25 μL agarose-bound *Galanthus nivalis* lectin (GNA) in HEPES buffer (10 mM HEPES, pH 7.5, containing 150 mM NaCl) and incubated overnight at 4°C. After centrifugation (14,000 rpm, 2 min, RT) the supernatants from the GNA-treated protein extracts were collected. The precipitates were washed three times in HEPES buffer and once in PBS. Glycoproteins were released from the glycoprotein-lectin-agarose complexes by boiling 10 min in 25 μL LSB containing β-ME at 100°C for 10 min. After final centrifugation the supernatants containing GNA-positive glycoproteins were collected and destined for SDS-PAGE separation followed by MS/MS analysis.

2.5. Lectin Blotting. GNA precipitates, the supernatant collected after GNA precipitation, and cell lysate proteins were separated on 10% SDS-PAGE under reducing conditions and then transferred to a PVDF membrane. To detect proteins carrying high-mannose N-oligosaccharides, the PVDF blots were blocked in Carbo-Free Blocking Solution overnight at 4°C. After washing three times in TBST and once in TBS with 1 mM $MgCl_2$, 1 mM $MnCl_2$, and 1 mM $CaCl_2$, the membranes were incubated with biotinylated GNA lectin (1:4000) in TBS with the ions for 1 h at RT. After further washing in TBST the membranes were incubated for 1 h at RT with AP-conjugated ExtrAvidin (1:4000). After final washing, the GNA-positive proteins were visualized using NBT/BCIP solution as substrate for AP.

2.6. MS/MS Analysis. GNA precipitates (20 μL from 25 μL total volume) were separated by SDS-PAGE. The gel was fixed with 7% acetic acid in 40% methanol (v/v) for 30 min and stained with Coomassie Brilliant Blue for 2 h. The gel bands corresponding to the GNA-positive proteins (separated on the same gel but destined for lectin reaction on a PVDF membrane; the 5 μL remainder from 25 μL total volume) were excised, subjected to trypsin digestion, and analyzed by tandem mass spectrometry MS/MS in the Mass Spectrometry Laboratory of the Institute of Biochemistry and Biophysics, Polish Academy of Sciences (Warsaw, Poland). Proteins were identified by matching the peptides with the Sprot nonredundant database (547357 sequences/194874700 residues) with a *Homo sapiens* filter (20274 sequences) from the Mascot Distiller software (version 2.4.2.0, MatrixScience). Scores higher than 46 were considered to be significant ($p < 0.0005$).

2.7. Endo H Digestion. The content of high-mannose and hybrid glycans in integrin subunits was determined using endo-β-N-acetylglucosaminidase H from *Streptomyces plicatus*. The cell glycoproteins (15 μg) were suspended in sodium phosphate buffer (pH 5.5) to 50 mM final concentration. Protein denaturation was carried out in the presence of 0.2% SDS and 1 M β-ME for 3 min. After cooling to RT, 25 mU Endo H was added and the samples were incubated overnight at 37°C. The reaction was stopped by heating at 100°C for 10 min. Both digested and nondigested samples were boiled in LSB with β-ME prior to SDS-PAGE on 10% polyacrylamide gels.

2.8. Immunoblotting. Equal amounts of proteins in LSB with β-ME (15 μg) were separated on 10% polyacrylamide gel and transferred to a PVDF membrane. After blocking in 1% BSA in TBST, integrin subunits were incubated for 1 h at RT with anti-β1 and anti-β3 antibody diluted 1:1000 in 1% BSA in TBST. Rabbit anti-GAPDH IgG was diluted 1:4000 and incubated on a membrane in the same conditions. Then anti-mouse IgG and anti-rabbit IgG were applied in a 1:4000 dilution and incubated at RT for 1 h. Integrin subunits were visualized by chemiluminescence in the GeneGnome Imaging System (Syngen) or with the colorimetric reaction by incubating the membranes with BCIP/NBT substrate for AP. The oligomannose/hybrid N-glycan amounts were calculated based on loss of molecular mass after Endo H digestion using UVImap Image Quantification software (UVItec).

3. Results

3.1. CsA Reduces GNA-Positive Cell Number, but the Synergistic Action of CsA and Rapa Increases the Amount of GNA-Positive Glycoproteins. Glycosylation of alloantigen-activated PBMCs from two individuals mixed together in two-way MLR cell culture was analyzed using FITC-labeled *Galanthus nivalis* agglutinin (GNA) in flow cytometry. We found that the number of leukocytes covered by oligomannose/hybrid-type N-glycans decreased dramatically in the presence of CsA applied alone or with Rapa (Figure 1). Mean fluorescence intensity (MFI) was reduced slightly by the drugs given separately but the combination of both drugs significantly raised the MFI value. CsA was responsible for removal of high-mannose/hybrid N-glycans from the surface of over 60% of the leukocytes, but the synergistic effect of both immunosuppressive drugs markedly increased the amount of oligomannose/hybrid-type N-glycans on the remaining cells.

3.2. Glycoproteins Bearing High-Mannose/Hybrid Structures Are Affected by CsA and Rapa. Lectin blotting (LB) with biotinylated GNA disclosed changes in the oligomannose/hybrid-type glycosylation of some proteins in samples with CsA given together with Rapa; the reaction was more intense in bands 1 and 2, while reduction of GNA binding was seen in band 3 (Figure 2(a)). Based on the GNA reaction, bands found to have been altered in intensity by immunosuppressive agents were excised from the gels (Figure 2(b)) and their content was analyzed using MS/MS. This assay showed 62 possible proteins in band 1, 151 in band 2, and 126 in band 3. The ten identified proteins with the highest scores for each band are listed in Table 1. Among them are transmembrane proteins (β integrins, HLA class I histocompatibility antigen, LAMPs) and cytoplasmic proteins (enzymes of various metabolic pathways, coagulation factors). The molecular mass of the identified monomeric glycoproteins, calculated based on the amino acid sequences, was lower than the mass determined in SDS-PAGE, due to the presence of N-glycan components. The theoretical molecular weight of multimeric glycoproteins is higher than that determined based on Protein Ladder standards, because the samples were resolved in reducing conditions.

3.3. Expression of β1 Precursor and β3 Integrin Subunits Is Changed by CsA and Rapa. In further analyses we focused on the β integrin subunits identified in the band 1 to verify the results obtained by MS/MS analysis. Immunodetection

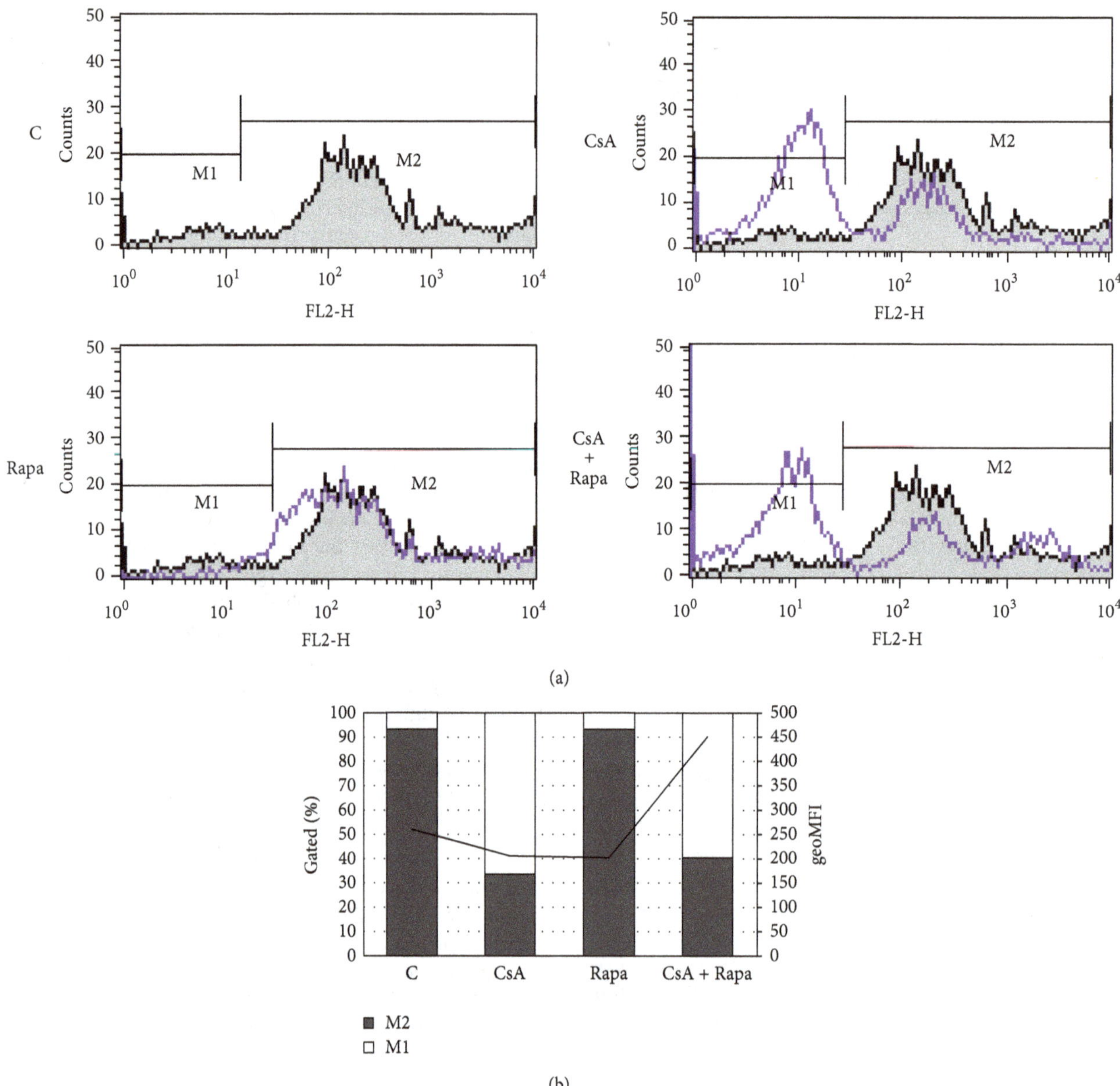

Figure 1: Immunosuppressive drugs alter the surface expression of high-mannose/hybrid N-glycans. Peripheral blood mononuclear cells were cultured for 6 days in the presence of CsA (200 ng per 1 mL medium), Rapa (20 ng per 1 mL medium), and the combination of CsA (150 ng per 1 mL medium) and Rapa (12 ng per 1 mL medium) in a two-way mixed leukocyte reaction (MLR). Immunosuppressive drug-treated and control cells were stained with biotinylated GNA (1 : 100), followed by incubation with FITC-conjugated ExtrAvidin. M2 region corresponds to GNA-positive leukocytes after allostimulation. Fluorescence was measured using a FACSCalibur flow cytometer (BD Biosciences). C: untreated cells, CsA: cyclosporin A, and Rapa: rapamycin.

of the $\beta1$ subunit after releasing the high-mannose/hybrid-type N-glycans with Endo H revealed that the $\beta1$ precursor, with lower molecular mass, mainly carries these types of N-glycans (Figure 3), but the mobility shift in the control and immunosuppressive drug-treated MLR cells was comparable. Comparable loss of molecular weight between the control and tested cells after Endo H digestion was also found in the $\beta3$ subunit. We observed, however, a significant increase of the intensity of the $\beta1$ (both forms) and $\beta3$ subunits in MLR cells cultured in the presence of Rapa alone or combined with CsA. GNA precipitation confirmed the results from Endo H digestion of the $\beta1$ subunit (Figure 4). GNA recognized mainly the $\beta1$ precursor form; the mature subunit remained unprecipitated in supernatants. Here we also observed higher intensity of the $\beta1$ subunit in MLR treated with Rapa and the combination of both drugs. These results indicate that high-mannose/hybrid-type glycosylation did not change on a single β integrin molecule but that the increased binding of GNA resulted from enhancement of β integrin expression (Figures 3 and 4) and that it contributed to the overall increase of high-mannose/hybrid-type glycans on the cell surface in the presence of CsA and Rapa (Figure 1).

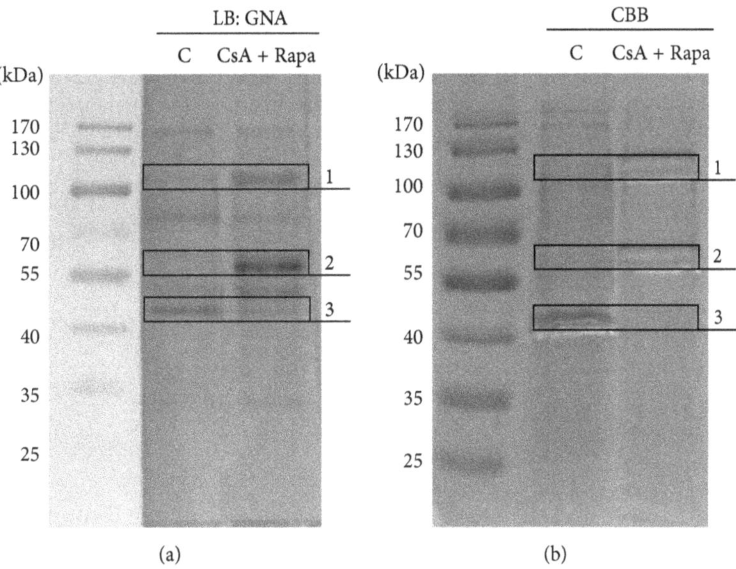

FIGURE 2: Immunosuppressive drugs change the intensity of bands containing GNA-positive proteins. Peripheral blood mononuclear cells were cultured for 6 days in the presence of the combination of CsA (150 ng per 1 mL medium) and Rapa (12 ng per 1 mL medium) in a two-way mixed leukocyte reaction (MLR) and then lysed in RIPA buffer. Whole-cell lysate proteins (500 μg) were precipitated with 25 μL agarose-bound *Galanthus nivalis* lectin (GNA). The captured glycoproteins were recovered by boiling in Laemmli sample buffer with β-ME and resolved by 10% SDS-PAGE under reducing conditions. One-fifth of the GNA precipitate was destined for Western blotting (WB) and after probing with biotinylated-GNA was visualized by AP colorimetric reaction (a). The remaining four-fifths of the precipitate, after resolving on the same gel, were stained with Coomassie Brilliant Blue (CBB) and the bands were excised for MS/MS analysis (b). Molecular weight of proteins was assigned using a PageRuler Prestained Protein Ladder (Thermo Scientific, 26616). LP: lectin precipitation, C: untreated cells, CsA: cyclosporin A, and Rapa: rapamycin.

4. Discussion

It is well documented that immunosuppressive drugs, designed to inhibit activation of the immune response [34], act by changing the expression of many proteins on immune cells [38–40], including integrins [41–44], but there are only few studies showing that they influence protein glycosylation [15, 45, 46]. For this reason we focused on determining the effects of the immunosuppressive drugs CsA and Rapa on N-glycosylation of leukocytes alloactivated *in vitro*. Flow cytometric analysis showed that CsA downregulated the amount of GNA-positive leukocytes, but both drugs acting synergistically increased the surface expression of high-mannose/hybrid-type N-glycans on the remaining leukocytes (Figure 1). Lectin blotting confirmed the enhancement of the reaction with GNA lectin of some SDS-PAGE-resolved glycoproteins (Figure 2(a)). The synergistic effects of CsA and Rapa, different from those of one-drug treatment, result from the various molecular mechanisms of these drugs [40]. They act at different stages of the T cell cycle: CsA at the G0 phase of the T lymphocyte cell cycle, and Rapa later at the transition from the G1 to the S phase. CsA interacts with calcineurin to block IL-2 gene transcription and then to inhibit T-cell proliferation, leading to decreased IL-2 production and secretion by T cells. Rapa blocks the intracellular signaling trigger by binding IL-2 to its receptor, thereby inhibiting T-cell responses to cytokines [38, 40, 47]. Most protocols use a combination of agents for induction and maintenance of immunosuppression to improve patient survival and graft survival rates and to reduce side effects [47].

In a proteomic study, Lee et al. [38] showed that most of the altered proteins from human T lymphocytes treated with CsA and a polysaccharopeptide have functional significance in protein degradation, the antioxidant pathway, energy metabolism, and immune cell regulation. Our MS/MS analysis revealed that among the human leukocyte glycoproteins affected by CsA and Rapa are HLA class I histocompatibility antigens (decreased reaction with GNA), enzymes of various metabolic pathways, coagulation factors, the adhesion protein LAMP1, and integrins of the β1 and β3 subfamilies (increased reaction with GNA) (Table 1). In further analyses we focused on the β1 and β3 integrin subunits. Immunodetection of β1 and β3 subunits after Endo H digestion showed that the more intense reaction with GNA in Rapa- and Rapa/CsA-treated leukocytes was not the result of changed oligomannose/hybrid glycosylation on these proteins, but rather increased expression of the integrins (Figure 3). Immunosuppressive agents usually act by decreasing protein expression, which leads to attenuation of the immune response and induces a state of tolerance [40]. From previous results it is known that the changes in integrin expression caused by immunosuppressive drugs or blocking antibodies depend on the target cells and on the type and even the dose of agents. In a recent study, Zal et al. [44] observed reduction of α2 and β1 integrin expression on kidney fibroblasts from CsA-treated rats. Sarnacki et al. [27] found that

Table 1: Cyclosporin A (CsA) and rapamycin- (Rapa-) affected GNA-positive glycoproteins identified by MS/MS. Proteins bearing high mannose/hybrid-type oligosaccharides expressed on MLR-activated leukocytes treated with a combination of CsA (150 ng per 1 mL medium) and Rapa (12 ng per 1 mL medium) were identified in MS/MS analysis by comparison of the results with the Sprot database. Ten glycoproteins with the highest protein score for each band are presented.

Band no.	Accession no.	Protein name	Mascot score	Number of significant peptide matches	Protein sequence coverage [%]	Mass based on amino acid sequence [kDa]	Relative mass calculated based on standard proteins [kDa]
1	P05106	Integrin beta-3	6117	145	34	90.2	102.4
	P14625	Endoplasmin	692	27	23	92.6	
	P05556	Integrin beta-1	618	19	16	91.7	
	Q9NZ08	Endoplasmic reticulum aminopeptidase 1	321	8	8	100.0	
	P19367	Hexokinase-1	315	7	7	100.0	
	P11279	Lysosome-associated membrane glycoprotein 1	275	7	6	45.4	
	O00462	Beta-mannosidase	236	9	9	101.8	
	P12259	Coagulation factor V	226	6	6	252.7	
	Q99467	CD180 antigen	205	2	2	75.2	
	Q8TB96	T-cell immunomodulatory protein	124	3	3	68.5	
2	P05164	Myeloperoxidase	2491	88	25	83.8	60.5
	P07237	Protein disulfide isomerase	502	18	14	57.1	
	P51688	N-Sulphoglucosamine sulphohydrolase	420	13	10	56.7	
	P16278	Beta-galactosidase	519	9	9	76.0	
	P00488	Coagulation factor XIII A chain	581	14	14	83.2	
	P01876	Ig alpha-1 chain C region	337	8	7	37.6	
	Q9Y4L1	Hypoxia upregulated protein 1	319	11	9	111.3	
	Q9NZK5	Adenosine deaminase CECR1	234	11	10	59.0	
	P08236	Beta-glucuronidase	208	6	5	74.7	
	Q9UHL4	Dipeptidyl peptidase 2	206	5	5	54.3	
3	Q6P4A8	Phospholipase B-like 1	596	18	8	63.2	42.6
	P15586	N-Acetylglucosamine-6-sulfatase	287	9	5	62.0	
	O14773	Tripeptidyl-peptidase 1	250	6	4	61.2	
	P01889	HLA class I histocompatibility antigen, B-7 alpha chain	172	3	3	40.4	
	Q9BS26	Endoplasmic reticulum resident protein 44	166	5	5	46.9	
	Q07000	HLA class I histocompatibility antigen, Cw-15 alpha chain	121	3	3	40.8	
	P05121	Plasminogen activator inhibitor 1	84	4	4	45.0	
	P04233	HLA class II histocompatibility antigen gamma chain	76	1	1	33.5	
	P10314	HLA class I histocompatibility antigen, A-32 alpha chain	73	3	3	41.0	
	P09326	CD48 antigen	67	2	2	27.7	

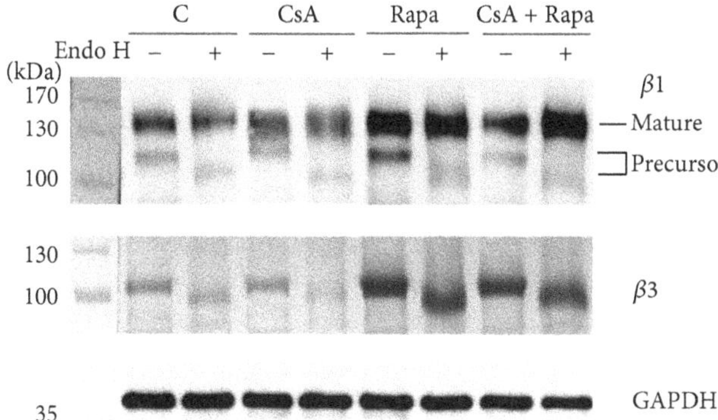

FIGURE 3: Rapamycin (Rapa) and the combination of cyclosporin A (CsA) and Rapa changes $\beta 1$ and $\beta 3$ integrin expression on MLR-activated cells. Peripheral blood mononuclear cells were cultured for 6 days in the presence of CsA (200 ng per 1 mL medium), Rapa (20 ng per 1 mL medium), and the combination of CsA (150 ng per 1 mL medium) and Rapa (12 ng per 1 mL medium) in a two-way mixed leukocyte reaction (MLR) and then lysed in RIPA buffer. Protein extracts (15 μg) were digested with endo-β-N-acetylglucosaminidase H (Endo H) from *Streptomyces plicatus*, SDS-PAGE-separated on 10% gel under reducing conditions, electroblotted onto a PVDF membrane, and probed with specific primary antibodies: mouse monoclonal anti-$\beta 1$ (Chemicon, MAB2251, clone B3B11) and rabbit polyclonal anti-$\beta 3$ (Chemicon, AB1932). Antibody-bound integrins were visualized by chemiluminescence. GAPDH was the endogenous control. C: untreated cells.

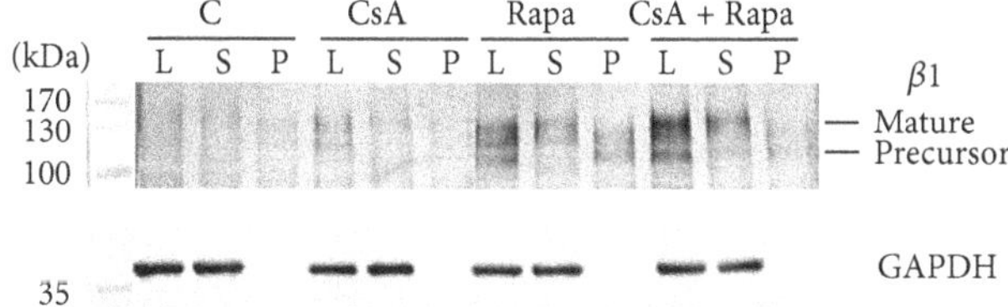

FIGURE 4: High-mannose/hybrid-type glycans are present mainly on premature $\beta 1$ integrin subunit. Cell lysate (L), glycoproteins precipitated with GNA-agarose (P), and supernatant collected after precipitation (S), containing proteins not recognized by GNA, were resolved on 10% SDS-PAGE gel under reducing conditions, electrotransferred to a PVDF membrane and destined for $\beta 1$ integrin subunit immunodetection. GAPDH was the endogenous control. C: untreated cells, CsA: cyclosporin A, and Rapa: rapamycin.

anti-LFA-1 protects against MHC-incompatible graft rejection of fetal small bowel grafts transplanted into mice, making this integrin a potential target for immunosuppression in intestinal transplantation. In turn, the effect of the novel immunosuppressive drug mycophenolate mofetil (MMF) on tumor cells was dose- and cell line-dependent. In kidney carcinoma Caki I cells and pancreatic carcinoma DanG cells treated with 0.1 μM and 1 μM MMF, the expression of integrins of the $\beta 1$ subfamily ($\alpha 1\beta 1$, $\alpha 2\beta 1$, $\alpha 3\beta 1$, $\alpha 4\beta 1$, $\alpha 5\beta 1$, and $\alpha 6\beta 1$) was downregulated; in colonic adenocarcinoma HT-29, $\alpha 3\beta 1$, and $\alpha 6\beta 1$ integrins were upregulated in the presence of 1 μM MMF; and in prostate carcinoma DU-145 most of the analyzed integrins ($\alpha 1\beta 1$, $\alpha 2\beta 1$, $\alpha 3\beta 1$, and $\alpha 5\beta 1$) were upregulated under both MMF doses [41]. Dexamethasone (DEX), a glucocorticoid used commonly for topical ocular application, upregulated $\alpha v\beta 3$ integrin expression in the N27TM-2 cell line derived from human ocular trabecular meshwork, due to an increase of both the half-life and transcription of $\beta 3$ integrin mRNA [42]. CsA also upregulated integrin $\beta 3$ expression but in a dose-dependent manner, resulting in enhanced murine embryonic adhesion and invasion, which promoted embryo implantation [43]. Our work also showed an increase of $\beta 1$ and $\beta 3$ integrin expression in the presence of a therapeutic dose of Rapa and under CsA and Rapa combined (Figures 3 and 4). An earlier study demonstrated that integrins $\beta 1$ and $\beta 3$ mediate adhesion of murine $CD8^+$ cytotoxic T lymphocytes (CTL) to fibronectin (FN), which increased signal triggering by an association of proline-rich tyrosine kinase-2 (Pyk2) with paxillin and the Src kinases, resulting in MHC I-peptide-driven CTL degranulation [48]. $\beta 1$ and $\beta 3$ integrins participate in adhesion of activated T cells to ECM proteins upon TCR triggering or, spontaneously, in secondary lymphoid organs or inflamed tissues, where they become highly exposed to ECM proteins [48, 49]. In this context it is difficult to explain the increase of $\beta 1$ and $\beta 3$ integrin expression we observed upon immunosuppressive drug treatment, but we note that the upregulation of integrin expression was accompanied by an increase of high-mannose/hybrid-type oligosaccharides on $\beta 1$ and $\beta 3$ integrins, as shown by the reaction with GNA (Figure 2(a)). The total surface expression of the high-mannose/hybrid-type N-glycans was also influenced by the immunosuppressive drugs we used; the combination of Rapa and CsA markedly increased the amount of those structures (Figure 1). Only a few previous studies have addressed the effect of immunosuppressive agents on leukocyte glycosylation. Paul et al. [46] showed that MMF inhibited IL-1-induced expression of GNA-recognized oligosaccharides with terminal mannose (Man) on rat endothelial cells. The ability of MMF to downregulate glycosylation results from MMF inhibition of inosine-monophosphate dehydrogenase, the enzyme that catalyses biosynthesis of (deoxy) guanosine nucleotides necessary for transfer of Man and fucose to glycoproteins [46, 50]. MMF-induced reduction of the expression and glycosylation of some adhesion molecules decreases the recruitment of lymphocytes and monocytes to sites of inflammation and graft rejection [50]. Itraconazole (Ita), one of the mTOR inhibitors, reduced poly-N-acetyllactosamine and tetra-antennary complex-type N-glycans in human umbilical vein endothelial cells (HUVEC) and caused an increase of Man5GlcNAc2 oligomannose structures on vascular endothelial growth factor receptor 2 (VEGFR2). Hypoglycosylation of VEGFR2 strongly inhibited its autophosphorylation after VEGF stimulation [15]. Induction of hypoglycosylation on VEGFR2 in HUVEC cells by Ita was similar to the effects of this drug in macrophages RAW 264.7. Glycosylphosphatidylinositol-anchored glycoprotein CD14 in RAW 264.7 became Endo H-sensitive in the presence of Ita. CD14 with altered glycosylation was delivered to the cell surface, as determined by binding of concanavalin A (Con-A) [51]. Alteration of glycan synthesis by immunosuppressive drugs has also been observed in cancer cells. Treatment of MDA-MB231 breast cancer cells with Rapa upregulated the sialylation of N-glycans on $\beta 1$ integrin

[45]. The clinically relevant concentration of CsA markedly decreased glucosylceramide levels in the multidrug-resistant human breast cancer MCF-7 cell line [52].

How does upregulation of GNA-positive glycoproteins, among the β integrins, driven by these anti-inflammatory immunosuppressive drugs, contribute to the development of immune tolerance against allogeneic antigens? We find a possible explanation in early studies by Muchmore et al. [13], which showed that mannose-rich oligosaccharide structures on uromodulin, ovalbumin, and soybean lectin (SBA) directly inhibit the antigen-driven T cell response in human mononuclear cell culture. What is more, treatment of endothelial cells with 1-deoxymannojirimycin (DMJ) and castanospermine (CAST), inhibitors which cause accumulation of high-mannose-type oligosaccharides, decreased interleukin 1-induced lymphocyte binding to endothelial cells; reduction of lymphocyte extravasation results in suppression of the immune response [53]. Similarly, the presence of immature high-mannose oligosaccharides on both subunits of FN receptor, integrin $\alpha 5\beta 1$ in the cell surface of human fibroblasts, led to attenuation of ligand binding under treatment with DMJ. Inhibition of oligosaccharide processing at the high-mannose N-glycan stage did not alter receptor assembly and insertion into the plasma membrane, but it significantly modified integrin binding ability [14]. What is interesting is that the content of immature N-glycans diminishes during lymphocyte maturation; half of the N-glycans on CD45 on thymocytes are high-mannose or hybrid-type, while the majority of N-glycans on CD45 on peripheral T cells are ST6GalI-modified complex-type structures [30]. Conversion of high-mannose to complex-type N-linked glycans is also necessary for differentiation of human B lymphocytes into cells secreting immunoglobulins (Ig), as determined by strong inhibition of Ig production in culture of human lymphocytes with DMJ or swainsonine (SW), which block conversion of high-mannose to complex-type glycans [54]. On the other hand, activation of alloantigen-reactive regulatory T cells (Treg) resulted in increased expression of $\alpha 1,2$-mannosidase, the enzyme that catalyzes removal of Man from Man9GlcNAc2 and generates Man5GlcNAc2. In mice, reduction of high-mannose structures was not required for the suppressive capacity of Treg but facilitated its migration to sites where it regulates the immune response [35]. The divergence of these results may indicate that the glycan-mediated effect is specific to the T cell type or organism. In view of the above-mentioned studies, we suggest that the abundant high-mannose/hybrid-type glycans on $\beta 1$ and $\beta 3$ integrins upregulated by CsA and Rapa may contribute to suppression of the immune response.

A variety of previous studies have shown that glycans play important roles in immune cell interactions during the immune response [5, 8, 33, 55], and now our results give further evidence that changes in oligosaccharide composition may shift the balance between the pro- and anti-inflammatory activities of leukocytes. Rapa and CsA have been shown to act synergistically for prolongation of allograft and xenograft survival [40, 47]. Possibly the changes in the glycosylation profile of leukocytes promote the development of tolerance in transplantation. New approaches aimed at developing better immunosuppressive strategies should incorporate the potential ability of drugs to alter glycosylation of target proteins.

5. Conclusions

Our study showed that these immunosuppressive drugs affect high-mannose/hybrid-type glycosylation of human leukocytes activated in an MLR reaction. CsA significantly reduced the number of leukocytes covered by high-mannose/hybrid N-glycans, and the synergistic action of CsA and Rapa led to an increase of these structures on the remaining leukocytes. This is the first study indicating that $\beta 1$ and $\beta 3$ integrins bearing high-mannose/hybrid structures are affected by Rapa and CsA. By regulating the protein amount, the immunosuppressive drugs increased the oligomannose/hybrid-type N-glycosylation on the leukocyte surface. This alteration of glycosylation on leukocytes may contribute to the development of immune tolerance. The functional consequences of changes in the glycosylation profile are an area for further study.

Conflict of Interests

The authors declare that there is no conflict of interests regarding the publication of this paper.

Acknowledgments

The authors thank Michael Jacobs for line-editing the paper for submission, Lidia Malchar for expert technical assistance, and Ewa Sitkiewicz (Mass Spectrometry Laboratory, Polish Academy of Sciences, Warsaw) for help in analysis of MS results. This work was supported by grants K/ZDS/004829 (Jagiellonian University) and Iuventus Plus IP2010003370 from the Ministry of Science and Higher Education (University of Warsaw).

References

[1] S. M. Haslam, S. Julien, J. M. Burchell et al., "Characterizing the glycome of the mammalian immune system," *Immunology and Cell Biology*, vol. 86, no. 7, pp. 564–573, 2008.

[2] J. L. Johnson, M. B. Jones, S. O. Ryan, and B. A. Cobb, "The regulatory power of glycans and their binding partners in immunity," *Trends in Immunology*, vol. 34, no. 6, pp. 290–298, 2013.

[3] J. D. Marth and P. K. Grewal, "Mammalian glycosylation in immunity," *Nature Reviews Immunology*, vol. 8, no. 11, pp. 874–887, 2008.

[4] P. M. Rudd, M. R. Wormald, and R. A. Dwek, "Sugar-mediated ligand-receptor interactions in the immune system," *Trends in Biotechnology*, vol. 22, no. 10, pp. 524–530, 2004.

[5] G. A. Rabinovich, Y. van Kooyk, and B. A. Cobb, "Glycobiology of immune responses," *Annals of the New York Academy of Sciences*, vol. 1253, no. 1, pp. 1–15, 2012.

[6] A. Kobata, "A journey to the world of glycobiology," *Glycoconjugate Journal*, vol. 17, no. 7–9, pp. 443–464, 2000.

[7] C. Boscher, J. W. Dennis, and I. R. Nabi, "Glycosylation, galectins and cellular signaling," *Current Opinion in Cell Biology*, vol. 23, no. 4, pp. 383–392, 2011.

[8] S. O. Ryan and B. A. Cobb, "Roles for major histocompatibility complex glycosylation in immune function," *Seminars in Immunopathology*, vol. 34, no. 3, pp. 425–441, 2012.

[9] S. Ringeard, J. Harb, F. Gautier, J. Menanteau, and K. Meflah, "Altered glycosylation of $\alpha(s)\beta1$ integrins from rat colon carcinoma cells decreases their interaction with fibronectin," *Journal of Cellular Biochemistry*, vol. 62, no. 1, pp. 40–49, 1996.

[10] Y. Zhang, J.-H. Zhao, X.-Y. Zhang, H.-B. Guo, F. Liu, and H.-L. Chen, "Relations of the type and branch of surface N-glycans to cell adhesion, migration and integrin expressions," *Molecular and Cellular Biochemistry*, vol. 260, no. 1, pp. 137–146, 2004.

[11] S. Ehlers, "DC-SIGN and mannosylated surface structures of *Mycobacterium tuberculosis*: a deceptive liaison," *European Journal of Cell Biology*, vol. 89, no. 1, pp. 95–101, 2010.

[12] Y. van Kooyk and G. A. Rabinovich, "Protein-glycan interactions in the control of innate and adaptive immune responses," *Nature Immunology*, vol. 9, no. 6, pp. 593–601, 2008.

[13] A. V. Muchmore, N. Sathyamoorthy, J. Decker, and A. P. Sherblom, "Evidence that specific high-mannose oligosaccharides can directly inhibit antigen-driven T-cell responses," *Journal of Leukocyte Biology*, vol. 48, no. 5, pp. 457–464, 1990.

[14] S. K. Akiyama, S. S. Yamada, and K. M. Yamada, "Analysis of the role of glycosylation of the human fibronectin receptor," *The Journal of Biological Chemistry*, vol. 264, no. 30, pp. 18011–18018, 1989.

[15] B. A. Nacev, P. Grassi, A. Dell, S. M. Haslam, and J. O. Liu, "The antifungal drug itraconazole inhibits vascular endothelial growth factor receptor 2 (VEGFR2) glycosylation, trafficking, and signaling in endothelial cells," *The Journal of Biological Chemistry*, vol. 286, no. 51, pp. 44045–44056, 2011.

[16] R. Evans, I. Patzak, L. Svensson et al., "Integrins in immunity," *Journal of Cell Science*, vol. 122, no. 2, pp. 215–225, 2009.

[17] N. Hogg, M. Laschinger, K. Giles, and A. McDowall, "T-cell integrins: more than just sticking points," *Journal of Cell Science*, vol. 116, no. 23, pp. 4695–4705, 2003.

[18] J. T. Pribila, A. C. Quale, K. L. Mueller, and Y. Shimizu, "Integrins and T cell-mediated immunity," *Annual Review of Immunology*, vol. 22, pp. 157–180, 2004.

[19] Y. Zhang and H. Wang, "Integrin signalling and function in immune cells," *Immunology*, vol. 135, no. 4, pp. 268–275, 2012.

[20] E. S. Harris, T. M. McIntyre, S. M. Prescott, and G. A. Zimmerman, "The leukocyte integrins," *The Journal of Biological Chemistry*, vol. 275, no. 31, pp. 23409–23412, 2000.

[21] T. N. Sims and M. L. Dustin, "The immunological synapse: integrins take the stage," *Immunological Reviews*, vol. 186, pp. 100–117, 2002.

[22] M. L. Dustin and J. A. Cooper, "The immunological synapse and the actin cytoskeleton: molecular hardware for T cell signaling," *Nature Immunology*, vol. 1, no. 1, pp. 23–29, 2000.

[23] G. M. Griffiths, A. Tsun, and J. C. Stinchcombe, "The immunological synapse: a focal point for endocytosis and exocytosis," *Journal of Cell Biology*, vol. 189, no. 3, pp. 399–406, 2010.

[24] D. M. Rose, R. Alon, and M. H. Ginsberg, "Integrin modulation and signaling in leukocyte adhesion and migration," *Immunological Reviews*, vol. 218, no. 1, pp. 126–134, 2007.

[25] A. Lacy-Hulbert, T. Ueno, T. Ito et al., "$\beta3$ integrins regulate lymphocyte migration and cytokine responses in heart transplant rejection," *American Journal of Transplantation*, vol. 7, no. 5, pp. 1080–1090, 2007.

[26] A. D. Luster, R. Alon, and U. H. von Andrian, "Immune cell migration in inflammation: present and future therapeutic targets," *Nature Immunology*, vol. 6, no. 12, pp. 1182–1190, 2005.

[27] S. Sarnacki, Y. Révillon, A. Fischer et al., "Blockade of the integrin $\alpha L\beta2$ but not of integrins $\alpha4$ and/or $\beta7$ significantly prolongs intestinal allograft survival in mice," *Gut*, vol. 47, no. 1, pp. 97–104, 2000.

[28] J. Gu and N. Taniguchi, "Potential of N-glycan in cell adhesion and migration as either a positive or negative regulator," *Cell Adhesion & Migration*, vol. 2, no. 4, pp. 243–245, 2008.

[29] M. A. Daniels, K. A. Hogquist, and S. C. Jameson, "Sweet 'n' sour: the impact of differential glycosylation on T cell responses," *Nature Immunology*, vol. 3, no. 10, pp. 903–910, 2002.

[30] M. C. Clark and L. G. Baum, "T cells modulate glycans on CD43 and CD45 during development and activation, signal regulation, and survival," *Annals of the New York Academy of Sciences*, vol. 1253, no. 1, pp. 58–67, 2012.

[31] P. M. Rudd, M. R. Wormald, R. L. Stanfield et al., "Roles for glycosylation of cell surface receptors involved in cellular immune recognition," *Journal of Molecular Biology*, vol. 293, no. 2, pp. 351–366, 1999.

[32] D. H. Dube and C. R. Bertozzi, "Glycans in cancer and inflammation—potential for therapeutics and diagnostics," *Nature Reviews Drug Discovery*, vol. 4, no. 6, pp. 477–488, 2005.

[33] K. Ohtsubo and J. D. Marth, "Glycosylation in cellular mechanisms of health and disease," *Cell*, vol. 126, no. 5, pp. 855–867, 2006.

[34] J. Chinen and R. H. Buckley, "Transplantation immunology: solid organ and bone marrow," *Journal of Allergy and Clinical Immunology*, vol. 125, no. 2, pp. S324–S335, 2010.

[35] E. T. Long, S. Baker, V. Oliveira, B. Sawitzkib, and K. J. Wood, "Alpha-1,2-mannosidase and hence N-glycosylation are required for regulatory T cell migration and allograft tolerance in mice," *PLoS ONE*, vol. 5, no. 1, Article ID e8894, 2010.

[36] K. Bocian, J. Borysowski, P. Wierzbicki et al., "Rapamycin, unlike cyclosporine A, enhances suppressive functions of in vitro-induced $CD4^{+}CD25+$ Tregs," *Nephrology Dialysis Transplantation*, vol. 25, no. 3, pp. 710–717, 2010.

[37] R. N. Saunders, M. S. Metcalfe, and M. L. Nicholson, "Rapamycin in transplantation: a review of the evidence," *Kidney International*, vol. 59, no. 1, pp. 3–16, 2001.

[38] C.-L. Lee, P.-P. Jiang, W.-H. Sit, and J. M.-F. Wan, "Proteome of human T lymphocytes with treatment of cyclosporine and polysaccharopeptide: analysis of significant proteins that manipulate T cells proliferation and immunosuppression," *International Immunopharmacology*, vol. 7, no. 10, pp. 1311–1324, 2007.

[39] K. Kędzierska, K. Sporniak-Tutak, K. Sindrewicz et al., "Effects of immunosuppressive treatment on protein expression in rat kidney," *Drug Design, Development and Therapy*, vol. 8, pp. 1695–1708, 2014.

[40] D. F. Martin, L. R. DeBarge, R. B. Nussenblatt, C.-C. Chan, and F. G. Roberge, "Synergistic effect of rapamycin and cyclosporin A in the treatment of experimental autoimmune uveoretinitis," *Journal of Immunology*, vol. 154, no. 2, pp. 922–927, 1995.

[41] T. Engl, J. Makarević, B. Relja et al., "Mycophenolate mofetil modulates adhesion receptors of the beta1 integrin family on tumor cells: impact on tumor recurrence and malignancy," *BMC Cancer*, vol. 5, article 4, 2005.

[42] J. A. Faralli, D. Gagen, M. S. Filla, T. N. Crotti, and D. M. Peters, "Dexamethasone increases $\alpha v\beta3$ integrin expression and

affinity through a calcineurin/NFAT pathway," *Biochimica et Biophysica Acta—Molecular Cell Research*, vol. 1833, no. 12, pp. 3306–3313, 2013.

[43] Y.-H. Huang, Y.-L. Ma, L. Ma et al., "Cyclosporine A improves adhesion and invasion of mouse preimplantation embryos via upregulating integrin $\beta3$ and matrix metalloproteinase-9," *International Journal of Clinical and Experimental Pathology*, vol. 7, no. 4, pp. 1379–1388, 2014.

[44] F. Zal, Z. Mostafavi-Pour, A. Moattari, A. Sardarian, and M. Vessal, "Altered expression of $alpha_2beta_1$ integrin in kidney fibroblasts: a potential mechanism for CsA-induced nephrotoxicity," *Archives of Iranian Medicine*, vol. 17, no. 8, pp. 556–562, 2014.

[45] T. Isaji, S. Im, W. Gu et al., "An oncogenic protein Golgi phosphoprotein 3 up-regulates cell migration via sialylation," *The Journal of Biological Chemistry*, vol. 289, no. 30, pp. 20694–20705, 2014.

[46] L. C. Paul, J.-F. Valentin, J. A. Bruijn, and S. Zhang, "Donor treatment with mycophenolate mofetil protects against ischemia-reperfusion injury," *Transplantation Proceedings*, vol. 31, no. 1-2, p. 1026, 1999.

[47] M. M. Aw, "Transplant immunology," *Journal of Pediatric Surgery*, vol. 38, no. 9, pp. 1275–1280, 2003.

[48] M.-A. Doucey, D. F. Legler, M. Faroudi et al., "The beta1 and beta3 integrins promote T cell receptor-mediated cytotoxic T lymphocyte activation," *The Journal of Biological Chemistry*, vol. 278, no. 29, pp. 26983–26991, 2003.

[49] M. L. Dustin and A. R. de Fougerolles, "Reprograming T cells: the role of extracellular matrix in coordination of T cell activation and migration," *Current Opinion in Immunology*, vol. 13, no. 3, pp. 286–290, 2001.

[50] A. C. Allison and E. M. Eugui, "Mycophenolate mofetil and its mechanisms of action," *Immunopharmacology*, vol. 47, no. 2-3, pp. 85–118, 2000.

[51] T. Frey and A. De Maio, "The antifungal agent itraconazole induces the accumulation of high mannose glycoproteins in macrophages," *Journal of Biological Chemistry*, vol. 284, no. 25, pp. 16882–16890, 2009.

[52] Y. Lavie, H.-T. Cao, A. Volner et al., "Agents that reverse multidrug resistance, tamoxifen, verapamil, and cyclosporin A, block glycosphingolipid metabolism by inhibiting ceramide glycosylation in human cancer cells," *The Journal of Biological Chemistry*, vol. 272, no. 3, pp. 1682–1687, 1997.

[53] R. Renkonen and J. Ustinov, "Carbohydrate synthesis inhibitors decrease interleukin 1-stimulated lymphocyte binding to endothelial cells," *European Journal of Immunology*, vol. 21, no. 3, pp. 777–781, 1991.

[54] A. Tulp, M. Barnhoorn, E. Bause, and H. Ploegh, "Inhibition of N-linked oligosaccharide trimming mannosidases blocks human B cell development," *The EMBO Journal*, vol. 5, no. 8, pp. 1783–1790, 1986.

[55] M. Sperandio, C. A. Gleissner, and K. Ley, "Glycosylation in immune cell trafficking," *Immunological Reviews*, vol. 230, no. 1, pp. 97–113, 2009.

3

A Heuristic Framework for Image Filtering and Segmentation: Application to Blood Vessel Immunohistochemistry

Chi-Hsuan Tsou,[1] Yi-Chien Lu,[2] Ang Yuan,[3] Yeun-Chung Chang,[2] and Chung-Ming Chen[1]

[1]*Institute of Biomedical Engineering, College of Medicine and College of Engineering, National Taiwan University, No. 1, Section 1, Jen-Ai Road, Taipei 100, Taiwan*
[2]*Department of Radiology, National Taiwan University College of Medicine and Department of Medical Imaging, National Taiwan University Hospital, No. 7, Chung-Shan South Road, Taipei 100, Taiwan*
[3]*Department of Internal Medicine, National Taiwan University College of Medicine, No. 7, Chung-Shan South Road, Taipei 100, Taiwan*

Correspondence should be addressed to Chung-Ming Chen; chung@ntu.edu.tw

Academic Editor: Giovanni Tuccari

The blood vessel density in a cancerous tissue sample may represent increased levels of tumor growth. However, identifying blood vessels in the histological (tissue) image is difficult and time-consuming and depends heavily on the observer's experience. To overcome this drawback, computer-aided image analysis frameworks have been investigated in order to boost object identification in histological images. We present a novel algorithm to automatically abstract the salient regions in blood vessel images. Experimental results show that the proposed framework is capable of deriving vessel boundaries that are comparable to those demarcated manually, even for vessel regions with weak contrast between the object boundaries and background clutter.

1. Introduction

Computer-aided diagnosis (CADx) for high-throughput tissue banks and digitized histological (tissue) images has shown promise for relieving pathologists' workload by assisting in differentiating cases of benign and difficult-to-diagnose suspicious tumor areas [1–5]. The CADx system is expected to improve clinical practice [1, 2] and the performance of human observers as they interpret histological images [3–5]. For example, the qualitative evaluation of the spatial distribution of vessels surrounding tumors may represent the increased levels of angiogenesis (the growth of new capillary blood vessels) in tumor growth [6–9]. To investigate the increased levels of tumorigenicity (the ability to give rise to tumors), the blood vessel density in a cancerous tissue sample can be determined by using immunohistochemical (IHC) staining methods. However, the interpretation of the histopathological image is relatively difficult and time-consuming, and the identification of blood vessels depends heavily on the observer's experience.

To overcome this drawback, computer-aided image analysis frameworks have been widely and intensively investigated in order to boost the performance of object identification in histological images [1]. Generally, a clinical decision support system starts with quality control and ends with predictive modeling for several cancer endpoints [10]. Nevertheless, it remains impractical to apply these computer-aided diagnostic algorithms in clinical applications. The primary difficulty lies in quantitatively characterizing the histological images, given the variety of imaging methods and disease-specific textures. Therefore, a pressing need exists for a computer-aided image analysis approach to quantify the useful factors for angiogenesis: area, spatial distribution, and density of blood vessels. Blood vessel region abstraction is a crucial step for achieving this goal. However, the development of robust algorithms for the automated analysis of blood vessel images has many challenges, including an extensive variation in blood vessel structure and features and missing blood vessel boundaries caused by weak contrast, background clutter, and stain contamination.

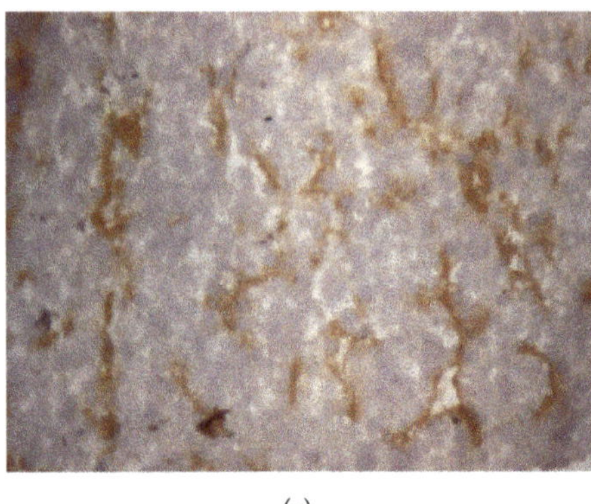

(a)

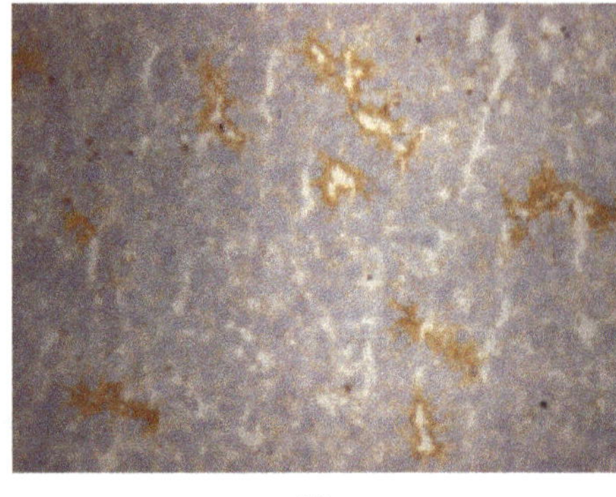

(b)

FIGURE 1: Immunostained vessel images.

Based on the image analysis methods used for blood vessel quantification, our proposed framework includes two main components:

(1) An image filtering algorithm that uses color, luminance, and spatial variations in pixel intensities in order to make a visual search more efficient.

(2) An image segmentation algorithm that incorporates the global feature information derived from measurements of pixel intensities into the curve evolution and the curvature flow component.

One important advantage of using image filtering over a segmentation method is the ability to improve the accuracy of image segmentation; the operator can more easily distinguish the location of the vascular area. For instance, some variations in staining and scanning conditions, such as image acquisition protocols, capturing-device properties, and lighting conditions, can reduce the accuracy of the quantifications, rendering them unusable.

Further, the structure and morphology of blood vessel images can be complicated, as shown in Figures 1(a) and 1(b). Traditional vessel image analysis methods [11–13] were unable to accurately detect the location of blood vessels. Therefore, we propose an image filtering algorithm allowing foreground (i.e., vessel) regions to be easily detected.

In this paper, we present a novel algorithm for automatically abstracting the blood vessel image that highlights the blood vessel regions and reduces the texture noise of the nonvessel regions. We examine the Gaussian color model of the original image to extract the large-scale layer and use the normalized color of the original color layer to extract the detailed layer. We then recombine the color layer of the original image, the large-scale layer, and the detailed layer to produce an image with two properties: salient blood vessel regions and a homogeneous background. Finally, we abstract this image using luminance quantization to generate the visually important blood vessel regions.

For vessel image quantification, the proposed image segmentation algorithm consists of two steps. In the first step, a region-based active contour method, namely, the graph partitioning active contours (GPAC) method, is used to derive a preliminary result. The GPAC incorporates global feature information into the curve evolution and the curvature flow component. Because misclassification is often inevitable in the GPAC segmentation of blood vessel images, owing to the weak contrast between the object boundaries and the background clutter, the second step further improves the segmentation accuracy using statistical intensity information. The essential concept of the second step is to employ local adaptive thresholding to discriminate between the subvessel regions formed in the first step and the background. It alleviates the interference caused by other structures within the subvessel regions, while preserving or introducing only tolerable distortion to the properties of the vessel objects of interest.

The remainder of this paper is organized as follows: We present the proposed framework in Section 2, discuss the results obtained from experiments in Section 3, and, finally, conclude the paper in Section 4. (Note: An earlier version of this work was presented as a conference paper [14]. This journal version extends the previous work with more concrete examples of complete theories, experiments, and comparisons.)

2. Materials and Methods

Three non-small cell lung-cancer cell lines, CL1-0 transfect, VEGF isoform 189, and A549, were used. All of them were cultured with the ATCC complete growth medium RPMI 1640, within a combination of 2 mM L-glutamine, 1.5 g/L sodium bicarbonate, 4.5 g/L glucose, 100 U/mL penicillin G sodium, 100 μg/mL streptomycin sulfate, and 10% fetal bovine serum, in a humidified atmosphere consisting of 5% CO_2 in air at 37°C. Immunohistochemical analysis of the cryostat sections and quantitative analysis of the blood vessel densities of tumor samples were performed. An anti-CD31 mouse monoclonal antibody (clone MEC 13.3, PharMingen) was used in the analysis. The proposed heuristic framework for histological vessel image analysis, based on the image filtering and segmentation algorithms, is detailed in the following sections.

2.1. Automatic Immunostained Vessel Image Filtering Algorithm. An algorithm for blood vessel abstraction [14] which

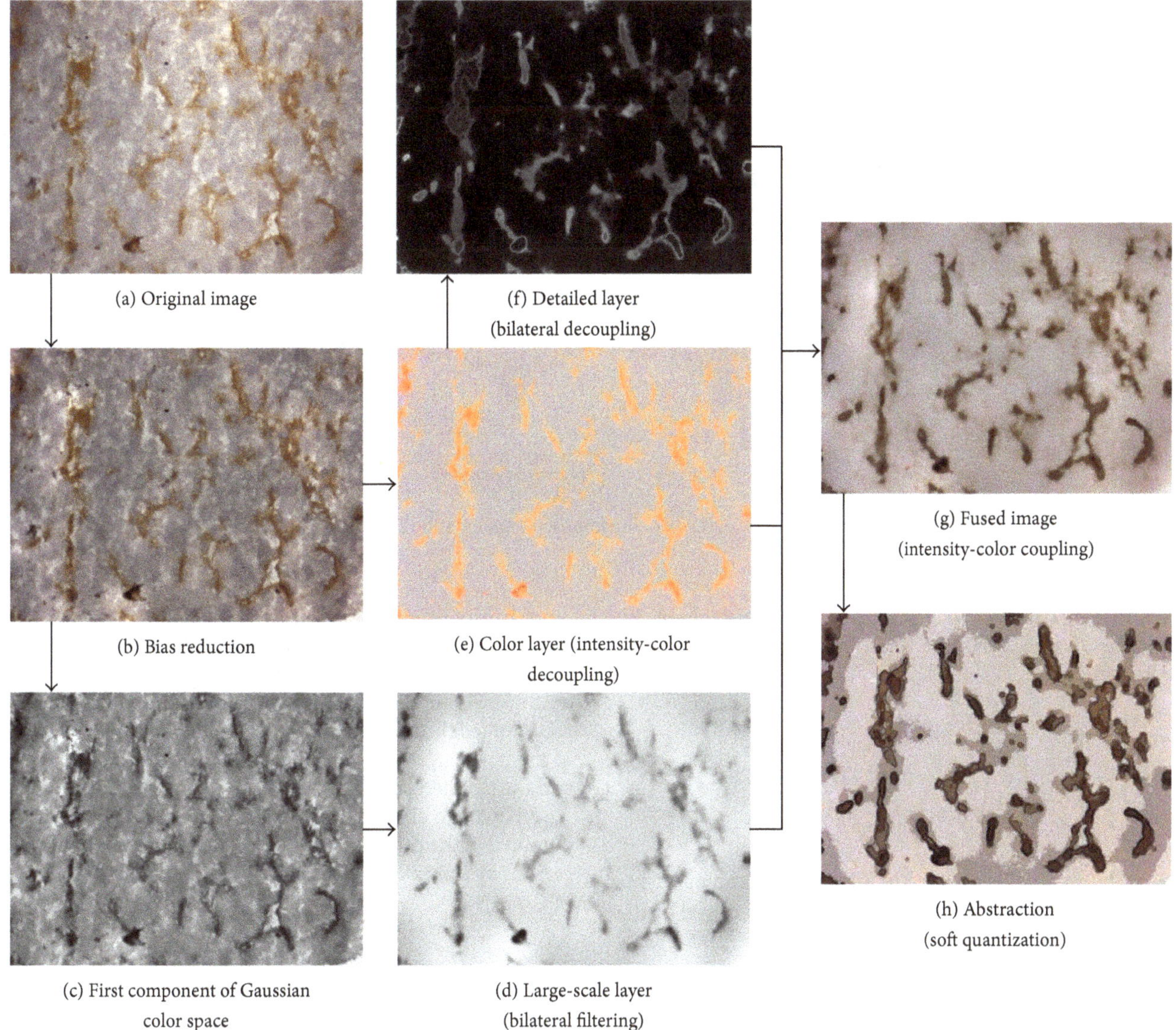

FIGURE 2: Flowchart of our proposed image filtering algorithm.

was based on computing salient maps of blood vessel regions was proposed. Our approach proceeded as follows. First, we examined the stain adhered to the objects, using the normalized color on the color layer of the original image, to extract the detail of the blood vessel regions. This procedure could reduce the texture noise due to large structural variations in the biological image. Second, in order to maintain the pattern distributions, we used bilateral filtering to smooth the first component of the Gaussian color model and emphasize sharp features. Thus, we could preserve the blood vessel regions and simultaneously enhance their sharpness by reconstructing the detailed and large-scale layers. An overview of the complete algorithm is summarized in Figure 2.

Due to platform illumination variations in image acquisition, Niblack's adaptive thresholding method was performed to remove the light bias [15]. The basic concept of Niblack's method is to build a threshold surface T, based on the local mean m and standard deviation s of gray values, computed over a small neighborhood around each pixel in the form of

$$T = m + k \cdot s, \tag{1}$$

where k is a negative constant. This method tends to produce the distribution of the light illumination. As a result, the light bias was reduced by dividing the intensity of the original by the threshold surface. The definition of the intensity and color channels is a linear weighted combination of R, G, and B for intensity estimation [16]:

$$I = \frac{R}{(R+G+B)}R + \frac{G}{(R+G+B)}G + \frac{B}{(R+G+B)}B. \tag{2}$$

The intensity distribution of blood vessel regions was heterogeneous and the background of the original image was also cluttered. Therefore, using perceptual uniform color

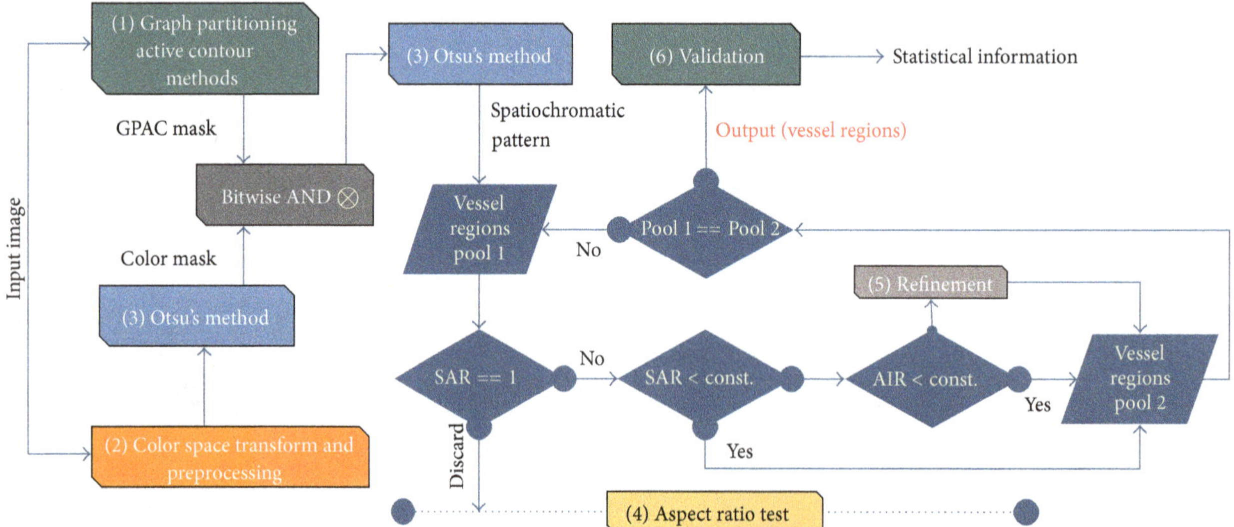

Figure 3: Overview of our proposed segmentation system.

spaces in such images was necessary. We transformed the original RGB image into the Gaussian color space [17] using the following:

$$\begin{bmatrix} \widehat{E} \\ \widehat{E}_{\lambda} \\ \widehat{E}_{\lambda\lambda} \end{bmatrix} = \begin{pmatrix} 0.06 & 0.63 & 0.27 \\ 0.3 & 0.04 & -0.35 \\ 0.34 & -0.6 & 0.17 \end{pmatrix} \begin{bmatrix} R \\ G \\ B \end{bmatrix}. \quad (3)$$

For human color vision, the first of three components $\widehat{E}$, $\widehat{E}_{\lambda}$, and $\widehat{E}_{\lambda\lambda}$ of the Gaussian color model, measured by the Taylor expansion of the Gaussian weighted spectral energy distribution at $\lambda_0 \simeq 520\,\text{nm}$ and scale $\sigma_{\lambda} \simeq 55\,\text{nm}$, was used as an input for large-scale calculation. The invariant $\widehat{C}_{\lambda} = \widehat{E}_{\lambda}/\widehat{E}$ (the object's reflectance property, independent of viewpoint, surface orientation, illumination direction, or illumination intensity) was represented using normalized color to obtain the detailed layer of the original image.

After acquiring the normalized color, we used a bilateral decoupling procedure [16] to decompose the image into layers corresponding to the sharp details within the blood vessel regions. The bilateral filter [18] combined domain and range filtering by replacing the pixel value with a weighted average of similar (weight r on the pixel difference) and nearby (weight s on the spatial location) pixel values. The objective of the bilateral filter was to group perceptually similar colors together and preserve only the perceptually visible edge. Given an image $f(\cdot)$, the output $J(\cdot)$ of the bilateral filter for a pixel x was

$$J_x = \frac{1}{k(x)} \sum_{n \in \Omega} s(n-x)\, r(f_n - f_x)\, f_n \quad (4)$$

with normalization

$$k(x) = \sum_{n \in \Omega} s(n-x)\, r(f_n - f_x). \quad (5)$$

We used a combination of the bilateral filters of the normalized color to deduce the detailed layer. The large-scale layer was derived from a single iteration of a bilateral filter of the first component of the Gaussian color model. Then, we recombined the image using the element-by-element product of the color layer of the original image, the large-scale layer, and the detailed layer.

In order to abstract the blood vessel regions in the image obtained in the previous step, we modeled the visually salient regions by luminance quantization as follows [19]:

$$Q(\widehat{s}, q, \kappa_q) = q_{\text{nearest}} + \frac{\Delta q}{2} \tanh\left(\kappa_q \cdot \left(h(\widehat{s}) - q_{\text{nearest}}\right)\right), \quad (6)$$

where $Q(\cdot)$ is the pseudoquantized image, Δq is the bin width, q_{nearest} is the bin boundary closest to $h(\widehat{s})$, and κ_q is a parameter controlling the sharpness of the transition from one bin to another. The result of our approach is shown in Figures 2(h) and 9.

2.2. Histological Image Segmentation Algorithm. The main stages of the proposed segmentation scheme are as follows: (1) the graph partitioning active contours (GPAC) method [20]; (2) color space transform and preprocessing; (3) Otsu's clustering method [21]; (4) aspect ratio test and refinement; and (5) validation. Figure 3 shows the overview diagram of the proposed segmentation scheme.

2.2.1. Graph Partitioning Active Contours Methods. The main objective of graph-based segmentation methods is to seek the best partition of the affinity graph, denoted as G, in which every image pixel is regarded as a graph node and every possible pairwise relation of image pixels is represented as a graph edge. The GPAC method [20] is a variational framework for pairwise-similarity-based segmentation which has an important characteristic called stability. This means it

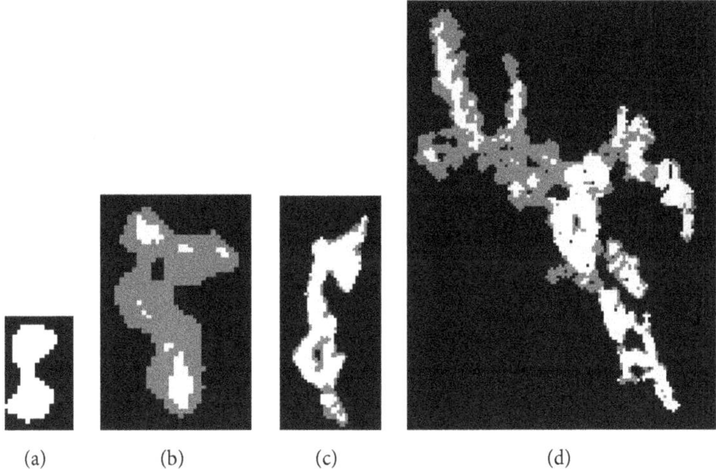

FIGURE 4: Four different spatiochromatic patterns. (a) Type 1; (b) Type 4; (c) Type 2; (d) Type 3.

TABLE 1: Five different region types derived according to their spatiochromatic patterns.

	Type 1	Type 2	Type 3	Type 4	Type 5
Vessel (white)	All	Almost	Half	Few	None
Surrounding tissue (gray)	None	Few	Half	Almost	All

usually converges to the same result despite varying curve initializations and noise. Partitioning was used to derive the approximation of vessel regions in the image as an input of local adaptive thresholding while reducing computational efforts.

2.2.2. Color Space Transform and Preprocessing. The intensity distribution of blood vessel regions was heterogeneous and the background of the original image was also cluttered. Therefore, using perceptual uniform color spaces in such images was necessary. As a result, we applied the transformation of the original RGB image into the YCbCr color space. Because of platform illumination variations in image acquisition, the process of image contrast enhancement using the sigmoid function in a spatial domain was used to correct the light bias.

2.2.3. Threshold Selection. Otsu's method [21] is a bimodal clustering technique based on intensity estimation for the analysis of histogram distribution. Subvessel regions formed in the first step are discriminated from the background by minimizing the within-class variance of the regions formed by thresholding.

2.2.4. Aspect Ratio Test and Refinement. Five different region types are derived, as shown in Table 1, according to their spatiochromatic patterns, as shown in Figure 4. The aspect ratio test comprises three criteria for distinguishing Type 3 regions from other type patterns. The definitions of these criteria are listed below.

Criterion 1. If the vessel-candidate region is Type 5 (i.e., all gray and no white tissue), then it will become part of the background (i.e., SAR = 1), thus eliminating unnecessary calculations.

Criterion 2. Calculate the surrounding area ratio (SAR) for each vessel-candidate region:

$$\text{SAR} = \frac{\text{surrounding tissue}}{\text{its vessel-candidate areas}}, \tag{7}$$

where the surrounding tissue represents the gray part of the vessel-candidate area, which includes both gray and white areas.

Criterion 3. Calculate the area image ratio (AIR) for each vessel-candidate region:

$$\text{AIR} = \frac{\text{its vessel-candidate areas}}{\text{image size}}. \tag{8}$$

The aspect ratio test was conducted in order to identify the Type 3 pattern (i.e., half gray and half white). The relative vessel region is then arranged for the refinement step procedure, as shown in Figure 5.

2.2.5. Validation. Our collaborating assistant manually calculated the vessel numbers in the images; we consider this to be the ground truth. We compared her numbers with the automatically generated numbers as follows:

$$\text{error} = \frac{\text{Number (computer XOR GT)}}{\text{Number (GT)}} \times 100\%, \tag{9}$$

where computer is the region number (based on the automatically detected border) and ground truth (GT) was defined above.

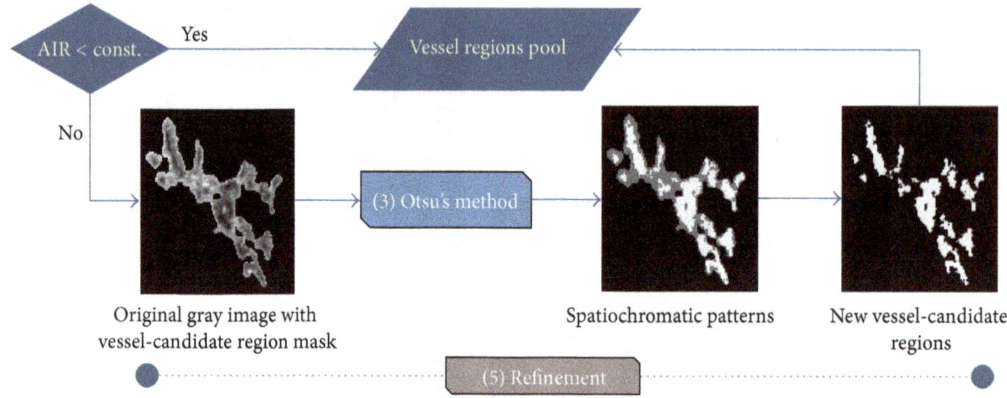

FIGURE 5: Refinement step process in the segmentation algorithm.

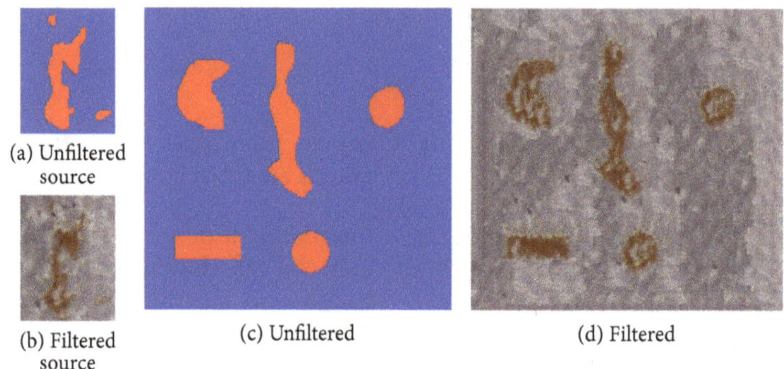

FIGURE 6: Synthetic vascular image. The unfiltered source image (a) was outlined manually to annotate (b). We created the unfiltered target image (c); then the filter learned from (a) and (b) was applied to (c) to get (d). The result is shown in (d).

3. Results and Discussion

3.1. Automatic Immunostained Vessel Image Filtering Algorithm. To create the synthetic vascular images with different complex vessel samples, we used "image analogies" [22] that effectively apply the statistics of a labeled image (Figure 6(a)) to a new unlabeled image (Figure 6(c)). Specifically, a synthetic vascular image (Figure 6(d)) was created by coating the given vessel samples (Figure 6(b)) with a labeling of the components of the vessel images. The experimental results of the synthetic vascular images in Figure 7 showed that filtering images within the nonvessel regions could improve the image segmentation accuracy using fuzzy c-means clustering, as shown in Figure 8, and preserve the vessel regions as well. We applied the three-class fuzzy c-means clustering to the synthetic vascular images and considered the first clustering as vessel pixels. The clustering error is defined as

$$\text{error} = \frac{\text{Area}\,(\text{computer XOR GT})}{\text{Area}\,(\text{GT})} \times 100\%, \quad (10)$$

where computer is the binary image obtained by filling the image segmentation by fuzzy c-means clustering, and the ground truth (GT) is obtained from Figure 6(c).

The experimental results of salient blood vessel region detection and abstraction using our method, shown in Figure 9, showed that the sharpness of the blood vessel borders was enhanced and the details of the blood vessel regions were also preserved. For instance, Figure 10(a) shows a detailed layer from Figure 2(a) with low contrast in the blood vessel regions while the background regions have high contrast and texture noise. The result of our proposed filtering method showed that our approach could increase the contrast in the blood vessel regions and also reduce the noise in the background regions, as shown in Figure 10(b).

In our experiment, if the margin of the blood vessel region was quite thin—for example, when the blood vessel cavity is surrounded by only a few blood vessel wall areas, as in Figure 10(c)—the final abstraction, as shown in Figure 10(d), would regard the cavity as background. This problem is currently under study, using machine learning techniques. In practice, we have gained promising abstraction results on a wide range of complex blood vessel images, as shown in Figure 9.

3.2. Histology Image Segmentation Algorithm

3.2.1. Calculation Results. Figures 11(a) and 11(c) show the segmentation results. Figures 11(b) and 11(d) show the annotated locations of the blood vessels, as provided by the expert. It can be observed in Figure 11(a) that the blood vessel regions in the upper right with lower contrast are relatively difficult to identify, while the background regions have high contrast

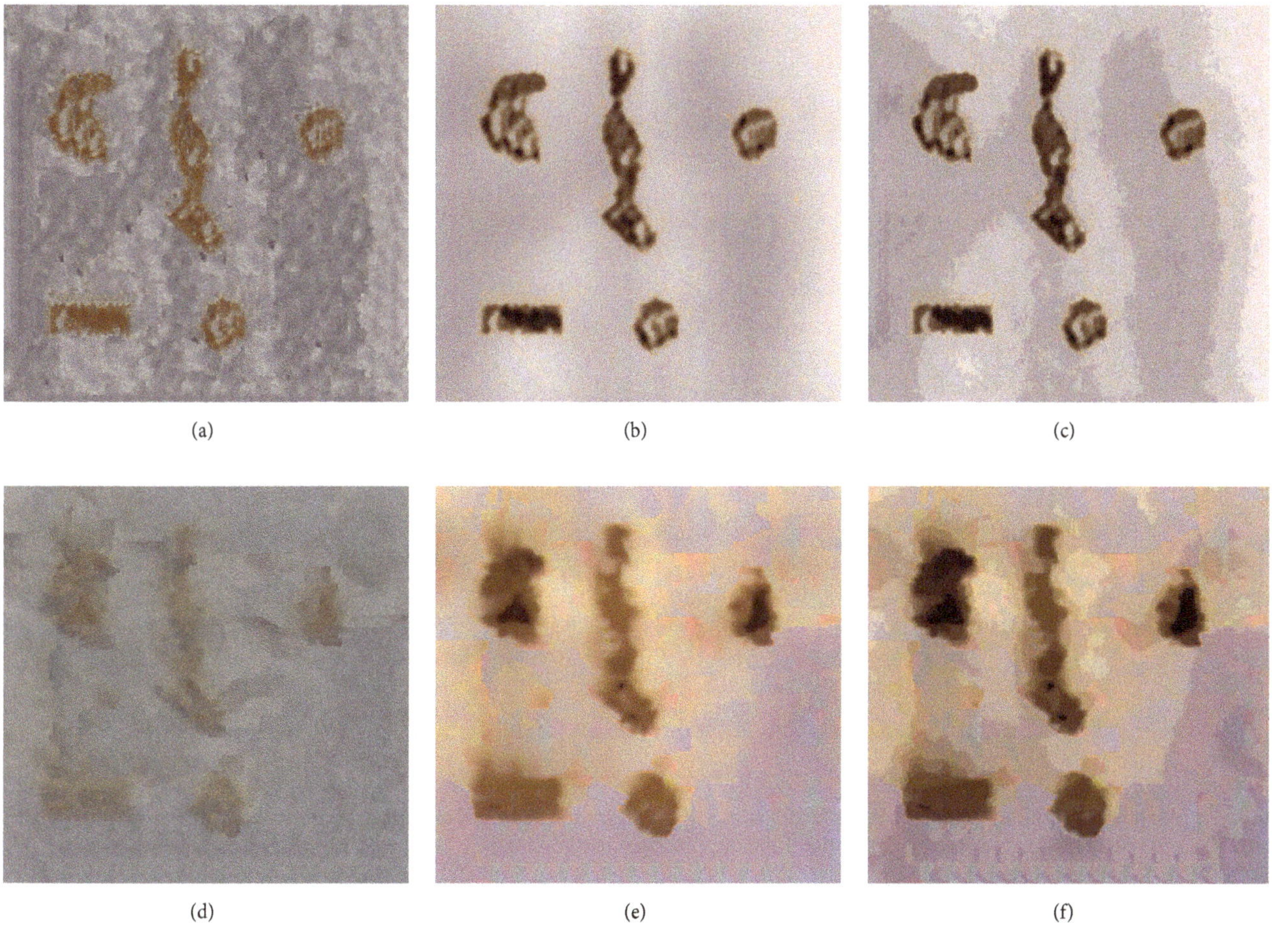

(a) (b) (c)

(d) (e) (f)

FIGURE 7: Synthetic vascular images. Abstraction results: original images (left), reconstructed images of the color layer of the original images, large-scale, and detailed layers (median), and salient blood vessel region abstraction from our proposed filtering method (right).

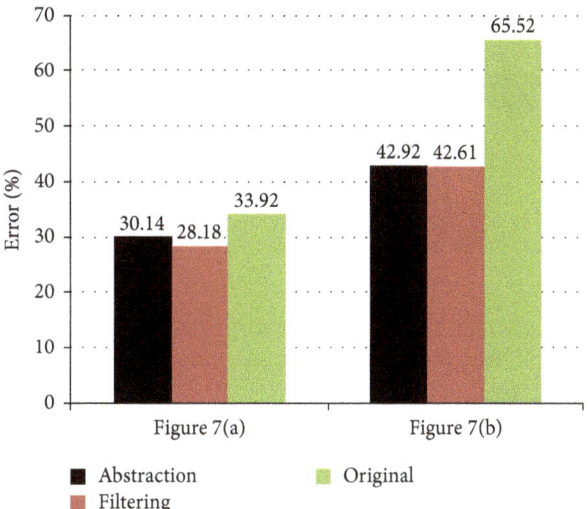

FIGURE 8: Error rates of image segmentation by fuzzy c-means clustering.

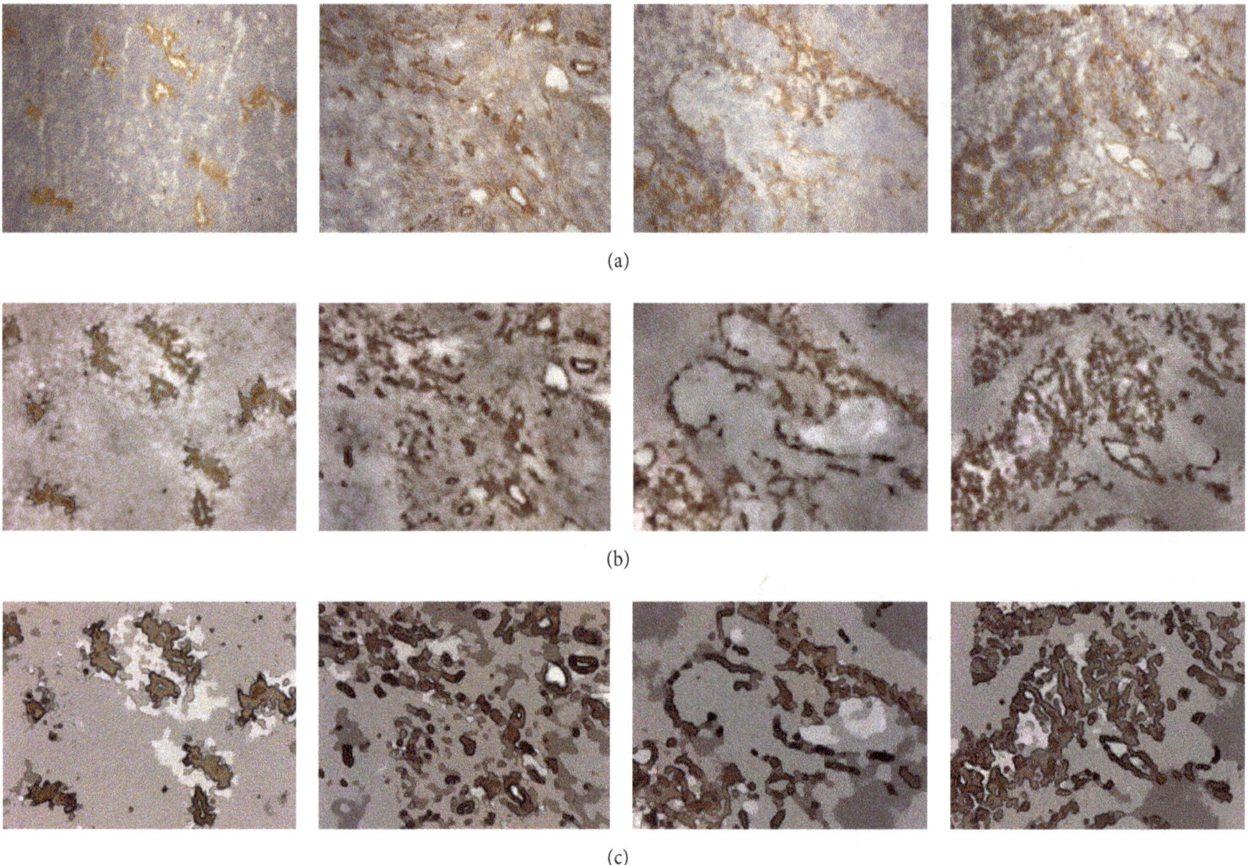

FIGURE 9: Abstraction results: original images (a); reconstructed images of the color layer of the original images, large-scale, and detailed layers (b); and salient blood vessel region abstraction from our proposed method (c).

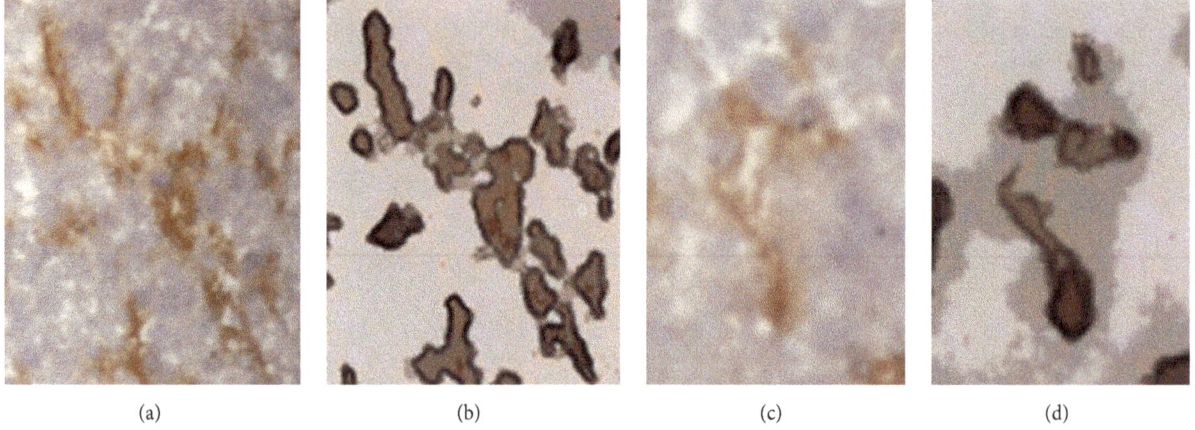

FIGURE 10: (a) Detail from Figure 2(a) with low contrast in the blood vessel regions. (b) Result of our proposed method with salient blood vessel regions. (c) Detail from Figure 2(a) with the cavity of the blood vessel surrounded by a few blood vessel wall areas. (d) Result of our proposed method with broken regions.

and texture noise. The result showed that our approach could delineate the major parts of the blood vessel regions and still do well in the blood vessel regions with the cavity, which is surrounded by few blood vessel wall areas.

3.2.2. Comparison of Results. Figure 12 compares the results of the proposed segmentation method with different spatiochromatic conditions. The results after applying the aspect ratio test were much better in some conditions in terms

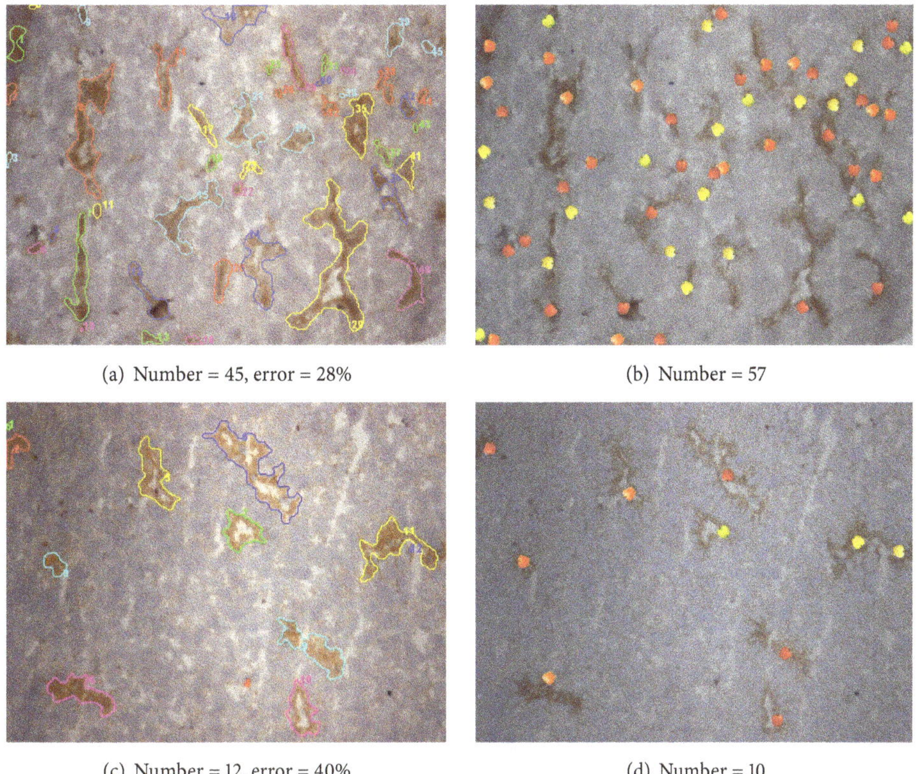

(a) Number = 45, error = 28%

(b) Number = 57

(c) Number = 12, error = 40%

(d) Number = 10

FIGURE 11: Calculation results. ((a), (c)) The boundaries are generated by our algorithm; ((b), (d)) those in apple dots are from the observer.

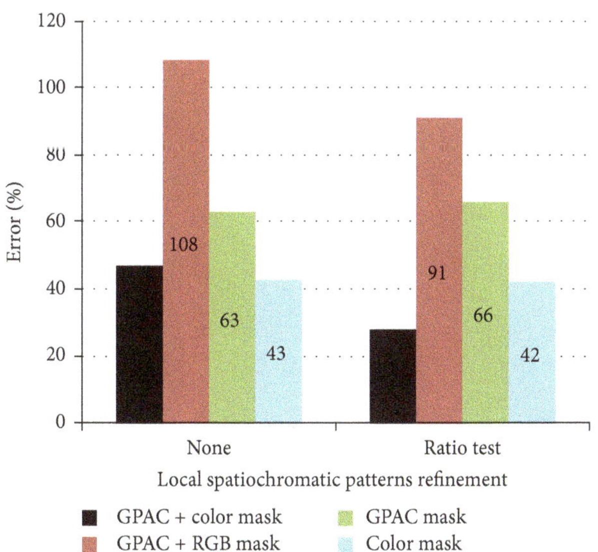

FIGURE 12: Comparison results.

of the relationships between color style and vessel regions. Clearly, the proposed algorithm can better demarcate the blood vessel regions.

4. Conclusion

This paper provides a framework for automatically detecting and abstracting blood vessel regions using color, luminance, and other details from the original image. Currently, we are exploiting various unsupervised classifications to deal with the problem caused by a cavity in the blood vessel regions and are focusing on the implementation of a fully automated, objective, computer based image analysis tool for the quantification of blood vessel images. We demonstrated that the implemented tool can calculate the vessel number and its area. The produced results were highly correlated with the human visual counts, conducted by an assistant from our department. Our next step is the exploration of various image textural features to achieve further quantification and automation in the assessment of vessel images.

Conflict of Interests

The authors declare that there is no conflict of interests regarding the publication of this paper.

References

[1] M. N. Gurcan, L. E. Boucheron, A. Can, A. Madabhushi, N. M. Rajpoot, and B. Yener, "Histopathological image analysis: a review," *IEEE Reviews in Biomedical Engineering*, vol. 2, pp. 147–171, 2009.

[2] P. Belhomme, M. Oger, J.-J. Michels, B. Plancoulaine, and P. Herlin, "Towards a computer aided diagnosis system dedicated to virtual microscopy based on stereology sampling and diffusion maps," *Diagnostic Pathology*, vol. 6, supplement 1, article S3, 2011.

[3] K. L. Weind, C. F. Maier, B. K. Rutt, and M. Moussa, "Invasive carcinomas and fibroadenomas of the breast: comparison of microvessel distributions—implications for imaging modalities," *Radiology*, vol. 208, no. 2, pp. 477–483, 1998.

[4] A. S.-Y. Leong, "Quantitation in immunohistology: fact or fiction? A discussion of variables that influence results," *Applied Immunohistochemistry and Molecular Morphology*, vol. 12, no. 1, pp. 1–7, 2004.

[5] P. J. Tadrous, "On the concept of objectivity in digital image analysis in pathology," *Pathology*, vol. 42, no. 3, pp. 207–211, 2010.

[6] L. T. G. Mikalsen, H. P. Dhakal, Ø. S. Bruland et al., "The clinical impact of mean vessel size and solidity in breast carcinoma patients," *PLoS ONE*, vol. 8, no. 10, Article ID e75954, 2013.

[7] P. Carmeliet and R. K. Jain, "Angiogenesis in cancer and other diseases," *Nature*, vol. 407, no. 6801, pp. 249–257, 2000.

[8] G. Bergers and L. E. Benjamin, "Tumorigenesis and the angiogenic switch," *Nature Reviews Cancer*, vol. 3, no. 6, pp. 401–410, 2003.

[9] J. Laitakari, V. Näyhä, and F. Stenbäck, "Size, shape, structure, and direction of angiogenesis in laryngeal tumour development," *Journal of Clinical Pathology*, vol. 57, no. 4, pp. 394–401, 2004.

[10] S. Kothari, J. H. Phan, T. H. Stokes, and M. D. Wang, "Pathology imaging informatics for quantitative analysis of whole-slide images," *Journal of the American Medical Informatics Association*, vol. 20, no. 6, pp. 1099–1108, 2013.

[11] K. A. Vermeer, F. M. Vos, H. G. Lemij, and A. M. Vossepoel, "A model based method for retinal blood vessel detection," *Computers in Biology and Medicine*, vol. 34, no. 4, pp. 209–219, 2004.

[12] J. J. Staal, M. D. Abramoff, M. Niemeijer, M. A. Viergever, and B. van Ginneken, "Ridge-based vessel segmentation in color images of the retina," *IEEE Transactions on Medical Imaging*, vol. 23, no. 4, pp. 501–509, 2004.

[13] B. S. Y. Lam and H. Yan, "Blood vessel extraction based on Mumford Shah model and skeletonization," in *Proceedings of the International Conference on Machine Learning and Cybernetics*, pp. 4227–4232, Dalian, China, August 2006.

[14] C.-H. Tsou, Y.-C. Lu, A. Yuan, Y.-C. Chang, and J.-H. Chen, "Automatic immunostaining vessel image filtering for visual search efficiency," in *Proceedings of the Annual International Conference of the IEEE Engineering in Medicine and Biology Society (EMBC '10)*, pp. 5653–5656, IEEE, Buenos Aires, Argentina, August-September 2010.

[15] W. Niblack, *An Introduction to Digital Image Processing*, Prentice Hall, Englewood Cliffs, NJ, USA, 1986.

[16] E. Eisemann and F. Durand, "Flash photography enhancement via intrinsic relighting," *ACM Transactions on Graphics*, vol. 23, no. 3, pp. 673–678, 2004.

[17] J.-M. Geusebroek, R. van den Boomgaard, A. W. M. Smeulders, and H. Geerts, "Color invariance," *IEEE Transactions on Pattern Analysis and Machine Intelligence*, vol. 23, no. 12, pp. 1338–1350, 2001.

[18] C. Tomasi and R. Manduchi, "Bilateral filtering for gray and color images," in *Proceedings of the IEEE 6th International Conference on Computer Vision*, pp. 839–846, IEEE, January 1998.

[19] H. Winnemoeller, S. C. Olsen, and B. Gooch, "Real-time video abstraction," *ACM Transactions on Graphics*, vol. 25, no. 3, pp. 1221–1226, 2006.

[20] B. Sumengen and B. S. Manjunath, "Graph partitioning active contours (GPAC) for image segmentation," *IEEE Transactions on Pattern Analysis and Machine Intelligence*, vol. 28, no. 4, pp. 509–521, 2006.

[21] N. Otsu, "A threshold selection method from gray-level histograms," *IEEE Transactions on Systems, Man, and Cybernetics*, vol. 9, no. 1, pp. 62–66, 1979.

[22] A. Hertzmann, C. E. Jacobs, N. Oliver, B. Curless, and D. H. Salesin, "Image analogies," in *Proceedings of the 28th Annual Conference on Computer Graphics and Interactive Techniques (SIGGRAPH '01)*, pp. 327–340, ACM, Los Angeles, Calif, USA, August 2001.

4

Quercetin Reduces Ehrlich Tumor-Induced Cancer Pain in Mice

Cassia Calixto-Campos,[1] Mab P. Corrêa,[1] Thacyana T. Carvalho,[1] Ana C. Zarpelon,[1] Miriam S. N. Hohmann,[1] Ana C. Rossaneis,[1] Leticia Coelho-Silva,[1] Wander R. Pavanelli,[1] Phileno Pinge-Filho,[1] Jefferson Crespigio,[1] Catia C. F. Bernardy,[2] Rubia Casagrande,[3] and Waldiceu A. Verri Jr.[1]

[1]*Department of Pathology, Biological Sciences Centre, Londrina State University, Rodovia Celso Garcia Cid KM480 PR445, Caixa Postal 10.011, 86057-970 Londrina, PR, Brazil*
[2]*Department of Nursing, Health Science Centre, Londrina State University, Avenue Robert Koch 60, 86038-350 Londrina, PR, Brazil*
[3]*Department of Pharmaceutical Sciences, Health Science Centre, Londrina State University, Avenue Robert Koch 60, 86038-350 Londrina, PR, Brazil*

Correspondence should be addressed to Waldiceu A. Verri Jr.; waldiceujr@yahoo.com.br

Academic Editor: Francesco A. Mauri

Cancer pain directly affects the patient's quality of life. We have previously demonstrated that the subcutaneous administration of the mammary adenocarcinoma known as Ehrlich tumor induces pain in mice. Several studies have shown that the flavonoid quercetin presents important biological effects, including anti-inflammatory, antioxidant, analgesic, and antitumor activity. Therefore, the analgesic effect and mechanisms of quercetin were evaluated in Ehrlich tumor-induced cancer pain in mice. Intraperitoneal (i.p.) treatments with quercetin reduced Ehrlich tumor-induced mechanical and thermal hyperalgesia, but not paw thickness or histological alterations, indicating an analgesic effect without affecting tumor growth. Regarding the analgesic mechanisms of quercetin, it inhibited the production of hyperalgesic cytokines IL-1β and TNFα and decreased neutrophil recruitment (myeloperoxidase activity) and oxidative stress. Naloxone (opioid receptor antagonist) inhibited quercetin analgesia without interfering with neutrophil recruitment, cytokine production, and oxidative stress. Importantly, cotreatment with morphine and quercetin at doses that were ineffective as single treatment reduced the nociceptive responses. Concluding, quercetin reduces the Ehrlich tumor-induced cancer pain by reducing the production of hyperalgesic cytokines, neutrophil recruitment, and oxidative stress as well as by activating an opioid-dependent analgesic pathway and potentiation of morphine analgesia. Thus, quercetin treatment seems a suitable therapeutic approach for cancer pain that merits further investigation.

1. Introduction

Approximately 50% of all cancer patients have pain [1] in early-state cancer or advanced cancer [1–4]. Cancer patients may present hyperalgesia, allodynia, and spontaneous pain, which account for poor life quality [5]. Cancer pain is a severe clinical health problem for these patients and currently the treatment for this pain is inadequate enhancing this problem [6]. In fact, at least half patients with cancer pain have received inadequate analgesic therapy [7]. One explanation for inadequate analgesic prescription could be a failure to identify pain mechanisms [2].

Several studies have demonstrated the participation of varied pathways and mediators involved in cancer pain development, such as cytokines [8–10], spinal glial activation [11–14], transient receptor potential vanilloid receptor 1 (TRPV1), acid-sensing ion channels (ASICs), bradykinin, adenosine triphosphate (ATP), endothelin [15], reactive oxygen species [16], and intracellular signaling pathway such as mitogen-activated protein kinases p38 [17] and JNK [18]. Cancer pain mechanisms are also dependent on the cancer type implicating that some slight variations in the mechanisms or role of a certain pathway may be greater depending on cancer type. Therefore, cancer pain is a complex condition and as already mentioned its control might also depend on adequate pharmacological tools. Opioids are effective clinically used analgesics in cancer pain; however, they have many side effects that increase with the dose of opioid and, in addition to tolerance, the dose regimen increases with the tumor growth [19]. Thus, it is important to find novel therapeutic approaches to reduce cancer pain and/or improve current clinical therapies.

Flavonoids such as quercetin present low toxicity [20], which together with its antinociceptive effect in models of inflammation [21] and neuropathic pain [22] suggests its usefulness as an analgesic drug. Moreover, cancer pain might present components of inflammatory pain related to the inflammatory response against the tumor cells and neuropathic pain related to neuronal damage and nerve compression. It has been demonstrated in models of inflammation that the mechanisms of quercetin are related to inhibition of oxidative stress and cytokine production [23, 24]. In models of diabetic neuropathic pain, quercetin induces an analgesic effect amenable by opioid receptor antagonist [22]. In fact, inhibition of oxidative stress, cytokine production, and opioid receptor-dependent effects seem to be major mechanisms of quercetin since they were also observed in models such as colitis [25], neuropathy [26], hepatic fibrosis [27], periodontitis-induced bone resorption [28], and allergic inflammation [29].

In the present study, the analgesic activity and mechanisms of quercetin were investigated in Ehrlich tumor-induced cancer pain in mice [30]. This is a model of murine mammary adenocarcinoma-induced pain presenting features like those of preoperative breast cancer with spontaneous pain and pain upon examination (pressure of the lump, hyperalgesia) [30–32] with the benefit of development in standard Swiss mice. Furthermore, Ehrlich tumor induces bone/cartilage destruction indicating the possible involvement of a bone pain component in its nociceptive mechanisms [30].

2. Material and Methods

2.1. General Experimental Procedures. The measurement of basal responses to mechanical and thermal stimuli and paw thickness was performed at day 0. Afterwards, mice received intraplantar (i.pl.) injection of Ehrlich tumor cells (1×10^6 or 1×10^7). Ehrlich's tumor cells are cultivated *in vivo*, by passages in the peritoneum of Swiss mice in ascitic form. Ten days after the intraperitoneal (i.p.) injection of 0.2 mL of ascitic peritoneal fluid containing Ehrlich tumor cells in mice, the ascitic fluid of tumor cells was collected and washed in phosphate-buffered saline (PBS, pH 7.4) followed by centrifugation (200 g, 10 min) three times. The cell viability was determined by 0.5% trypan blue exclusion method in Neubauer chamber. Ehrlich tumor cells were suspended to the final concentrations of 1×10^6 or 1×10^7 in 25 μL of saline and injected into the subcutaneous tissue of mice, which passes from ascitic form to solid form [30]. Mice received the Ehrlich tumor cells (1×10^6 or 1×10^7 in 25 μL of saline) and received the acute treatment with quercetin (10–100 mg/kg, i.p.) or vehicle (2% DMSO in saline) on the 8th day after injection of the cells, and mechanical and thermal hyperalgesia and paw thickness were determined after 1, 3, 5, and 7 h. For chronic treatment, mice were treated with quercetin (10–100 mg/kg, i.p) 10 min after Ehrlich tumor cells injection followed by daily treatment. Mechanical and thermal hyperalgesia and paw thickness were evaluated on days 2, 4, 6, 8, 10, and 12 after the injection of 1×10^6 cells and 3 h after treatment with quercetin. A control group received saline (25 μL/paw, vehicle of Ehrlich tumor cells) and quercetin (100 mg/kg, i.p) treatment. On the 12th day of the injection of tumor cells, 3 h after the daily treatment with quercetin (100 mg/kg i.p., both tumor and saline group) or vehicle, paw samples were collected for histological analysis and microscopic observation. Paw skin and spinal cord samples were collected to determine myeloperoxidase (MPO) activity, interleukin-1β (IL-1β), and tumor necrosis factor α (TNFα) concentration by ELISA, FRAP, ABTS, and GSH levels. In another set of experiments, mice received 1×10^7 Ehrlich tumor cells or saline and were treated with quercetin (100 mg/kg, i.p.) or vehicle starting 10 min after Ehrlich tumor cells injection and followed by daily treatment during 8 days. On the 8th day, 3 h after treatment, the overt pain-like behavior was assessed. In other experiments, mice received Ehrlich tumor cells (1×10^6 or 1×10^7) and were treated with quercetin (100 mg/kg, i.p.) or vehicle daily during 8 days; on the 8th day, mice received the treatment with naloxone (1 mg/kg i.p.) (an opioid receptor antagonist) followed by evaluation of mechanical and thermal hyperalgesia, paw thickness, overt pain, and collection of spinal cord and paw skin and samples for evaluation of myeloperoxidase (MPO) activity (only paw skin), IL-1β and TNFα concentration, FRAP, ABTS, and GSH levels. Lastly, we assessed the effect of cotreatment with quercetin (10 mg/kg, i.p.) and morphine (1 mg/kg, i.p.) (at doses that were not effectively analgesic as single treatment) over Ehrlich tumor-induced (1×10^6 or 1×10^7 cells) mechanical hyperalgesia, thermal hyperalgesia, paw thickness, and overt pain-like behavior. Time points of the analyzed parameters were standardized in our laboratory [30].

2.2. Test Compound. The compounds used in this study were PBS pH 7.4, saline (NaCl 0.9%, Fresenius Kabi Brasil Ltda., Aquiraz, CE, Brazil), Tween, and DMSO 2%, and quercetin at 95% purity was purchased from Acros Organics (Fair Lawn, NJ, USA).

2.3. Ehrlich Tumor Cells. Peritoneal ascitic fluid of mice that received Ehrlich tumor cells i.p. was collected and injected in other mice. Ten days after the injection of ascitic fluid containing Ehrlich tumor cells, the ascitic fluid was collected for experiments. Ehrlich tumor cells were developed by Paul Ehrlich in 1896 and described as a spontaneous breast adenocarcinoma of female mice. It was originally developed as an ascitic form but can be converted to solid form when inoculated into tissues. Injection of Ehrlich tumor cells in the paw induces mechanical hyperalgesia, thermal hyperalgesia, increase of paw thickness, and overt pain-like behavior [30].

2.4. Animals. Male Swiss mice (25–30 g), from the Universidade Estadual de Londrina, Londrina, Parana, Brazil, were used in this study. Mice were housed in standard clear plastic cages with free access to food and water and a light/dark cycle of 12 : 12 h and kept at 21°C. All behavioral testing was performed between 9 a.m. and 5 p.m. in a temperature-controlled room. Animal care and handling procedures were approved by the Ethics Committee of the Universidade Estadual de Londrina (13279.2011.76). Every effort was made to minimize the number of animals used and their suffering.

2.5. Mechanical Hyperalgesia. Mechanical hyperalgesia was evaluated as previously reported [30]. In a quiet room, mice were placed in acrylic cages (12 × 10 × 17 cm) with wire grid floors, 15–30 min before the start of testing. The test consisted of evoking a hindpaw flexion reflex with a hand-held force transducer (electronic anesthesiometer, Insight, Ribeirão Preto, SP, Brazil) adapted with a 0.5 mm^2 polypropylene tip. The investigator was trained to apply the tip perpendicularly to the central area of the hindpaw with a gradual increase in pressure. The end point was characterized by the removal of the paw followed by clear flinching movements. After the paw withdrawal, the intensity of the pressure was recorded automatically. The value for the response was an average of three measurements. The animals were tested before and after treatment. The results are expressed by delta (Δ) withdrawal threshold (in g) calculated by subtracting the mean measurements at 1, 3, 5, and 7 h after acute treatment on the 8th day after injection of the Ehrlich tumor cells or 3 h after each daily treatment with quercetin in the chronic protocol on days 2, 4, 6, 8, 10, and 12 after injection of the cells from the zero-time mean measurements.

2.6. Thermal Hyperalgesia. Mice were placed in a 10 cm-wide glass cylinder on a hot plate (IITC Life Science, Inc., Woodland Hills, CA, United States) maintained at 55°C. Two control latencies of at least 10 min apart were determined for each mouse. The normal latency (reaction time) was 10–15 s. The reaction time was scored when the animal jumped or licked its paws. A maximum latency (cut-off) was set at 20 s to avoid tissue damage [30]. The results are expressed as thermal threshold.

2.7. Paw Thickness or Tumor Growth. Paw thickness was determined before and at indicated time points (at 48 h intervals) after the injection of Ehrlich tumor cells using an analog caliper. Paw thickness/tumor growth was presented as Δ mm [30].

2.8. Overt Pain-Like Behavior Evaluation. Mice received 1 × 10^7 cells/paw in 25 μL and were placed in clear glass compartments at room temperature. After an acclimation period of 10 min, mice were observed during 10 min, and the cumulative number of flinches was determined [30].

2.9. Histopathological Analyses. Twelve days after the injection of the Ehrlich tumor cells, mice were euthanized and the paw was removed and decalcified in EDTA solution during 35 days. Samples were embedded in paraffin, sectioned into 5 μm section, and stained with hematoxylin and eosin for light microscopic analysis [30].

2.10. Myeloperoxidase (MPO) Activity. Neutrophil recruitment to the paw skin was evaluated by the MPO kinetic-colorimetric assay [25]. Paw skin samples were collected in 50 mM K_2PO_4 buffer (pH 6.0) containing 0.5% HTAB and were homogenized using a Polytron (PT3100). After the homogenates were centrifuged at 16.100 g for 2 min, the resulting supernatant was assayed for MPO activity at 450 nm (Multiskan GO Microplate Spectrophotometer) with three readings within 1 min. The MPO activity of the samples was compared with a standard curve of neutrophils. The results were presented as the MPO activity (number of neutrophils × 10^5/mg of tissue).

2.11. Cytokine Measurement. Mice spinal cord (L4–L6) and paw skin samples were collected and homogenized in 500 μL of buffer containing protease inhibitors, and IL-1β and TNFα levels were determined as described previously by an enzyme-linked immunosorbent assay (ELISA) using eBioscience kits. The results were expressed as picograms (pg) of cytokine/mg of spinal cord or paw skin. As a control, the concentrations of these cytokines were determined in animals injected with saline and treated with vehicle [25].

2.12. Antioxidants Tests. Spinal cord and paw skin tissue samples were collected and immediately homogenized with 500 μL of 1.15% KCl. Samples were centrifuged (10 min, 0.2 g, and 4°C) and the total antioxidant capacity was determined by the FRAP (ferric reducing ability potential) and ABTS (ability to scavenge ABTS radical) assays [25]. For FRAP assay, 50 μL of supernatant was mixed with 150 μL of deionized water and 1.5 mL of FRAP reagent freshly prepared. The reaction mixture was incubated at 37°C for 30 min and absorbance was measured at 595 nm. For ABTS assay, ABTS solution was diluted with phosphate buffer saline pH 7.4 (PBS) to an absorbance of 0.80 at 730 nm. Then, 1.0 mL of diluted ABTS solution was mixed with 20 μL of supernatant. After 6 min, the absorbance was measured at 730 nm. The results were equated against a Trolox standard curve (1.5–30 μmol/L, final concentrations). The results were expressed as Trolox equivalents per gram of spinal cord or paw skin in both assays. For GSH measurement, spinal cord and paw skin samples were collected and maintained at −80°C for at least 48 h. Samples were homogenized with 200 μL of 0.02 M EDTA. The homogenate was mixed with 25 μL of 50% trichloroacetic acid and was homogenized three times during 15 min. The mixture was centrifuged (15 min, 1.5 g, and 4°C). The supernatant was added to 200 μL of 0.2 M TRIS buffer, pH 8.2, and 10 μL of 0.01 M DTNB. After 5 min, the absorbance was measured at 412 nm against a reagent blank with no supernatant. A standard curve with GSH was performed. The results are expressed as GSH per mg of protein of spinal cord or paw skin [25]. For protein determination, 60 μL of supernatant was mixed with 60 μL of copper reagent freshly prepared. After 10 min, 180 μL of Folin solution was added. The resulting solution was incubated at 50°C for 10 min. The absorbance was measured at 660 nm and the results equated to a standard curve of bovine serum albumin [33].

2.13. Statistical Analysis. Results are presented as means ± SEM of measurements made on six mice in each group per experiment and are representative of two independent experiments. Two-way analysis of variance (ANOVA) was used to compare the groups and doses at all times (curves) when the hyperalgesic responses were measured at different times after the administration or enforcement of the stimuli. The factors analyzed were treatment, time, and time versus treatment interaction. When there was a significant time versus treatment interaction, one-way ANOVA followed by Tukey's t-test was performed on each occasion. Statistical differences were considered to be significant at $p < 0.05$.

3. Results and Discussion

3.1. Quercetin Inhibits Pain-Like Behavior and Neutrophil Recruitment Induced by Ehrlich Tumor Cells. Ehrlich tumor cells induced significant mechanical hyperalgesia starting at the 4th day up to the 12th day and thermal hyperalgesia starting at the 2nd day up to the 12th day confirming previous standardization [30]. The acute analgesic effect of quercetin (10–100 mg/kg, i.p. 2% DMSO diluted in saline) was assessed on the 8th day after injection of the Ehrlich tumor cells at 1, 3, 5, and 7 h after treatment. Quercetin (100 mg/kg, i.p.) treatment significantly reduced the mechanical and thermal hyperalgesia at 3 and 5 h after treatment (Figures 1(a) and 1(b), resp.) but did not alter the paw thickness (Figure 1(c)). The chronic posttreatment with quercetin (10–100 mg/kg, 2% DMSO diluted in saline) significantly reduced the mechanical hyperalgesia from days 6 to 12 (Figure 2(a)) and thermal hyperalgesia between 4 and 12 days (Figure 2(b)) in a dose-dependent manner. The inhibition of Ehrlich tumor-induced mechanical and thermal hyperalgesia was not accompanied by alteration of paw thickness, indicating that quercetin did not affect tumor growth (Figure 2(c)). The treatment with quercetin (100 mg/kg, i.p) of mice that received Ehrlich tumor vehicle (saline) did not alter the basal mechanical or thermal hyperalgesia, or paw thickness (Figures 2(a)–2(c)) indicating that quercetin did not present *per se* effects.

In the present model, Ehrlich tumor cells induced overt pain-like behavior, such as paw flinching, at the dose of 1×10^7 cells with peak of response at the 8th day after injection [30]. At this time point, the daily treatment with quercetin also inhibited Ehrlich tumor-induced paw flinching (Figure 2(d)) with significant analgesic effect with the dose of 100 mg/kg of quercetin over 10 and 30 mg/kg. There was no effect on mice that received Ehrlich tumor vehicle (saline) plus quercetin treatment (100 mg/kg, i.p.). Considering the results of Figures 1 and 2, the dose of 100 mg/kg of quercetin was selected for the next experiments. Corroborating the present data, quercetin also inhibited mechanical hyperalgesia, thermal hyperalgesia, and overt pain-like behavior induced by varied stimuli in other models of inflammatory and neuropathic pain [21, 22, 34, 35], and the dose of 100 mg/kg of quercetin was also selected [21, 22, 25, 36].

In agreement with the results of Figure 2(c), hematoxylin/eosin staining of paw samples revealed no histological differences between mice with tumor treated with quercetin and vehicle control group. Mice that received saline in the paw and were treated with the vehicle of quercetin (Figure 3(a)) or quercetin (100 mg/kg i.p.) (Figure 3(b)) showed normal tissue. The arrows show the presence of epidermis, dermis, skeletal muscle fibers, and intact bone and cartilage. On the other hand, mice that received Ehrlich tumor cells and were treated with the vehicle of quercetin (Figures 3(c) and 3(e)) or with quercetin (100 mg/kg i.p) (Figures 3(d) and 3(f)) presented cartilage destruction, tissue necrosis, and intense tumor proliferation. This could be seen as a drawback data in the sense that quercetin does not inhibit Ehrlich tumor cells growth and, therefore, quercetin does not present an antitumor effect at this analgesic dose. On the other hand, the positive side is that quercetin exerts an analgesic effect without affecting tumor growth; thus, it is suitable for treatment of cancer pain and does not promote tumor growth. Nevertheless, some studies have shown the antitumor effect of quercetin. For instance, treatment with quercetin induced apoptosis and/or inhibited the growth of human breast carcinoma MCF-7 cells [37], K562 human chronic myeloid leukemia, Molt-4 acute T-lymphocytic leukemia, Raji Burkitt lymphoma [38], nasopharyngeal carcinoma cells [39], and other cancer cell lines [40, 41]. Dose of treatment, *in vivo* versus *in vitro* contexts, and cancer cell lines are some possible explanations for this divergent data. Nevertheless, it is possible that higher doses of quercetin would present antitumor effect with improved analgesia since it would present an intrinsic analgesic effect plus reduction of tumor and the immune response against the tumor.

There is evidence that ascitic Ehrlich tumor induces the recruitment to the peritoneal cavity of mice of cellular populations consistent with dendritic cells, monocytes, and neutrophils [42]. In the present study, it was observed that Ehrlich tumor injection in the paw induces an increase of myeloperoxidase (MPO) activity and daily treatment with quercetin (100 mg/kg, i.p.) inhibited this increase of MPO activity (Figure 4). The saline group treated with quercetin (100 mg/kg, i.p) did not present alteration of MPO activity compared to quercetin vehicle. MPO is an important enzyme of neutrophil microbicidal activity and is used as a marker of inflammation and neutrophil recruitment [43]. The inhibition of neutrophil recruitment or activation is an analgesic mechanism since recruited neutrophils contribute to hyperalgesia by further producing nociceptive molecules [43]. Therefore, inhibiting neutrophil recruitment might be accounting for the analgesic effect of quercetin. In addition to neutrophils, macrophages express MPO, suggesting that the inhibition of MPO activity by quercetin treatment could also involve the reduction of macrophage counts. This is consistent with the demonstration that Ehrlich tumor cells induce the recruitment of monocytes, which

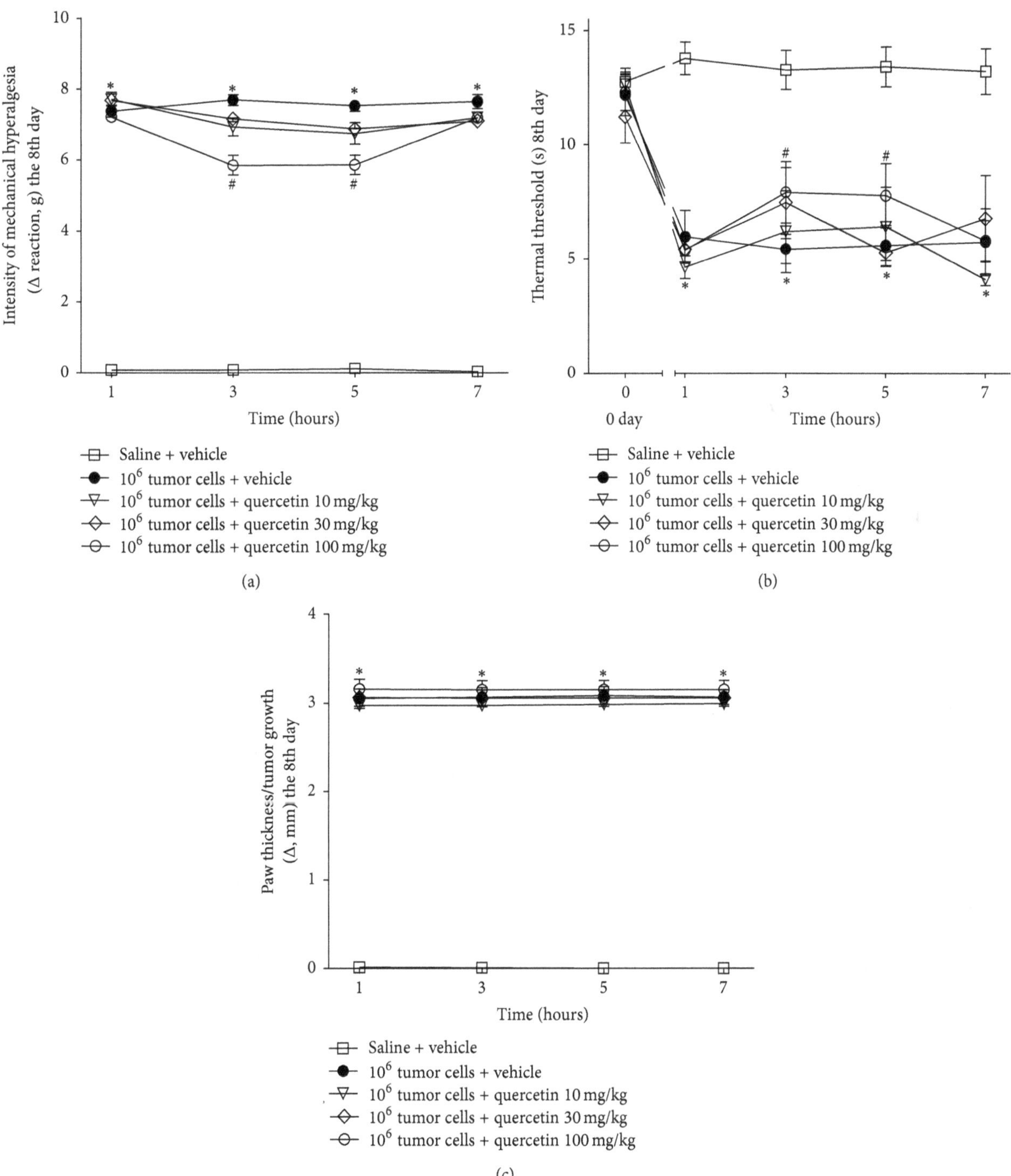

FIGURE 1: Acute treatment with quercetin inhibits Ehrlich tumor-induced pain-like behavior in mice. Mice received the intraplantar (i.pl.) administration of Ehrlich tumor cells 1×10^6 (a–c), and in the 8th day after injection, the tumor cells mice received the acute treatment with quercetin (10, 30, and 100 mg/kg i.p.). Mechanical hyperalgesia (a), thermal hyperalgesia (b), and paw thickness (c) were accessed at 1, 3, 5, and 7 hours after the treatment. Data are presented as means ± SEM of six mice per group per experiment and are representative of two separated experiments: $^*p < 0.05$ compared to the saline group and $^{\#}p < 0.05$ compared to the tumor group. One-way ANOVA followed by Tukey's test.

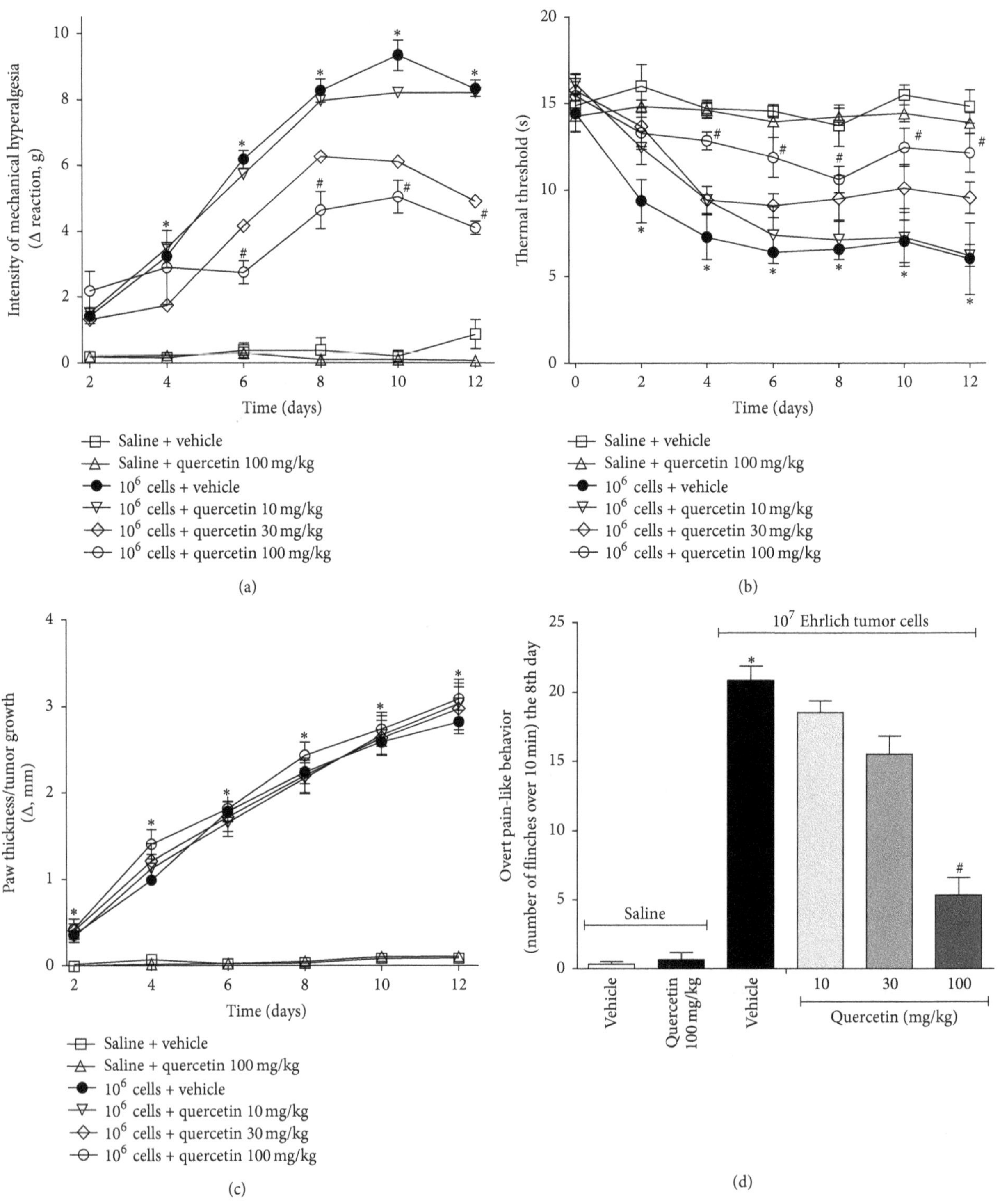

FIGURE 2: The chronic treatment with quercetin inhibits in a dose-dependent manner Ehrlich tumor-induced pain-like behavior in mice. Mice received the intraplantar (i.pl.) administration of Ehrlich tumor cells (1×10^6 (a–c) or 1×10^7 (d)) and were treated daily with quercetin (10, 30, and 100 mg/kg i.p.) during 12 days (a–c) or 8 days (d) starting 10 min after tumor injection. The control group of Ehrlich tumor vehicle was saline and saline plus quercetin group was a control of possible *per se* effects of quercetin. Mechanical hyperalgesia (a), thermal hyperalgesia (b), paw thickness (c), and overt pain-like behavior (d) were evaluated 3 h after the treatment. Data are presented as means ± SEM of six mice per group per experiment and representative of two separated experiments: $^{*}p < 0.05$ compared to the saline group and $^{\#}p < 0.05$ compared to the tumor group. One-way ANOVA followed by Tukey's test.

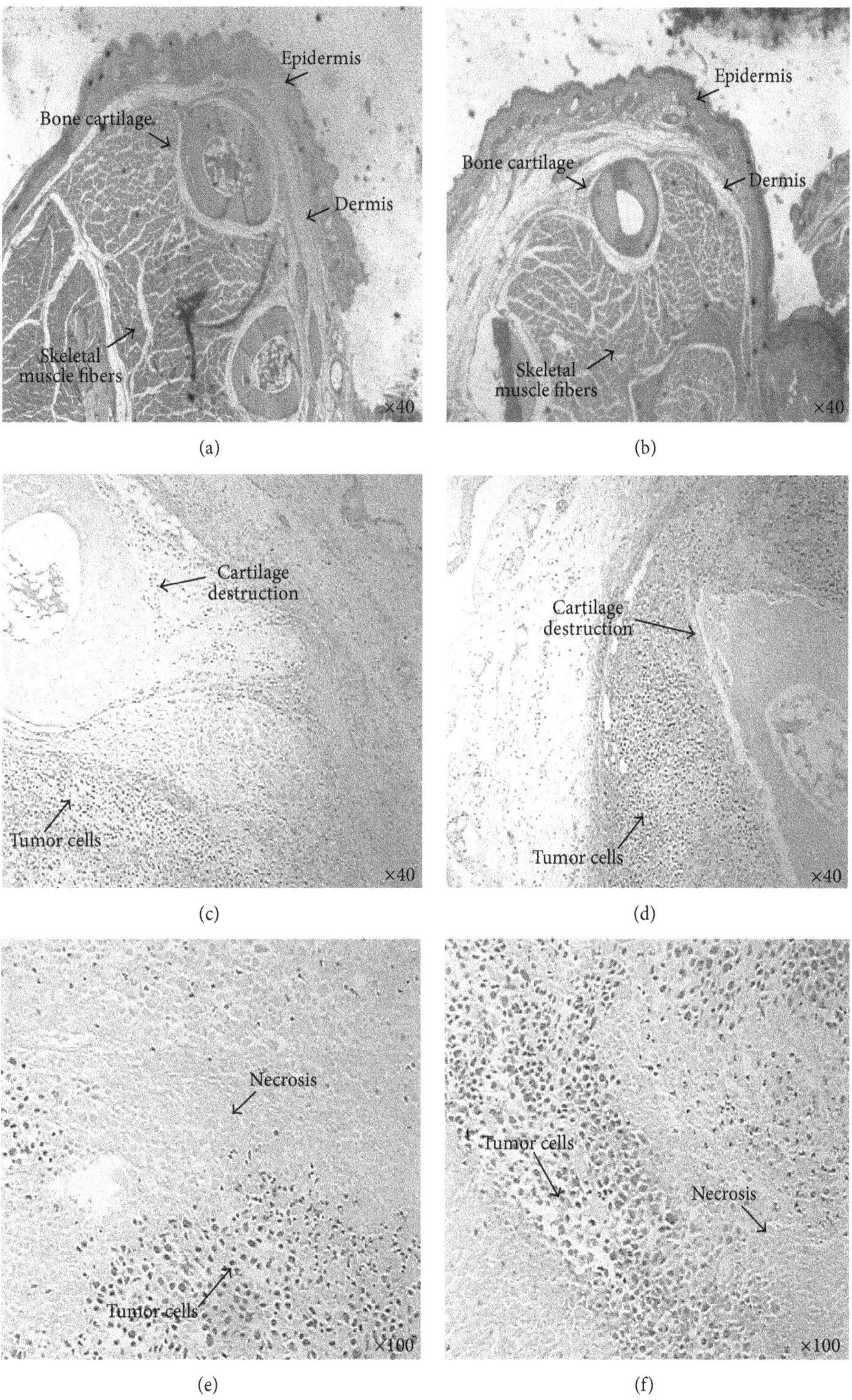

FIGURE 3: Quercetin does not alter Ehrlich tumor-induced histological modifications. Mice received saline (25 μL) or Ehrlich tumor cells ($1 \times 10^6/25\,\mu$L) and were treated i.p. with quercetin (100 mg/kg, 2% DMSO diluted in saline) or vehicle (2% DMSO) 10 min after the i.pl. injection. The treatment continued daily during 12 days. In the 12th day, mice were euthanized and the paw was collected for histological analysis performed with hematoxylin/eosin staining. Panel (a) shows the histology of saline i.pl. plus quercetin vehicle group, (b) saline i.pl. plus quercetin (100 mg/kg i.p.), (c and e) tumor animal treated with vehicle, and (d and f) tumor animal treated with quercetin (100 mg/kg i.p.). Arrows indicate intact bone cartilage, presence of skeletal muscle fibers, dermis and epidermis: (a-b) bone/cartilage destruction (c-d), tissue necrosis (e-f), and presence of tumor cells (c–f).

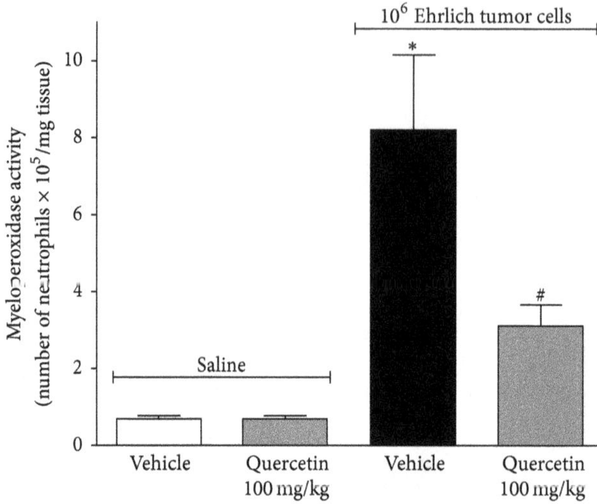

FIGURE 4: Quercetin inhibits neutrophil recruitment induced by Ehrlich tumor cells. Mice were treated i.p. with quercetin (100 mg/kg, 2% DMSO diluted in saline) or vehicle (2% DMSO) 10 min after the injection of Ehrlich tumor cell ($1 \times 10^6/25\,\mu$L) or saline (25 μL). The neutrophil recruitment was evaluated in samples of paw skin collected after 12 days of treatment using the myeloperoxidase (MPO) activity assay. Data are presented as means ± SEM of six mice per group per experiment and representative of two separated experiments: $^*p < 0.05$ compared to the saline group and $^\#p < 0.05$ compared to the tumor group. One-way ANOVA followed by Tukey's test.

could differentiate into macrophages [42]. Treatment with quercetin also inhibits MPO activity *in vitro* [44] and also the neutrophil recruitment *in vivo* and neutrophil chemotaxis *in vitro* induced by chemokines, fMLP (formyl-methionyl-leucyl-phenylalanine) and leukotriene B_4 [40]. Therefore, quercetin is able to inhibit the MPO enzyme as well as the recruitment of cells expressing MPO. In addition to inhibiting the chemotactic effects of cytokines, peptides, and lipid mediators, quercetin also inhibits the production of such molecules. Thus, in the next set of experiments, whether quercetin would inhibit the production of cytokines with hyperalgesic and chemotactic functions such as IL-1β and TNFα was investigated [45].

3.2. Quercetin Inhibits IL-1β and TNFα Production Induced by Ehrlich Tumor Cells in the Spinal Cord and Paw Skin. Mice received daily treatment during 12 days with quercetin (100 mg/kg, i.p.) starting 10 min after the injection of saline or Ehrlich tumor (1×10^6, i.pl.) injection as described at Figure 2, and samples were collected in the 12th day (Figure 5). Ehrlich tumor cells induced significant production of IL-1β in the spinal cord (Figure 5(a)) and in the paw skin (Figure 5(b)). TNFα levels were also increased in spinal cord (Figure 5(c)) and paw skin (Figure 5(d)). Quercetin treatment inhibited Ehrlich tumor-induced IL-1β and TNFα production in the spinal cord and paw skin (Figure 5). The daily treatment with quercetin (100 mg/kg i.p.) in mice that received i.pl. control saline did not alter the production of cytokines compared to naive group. Cytokines including IL-1β and TNFα have spinal cord and peripheral nociceptive roles as observed in inflammation and neuropathic and cancer models. Therefore, inhibiting IL-1β and/or TNFα production or action at the central spinal cord or peripheral levels is a promising analgesic approach [45]. In fact, the intrathecal treatment with IL-ra (an IL-1 receptor antagonist) inhibited the hyperalgesia induced by AT-3.1 prostate cancer cells into the tibia of rats [46] and systemic treatment with anakinra (an IL-1 receptor antagonist) reduced the hyperalgesia induced by osteosarcoma model of bone cancer pain [47]. The i.pl. injection of lung carcinoma cells induces hyperalgesia in mice accompanied by high peripheral production of IL-1β and TNFα, and the treatment with etanercept (a TNF-neutralizing soluble receptor) prevented the development of heat hyperalgesia. Furthermore, TNF-induced cancer-related heat hyperalgesia through nociceptor sensitization is linked to upregulation of transient receptor potential vanilloid 1 (TRPV1) [8]. Similarly, etanercept also reduced the mechanical hyperalgesia in a bone cancer model [13, 48]. The nociception triggered by IL-1β and TNFα presents peripheral and central spinal cord mechanisms. For instance, TNFα triggers acute inflammatory hyperalgesia by inducing IL-1β production, which in turn induces prostaglandin E_2 production. Prostaglandin E_2 is ultimately responsible for sensitization of nociceptive neurons [45]. After the first inflammatory stimulus, there is a condition named hyperalgesic priming representing prolonged inflammation in which TNFR1 expression is induced in nociceptive neurons and, therefore, TNFα can exert a direct sensitizing effect [49]. *In vitro*, dorsal root ganglia (DRG) neurons express TNFR1 receptors possibly due to the collection procedure of the DRG, which resembles axotomy. In this condition, TNFα induces p38 mitogen-activated protein (MAP) kinase activation that phosphorylates tetrodotoxin-resistant sodium

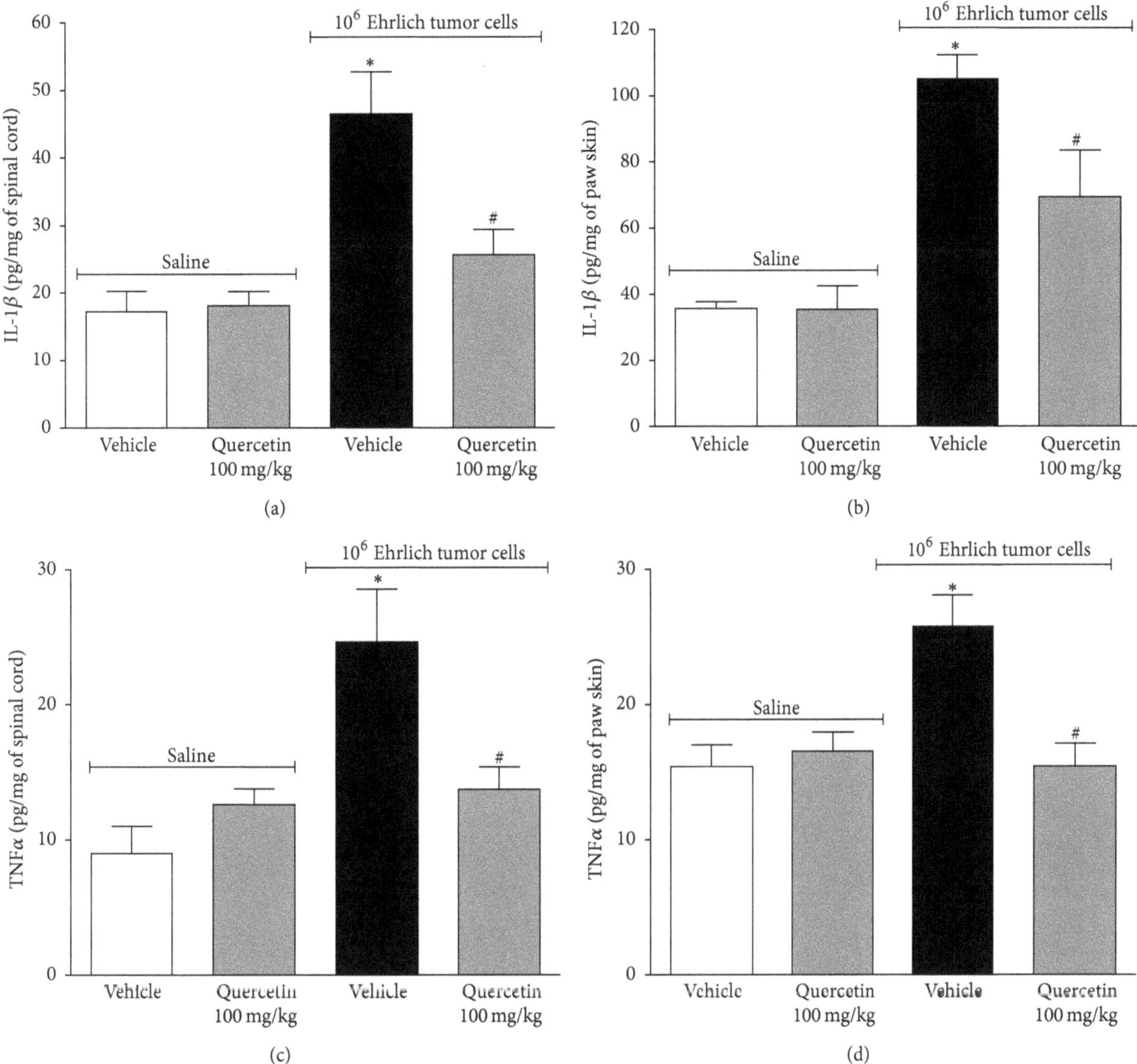

FIGURE 5: Quercetin inhibits IL-1β and TNFα production induced by Ehrlich tumor cells in the spinal cord and paw skin. Mice were treated i.p. with quercetin (100 mg/kg, 2% DMSO diluted in saline) or vehicle (2% DMSO) 10 min after the injection of Ehrlich tumor cell ($1 \times 10^6/25\,\mu$L) or saline (25 μL). The treatment continued daily. In the 12th day after injection, the Ehrlich tumor cells, the spinal cord, and the paw skin samples were collected for cytokine measurement. IL-1β in spinal cord (a) or paw skin (b) and TNFα in spinal cord (c) or paw skin (d) were determined by ELISA. Data are presented as means ± SEM of six mice per group per experiment and representative of two separated experiments: $^*p < 0.05$ compared to the saline group and $^\#p < 0.05$ compared to the tumor group. One-way ANOVA followed by Tukey's test.

channels resulting in neuronal depolarization [50]. TNFR1 and TNFR2 also participate in the spinal cord activation of astrocytes and pain [13]. In cancer, the inhibition of p38-MAPK signaling pathway attenuates breast cancer-induced bone pain [17]. TNFR2 also plays a pronounced role in lung carcinoma cells-induced heat hyperalgesia [8]. Therefore, cytokines such as IL-1β and TNFα are involved in the neuronal activation at peripheral sites, DRG, and spinal cord in varied painful conditions and targeting these cytokines is one of the efficient analgesic approaches in cancer pain.

3.3. Quercetin Inhibits the Oxidative Stress Induced by Ehrlich Tumor Cells. There is close relation between cytokines and oxidative stress in pain induction. IL-1β and TNFα can activate nicotinamide adenine dinucleotide phosphate-(NADPH-) oxidase, resulting in the production of superoxide anion. In turn, superoxide anion activates nuclear factor kappa B (NFκB) and enhances cytokine production [23, 51, 52]. In this sense, the effect of quercetin on Ehrlich tumor-induced oxidative stress was accessed by the total antioxidant capacity depletion in the spinal cord and paw skin using

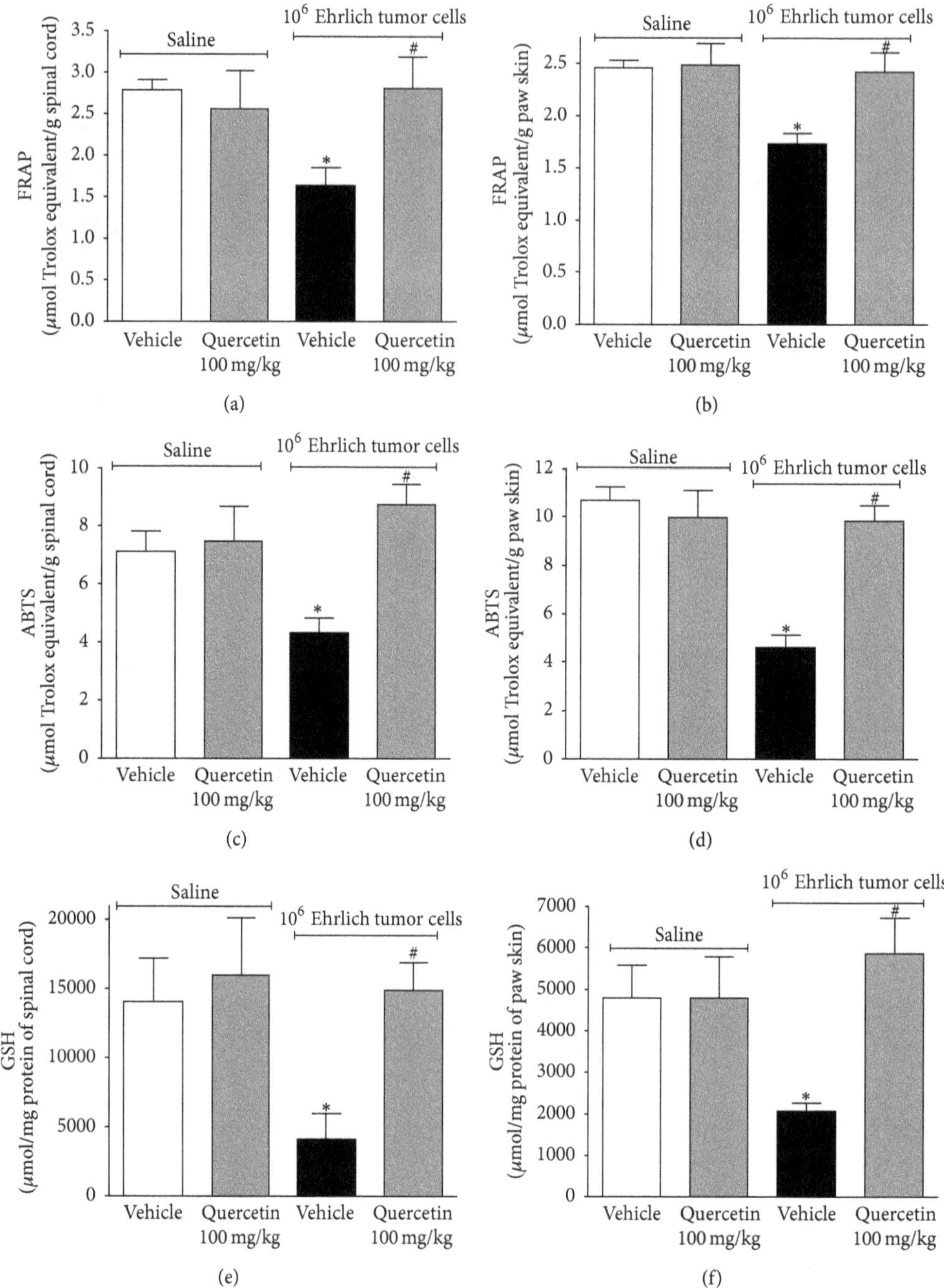

FIGURE 6: Quercetin inhibits the oxidative stress induced by Ehrlich tumor cells. Mice were treated with quercetin (100 mg/kg, i.p.) or vehicle 10 min after the injection of Ehrlich tumor cells ($1 \times 10^6/25\,\mu$L) or saline. The treatment continued daily during 12 days, and, in the 12th day, 3 h after the treatment, samples of spinal cord and paw skin were collected for the oxidative stress assays. The FRAP and ABTS ability of spinal cord ((a) and (c), resp.) and paw skin ((b) and (d), resp.) tissues and GSH levels in spinal cord (e) and paw skin (f) were accessed. Data are presented as means ± SEM of six mice per group per experiment and representative of two separated experiments: $^{*}p < 0.05$ compared to the saline group and $^{\#}p < 0.05$ compared to the tumor group. One-way ANOVA followed by Tukey's test.

the ability to ferric reducing potential (FRAP) assay, scavenge 2,2′-azinobis-(3-ethylbenzothiazoline 6-sulfonic acid radical) (ABTS) assay, and reduced glutathione (GSH) levels. Mice were divided and treated as in Figure 2 and samples were collected in the 12th day. Ehrlich tumor cells induced oxidative stress (Figure 6). The quercetin treatment showed a significant increase in FRAP at both the spinal cord (Figure 6(a)) and paw skin (Figure 6(b)) and ABTS in the spinal cord (Figure 6(c)) and paw skin (Figure 6(d)). It is known that quercetin is an antioxidant flavonoid and its

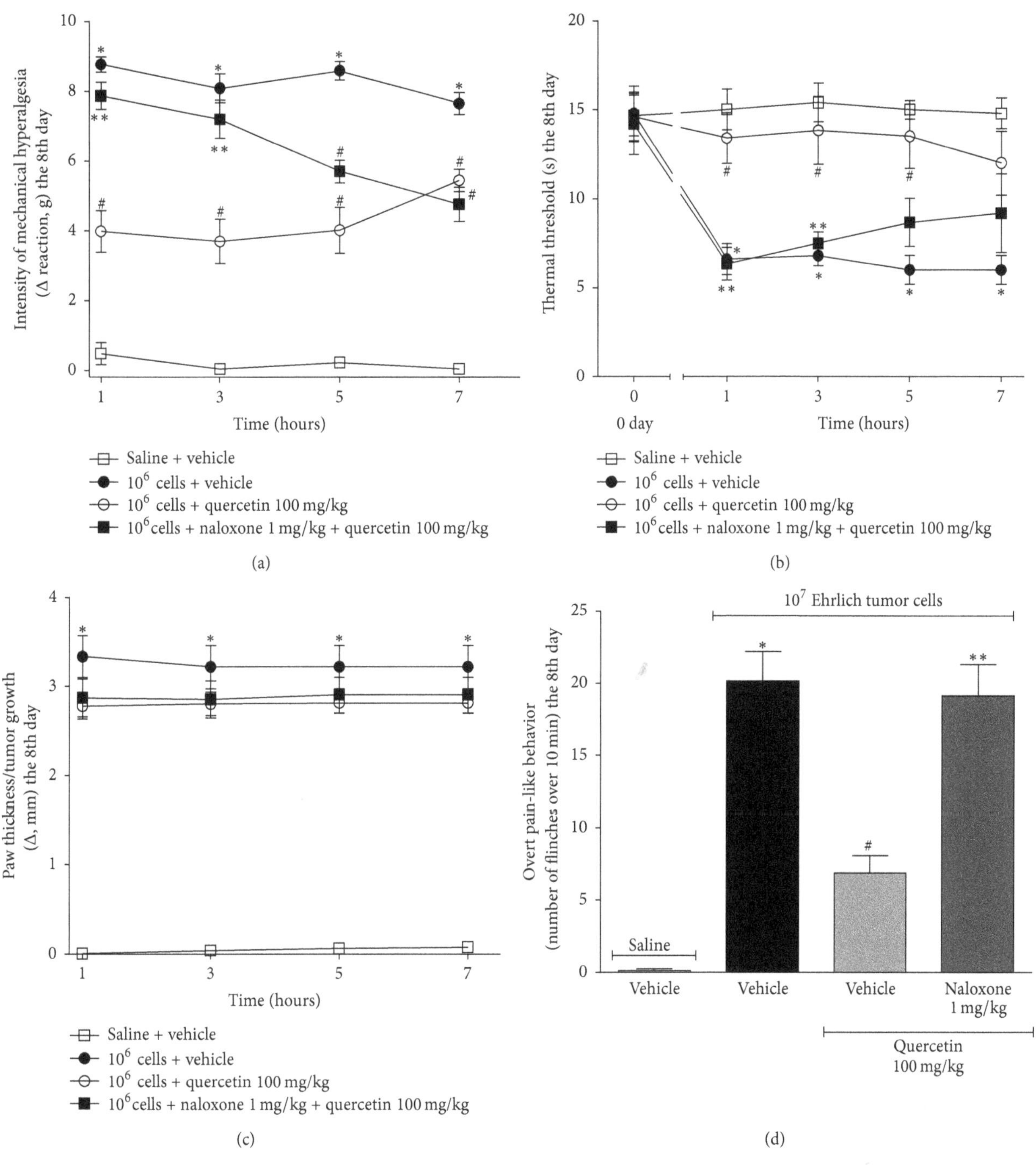

FIGURE 7: The opioid receptor antagonist, naloxone, inhibits quercetin analgesia in the Ehrlich tumor-induced pain model. Mice were treated with quercetin (100 mg/kg, i.p., starting 10 min after tumor administration) during 8 days after the injection of Ehrlich tumor cells (1×10^6 or 1×10^7 cells/25 μL) or saline and, in the 8th day, one group of mice that received quercetin was also treated with naloxone (1 mg/kg i.p. diluted in saline) 1 h before the treatment with quercetin. The evaluation of mechanical hyperalgesia (a), thermal hyperalgesia (b), and paw thickness (c) was performed 1, 3, 5, and 7 h after the treatments, and the overt pain-like behavior (d) was evaluated 1 h after the treatment. Data are presented as means ± SEM of six mice per group per experiment and representative of two separated experiments: $^{*}p < 0.05$ compared to the saline group, $^{\#}p < 0.05$ compared to the tumor group, and $^{**}p < 0.05$ compared to the quercetin group. One-way ANOVA followed by Tukey's test.

effects could be explained by the presence of structural antioxidant chemical groups [53]. However, there is no antioxidant structural relationship of flavonoids and the inhibition of intracellular signaling pathways such as mitogen-activated protein kinases [23]. Therefore, the presence of structural antioxidant chemical groups does not fully explain the activities of quercetin.

In cancer and during chemotherapy treatment, there is increased production of reactive species [54], which can result in antioxidant depletion and, consequently, oxidative stress. The main consequence of rapid cellular division in cancer is the increase of the metabolic by products, such as excessive production of reactive oxygen species (ROS) [55]. Decreased levels of GSH have been reported in patients with breast cancer [56, 57]. The increased oxidative stress gives rise to inflammation, which could further aggravates the pain [57]. In this sense, quercetin may present an important applicability in reducing cancer-induced oxidative stress. It is noteworthy that the inhibition of peripheral oxidative stress observed may also be attributed to the reduction in neutrophil recruitment by quercetin (Figure 4), because activated neutrophils are important sources of reactive oxygen and nitrogen species in the tissue. Quercetin also inhibited Ehrlich tumor-induced GSH depletion in the spinal cord (Figure 6(e)) and paw skin (Figure 6(f)). This is in agreement with previous studies demonstrating that quercetin presents beneficial effects through antioxidant activities in other experimental models such as colitis [25] and inflammatory pain [21]. It has been suggested that the prevention of GSH depletion may be an important analgesic mechanism [58]. GSH can reduce reactive species and is an important molecule of the endogenous antioxidant system. In this sense, the preservation of GSH levels by quercetin may also prevent total antioxidant capacity depletion and oxidative stress [54]. Therefore, the antinociceptive activity of quercetin could also be associated with the inhibition of oxidative stress in this model.

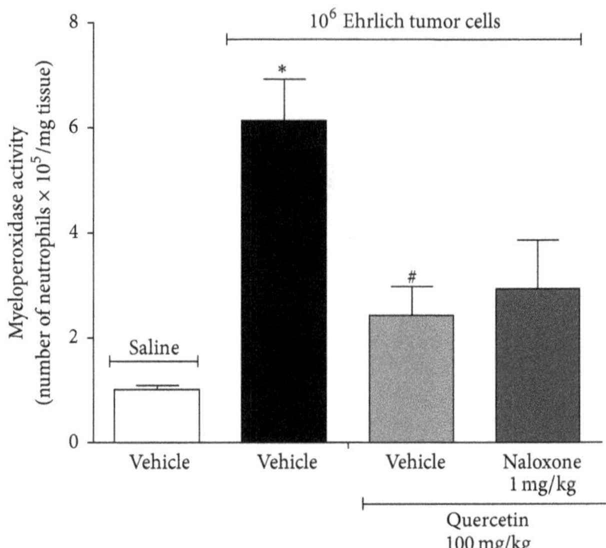

FIGURE 8: Naloxone did not reverse the effect of quercetin in reducing Ehrlich tumor cells-induced neutrophil recruitment. Mice were treated with quercetin (100 mg/kg, i.p., starting 10 min after tumor administration) during 8 days after the injection of Ehrlich tumor cells (1×10^6 or 1×10^7 cells/25 μL) or saline and, in the 8th day, one group of mice that received quercetin was also treated with naloxone (1 mg/kg i.p. diluted in saline) or its vehicle 1 h before the treatment with quercetin. The neutrophil recruitment was evaluated in samples of paw skin collected after 3 h of the treatment with quercetin by the myeloperoxidase (MPO) activity assay. Data are presented as means ± SEM of six mice per group per experiment and representative of two separated experiments: $^*p < 0.05$ compared to the saline group and $^\#p < 0.05$ compared to the tumor group. One-way ANOVA followed by Tukey's test.

3.4. Quercetin Analgesia, but Not the Anti-Inflammatory Effect, Depends on Endogenous Opioids. Mice were treated with quercetin as in Figure 2 daily during 8 days. In the 8th day, one group was treated with naloxone (an opioid receptor antagonist, 1 mg/kg, diluted in saline, i.p.) 1 h before the treatment with quercetin (Figure 7) and mechanical hyperalgesia, thermal hyperalgesia, and paw thickness were assessed after 1, 3, 5, and 7 h (Figures 7(a)–7(c)). Quercetin significantly reduced Ehrlich tumor-induced mechanical and thermal hyperalgesia at all time points. The analgesic effect of quercetin was inhibited by naloxone at 1 and 3 h after treatment (Figures 7(a) and 7(b)). As observed in Figure 2, quercetin did not affect paw thickness and naloxone did not alter this absence of effect of quercetin over Ehrlich tumor growth (Figure 7(c)). The same treatment regimen was performed on mice that receive 1×10^7 Ehrlich tumor cells to induce paw flinching. In the 8th day, 1 h after treatment with quercetin, Ehrlich tumor cell-induced paw flinches were evaluated. Quercetin significantly decreased Ehrlich tumor-induced paw flinches and treatment with naloxone inhibited the analgesic effect of quercetin (Figure 7(d)). The dose of naloxone was selected in previous studies [30]. These results indicate that the analgesic effect of quercetin in Ehrlich tumor-induced pain depends on opioid mechanisms. In agreement with our study, the analgesic effect of quercetin in a model of streptozotocin-induced diabetic neuropathic pain [22] and lipopolysaccharide-induced hyperalgesia [59] also depends on opioid mechanisms and is reversible by treatment with naloxone. On the other hand, using the same protocol as for Figure 7, we observed that naloxone did not alter the quercetin inhibition of Ehrlich tumor cells-induced MPO activity in the paw skin (Figure 8). Furthermore, following the same protocol of Figure 7, the effect of naloxone on quercetin inhibition of Ehrlich tumor cells-induced spinal cord and paw skin production of IL-1β (Figures 9(a) and 9(b)), TNFα (Figures 9(c) and 9(d)), FRAP, ABTS, and GSH (Figures 10(a)–10(f)) were determined. The treatment with naloxone did not alter the anti-inflammatory and antioxidant effects of quercetin (Figures 9 and 10). The anti-inflammatory effect of opioids has already been described. For instance, kappa-opioid agonist exerts anti-inflammatory actions by reduction of adhesion molecule expression, inhibition of cell trafficking, and TNF release and expression [60]. Our data

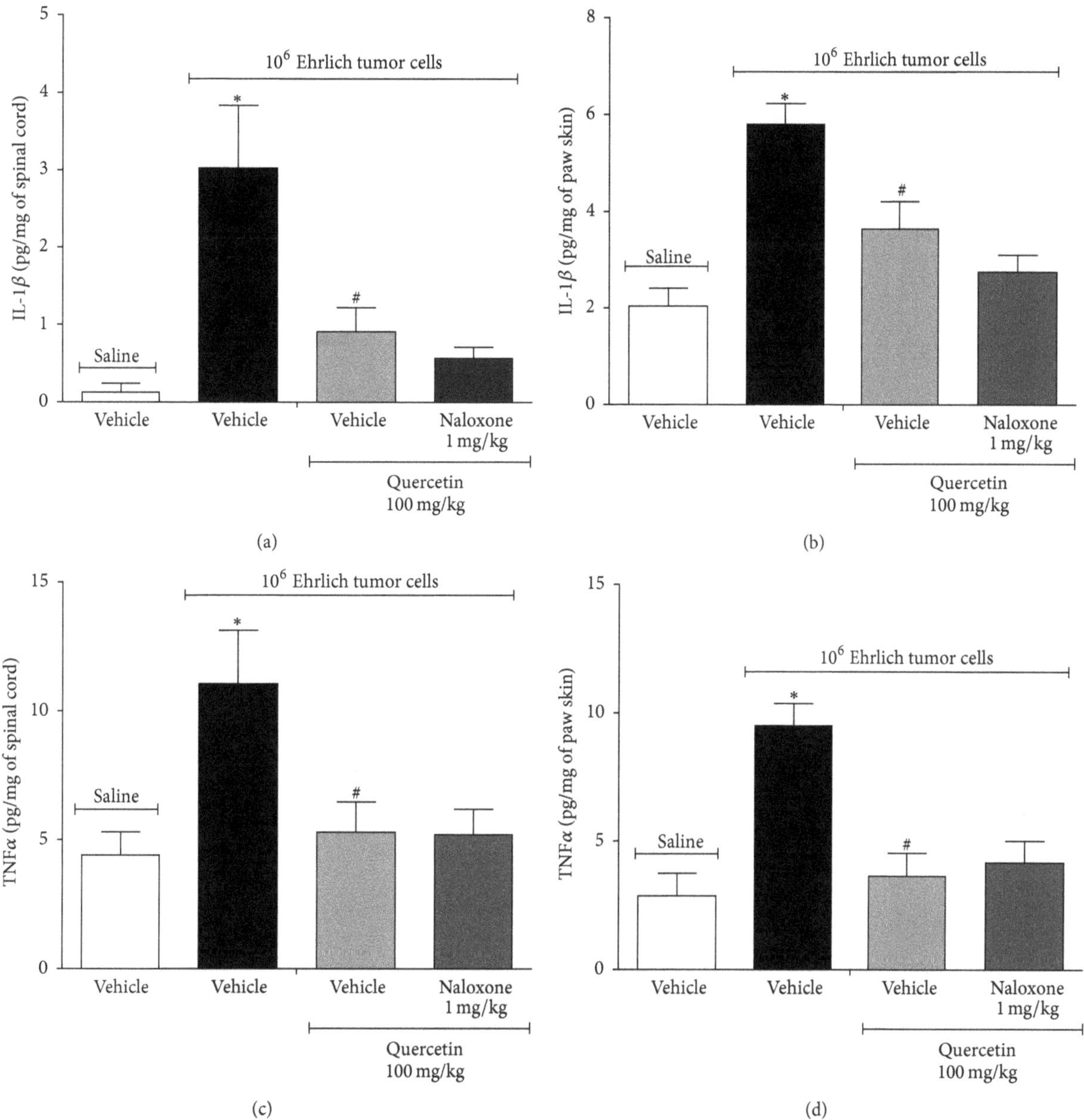

FIGURE 9: Naloxone did not reverse the effect of quercetin in reducing Ehrlich tumor cells-induced cytokine production. Mice were treated with quercetin (100 mg/kg, i.p., starting 10 min after tumor administration) during 8 days after the injection of Ehrlich tumor cells (1×10^6 or 1×10^7 cells/25 μL) or saline and, in the 8th day, one group of mice that received quercetin was also treated with naloxone (1 mg/kg i.p. diluted in saline) or its vehicle 1 h before the treatment with quercetin. IL-1β concentration in spinal cord (a) or paw skin (b) and TNFα concentration in spinal cord (c) or paw skin (d) were determined by ELISA 3 h after the treatment with quercetin. Data are presented as means ± SEM of six mice per group per experiment and representative of two separated experiments: $^*p < 0.05$ compared to the saline group and $^{\#}p < 0.05$ compared to the tumor group. One-way ANOVA followed by Tukey's test.

suggest that the analgesic effect of quercetin in Ehrlich tumor-induced cancer pain is dependent on endogenous opioid mechanisms; however, these opioid-dependent mechanisms are not responsible for the anti-inflammatory and antioxidant actions of quercetin observed as reduction of MPO activity, cytokine production, and oxidative stress in the current protocol.

3.5. Combined Treatment with Quercetin and Morphine at Doses That Are Ineffective as Single Treatment Reduces Ehrlich Tumor-Induced Pain-Like Responses. Mice were treated with quercetin (10 mg/kg i.p., a dose without significant analgesic effect *per se*, Figure 2) 10 min after administration of Ehrlich tumor cells (1×10^6 or 1×10^7 cells, i.pl.). Mice were treated daily during 8 days. In the 8th day, mice were treated with

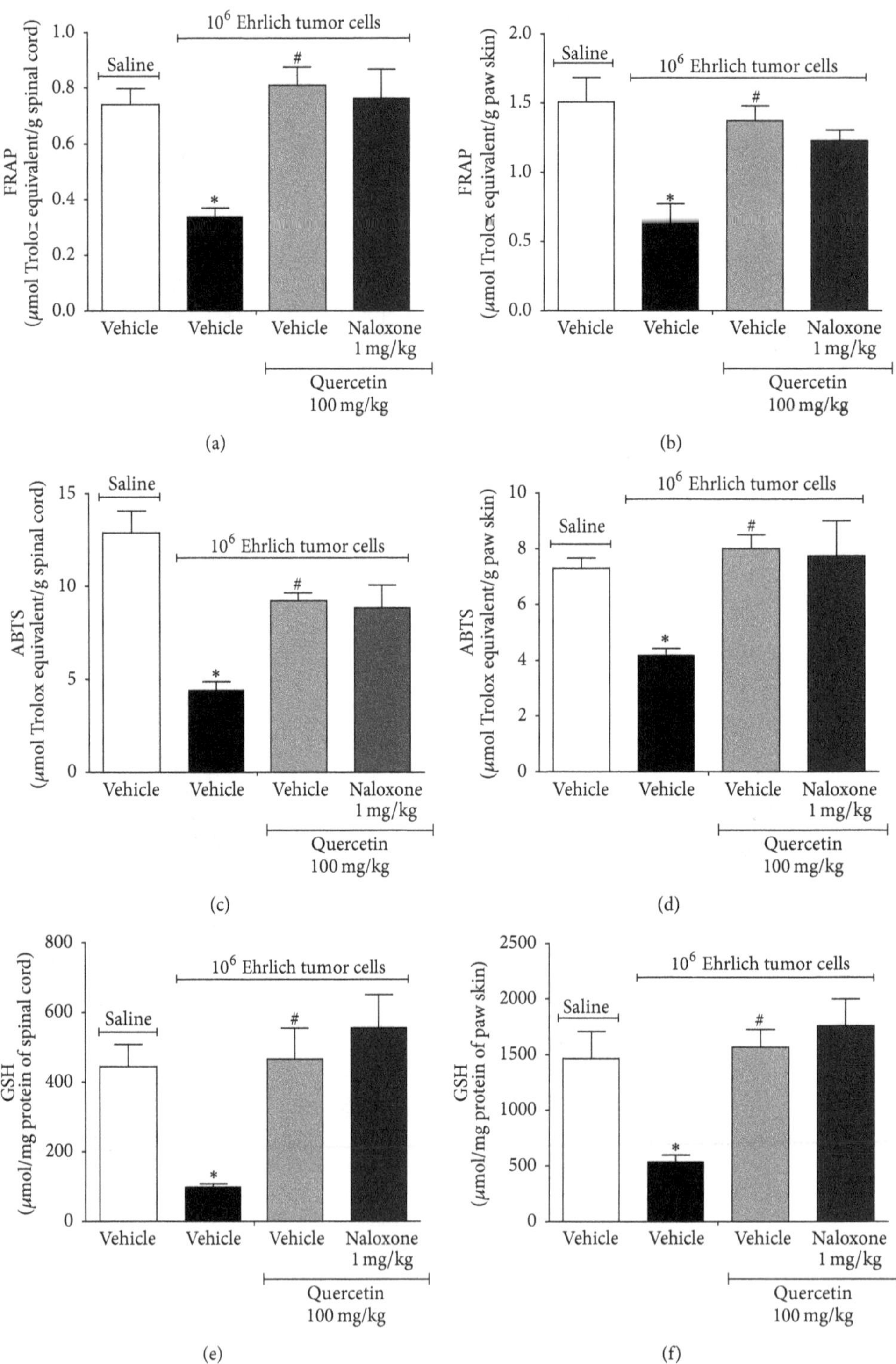

FIGURE 10: Naloxone did not reverse the effect of quercetin in reducing Ehrlich tumor cells-induced oxidative stress. Mice were treated with quercetin (100 mg/kg, i.p., starting 10 min after tumor administration) during 8 days after the injection of Ehrlich tumor cells (1×10^6 or 1×10^7 cells/25 μL) or saline and, in the 8th day, one group of mice that received quercetin was also treated with naloxone (1 mg/kg i.p. diluted in saline) or its vehicle 1 h before the treatment with quercetin. Three hours after the treatment with quercetin, samples of spinal cord and paw skin were collected for the oxidative stress assays. The FRAP and ABTS ability of spinal cord ((a) and (c), resp.) and paw skin ((b) and (d), resp.) tissues and GSH levels in the spinal cord (e) and paw skin (f) were accessed. Data are presented as means ± SEM of six mice per group per experiment and representative of two separated experiments: $^*p < 0.05$ compared to the saline group and $^\#p < 0.05$ compared to the tumor group. One-way ANOVA followed by Tukey's test.

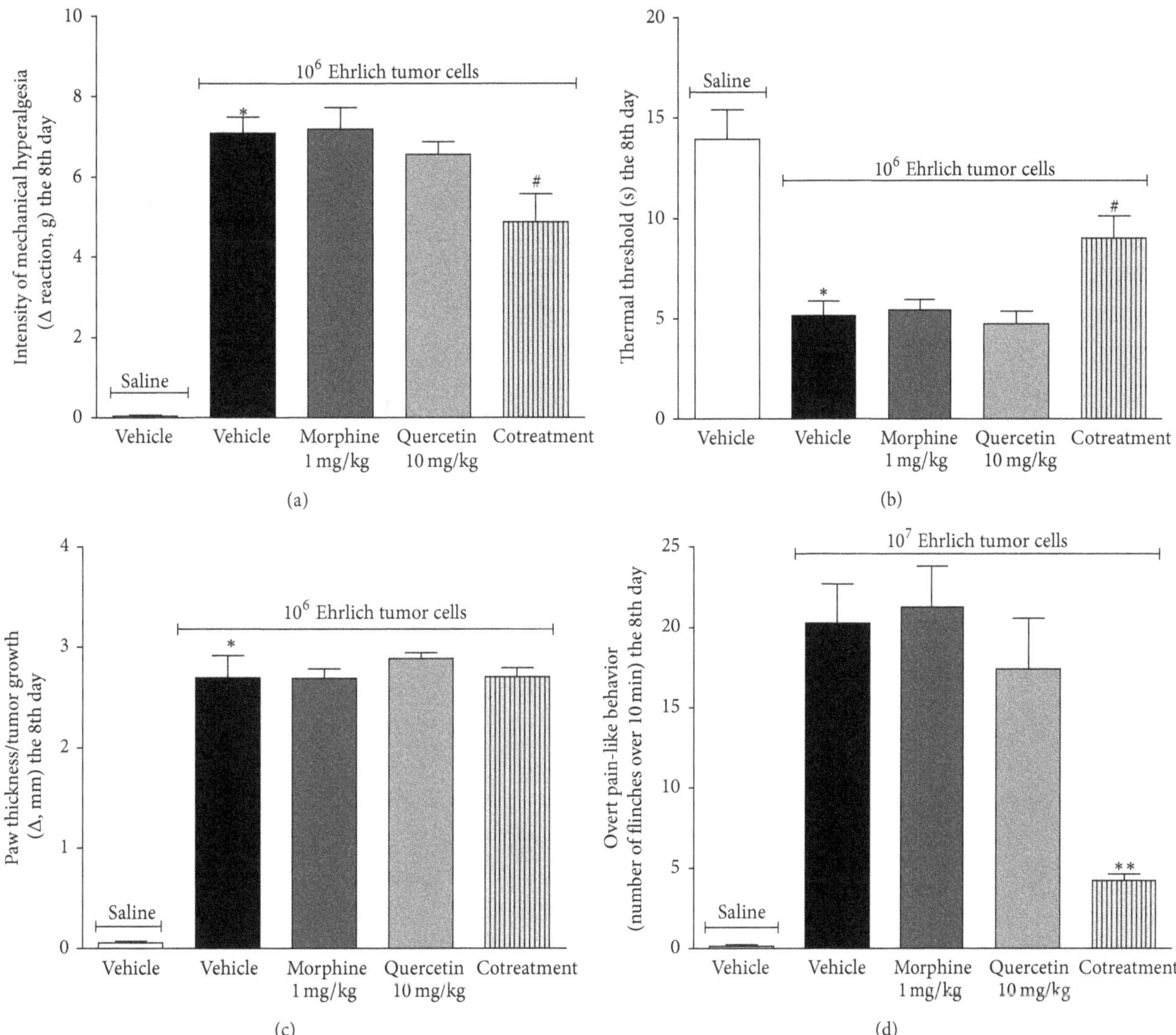

FIGURE 11: Combined treatment with quercetin and morphine at doses that are ineffective as single treatment reduces Ehrlich tumor-induced pain-like responses. Mice were treated with quercetin (10 mg/kg i.p., a dose without significant analgesic effect *per se*), before the injection of Ehrlich tumor cells (1×10^6 or 1×10^7 cells, i.pl.). Mice were treated daily during 8 days and, in the 8th day, mice were treated with quercetin and after 2 h and 15 min received morphine (1 mg/kg i.p., a dose without significant analgesic effect *per se*). Mechanical (a) and thermal hyperalgesia (b), paw thickness (c), and overt pain-like behavior (d) were evaluated 3 h after the last quercetin treatment. Data are presented as means ± SEM of six mice per group per experiment and representative of two separated experiments: $^*p < 0.05$ compared to the saline group, $^\#p < 0.05$ compared to the tumor group, and $^{**}p < 0.05$ compared to the quercetin 10 mg/kg and morphine 1 mg/kg. One-way ANOVA followed by Tukey's test.

morphine (1 mg/kg i.p., a dose without significant analgesic effect *per se*) 2 h and 15 min after quercetin administration. Mechanical hyperalgesia, thermal hyperalgesia, paw thickness (1×10^6 Ehrlich tumor cells), and paw flinching (1×10^7 Ehrlich tumor cells) were assessed 45 min after morphine treatment or 3 h after quercetin treatment (Figures 11(a)–11(d)). Ehrlich tumor-induced mechanical and thermal hyperalgesia were not reduced by treatment with quercetin (10 mg/kg, i.p.) or morphine (1 mg/kg, i.p.) alone. However, the cotreatment with quercetin and morphine significantly reduced the mechanical (Figure 11(a)) and thermal hyperalgesia (Figure 11(b)). Ehrlich tumor-induced increase in the paw thickness was not altered by quercetin, morphine, or cotreatment with both molecules (Figure 11(c)). Finally, Ehrlich tumor-induced paw flinches were also reduced by cotreatment with quercetin and morphine, but not by quercetin or morphine alone (Figure 11(d)). These results suggest a synergic analgesic effect of quercetin and morphine over Ehrlich tumor-induced pain. Moreover, this synergy was more evident in the overt pain-like response, which clearly showed a potentiation of analgesia (Figure 11(d)). Therefore, these results on synergy or even potentiation of analgesia by cotreatment with quercetin and morphine at doses without analgesic effect as single treatment are important in the sense that indicates possible reduction of morphine dosage by combination with quercetin treatment to control cancer pain.

Evidence supports a synergy/potentiation between quercetin and opioids/morphine in other models, indicating that this effect should be addressed. For instance, quercetin reduces the morphine tolerance [61], reduces naloxone-precipitated withdrawal contracture of the acute morphine-dependent guinea-pig ileum [62], and exhibits morphine-like inhibition of acetylcholine release in the coaxially stimulated ileum [63]. Therefore, the opioid-related actions of quercetin are consistent in varied systems and may contribute to reduce morphine dosage ([22, 61] and present data) as well as morphine tolerance [62]. Mechanistically, quercetin inhibits morphine tolerance by inhibiting nitric oxide synthase activity [61]. Therefore, it is likely that quercetin potentiates opioid activity indirectly by inhibiting mechanisms that would limit opioid effects and not by inducing opioid release or binding to and activating opioid receptors, which explain a synergic/potentiating effect of quercetin and morphine.

In addition to the analgesic effects, opioids also present anti-inflammatory actions *in vitro* and *in vivo* [64, 65]. The present results suggest that quercetin inhibits Ehrlich tumor cells-induced pain by two independent mechanisms: (a) an opioid-related analgesic mechanism and (b) an anti-inflammatory/antioxidant mechanism. The opioid-related mechanism might present central analgesic effects since per oral treatment with quercetin inhibited diabetic neuropathic pain in mice in the tail-immersion in warm water test, which evaluates the involvement of central nociceptive responses, in a naloxone sensitive manner [22]. The anti-inflammatory/antioxidant mechanism of quercetin is related to the inhibition of proinflammatory signaling pathways and intrinsic structural antioxidant chemical groups of quercetin [23].

In conclusion, the present study demonstrates that quercetin inhibits Ehrlich tumor-induced pain by mechanisms targeting peripheral and spinal cord oxidative stress and hyperalgesic cytokine production as well as inducing an opioid-related analgesic mechanism, resulting in potentiation of morphine analgesia. The analgesic dose of quercetin did not alter tumor growth demonstrating; therefore, its analgesia does not depend on reducing tumor mass.

Conflict of Interests

The authors declare that they have no conflict of interests.

Acknowledgments

This work was supported by grants from Conselho Nacional de Desenvolvimento Científico e Tecnológico (CNPq, Brazil), Coordenadoria de Aperfeiçoamento de Pessoal de Nível Superior (CAPES, Brazil), Ministério da Ciência, Tecnologia e Inovação (MCTI, Brazil), Secretaria da Ciência, Tecnologia e Ensino Superior (SETI, Brazil)/Fundação Araucária (Brazil), and Parana State Government (Brazil). Ana C. Zarpelon received a post doc fellowship from CAPES/ Fundação Araucária.

References

[1] W. L. Peng, G. J. Wu, W. Z. Sun, J. C. Chen, and A. T. Huang, "Multidisciplinary management of cancer pain: a longitudinal retrospective study on a cohort of end-stage cancer patients," *Journal of Pain and Symptom Management*, vol. 32, no. 5, pp. 444–452, 2006.

[2] M. I. Bennett, C. Rayment, M. Hjermstad, N. Aass, A. Caraceni, and S. Kaasa, "Prevalence and aetiology of neuropathic pain in cancer patients: a systematic review," *Pain*, vol. 153, no. 2, pp. 359–365, 2012.

[3] M. H. J. van den Beuken-van Everdingen, J. M. de Rijke, A. G. Kessels, H. C. Schouten, M. van Kleef, and J. Patijn, "Prevalence of pain in patients with cancer: a systematic review of the past 40 years," *Annals of Oncology*, vol. 18, no. 9, pp. 1437–1449, 2007.

[4] J. Hearn and I. J. Higginson, "Cancer pain epidemiology: a systematic review," in *Cancer Pain: Assessment and Management*, E. D. Bruera and R. K. Portenoy, Eds., pp. 19–37, Cambridge University Press, London, UK, 2003.

[5] J. M. Regan and P. Peng, "Neurophysiology of cancer pain," *Cancer Control*, vol. 7, no. 2, pp. 111–119, 2000.

[6] R. Zhang, Y. Liu, J. Zhang, Y. Zheng, X. Gu, and Z. Ma, "Intrathecal administration of roscovitine attenuates cancer pain and inhibits the expression of NMDA receptor 2B subunit mRNA," *Pharmacology Biochemistry and Behavior*, vol. 102, no. 1, pp. 139–145, 2012.

[7] S. Deandrea, M. Montanari, L. Moja, and G. Apolone, "Prevalence of undertreatment in cancer pain. A review of published literature," *Annals of Oncology*, vol. 19, no. 12, pp. 1985–1991, 2008.

[8] C. E. Constantin, N. Mair, C. A. Sailer et al., "Endogenous tumor necrosis factor α (TNFα) requires TNF receptor type 2 to generate heat hyperalgesia in a mouse cancer model," *The Journal of Neuroscience*, vol. 28, no. 19, pp. 5072–5081, 2008.

[9] M. Kress, "Cytokines and cancer pain," in *Cancer Pain: From Molecules to Suffering*, A. J. Paice, R. F. Bell, E. A. Kalso, O. A. Soyannwo, and O. A. Soyannwo, Eds., chapter 4, pp. 63–84, IASP Press, Washington, DC, USA, 1st edition, 2010.

[10] X. Gu, Y. Zheng, B. Ren et al., "Intraperitoneal injection of thalidomide attenuates bone cancer pain and decreases spinal tumor necrosis factor-α expression in a mouse model," *Molecular Pain*, vol. 6, article 64, 10 pages, 2010.

[11] M. J. Schwei, P. Honore, S. D. Rogers et al., "Neurochemical and cellular reorganization of the spinal cord in a murine model of bone cancer pain," *The Journal of Neuroscience*, vol. 19, no. 24, pp. 10886–10897, 1999.

[12] S. J. Medhurst, K. Walker, M. Bowes et al., "A rat model of bone cancer pain," *Pain*, vol. 96, no. 1-2, pp. 129–140, 2002.

[13] C. Geis, M. Graulich, A. Wissmann et al., "Evoked pain behavior and spinal glia activation is dependent on tumor necrosis factor receptor 1 and 2 in a mouse model of bone cancer pain," *Neuroscience*, vol. 169, no. 1, pp. 463–474, 2010.

[14] J. Xu, M.-D. Zhu, X. Zhang et al., "NFκB-mediated CXCL1 production in spinal cord astrocytes contributes to the maintenance of bone cancer pain in mice," *Journal of Neuroinflammation*, vol. 11, no. 38, pp. 1–13, 2014.

[15] P. W. Mantyh, "Cancer pain and its impact on diagnosis, survival and quality of life," *Nature Reviews Neuroscience*, vol. 7, no. 10, pp. 797–809, 2006.

[16] M. G. Nashed, M. D. Balenko, and G. Singh, "Cancer-induced oxidative stress and pain," *Current Pain and Headache Reports*, vol. 18, article 384, 2014.

[17] D. Sukhtankar, A. Okun, A. Chandramouli et al., "Inhibition of p38-MAPK signaling pathway attenuates breast cancer induced bone pain and disease progression in a murine model of cancer-induced bone pain," *Molecular Pain*, vol. 7, article 81, 2011.

[18] Y.-J. Gao, J.-K. Cheng, Q. Zeng et al., "Selective inhibition of JNK with a peptide inhibitor attenuates pain hypersensitivity and tumor growth in a mouse skin cancer pain model," *Experimental Neurology*, vol. 219, no. 1, pp. 146–155, 2009.

[19] J. Devulder, A. Jacobs, U. Richarz, and H. Wiggett, "Impact of opioid rescue medication for breakthrough pain on the efficacy and tolerability of long-acting opioids in patients with chronic non-malignant pain," *British Journal of Anaesthesia*, vol. 103, no. 4, pp. 576–585, 2009.

[20] T. Okamoto, "Safety of quercetin for clinical application," *International Journal of Molecular Medicine*, vol. 16, no. 2, pp. 275–278, 2005.

[21] D. A. Valério, S. R. Georgetti, D. A. Magro et al., "Quercetin reduces inflammatory pain: inhibition of oxidative stress and cytokine production," *Journal of Natural Products*, vol. 72, no. 11, pp. 1975–1979, 2009.

[22] M. Anjaneyulu and K. Chopra, "Quercetin, a bioflavonoid, attenuates thermal hyperalgesia in a mouse model of diabetic neuropathic pain," *Progress in Neuro-Psychopharmacology & Biological Psychiatry*, vol. 27, no. 6, pp. 1001–1005, 2003.

[23] W. A. Verri Jr., F. T. M. C. Vicentini, M. M. Baracat et al., "Flavonoids as anti-inflammatory and analgesic drugs: mechanisms of action and perspectives in the development of pharmaceutical forms," in *Studies in Natural Products Chemistry*, Atta-ur-Rahman, Ed., vol. 36, chapter 9, pp. 297–330, Elsevier, Amsterdam, The Netherlands, 2012.

[24] F. T. M. C. Vicentini, T. He, Y. Shao et al., "Quercetin inhibits UV irradiation-induced inflammatory cytokine production in primary human keratinocytes by suppressing NF-κB pathway," *Journal of Dermatological Science*, vol. 61, no. 3, pp. 162–168, 2011.

[25] C. F. S. Guazelli, V. Fattori, B. B. Colombo et al., "Quercetin-loaded microcapsules ameliorate experimental colitis in mice by anti-inflammatory and antioxidant mechanisms," *Journal of Natural Products*, vol. 76, no. 2, pp. 200–208, 2013.

[26] M. I. Azevedo, A. F. Pereira, R. B. Nogueira et al., "The antioxidant effects of the flavonoids rutin and quercetin inhibit oxaliplatin-induced chronic painful peripheral neuropathy," *Molecular Pain*, vol. 9, article 53, 14 pages, 2013.

[27] Y. Wan, M. H. Tang, X. C. Chen, L. J. Chen, Y. Q. Wei, and Y. S. Wang, "Inhibitory effect of liposomal quercetin on acute hepatitis and hepatic fibrosis induced by concanavalin A," *Brazilian Journal of Medical and Biological Research*, vol. 47, no. 8, pp. 655–661, 2014.

[28] M. H. Napimoga, J. T. Clemente-Napimoga, C. G. Macedo et al., "Quercetin inhibits inflammatory bone resorption in a mouse periodontitis model," *Journal of Natural Products*, vol. 76, no. 12, pp. 2316–2321, 2013.

[29] A. P. Rogerio, C. L. Dora, E. L. Andrade et al., "Anti-inflammatory effect of quercetin-loaded microemulsion in the airways allergic inflammatory model in mice," *Pharmacological Research*, vol. 61, no. 4, pp. 288–297, 2010.

[30] C. Calixto-Campos, A. C. Zarpelon, M. Corrêa et al., "The ehrlich tumor induces pain-like behavior in mice: a novel model of cancer pain for pathophysiological studies and pharmacological screening," *BioMed Research International*, vol. 2013, Article ID 624815, 12 pages, 2013.

[31] W. G. Harris, E. A. Benson, D. Cartwright et al., "Symptoms and signs of operable breast cancer," *The Journal of the Royal College of General Practitioners*, vol. 33, pp. 473–476, 1983.

[32] K. Krøner, B. Krebs, J. Skov, and H. S. Jørgensen, "Immediate and long-term phantom breast syndrome after mastectomy: incidence, clinical characteristics and relationship to pre-mastectomy breast pain," *Pain*, vol. 36, no. 3, pp. 327–334, 1989.

[33] O. H. Lowry, N. J. Rosebrough, A. L. Farr, and R. J. Randall, "Protein measurement with the Folin phenol reagent," *The Journal of Biological Chemistry*, vol. 193, no. 1, pp. 265–275, 1951.

[34] A. W. Filho, V. C. Filho, L. Olinger, and M. M. De Souza, "Quercetin:further investigation of its antinociceptive properties and mechanisms of action," *Archives of Pharmacal Research*, vol. 31, no. 6, pp. 713–721, 2008.

[35] M. Anjaneyulu and K. Chopra, "Quercetin attenuates thermal hyperalgesia and cold allodynia in STZ-induced diabetic rats," *Indian Journal of Experimental Biology*, vol. 42, no. 8, pp. 766–769, 2004.

[36] F. O. Souto, A. C. Zarpelon, L. Staurengo-Ferrari et al., "Quercetin reduces neutrophil recruitment induced by CXCL8, LTB_4, and fMLP: inhibition of actin polymerization," *Journal of Natural Products*, vol. 74, no. 2, pp. 113–118, 2011.

[37] J. A. Choi, J. Y. Kim, J. Y. Lee et al., "Induction of cell cycle arrest and apoptosis in human breast cancer cells by quercetin," *International Journal of Oncology*, vol. 19, no. 4, pp. 837–844, 2001.

[38] Y.-Q. Wei, X. Zhao, Y. Kariya, H. Fukata, K. Teshigawara, and A. Uchida, "Induction of apoptosis by quercetin: involvement of heat shock protein," *Cancer Research*, vol. 54, no. 18, pp. 4952–4957, 1994.

[39] C. S. Ong, E. Tran, T. T. T. Nguyen et al., "Quercetin-induced growth inhibition and cell death in nasopharyngeal carcinoma cells are associated with increase in Bad and hypophosphorylated retinoblastoma expressions," *Oncology Reports*, vol. 11, no. 3, pp. 727–733, 2004.

[40] T.-B. Kang and N.-C. Liang, "Studies on the inhibitory effects of quercetin on the growth of HL-60 leukemia cells," *Biochemical Pharmacology*, vol. 54, no. 9, pp. 1013–1018, 1997.

[41] T. Kobayashi, T. Nakata, and T. Kuzumaki, "Effect of flavonoids on cell cycle progression in prostate cancer cells," *Cancer Letters*, vol. 176, no. 1, pp. 17–23, 2002.

[42] P. D. Fernandes, F. S. Guerra, N. M. Sales, T. B. Sardella, S. Jancar, and J. S. Neves, "Characterization of the inflammatory response during Ehrlich ascitic tumor development," *Journal of Pharmacological and Toxicological Methods*, vol. 71, pp. 83–89, 2015.

[43] W. A. Verri Jr., T. M. Cunha, D. A. Magro et al., "Targeting endothelin ETA and ETB receptors inhibits antigen-induced neutrophil migration and mechanical hypernociception in mice," *Naunyn-Schmiedeberg's Archives of Pharmacology*, vol. 379, no. 3, pp. 271–279, 2009.

[44] J. Pincemail, C. Deby, A. Thirion, M. de Bruyn-Dister, and R. Goutier, "Human myeloperoxidase activity is inhibited *in vitro* by quercetin. Comparison with three related compounds," *Experientia*, vol. 44, no. 5, pp. 450–453, 1988.

[45] W. A. Verri Jr., T. M. Cunha, C. A. Parada, S. Poole, F. Q. Cunha, and S. H. Ferreira, "Hypernociceptive role of cytokines

and chemokines: targets for analgesic drug development?" *Pharmacology & Therapeutics*, vol. 112, no. 1, pp. 116–138, 2006.

[46] R.-X. Zhang, B. Liu, A. Li et al., "Interleukin 1β facilitates bone cancer pain in rats by enhancing NMDA receptor NR-1 subunit phosphorylation," *Neuroscience*, vol. 154, no. 4, pp. 1533–1538, 2008.

[47] A. Baamonde, V. Curto-Reyes, L. Juárez, Á. Meana, A. Hidalgo, and L. Menéndez, "Antihyperalgesic effects induced by the IL-1 receptor antagonist anakinra and increased IL-1β levels in inflamed and osteosarcoma-bearing mice," *Life Sciences*, vol. 81, no. 8, pp. 673–682, 2007.

[48] P. W. Wacnik, L. J. Eikmeier, D. A. Simone, G. L. Wilcox, and A. J. Beitz, "Nociceptive characteristics of tumor necrosis factor-alpha in naive and tumor-bearing mice," *Neuroscience*, vol. 132, no. 2, pp. 479–491, 2005.

[49] C. A. Parada, J. J. Yeh, E. K. Joseph, and J. D. Levine, "Tumor necrosis factor receptor type-1 in sensory neurons contributes to induction of chronic enhancement of inflammatory hyperalgesia in rat," *European Journal of Neuroscience*, vol. 17, no. 9, pp. 1847–1852, 2003.

[50] X. Jin and R. W. Gereau IV, "Acute p38-mediated modulation of tetrodotoxin-resistant sodium channels in mouse sensory neurons by tumor necrosis factor-α," *The Journal of Neuroscience*, vol. 26, no. 1, pp. 246–255, 2006.

[51] Z.-Q. Wang, F. Porreca, S. Cuzzocrea et al., "A newly identified role for superoxide in inflammatory pain," *The Journal of Pharmacology and Experimental Therapeutics*, vol. 309, no. 3, pp. 869–878, 2004.

[52] L. E. Kilpatrick, S. Sun, H. Li, T. C. Vary, and H. M. Korchak, "Regulation of TNF-induced oxygen radical production in human neutrophils: role of δ-PKC," *Journal of Leukocyte Biology*, vol. 87, no. 1, pp. 153–164, 2010.

[53] P. Pietta, P. Simonetti, C. Gardana, and P. Mauri, "Trolox equivalent antioxidant capacity (TEAC) of *Ginkgo biloba* flavonol and *Camellia sinensis* catechin metabolites," *Journal of Pharmaceutical and Biomedical Analysis*, vol. 23, no. 1, pp. 223–226, 2000.

[54] M. Valko, D. Leibfritz, J. Moncol, M. T. D. Cronin, M. Mazur, and J. Telser, "Free radicals and antioxidants in normal physiological functions and human disease," *International Journal of Biochemistry & Cell Biology*, vol. 39, no. 1, pp. 44–84, 2007.

[55] B. Halliwell, "Oxidative stress and cancer: have we moved forward?" *The Biochemical Journal*, vol. 401, no. 1, pp. 1–11, 2007.

[56] E. Beutler and T. Gelbart, "Plasma glutathione in health and in patients with malignant disease," *The Journal of Laboratory and Clinical Medicine*, vol. 105, no. 5, pp. 581–584, 1985.

[57] M. Mahajan, N. Tiwari, R. Sharma, S. Kaur, and N. Singh, "Oxidative stress and its relationship with adenosine deaminase activity in various stages of breast cancer," *Indian Journal of Clinical Biochemistry*, vol. 28, no. 1, pp. 51–54, 2013.

[58] S. M. Borghi, T. T. Carvalho, L. Staurengo-Ferrari et al., "Vitexin inhibits inflammatory pain in mice by targeting TRPV1, oxidative stress, and cytokines," *Journal of Natural Products*, vol. 76, no. 6, pp. 1141–1146, 2013.

[59] M. Anjaneyulu and K. Chopra, "Reversal of lipopolysaccharide-induced thermal and behavioural hyperalgesia by quercetin," *Drug Development Research*, vol. 58, no. 3, pp. 248–252, 2003.

[60] J. S. Walker, "Anti-inflammatory effects of opioids," *Advances in Experimental Medicine and Biology*, vol. 521, pp. 148–160, 2003.

[61] P. S. Naidu, A. Singh, D. Joshi, and S. K. Kulkarni, "Possible mechanisms of action in quercetin reversal of morphine tolerance and dependence," *Addiction Biology*, vol. 8, no. 3, pp. 327–336, 2003.

[62] A. Capasso, S. Piacente, C. Pizza, and L. Sorrentino, "Flavonoids reduce morphine withdrawal in-vitro," *The Journal of Pharmacy and Pharmacology*, vol. 50, no. 5, pp. 561–564, 1998.

[63] G. D. Lutterodt, "Inhibition of gastrointestinal release of acetylchoune byquercetin as a possible mode of action of *Psidium guajava* leaf extracts in the treatment of acute diarrhoeal disease," *Journal of Ethnopharmacology*, vol. 25, no. 3, pp. 235–247, 1989.

[64] P. K. Peterson, B. Sharp, G. Gekker, C. Brummitt, and W. F. Keane, "Opioid-mediated suppression of interferon gamma production by cultured peripheral blood mononuclear cells," *The Journal of Clinical Investigation*, vol. 80, no. 3, pp. 824–831, 1987.

[65] T. K. Eisenstein, J. L. Bussiere, T. J. Rogers, and M. W. Adler, "Immunosuppressive effects of morphine on immune responses in mice," *Advances in Experimental Medicine and Biology*, vol. 335, pp. 41–52, 1993.

5

The Role of Organelle Stresses in Diabetes Mellitus and Obesity: Implication for Treatment

Yi-Cheng Chang,[1,2,3] Siow-Wey Hee,[2] Meng-Lun Hsieh,[1]
Yung-Ming Jeng,[4,5] and Lee-Ming Chuang[2,6,7]

[1] *Graduate Institute of Medical Genomics and Proteomics, National Taiwan University, Taipei 100, Taiwan*
[2] *Department of Internal Medicine and Center for Obesity, Lifestyle and Metabolic Surgery, National Taiwan University Hospital, Taipei 100, Taiwan*
[3] *Institute of Biomedical Science, Academia Sinica, Taipei 100, Taiwan*
[4] *Graduate Institute of Pathology, National Taiwan University, Taipei 100, Taiwan*
[5] *Department of Pathology, National Taiwan University Hospital, Taipei 100, Taiwan*
[6] *College of Medicine, National Taiwan University, Taipei 100, Taiwan*
[7] *Institute of Preventive Medicine, College of Public Health, National Taiwan University, Taipei 100, Taiwan*

Correspondence should be addressed to Lee-Ming Chuang; leeming@ntu.edu.tw

Academic Editor: Poornima Mahavadi

The type 2 diabetes pandemic in recent decades is a huge global health threat. This pandemic is primarily attributed to the surplus of nutrients and the increased prevalence of obesity worldwide. In contrast, calorie restriction and weight reduction can drastically prevent type 2 diabetes, indicating a central role of nutrient excess in the development of diabetes. Recently, the molecular links between excessive nutrients, organelle stress, and development of metabolic disease have been extensively studied. Specifically, excessive nutrients trigger endoplasmic reticulum stress and increase the production of mitochondrial reactive oxygen species, leading to activation of stress signaling pathway, inflammatory response, lipogenesis, and pancreatic beta-cell death. Autophagy is required for clearance of hepatic lipid clearance, alleviation of pancreatic beta-cell stress, and white adipocyte differentiation. ROS scavengers, chemical chaperones, and autophagy activators have demonstrated promising effects for the treatment of insulin resistance and diabetes in preclinical models. Further results from clinical trials are eagerly awaited.

1. Introduction

Type 2 Diabetes Mellitus and Obesity: The Role of Nutrient Oversupply. Type 2 diabetes mellitus (T2DM) has become a global pandemic with huge health impact in recent decades. T2DM is a chronic progressive disorder characterized by peripheral insulin resistance in skeletal muscle, liver, and adipose tissue and the failure of pancreatic beta-cells to compensate for peripheral insulin resistance. Peripheral insulin resistance usually appears before the onset of hyperglycemia. Attenuated insulin action leads to reduced glucose uptake in skeletal muscle, reduced glucose uptake and increased lipolysis in adipose tissue, and decreased glycogen synthesis and increased glucose output of the liver, resulting in elevated plasma glucose and fatty acid levels [1]. To compensate for peripheral insulin resistance, pancreatic β-cells, which constitute only ~1% of pancreatic mass, have to dramatically increase proinsulin synthesis, imposing heavy biosynthesis burden on β-cells. Ultimately, pancreatic β-cells fail to overcome the resistance and frank hyperglycemia develops.

Obesity is the major driver of insulin resistance and T2DM. Obesity results from chronic imbalance of energy intake in excess of energy expenditure. Large prospective studies showed that lifestyle modification including diet restriction and exercise prevented the progression from prediabetes to diabetes by ~60% [2, 3]. In rhesus monkeys, long-term caloric-restricted diet drastically reduces incident diabetes or prediabetes [4]. These data clearly demonstrate excessive nutrient is critical for the development of obesity, leading to insulin resistance and T2DM.

Molecular Mechanism of Insulin Resistance. The molecular mechanism of insulin resistance is still not fully elucidated. Binding of insulin to insulin receptor triggers tyrosine autophosphorylation of the insulin receptor, which in turn phosphorylates the adaptor proteins insulin receptor substrate (IRS) proteins on tyrosine residues [5]. Tyrosine-phosphorylated IRS proteins recruit phosphoinositide-3-kinase (PI3K), a heterodimer consisting of a regulatory subunit p85 and a tightly associated catalytic subunit p110. Binding of the p85 regulatory subunit to phosphorylated IRS relieves catalytic subunit p110 and initiates a complex of signaling cascades that mediates downstream insulin action.

IRS proteins harbor several serine/threonine phosphorylation sites, which served as negative regulatory nodes that block insulin signaling triggered by tyrosine phosphorylation [6]. Several serine/threonine kinases including the cellular nutrient sensor mammalian target of rapamycin (mTOR) and ribosomal S6 kinase 1 (S6K1), the stress mediators c-Jun NH2-terminal kinases (JNK), and the proinflammatory IκB kinase β (IKKβ) and protein kinase θ (PKC-θ) block insulin signaling by serine-phosphorylation of IRS [6].

2. The Role of Endoplasmic Reticulum Stress and Unfolded Protein Response (UPR) in Diabetes and Obesity

The ER is a specialized organelle essential for synthesis and folding of secreted and ER-resident proteins, maintenance of intracellular calcium homeostasis, and lipid synthesis. The protein concentration in ER lumen is very high. Therefore, increased demand for protein synthesis or accumulation of misfolded protein in the ER luminal causes "ER stress," which triggers conserved transcriptional and translation programs, termed unfolded protein response (UPR), to cope with the ER stress [7]. The UPR are mediated by three ER membrane-bound mediators including inositol-requiring enzyme-1 (IRE-1), PKR-like endoplasmic reticulum kinase (PERK), and activating transcription factor 6 (ATF6), which are bound by the abundant ER chaperones glucose-regulated protein 78 (GRP78) in unstressed conditions. In stressful conditions when misfolded proteins accumulated, GRP78 chaperones are sequestered by misfolded proteins, releasing these UPR mediators. IRE1, an ancient ribonuclease and the oldest branch of UPR, cleaves 26-bp segment from the mRNA of x-box binding-1 (*XBP-1*) gene, creating an active/splice form of XBP-1 (XBP-1s). XBP-1s launches transcriptional programs to increase chaperone production, membrane biosynthesis, and gradation of misfolded proteins. Release of ATF6 from ER membrane unmasks its Golgi localization sequence. After processing by two proteases in Golgi, ATF6 is translocated to the nucleus to regulate the expression of genes encoding chaperones, enzymes for protein degradation, and ER membrane biogenesis. The release of PERK form membrane leads to its oligomerization and autophosphorylation. Activated PERK phosphorylates the eukaryotic initiation factor 2α (eIF2α), thereby suppressing general mRNA translation. However, specific mRNAs are preferentially translated when eIF2α is inhibited, including the transcriptional factor ATF4. Two downstream genes of ATF4 are the proapoptotic transcription factor C/EBP homologous protein (CHOP) and the growth arrest and DNA damage-inducible 34 (GADD34) which counteracts PERK's action by dephosphorylating eIF2α, thus promoting translational recovery. Collectively, the UPR relieves ER stress by decreased global protein synthesis, increased degradation of misfolded proteins, promoting chaperone synthesis, expansion of ER membrane volume, and triggering cell death [7].

2.1. Nutrient Excess, ER Stress, and Insulin Signaling. Several lines of evidence in human and mice indicate that chronic nutrient excess causes ER stress [8]. In contrast, ER stress is reduced by weight loss [9, 10]. Genetically manipulated mice models clearly demonstrate that ER stress and UPR influence insulin signaling and glucose homeostasis (Table 1, Figure 1(a)). *Xbp1* haploinsufficient mice show abnormal glucose intolerance and impaired insulin signaling in adipose tissue and liver on high-fat diet (HFD) [11]. The increased insulin resistance is mediated, at least in part, through IRE1-dependent activation of JNK. Conversely, hepatic overexpression of *Xbp1* lowers glucose in mice through interaction with FoxO1, a key transcriptional factor of gluconeogenesis [12], or uridine diphosphate (UDP) galactose-4-epimerase, an enzyme involved in galactose metabolism [13]. Mice with homozygous mutation at the eIF2α phosphorylation site (Ser51Ala) died at neonatal stage with defective gluconeogenesis [14]. Intriguingly, hepatic overexpression of *Gadd34*, which encodes an eIF2α-specific phosphatase that selectively counteracts PERK-eIF2α action, results in improved insulin sensitivity and diminished hepatic steatosis on HFD [15]. Hepatic overexpression of *Atf6* reduces gluconeogenesis [16] while silencing of hepatic *Atf6* increases gluconeogenesis [16]. The effect of ATF6 to suppress gluconeogenesis is mediated by disrupting the interaction between cAMP response element-binding protein (CREB) and transducer of regulated CREB protein 2 (TORC2), thereby decreasing the expression of gluconeogenic genes [16]. In addition, overexpression of chaperone GRP78 alleviates ER stress, restores insulin sensitivity, and resolves fatty liver in obese mice [17]. Similarly, deficiency of ER chaperone ORP150 results in impaired insulin signaling and impaired glucose tolerance, while overexpression of *Orp150* improves glucose tolerance and insulin signaling in obese mice [18]. These pieces of evidence strongly support that UPR modulates glucose homeostasis.

Mechanistically, all three canonical branches of UPR have been shown to promote inflammatory pathways. The activated IRE-1 recruits the tumor necrosis factor receptor associated factor 2 (TRAF2) and the apoptosis signal-regulating kinase 1 (ASK1) to the ER membrane, thereby activating JNK [19]. The PERK signaling has been shown to inhibit the translation of IKKβ, the main negative regulator of NF-κB, through phosphorylation of eIF2α [20]. ATF6 has also been shown to activate the NF-κB pathway [21].

Table 1: Genetically modified mice model linking organelle stress to metabolic diseases.

Model	Gene function	Tissue	Phenotypes
Xbp1	UPR	Global haploinsufficiency	Weight gain, glucose intolerance, and insulin resistance on HFD [11]
Xbp1	UPR	Liver-specific KO	Diminished hepatic cholesterol and triglyceride secretion and hepatic lipogenesis [22]
Xbp1	UPR	Liver-specific OE	Reducing serum glucose concentrations and increasing glucose tolerance [12] Fasting and postprandial hypoglycemia; increased hepatic triglyceride content [13]
Xbp1	UPR	β-cell-specific KO	Hyperglycemia and glucose intolerance resulting from decreased insulin secretion [14]
Perk	UPR	Mammary epithelium-specific KO	Reduced accumulation of lipid content and the milk produced [23]
Perk	UPR	β-cell-specific KO	Hyperglycemia associated with loss of islet and β-cell architecture [29, 30]
eIF2α	UPR	Phosphorylation site mutation	Defective gluconeogenesis and deficiency of pancreatic beta-cell [14]
Gadd34	UPR	Liver-specific OE	Lower liver glycogen levels, fasting hypoglycemia, diminished hepatics steatosis [15]
Atf6	UPR	Liver-specific OE/silencing	Increased hepatic glucose output/lowered hepatic glucose output [16]
Atf6	UPR	Global KO	Hepatic steatosis [24]
Atf6, eIF2α, Ire1	UPR	Global KO/phosphorylation site mutation	Hepatic steatosis [25]
Chop	UPR	Global KO	Delayed the onset of diabetes and beta-cell apoptosis [32]
Grp78	Chaperone	Liver-specific OE	Reduced hepatic triglyceride and cholesterol contents and improved insulin sensitivity improved [17]
Orp150	Chaperone	Liver-specific OE/Silencing	Improved insulin resistance and ameliorated glucose tolerance/increased insulin resistance [18]
Aif	Mitochondrion-localized flavoprotein	Muscle and liver-specific KO	Improved glucose tolerance, reduced fat mass, and increased insulin sensitivity [49]
Pgc-1α	Mitochondrial biogenesis	Global KO	Resistance to diet-induced obesity and insulin resistance [50, 51]
Tfam	Mitochondrial DNA transcription	Muscle-specific and adipose-specific KO	Improved glucose disposal [52, 53]
Tfam	Mitochondrial DNA transcription	β-cell-specific KO	Reduced β-cell mass and insulin secretion [61]
Cisd1	Mitochondrial iron transport	Global and liver-specific OE	Massive expansion of adipose tissue but improved insulin sensitivity [54]
Fxn	Assembly of iron-sulfur cluster in mitochondria	β-cell-specific KO	Increased islet oxidative stress, reduced islet mass, and diabetes [62]
Atg5	Autophagy	Adipose-specific KO	Impaired adipocyte differentiation [124]
Atg5	Autophagy	Global OE	Lean, enhanced glucose tolerance, insulin sensitivity, and extended lifespan [125]
Atg7	Autophagy	Global KO	Increased hepatic ER stress and impaired insulin sensitivity [69]
Atg7	Autophagy	β-cell-specific KO	Reduction of β-cells mass, reduced insulin secretion, mitochondria swelling, and lower ATP production [74, 75]
Atg7	Autophagy	Adipose-specific KO	Lean, browning of white adipose tissue, increased fatty acid oxidation, and improved insulin sensitivity [82, 83]
Atg7	Autophagy	Muscle-specific KO	Reduced weight and body fat, enhanced glucose tolerance and insulin sensitivity, enhanced lipolysis and fatty acid oxidation, and increased FGF21 level [85]

Table 1: Continued.

Model	Gene function	Tissue	Phenotypes
Atg7	Autophagy	AgRP neuron-specific KO	Lean with decreased food intake [126]
Atg7	Autophagy	POMC neuron-specific KO	Increased body weight and food intake, impaired glucose tolerance [127, 128]
Atg7	Autophagy	*Myf*5+ progenitors-specific KO	Impaired brown adipose tissue and skeletal muscle differentiation, browning of white adipose tissue, increased energy expenditure, increased body temperature, impaired glucose tolerance [129]
Atg7	Autophagy	β-cell-specific KO in hIAPP transgenics	Decreased β-cell mass and diabetes [77–79]
Atg7	Autophagy	Global haploinsufficiency in *ob/ob* mice	Reduces ER stress; improves insulin sensitivity and glucose tolerance *ob/ob* mice [84]
Atg7	Autophagy	Liver-specific OE in *ob/ob* mice	Improved insulin sensitivity and glucose tolerance [69]
Atg12	Autophagy	POMC neuron-specific KO	Weight gain, adiposity, and impaired glucose tolerance under HFD [130]

KO: knockout; OE: overexpression; UPR: unfolded protein response; HFD: high-fat diet; AgRP: agouti-related peptide; POMC: proopiomelanocortin; hIAPP: human islet amyloid polypeptide.

Both NF-κB and JNK pathways are critical mediators of inflammatory response that impairs insulin signaling by serine phosphorylation of IRS1.

2.2. ER Stress and Lipid Synthesis. In addition to glucose homeostasis, the three UPR branches also regulate lipid synthesis (Table 1, Figure 1(a)). Selective deletion of *Xbp-1s* in the liver resulted in marked diminished hepatic cholesterol and triglyceride secretion and hepatic lipogenesis by downregulating genes involved in fatty acid synthesis [22], whereas liver-specific overexpression of *Xbp-1s* increases hepatic triglycerides content [13]. Targeted deletion of *Perk* in mammary gland inhibits lipogenic enzymes expression, resulting in reduced lipid content and milk production [23]. *Atf6* knockout mice developed hepatic steatosis upon ER stress through regulation of genes involved in lipogenesis [24]. Similar phenotypes were observed in liver-specific *Ire1*-knockout mice and *eIF2α* loss-of-function mutation [25].

2.3. ER Stress and Insulin Secretion. Pancreas is exocrine and endocrine organ with heavy protein synthesis load. A transgenic green fluorescent mouse model for dynamic monitoring of ER stress detects significant ER stress signal (*Xbp1* mRNA splicing) in the pancreas 16 days after birth [26]. Several lines of evidence showed that UPR affect pancreatic islet survival and function (Table 1, Figure 1(a)). For example, mice with β-cell-specific deletion of *Xbp-1* displayed hyperglycemia and glucose intolerance resulting from decreased insulin secretion [27]. Translation attenuation through eIF2α phosphorylation prevents the oxidative stress and maintains the differentiated state of β-cells [28]. Preventing eIF2α phosphorylation in β-cells also causes hyperglycemia, indicating a significant role in PERK-eIF2α for islet survival [14]. *Perk*-deficient mice develop severe hyperglycemia due to reduced islet mass [29, 30]. In human, a loss-of-function mutation in *Perk* causes a heritable form of juvenile diabetes (the Wolcott-Rallison syndrome) (Table 2), characterized by severe defects in pancreatic β-cells [31]. Furthermore, loss of CHOP, a downstream proapoptotic transcription factor of PERK-eIF2α arm, protects islets from apoptosis in the diabetic mice [32]. Hence, the two major pathological features of type 2 diabetes including peripheral insulin resistance and defective insulin secretion are both affected by ER stress and UPR.

3. The Role of Mitochondrial Dysfunction in Diabetes and Obesity

3.1. Mitochondrial Dysfunction and Insulin Resistance. Mitochondrion is a specialized organelle where tricarboxylic acid cycle, oxidative phosphorylation, and fatty acid β-oxidation occur. Reduced mitochondrial phosphorylation and fatty acid β-oxidation are consistently observed in skeletal muscle and liver of insulin-resistant human [33–35]. Furthermore, expression of genes involved in mitochondrial oxidative phosphorylation is coordinately reduced in insulin-resistant or type 2 diabetic subjects [36, 37]. Therefore, it is long hypothesized that, in the presence of excessive nutrient flux, defective mitochondria lead to increased superoxide production and fatty acid accumulation in skeletal muscle and liver, leading to insulin resistance.

In support of these findings, HFD has been shown to increase mitochondrial reactive oxygen species (ROS) emission and shift the cellular environment to oxidized state in muscle in mice and human [38–40]. Mitochondrion-targeted overexpression of catalase reduces mitochondrial ROS emission and prevents diet-induced insulin resistance in mice [38]. ROS has been shown to activate the proinflammatory JNK and through modulation of cysteine residue or IKKβ [41–43], which in turn impairs insulin signaling via serine phosphorylation of IRS-1 (Figure 1(b)).

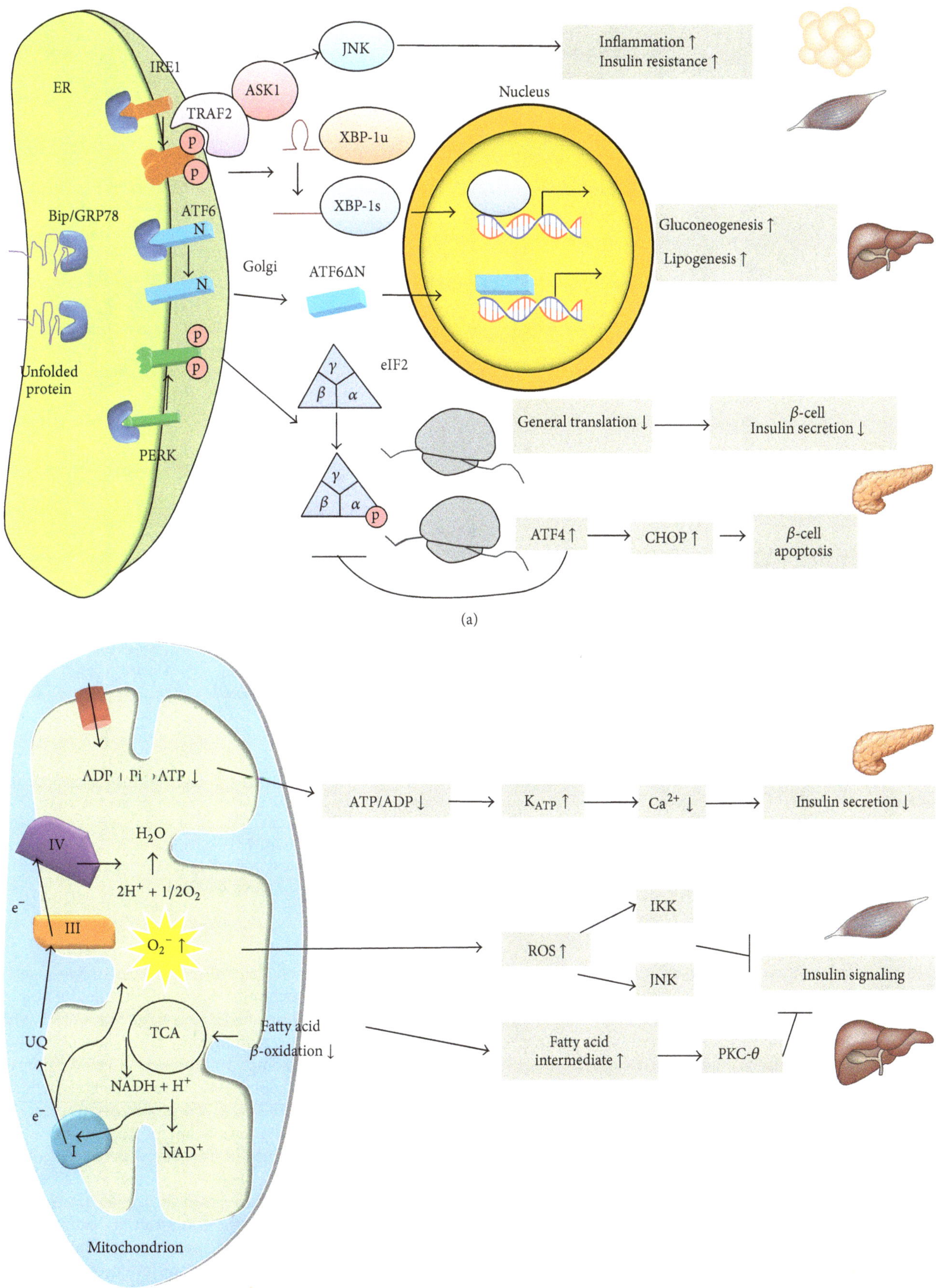

Figure 1: Continued.

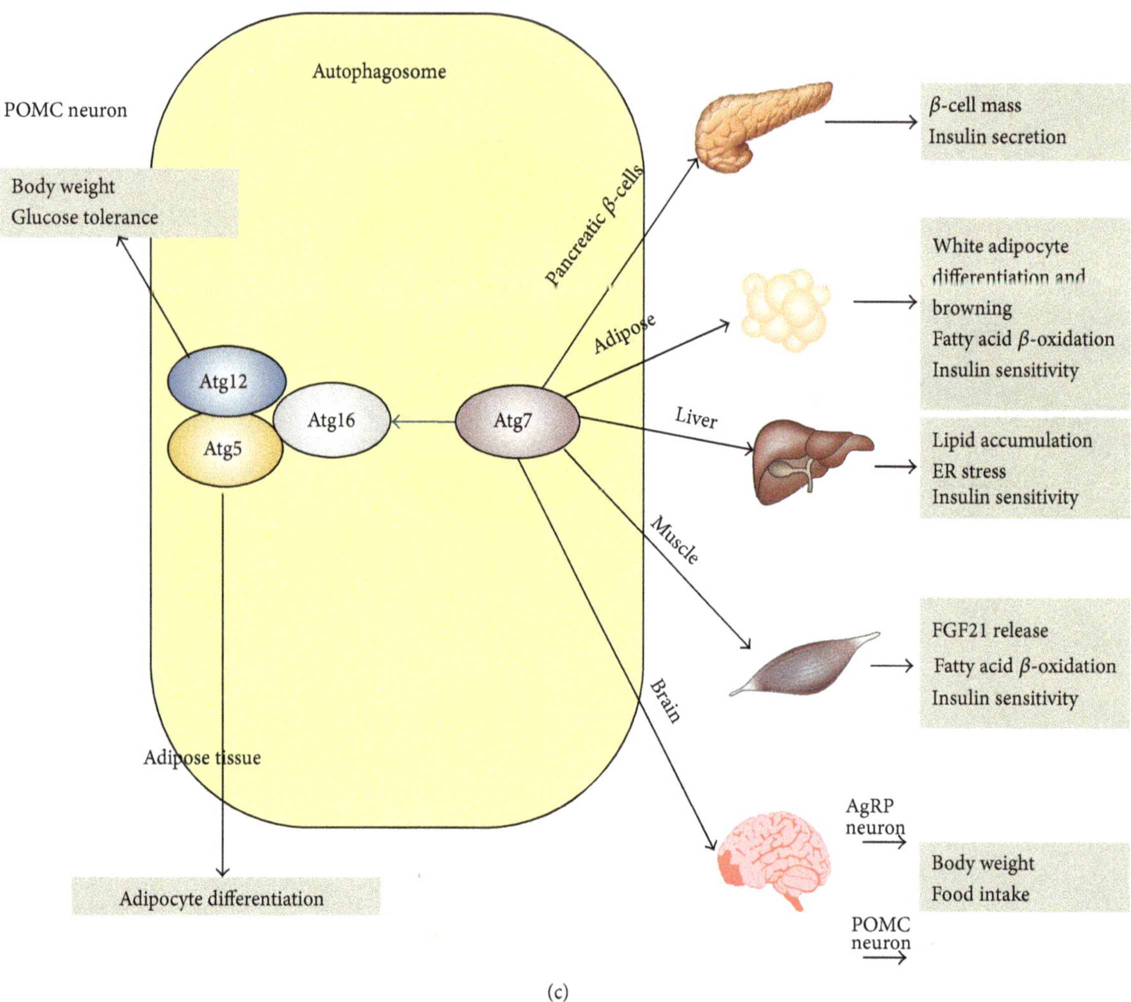

(c)

FIGURE 1: (a) Endoplasmic reticulum (ER) stress response and unfolded protein response (UPR) are linked to insulin resistance, inflammation lipogenesis, and pancreatic beta-cell survival. (b) Defective mitochondrial function leads to inflammation, insulin resistance, and reduced insulin secretion. (c) Autophagy regulates hepatic lipogenesis, adipocyte physiology, pancreatic beta-cell function, and appetite control. UPR: unfolded protein response; ROS: reactive oxygen species; NAD: nicotinamide adenine dinucleotide; NADH: reduced nicotinamide adenine dinucleotide; ADP: adenosine diphosphate; ATP: adenosine triphosphate; TCA: tricarboxylic acid cycle; K_{ATP}: ATP-dependent potassium channel; UQ: ubiquinol; FGF21: fibroblast growth factor-21; AgRP: agouti-related peptide; POMC: proopiomelanocortin.

In addition to ROS, defective mitochondrial fatty acid β-oxidation leads to accumulation of triglycerides and fatty acids intermediates (e.g., diacylglycerol or ceramide) that activate PKC-θ, a serine/threonine kinase, thus attenuating insulin signaling [44, 45] (Figure 1(b)). Knockout of acetyl-CoA carboxylase 2 (*Acc2*), an enzyme generating malonyl-CoA which is a strong inhibitor of fatty acid oxidation, resulted in increased fatty acid oxidation, reduced adiposity, and improved insulin sensitivity [46]. Fat infusion increases fatty acids intermediates accumulation in muscle and induces insulin resistance in humans [47]. In contrast, pharmacological inhibition of ceramide (a fatty acid intermediate) production prevented fat-induced insulin resistance in mice and human [48] (Figure 1(b)).

However, whether the observed reduced mitochondrial function in insulin-resistant human is causative or compensatory for the development of insulin resistance is not certain in experimental mice model. Muscle- or liver-specific deletion of *Aif*, a mitochondrial protein essential for respiratory chain function, leads to decreased mitochondrial oxidative phosphorylation but improves insulin sensitivity [49]. Knockout of peroxisome proliferator-activated receptor-gamma coactivator 1-alpha (*Pgc1α*), a master regulator of mitochondrial biogenesis, resulted in decreased mitochondrial oxidative phosphorylation but protection from diet-induced obesity and insulin resistance in mice [50, 51]. Similarly, muscle- or adipose-specific knockout of the transcription factor A, mitochondria (*Tfam*), a key transcription factor for mitochondrial DNA transcription, causes abnormal mitochondrial morphology and function but improved glucose disposal [52, 53]. Furthermore, lower rate of fatty acid beta-oxidation and compromised mitochondrial oxidative phosphorylation caused by overexpression of the CDGSH iron sulfur domain 1 protein (*Cisd1*), which encodes an outer

TABLE 2: Human hereditary syndrome linking organelle stress and diabetes mellitus.

Disease	Gene	Function	Phenotypes
Wolcott-Rallison syndrome	*PERK*	UPR	Neonatal or early-infancy diabetes, epiphyseal dysplasia, osteoporosis, and growth retardation [31]
Wolfram syndrome	*WFS1*	Negative regulator of UPR	Neurological dysfunctions and diabetes [131]
Friedreich's ataxia	*FXN*	Assembly of iron-sulfur cluster in mitochondria	Ataxia, cardiac dysfunction, and diabetes [63]
Kearns-Sayre syndrome	Large deletion of mitochondrial DNA	Respiratory chain	Ataxia, weakness, ptosis, pigmentary retinopathy, and diabetes [58]
MELAS (Mitochondrial encephalomyopathy, lactic acidosis, and stroke-like episodes)	Mitochondrial tRNA	tRNA	Seizure, ataxia, hemiparesis, cortical blindness, diabetes, and short stature [58]

mitochondrial membrane protein blocking iron transport iron into the mitochondria, resulted in massive fat accumulation but improved insulin sensitivity [54] (Table 1). These data suggest that mitochondrial dysfunction does not cause insulin resistance.

From electrochemical point of view, mitochondrial superoxide (mostly from complex I) is generated when complex I is fully reduced with electrons but downstream electron transfer components are also fully reduced and thus cannot accept any more electrons ("electron jam"). In this situation, the saturated electrons in complex I leak and react prematurely with oxygen to form superoxide, a partially reduced form of molecular oxygen. This occurs when adenosine triphosphate (ATP) synthesis is not required or when the reduced nicotinamide adenine dinucleotide (NADH)/nicotinamide adenine dinucleotide (NAD^+) ratio is high [55]. For mitochondria that are actively making ATP, the electrons are passed smoothly in the electron transfer train and hence the extent of superoxide production is low. When the ratio of $NADH/NAD^+$ is low (such as diet restriction), complex I is not reduced so that electron leak is also low [55]. It is actually not certain whether reduced mitochondrial biogenesis or reduced oxidative phosphorylation rate by genetic manipulation would actually decrease or increase ROS production. This may explain the controversies between insulin resistance and various mitochondrial dysfunction models.

Another point of view, termed "mitohormesis" holds that increased ROS production from mitochondria may act as downstream effectors that trigger nuclear compensatory response including antioxidant defense and metabolic adaptation. An example comes from the observation that antioxidant treatment blocks the extension of life induced by nutrient deprivation in worm [56]. Mild mitochondrial stress appears to be beneficial for organism to adapt for subsequent metabolic perturbations [57].

3.2. Mitochondrial Dysfunction and Insulin Secretion. Mitochondrial ATP generation plays a pivotal role in insulin secretion of pancreatic β-cell. Increased mitochondrial ATP production in response to hyperglycemia closes the ATP-sensitive potassium channel, leading to membrane depolarization, opening of voltage-sensitive calcium channel, calcium ion influx, and insulin granule exocytosis (Figure 1(b)). Several forms of syndromic mitochondrial diseases are characterized with diabetes [58] (Table 2). Mutations in the mitochondrial DNA (mtDNA), especially those in tRNA genes such as A3243G mutation, cause approximately 0.5–1% of all types of diabetes [59, 60]. Consistently, β-cell-specific disruption of *Tfam* causes severe mtDNA depletion, deficient oxidative phosphorylation, abnormal appearing mitochondria in islets, and impaired insulin secretion [61]. Similarly, targeted disruption of frataxin, a mitochondrial iron-binding protein in pancreatic β-cell, causes increased islet ROS, decreased islet mass, and diabetes in mice [62]. Furthermore, patients with mutations in the frataxin gene develop diabetes in 23% of cases [63] (Table 2).

4. The Role of Autophagy in Diabetes and Obesity

Autophagy is a cellular housekeeping process which trafficked cytoplasmic misfolded protein and damaged organelles for lytic degradation and recycle, hence maintaining a normal cellular function [64]. During autophagy, part of the cytoplasm containing sequestered materials is bounded by a double membrane to form an autophagolysosome, which further fuses with lysosome for degradation. This process involves induction, cargo recognition, and nucleation that are tightly controlled by a group of over 30 autophagy-related (ATG) proteins [65].

Autophagy is originally considered as a protein turnover process to replenish amino acid pool during starvation. This signaling process is converged to the mammalian target of rapamycin complex 1 (mTORC1) pathway and is strongly affected by the nutrient level or growth factors such as insulin. During nutrient-rich condition, mTORC1 is activated to phosphorylate Atg1/UNC51-like kinase 1 (ULK-1) complex and inactivate the autophagy process. Conversely, during starvation, the adenosine monophosphate (AMP) to

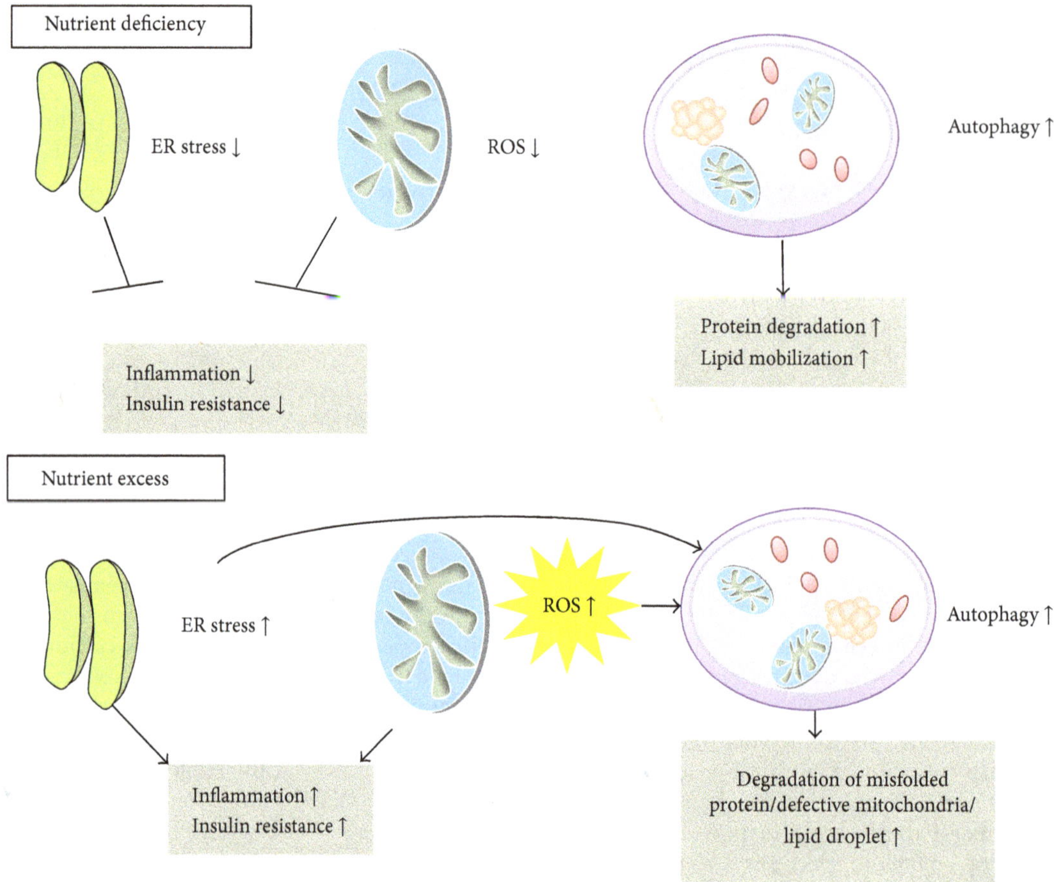

Figure 2: Interactions between endoplasmic reticulum (ER) stress, mitochondrial reactive oxygen species (ROS), and autophagy during nutrient deficiency and excess.

ATP increases. The energy depletion is sensed by AMP-activated protein kinase (AMPK) which activates autophagy by blocking mTORC1 activity and direct phosphorylation of Atgl/ULK1 [66]. A study using transgenic mouse model expressing a fluorescent marker of autophagy revealed that starvation activates autophagy in liver, heart, skeletal muscle, and kidney [67]. During starvation, autophagy provides amino acid for cellular fueling, protein synthesis, gluconeogenesis, and lipid mobilization.

In stressful condition such as increased mitochondrial ROS, ER stress, or accumulation of excessive lipid droplet, autophagy is activated to degrade defective mitochondria (mitophagy), stressed ER (ER-phagy), or accumulated lipid (lipophagy) to remove excessive ROS, ER stress, or lipid [68] (Figure 2).

4.1. Autophagy and Hepatic Lipid Metabolism. Obesity is associated with downregulation of autophagy in the liver [69]. Autophagy of lipid droplet (lipophagy) in hepatocyte facilitates the degradation of lipid in the liver and defective autophagy leads to massive accumulation of triglyceride, ER stress, and insulin resistance in the liver [69, 70]. In contrast, restoration of the *Atg7* expression in liver resulted in alleviated ER stress and improved hepatic sensitivity in obese mice [69].

4.2. Autophagy and Insulin Secretion. Pancreatic β-cells keep on synthesizing large amount of insulin to maintain normoglycemia. When the protein folding cannot keep pace with the massive synthesis rate such as during hyperglycemia, UPR occurred to halt the process [71]. ER-phagy is the specific term for autophagic control to degrade excessive misfolded protein to the lysosome for degradation and prevent insulin secretory defects [72, 73]. Disruption of *Atg7* in pancreatic β-cells causes ER stress, reduction of β-cells mass, and increase in β-cells apoptosis [74, 75]. IAPP is another peptide hormone released from β-cells, which normally are cosecreted with insulin [76]. Intracellular oligomer accumulation of human islet amyloid polypeptide (hIAPP) is toxic to β-cells, which is a typical morphological change in T2DM. Abnormal hIAPP aggregates are primary degraded by autophagy. Transgenic mice expressing hIAPP with β-cell-specific *Atg7* deletion accumulate hIAPP oligomers and develop diabetes with increased oxidative damage and decreased β-cell mass [77–79] (Table 1, Figure 1(c)). Density volume of autophagic vacuoles and autophagosomes was significantly higher in β-cells of diabetic human [80].

Mitophagy also acts to prevent the accumulation of depolarized mitochondria and maintain optimal β-cells mitochondrial function [81]. β-cells-specific *Atg7* knockout mice showed swollen mitochondria and reduced insulin secretion (Table 1, Figure 1(c)) [75].

TABLE 3: Treatment targeting organelle stress for diabetes mellitus and obesity.

Agent	Specific mechanism	Highest level of studies	Result
Tauroursodeoxycholic acid	Chemical chaperone	Randomized controlled trials	Improved insulin sensitivity in muscle and liver in obese individuals [86]
Phenylbutyrate	Chemical chaperone	Randomized controlled trials	Improved insulin sensitivity and beta-cell function in lipid-infused individuals [87]
Azoramide	ATF6 activators	Rodents	Improves insulin sensitivity and beta-cell function in obese mice [89]
Valproate	Increasing GRPP78	Rodents	Ameliorates atherosclerosis and hepatic steatosis in *Apoe*$^{-/-}$mice [90]
L-Carnitine or carnitine-orotate	Fatty acid transfer for beta-oxidation	Randomized controlled trials	Twelve of 17 studies showing improved insulin sensitivity or glycemic control in type 2 diabetic patients or alleviation of hepatic steatosis [98, 99]
Co-enzyme Q_{10}	Electron carrier from complex I and II to complex III	Randomized controlled trials	No net effect on glycemic control in type 2 diabetic patients [100]
α-lipoic acid	Antioxidant	Randomized controlled trials; rodent	Weight-reducing, glucose-lowering, and insulin-sensitizing effect; prevention of hepatic steatosis [101–110]
Vitamin E	Antioxidant	Randomized controlled trials	Inconsistent results on glycemic control [111–115]; reduced hepatic steatosis [122]
N-acetylcysteine	Antioxidant	Rodents	Prevents diet-induced obesity [116–118]
Peptide SS31	Mitochondria-targeted antioxidant peptide	Rodent	Improved glucose tolerance in diet-induced obese mice [38]
Resveratrol	SIRT1 agonist	Randomized controlled trials	Improved insulin sensitivity and glycemic control in diabetic patients; no effect in nondiabetic patients [120];
GSK5182	Estrogen-related receptor gamma inverse agonist	Rodents	Reduces hyperglycemia due to inhibition of hepatic gluconeogenesis [121]
Trehalose, imanitib	Enhance autophagy	Rodents	Improved glucose tolerance and insulin sensitivity in obese mice [84]
Dh404	Nrf2 activator	Rodents	Increased viability of islet by enhancing autophagy [123]

4.3. Autophagy, Adipose Tissue, and Skeletal Muscle. In contrast to the role of autophagy in hepatic lipid clearance and alleviating stress of pancreatic β-cells, the function of autophagy in adipose tissue and skeletal muscle deserves separate mention. Mice targeted with *Atg7* disruption in adipose tissue have reduced body fat, increased fatty acid β-oxidation, and improved insulin sensitivity [82, 83], indicating that autophagy is required for the production of large lipid droplets characteristic of white adipose tissue. However, *Atg7*$^{+/-}$-*ob/ob* mice showed exacerbated insulin resistance with elevated lipid levels [84] (Table 1, Figure 1(c)). Muscle-specific *Atg7* knockout mice exhibit lean phenotype with increased lipolysis and β-oxidation rate in adipose tissue, enhanced glucose tolerance, and improved insulin sensitivity [85]. This is due to the impairment of autophagy to degrade defective mitochondria, which leads to the fibroblast growth factor (FGF21) release, causing lipolysis and β-oxidation rate in adipose tissue [85]. These diverse results of the same gene exerting different function in different organs may be a result of noncell autonomous function.

4.4. Autophagy and Appetite Control. Furthermore, food intake in mice with agouti-related peptide (AgRP) neuron-specific *Atg7* deletion was decreased while it increased in proopiomelanocortin (POMC) neuron-specific *Atg7* deletion. The changes of the functional consequences converge on the controlling of a common neuropeptide, α-melanocyte-stimulating hormone (α-MSH), level (Table 1, Figure 1(c)).

5. Targeting Organelle Stress for Treating Metabolic Diseases

Chemical chaperones including tauroursodeoxycholate (TUDCA) and 4-phenylbutyrate (PBA) have been shown to reduce ER stress and improve insulin sensitivity in rodents and human [86, 87] (Table 3). These two drugs have been approved by the US Food and Drug Administration for the treatment of primary biliary cirrhosis. Numerous small molecules are identified to increase chaperone expression or to modulate specific arm of UPR *in vitro* using various screening strategies. For example, GSK2606414 has been shown to inhibit PERK kinase activity [88], azoramide to activate ATF6 [89], valproate to increase GRP78 expression [90], salubrinal and guanabenz to inhibit eIF2α dephosphorylation [91, 92], and 3-ethoxy-5,6-dibromosalicylaldehyde [93], STF-083010 [94], MKC-3946 [95], 4μ8C [96], and KIRA6 to inhibit IRE1 RNase activity [97]. Among them, valproate has been shown to attenuate atherosclerosis and alleviate hepatic steatosis [90] and azoramide has been shown to improve insulin sensitivity and pancreatic β-cell function in rodent models [89].

Pharmacological approaches to alleviate mitochondrial stress include carnitine [98, 99], Coenzyme Q_{10} [100], ROS scavengers (peptide SS31 [38], α-lipoic acid [101–110], vitamin E, beta-carotene, vitamin C [111–114], *N*-acetylcysteine [115–118], and mitoQ [119]), stimulators of mitochondrial biogenesis (resveratrol and other sirtuin activators [120], and estrogen-related receptor modulators [121]). Specifically, carnitine or carnitine-orotate complex, which promotes fatty acid β-oxidation, improves insulin sensitivity or attenuates hepatic steatosis in most randomized clinical trials [98, 99]. Coenzyme Q1, however, showed no net effect on glycemic control in most type 2 diabetic patients [100]. Most evidence demonstrated that α-lipoic acid is a potent weight-reducing and insulin sensitizing agent in human clinical trials and rodent models [101–110]. Multiple small clinical trials investigating the effect of antioxidant vitamin E, vitamin C, and beta-carotene on glycemic control in diabetic patients yielded inconsistent results [111–115]. However, in a randomized clinical trial of 247 adults with nonalcoholic steatohepatitis, vitamin E use, as compared with placebo, was associated with a significantly higher rate of improvement in nonalcoholic steatohepatitis [122]. N-acetylcysteine, an approved drug for acetaminophen intoxication and mucolysis, has been demonstrated to prevent diet-induced obesity in rodent models [116–118]. Significant controversies remained regarding the metabolic action of resveratrol in human; a meta-analysis of 11 randomized controlled trials revealed that resveratrol significantly reduces glucose, insulin, and insulin resistance in diabetic patients but not in nondiabetics [120] (Table 3). Further results from clinical trials and more potent SIRT1-activating compounds (STAC) such as SRT1720 and SRT2104 are awaited.

Various therapeutic agents may be used to enhance autophagy. Trehalose is an autophagy enhancer which improves the glucose intolerance of hIAPP transgenic mice fed a HFD and further reduced hIAPP oligomer accumulation and improved β-cells function [77]. Both Imatinib and trehalose were reported to improve metabolic parameters of *Atg7*$^{-/-}$-*ob/ob* mice by enhanced autophagic flux [84]. Dihydro-CDDO-trifluoroethyl amide (dh404) is an Nrf2 activator which can reduce oxidative stress in isolated rat islet by enhancing autophagy [123] (Table 3).

6. Future Perspectives

The interaction between ER stress, mitochondrial oxidative stress, and autophagy is complex. Most small molecules used to date do not have the required specificity. Furthermore, the multiple intrinsic feedback pathways, the cross-organ communication, and the interplay between autophagy and carcinogenesis make it difficult to target a single pathway to treat metabolic diseases without triggering unwanted side effects. Currently, the most efficient and safe way to reduce organelle stress and to treat metabolic disease is probably prevention of overnutrition.

Conflict of Interests

The authors declare that there is no conflict of interests regarding the publication of this paper.

Authors' Contribution

Yi-Cheng Chang and Siow-Wey Hee contributed equally to this work.

References

[1] A. R. Saltiel, "Series introduction: the molecular and physiological basis of insulin resistance: emerging implications for metabolic and cardiovascular diseases," *The Journal of Clinical Investigation*, vol. 106, no. 2, pp. 163–164, 2000.

[2] W. C. Knowler, E. Barrett-Connor, S. E. Fowler et al., "Reduction in the incidence of type 2 diabetes with lifestyle intervention or metformin," *The New England Journal of Medicine*, vol. 346, no. 6, pp. 393–403, 2002.

[3] J. Tuomilehto, J. Lindström, J. G. Eriksson et al., "Prevention of type 2 diabetes mellitus by changes in lifestyle among subjects with impaired glucose tolerance," *The New England Journal of Medicine*, vol. 344, no. 18, pp. 1343–1350, 2001.

[4] R. J. Colman, R. M. Anderson, S. C. Johnson et al., "Caloric restriction delays disease onset and mortality in rhesus monkeys," *Science*, vol. 325, no. 5937, pp. 201–204, 2009.

[5] A. R. Saltiel and C. R. Kahn, "Insulin signalling and the regulation of glucose and lipid metabolism," *Nature*, vol. 414, no. 6865, pp. 799–806, 2001.

[6] K. D. Copps and M. F. White, "Regulation of insulin sensitivity by serine/threonine phosphorylation of insulin receptor substrate proteins IRS1 and IRS2," *Diabetologia*, vol. 55, no. 10, pp. 2565–2582, 2012.

[7] D. Ron and P. Walter, "Signal integration in the endoplasmic reticulum unfolded protein response," *Nature Reviews Molecular Cell Biology*, vol. 8, no. 7, pp. 519–529, 2007.

[8] N. K. Sharma, S. K. Das, A. K. Mondal et al., "Endoplasmic reticulum stress markers are associated with obesity in nondiabetic subjects," *Journal of Clinical Endocrinology and Metabolism*, vol. 93, no. 11, pp. 4532–4541, 2008.

[9] M. F. Gregor, L. Yang, E. Fabbrini et al., "Endoplasmic reticulum stress is reduced in tissues of obese subjects after weight loss," *Diabetes*, vol. 58, no. 3, pp. 693–700, 2009.

[10] A. Tsutsumi, H. Motoshima, T. Kondo et al., "Caloric restriction decreases ER stress in liver and adipose tissue in ob/ob mice," *Biochemical and Biophysical Research Communications*, vol. 404, no. 1, pp. 339–344, 2011.

[11] U. Özcan, Q. Cao, E. Yilmaz et al., "Endoplasmic reticulum stress links obesity, insulin action, and type 2 diabetes," *Science*, vol. 306, no. 5695, pp. 457–461, 2004.

[12] Y. Zhou, J. Lee, C. M. Reno et al., "Regulation of glucose homeostasis through a XBP-1-FoxO1 interaction," *Nature Medicine*, vol. 17, no. 3, pp. 356–365, 2011.

[13] Y. Deng, Z. V. Wang, C. Tao et al., "The Xbp1s/GalE axis links ER stress to postprandial hepatic metabolism," *The Journal of Clinical Investigation*, vol. 123, no. 1, pp. 455–468, 2013.

[14] D. Scheuner, B. Song, E. McEwen et al., "Translational control is required for the unfolded protein response and in vivo glucose homeostasis," *Molecular Cell*, vol. 7, no. 6, pp. 1165–1176, 2001.

[15] S. Oyadomari, H. P. Harding, Y. Zhang, M. Oyadomari, and D. Ron, "Dephosphorylation of translation initiation factor 2α enhances glucose tolerance and attenuates hepatosteatosis in mice," *Cell Metabolism*, vol. 7, no. 6, pp. 520–532, 2008.

[16] Y. Wang, L. Vera, W. H. Fischer, and M. Montminy, "The CREB coactivator CRTC2 links hepatic ER stress and fasting gluconeogenesis," *Nature*, vol. 460, no. 7254, pp. 534–537, 2009.

[17] H. L. Kammoun, H. Chabanon, I. Hainault et al., "GRP78 expression inhibits insulin and ER stress-induced SREBP-1c activation and reduces hepatic steatosis in mice," *The Journal of Clinical Investigation*, vol. 119, no. 5, pp. 1201–1215, 2009.

[18] Y. Nakatani, H. Kaneto, D. Kawamori et al., "Involvement of endoplasmic reticulum stress in insulin resistance and diabetes," *The Journal of Biological Chemistry*, vol. 280, no. 1, pp. 847–851, 2005.

[19] M. Kaneko, Y. Niinuma, and Y. Nomura, "Activation signal of nuclear factor-κB in response to endoplasmic reticulum stress is transduced via IRE1 and tumor necrosis factor receptor-associated factor 2," *Biological and Pharmaceutical Bulletin*, vol. 26, no. 7, pp. 931–935, 2003.

[20] J. Deng, P. D. Lu, Y. Zhang et al., "Translational repression mediates activation of nuclear factor kappa B by phosphorylated translation initiation factor 2," *Molecular and Cellular Biology*, vol. 24, no. 23, pp. 10161–10168, 2004.

[21] H. Yamazaki, N. Hiramatsu, K. Hayakawa et al., "Activation of the Akt-NF-κB pathway by subtilase cytotoxin through the ATF6 branch of the unfolded protein response," *The Journal of Immunology*, vol. 183, no. 2, pp. 1480–1487, 2009.

[22] A.-H. Lee, E. F. Scapa, D. E. Cohen, and L. H. Glimcher, "Regulation of hepatic lipogenesis by the transcription factor XBP1," *Science*, vol. 320, no. 5882, pp. 1492–1496, 2008.

[23] E. Bobrovnikova-Marjon, G. Hatzivassiliou, C. Grigoriadou et al., "PERK-dependent regulation of lipogenesis during mouse mammary gland development and adipocyte differentiation," *Proceedings of the National Academy of Sciences of the United States of America*, vol. 105, no. 42, pp. 16314–16319, 2008.

[24] K. Yamamoto, K. Takahara, S. Oyadomari et al., "Induction of liver steatosis and lipid droplet formation in ATF6α-knockout mice burdened with pharmacological endoplasmic reticulum stress," *Molecular Biology of the Cell*, vol. 21, no. 17, pp. 2975–2986, 2010.

[25] D. T. Rutkowski, J. Wu, S.-H. Back et al., "UPR pathways combine to prevent hepatic steatosis caused by ER stress-mediated suppression of transcriptional master regulators," *Developmental Cell*, vol. 15, no. 6, pp. 829–840, 2008.

[26] T. Iwawaki, R. Akai, K. Kohno, and M. Miura, "A transgenic mouse model for monitoring endoplasmic reticulum stress," *Nature Medicine*, vol. 10, no. 1, pp. 98–102, 2004.

[27] A.-H. Lee, K. Heidtman, G. S. Hotamisligil, and L. H. Glimcher, "Dual and opposing roles of the unfolded protein response regulated by IRE1α and XBP1 in proinsulin processing and insulin secretion," *Proceedings of the National Academy of Sciences of the United States of America*, vol. 108, no. 21, pp. 8885–8890, 2011.

[28] S. H. Back, D. Scheuner, J. Han et al., "Translation attenuation through eIF2α phosphorylation prevents oxidative stress and maintains the differentiated state in β cells," *Cell Metabolism*, vol. 10, no. 1, pp. 13–26, 2009.

[29] Y. Gao, D. J. Sartori, C. Li et al., "PERK is required in the adult pancreas and is essential for maintenance of glucose homeostasis," *Molecular and Cellular Biology*, vol. 32, no. 24, pp. 5129–5139, 2012.

[30] W. Zhang, D. Feng, Y. Li, K. Iida, B. McGrath, and D. R. Cavener, "PERK EIF2AK3 control of pancreatic beta cell differentiation and proliferation is required for postnatal glucose homeostasis," *Cell Metabolism*, vol. 4, no. 6, pp. 491–497, 2006.

[31] M. Delépine, M. Nicolino, T. Barrett, M. Golamaully, G. M. Lathrop, and C. Julier, "EIF2AK3, encoding translation initiation factor 2-α kinase 3, is mutated in patients with Wolcott-Rallison syndrome," *Nature Genetics*, vol. 25, no. 4, pp. 406–409, 2000.

[32] S. Oyadomari, A. Koizumi, K. Takeda et al., "Targeted disruption of the *Chop* gene delays endoplasmic reticulum stress-mediated diabetes," *Journal of Clinical Investigation*, vol. 109, no. 4, pp. 525–532, 2002.

[33] K. F. Petersen, S. Dufour, D. Befroy, R. Garcia, and G. I. Shulman, "Impaired mitochondrial activity in the insulin-resistant offspring of patients with type 2 diabetes," *TheNew England Journal of Medicine*, vol. 350, no. 7, pp. 664–671, 2004.

[34] K. F. Petersen, D. Befroy, S. Dufour et al., "Mitochondrial dysfunction in the elderly: possible role in insulin resistance," *Science*, vol. 300, no. 5622, pp. 1140–1142, 2003.

[35] D. E. Befroy, K. F. Petersen, S. Dufour et al., "Impaired mitochondrial substrate oxidation in muscle of insulin-resistant offspring of type 2 diabetic patients," *Diabetes*, vol. 56, no. 5, pp. 1376–1381, 2007.

[36] V. K. Mootha, C. M. Lindgren, K.-F. Eriksson et al., "PGC-1α-responsive genes involved in oxidative phosphorylation are coordinately downregulated in human diabetes," *Nature Genetics*, vol. 34, no. 3, pp. 267–273, 2003.

[37] M. E. Patti, A. J. Butte, S. Crunkhorn et al., "Coordinated reduction of genes of oxidative metabolism in humans with insulin resistance and diabetes: potential role of PGC1 and NRF1," *Proceedings of the National Academy of Sciences of the United States of America*, vol. 100, no. 14, pp. 8466–8471, 2003.

[38] E. J. Anderson, M. E. Lustig, K. E. Boyle et al., "Mitochondrial H_2O_2 emission and cellular redox state link excess fat intake to insulin resistance in both rodents and humans," *The Journal of Clinical Investigation*, vol. 119, no. 3, pp. 573–581, 2009.

[39] C. Bonnard, A. Durand, S. Peyrol et al., "Mitochondrial dysfunction results from oxidative stress in the skeletal muscle of diet-induced insulin-resistant mice," *Journal of Clinical Investigation*, vol. 118, no. 2, pp. 789–800, 2008.

[40] S. Furukawa, T. Fujita, M. Shimabukuro et al., "Increased oxidative stress in obesity and its impact on metabolic syndrome," *The Journal of Clinical Investigation*, vol. 114, no. 12, pp. 1752–1761, 2004.

[41] H. Ichijo, E. Nishida, K. Irie et al., "Induction of apoptosis by ASK1, a mammalian MAPKKK that activates SAPK/JNK and

p38 signaling pathways," *Science*, vol. 275, no. 5296, pp. 90–94, 1997.

[42] K. Imoto, D. Kukidome, T. Nishikawa et al., "Impact of mitochondrial reactive oxygen species and apoptosis signal-regulating kinase 1 on insulin signaling," *Diabetes*, vol. 55, no. 5, pp. 1197–1204, 2006.

[43] K. Asehnoune, D. Strassheim, S. Mitra, J. Y. Kim, and E. Abraham, "Involvement of reactive oxygen species in Toll-like receptor 4-dependent activation of NF-κB," *The Journal of Immunology*, vol. 172, no. 4, pp. 2522–2529, 2004.

[44] M. E. Griffin, M. J. Marcucci, G. W. Cline et al., "Free fatty acid-induced insulin resistance is associated with activation of protein kinase C theta and alterations in the insulin signaling cascade," *Diabetes*, vol. 48, no. 6, pp. 1270–1274, 1999.

[45] J. K. Kim, J. J. Fillmore, M. J. Sunshine et al., "PKC-θ knockout mice are protected from fat-induced insulin resistance," *Journal of Clinical Investigation*, vol. 114, no. 6, pp. 823–827, 2004.

[46] S. C. Cheol, D. B. Savage, L. Abu-Elheiga et al., "Continuous fat oxidation in acetyl-CoA carboxylase 2 knockout mice increases total energy expenditure, reduces fat mass, and improves insulin sensitivity," *Proceedings of the National Academy of Sciences of the United States of America*, vol. 104, no. 42, pp. 16480–16485, 2007.

[47] S. I. Itani, N. B. Ruderman, F. Schmieder, and G. Boden, "Lipid-induced insulin resistance in human muscle is associated with changes in diacylglycerol, protein kinase C, and IkappaB-alpha," *Diabetes*, vol. 51, no. 7, pp. 2005–2011, 2002.

[48] W. L. Holland, J. T. Brozinick, L.-P. Wang et al., "Inhibition of ceramide synthesis ameliorates glucocorticoid-, saturated-fat-, and obesity-induced insulin resistance," *Cell Metabolism*, vol. 5, no. 3, pp. 167–179, 2007.

[49] J. A. Pospisilik, C. Knauf, N. Joza et al., "Targeted deletion of AIF decreases mitochondrial oxidative phosphorylation and protects from obesity and diabetes," *Cell*, vol. 131, no. 3, pp. 476–491, 2007.

[50] J. Lin, P.-H. Wu, P. T. Tarr et al., "Defects in adaptive energy metabolism with CNS-linked hyperactivity in PGC-1α null mice," *Cell*, vol. 119, no. 1, pp. 121–135, 2004.

[51] T. C. Leone, J. J. Lehman, B. N. Finck et al., "PGC-1alpha deficiency causes multi-system energy metabolic derangements: muscle dysfunction, abnormal weight control and hepatic steatosis," *PLoS Biology*, vol. 3, no. 4, article e101, 2005.

[52] A. Wredenberg, C. Freyer, M. E. Sandström et al., "Respiratory chain dysfunction in skeletal muscle does not cause insulin resistance," *Biochemical and Biophysical Research Communications*, vol. 350, no. 1, pp. 202–207, 2006.

[53] C. Vernochet, A. Mourier, O. Bezy et al., "Adipose-specific deletion of TFAM increases mitochondrial oxidation and protects mice against obesity and insulin resistance," *Cell Metabolism*, vol. 16, no. 6, pp. 765–776, 2012.

[54] C. M. Kusminski, W. L. Holland, K. Sun et al., "MitoNEET-driven alterations in adipocyte mitochondrial activity reveal a crucial adaptive process that preserves insulin sensitivity in obesity," *Nature Medicine*, vol. 18, no. 10, pp. 1539–1551, 2012.

[55] M. P. Murphy, "How mitochondria produce reactive oxygen species," *Biochemical Journal*, vol. 417, no. 1, pp. 1–13, 2009.

[56] T. J. Schulz, K. Zarse, A. Voigt, N. Urban, M. Birringer, and M. Ristow, "Glucose restriction extends *Caenorhabditis elegans* life span by inducing mitochondrial respiration and increasing oxidative stress," *Cell Metabolism*, vol. 6, no. 4, pp. 280–293, 2007.

[57] J. Yun and T. Finkel, "Mitohormesis," *Cell Metabolism*, vol. 19, no. 5, pp. 757–766, 2014.

[58] P. Maechler and C. B. Wollheim, "Mitochondrial function in normal and diabetic β-cells," *Nature*, vol. 414, no. 6865, pp. 807–812, 2001.

[59] S. DiMauro and E. A. Schon, "Mitochondrial respiratory-chain diseases," *The New England Journal of Medicine*, vol. 348, no. 26, pp. 2656–2668, 2003.

[60] T. Kadowaki, H. Kadowaki, Y. Mori et al., "A subtype of diabetes mellitus associated with a mutation of mitochondrial DNA," *The New England Journal of Medicine*, vol. 330, no. 14, pp. 962–968, 1994.

[61] J. P. Silva, M. Köhler, C. Graff et al., "Impaired insulin secretion and beta-cell loss in tissue-specific knockout mice with mitochondrial diabetes," *Nature Genetics*, vol. 26, no. 3, pp. 336–340, 2000.

[62] M. Ristow, H. Mulder, D. Pomplun et al., "Frataxin deficiency in pancreatic islets causes diabetes due to loss of β cell mass," *Journal of Clinical Investigation*, vol. 112, no. 4, pp. 527–534, 2003.

[63] R. L. Hewer, "Study of fatal cases of Friedreich's ataxia," *British Medical Journal*, vol. 3, no. 619, pp. 649–652, 1968.

[64] N. Mizushima and M. Komatsu, "Autophagy: renovation of cells and tissues," *Cell*, vol. 147, no. 4, pp. 728–741, 2011.

[65] Y. Feng, D. He, Z. Yao, and D. J. Klionsky, "The machinery of macroautophagy," *Cell Research*, vol. 24, no. 1, pp. 24–41, 2014.

[66] J. Kim, M. Kundu, B. Viollet, and K.-L. Guan, "AMPK and mTOR regulate autophagy through direct phosphorylation of Ulk1," *Nature Cell Biology*, vol. 13, no. 2, pp. 132–141, 2011.

[67] N. Mizushima, A. Yamamoto, M. Matsui, T. Yoshimori, and Y. Ohsumi, "In vivo analysis of autophagy in response to nutrient starvation using transgenic mice expressing a fluorescent autophagosome marker," *Molecular Biology of the Cell*, vol. 15, no. 3, pp. 1101–1111, 2004.

[68] C. He and D. J. Klionsky, "Regulation mechanisms and signaling pathways of autophagy," *Annual Review of Genetics*, vol. 43, pp. 67–93, 2009.

[69] L. Yang, P. Li, S. Fu, E. S. Calay, and G. S. Hotamisligil, "Defective hepatic autophagy in obesity promotes ER stress and causes insulin resistance," *Cell Metabolism*, vol. 11, no. 6, pp. 467–478, 2010.

[70] R. Singh, S. Kaushik, Y. Wang et al., "Autophagy regulates lipid metabolism," *Nature*, vol. 458, no. 7242, pp. 1131–1135, 2009.

[71] J. Lee and U. Ozcan, "Unfolded protein response signaling and metabolic diseases," *The Journal of Biological Chemistry*, vol. 289, no. 3, pp. 1203–1211, 2014.

[72] S. Bernales, K. L. McDonald, and P. Walter, "Autophagy counterbalances endoplasmic reticulum expansion during the unfolded protein response," *PLoS Biology*, vol. 4, no. 12, article e423, 2006.

[73] T. Yorimitsu, U. Nair, Z. Yang, and D. J. Klionsky, "Endoplasmic reticulum stress triggers autophagy," *Journal of Biological Chemistry*, vol. 281, no. 40, pp. 30299–30304, 2006.

[74] C. Ebato, T. Uchida, M. Arakawa et al., "Autophagy is important in islet homeostasis and compensatory increase of beta cell mass in response to high-fat diet," *Cell Metabolism*, vol. 8, no. 4, pp. 325–332, 2008.

[75] H. S. Jung, K. W. Chung, J. W. Kim et al., "Loss of autophagy diminishes pancreatic β cell mass and function with resultant hyperglycemia," *Cell Metabolism*, vol. 8, no. 4, pp. 318–324, 2008.

[76] P. Westermark, C. Wernstedt, E. Wilander, and K. Sletten, "A novel peptide in the calcitonin gene related peptide family as an amyloid fibril protein in the endocrine pancreas," *Biochemical and Biophysical Research Communications*, vol. 140, no. 3, pp. 827–831, 1986.

[77] J. Kim, H. Cheon, Y. T. Jeong et al., "Amyloidogenic peptide oligomer accumulation in autophagy-deficient β cells induces diabetes," *Journal of Clinical Investigation*, vol. 124, no. 8, pp. 3311–3324, 2014.

[78] J. F. Rivera, S. Costes, T. Gurlo, C. G. Glabe, and P. C. Butler, "Autophagy defends pancreatic β cells from human islet amyloid polypeptide-induced toxicity," *Journal of Clinical Investigation*, vol. 124, no. 8, pp. 3489–3500, 2014.

[79] N. Shigihara, A. Fukunaka, A. Hara et al., "Human IAPP-induced pancreatic β cell toxicity and its regulation by autophagy," *Journal of Clinical Investigation*, vol. 124, no. 8, pp. 3634–3644, 2014.

[80] M. Masini, M. Bugliani, R. Lupi et al., "Autophagy in human type 2 diabetes pancreatic beta cells," *Diabetologia*, vol. 52, no. 6, pp. 1083–1086, 2009.

[81] G. Ashrafi and T. L. Schwarz, "The pathways of mitophagy for quality control and clearance of mitochondria," *Cell Death & Differentiation*, vol. 20, no. 1, pp. 31–42, 2013.

[82] Y. Zhang, S. Goldman, R. Baerga, Y. Zhao, M. Komatsu, and S. Jin, "Adipose-specific deletion of autophagy-related gene 7 (atg7) in mice reveals a role in adipogenesis," *Proceedings of the National Academy of Sciences of the United States of America*, vol. 106, no. 47, pp. 19860–19865, 2009.

[83] R. Singh, Y. Xiang, Y. Wang et al., "Autophagy regulates adipose mass and differentiation in mice," *Journal of Clinical Investigation*, vol. 119, no. 11, pp. 3329–3339, 2009.

[84] Y. M. Lim, H. Lim, K. Y. Hur et al., "Systemic autophagy insufficiency compromises adaptation to metabolic stress and facilitates progression from obesity to diabetes," *Nature Communications*, vol. 5, article 4934, 2014.

[85] K. H. Kim, Y. T. Jeong, H. Oh et al., "Autophagy deficiency leads to protection from obesity and insulin resistance by inducing Fgf21 as a mitokine," *Nature Medicine*, vol. 19, no. 1, pp. 83–92, 2013.

[86] M. Kars, L. Yang, M. F. Gregor et al., "Tauroursodeoxycholic Acid may improve liver and muscle but not adipose tissue insulin sensitivity in obese men and women," *Diabetes*, vol. 59, no. 8, pp. 1899–1905, 2010.

[87] C. Xiao, A. Giacca, and G. F. Lewis, "Sodium phenylbutyrate, a drug with known capacity to reduce endoplasmic reticulum stress, partially alleviates lipid-induced insulin resistance and β-cell dysfunction in humans," *Diabetes*, vol. 60, no. 3, pp. 918–924, 2011.

[88] J. M. Axten, J. R. Medina, Y. Feng et al., "Discovery of 7-methyl-5-(1-[3-(trifluoromethyl)phenyl]acetyl-2,3-dihydro-1*H*-indol-5-yl)-7*H*-pyrrolo[2,3-*d*]pyrimidin-4-amine (GSK2606414), a potent and selective first-in-class inhibitor of protein kinase R (PKR)-like endoplasmic reticulum kinase (PERK)," *Journal of Medicinal Chemistry*, vol. 55, no. 16, pp. 7193–7207, 2012.

[89] S. Fu, A. Yalcin, G. Y. Lee et al., "Phenotypic assays identify azoramide as a small-molecule modulator of the unfolded protein response with antidiabetic activity," *Science Translational Medicine*, vol. 7, no. 292, Article ID 292ra98, 2015.

[90] C. S. McAlpine, A. J. Bowes, M. I. Khan, Y. Shi, and G. H. Werstuck, "Endoplasmic reticulum stress and glycogen synthase kinase-3β activation in apolipoprotein E-deficient mouse models of accelerated atherosclerosis," *Arteriosclerosis, Thrombosis, and Vascular Biology*, vol. 32, no. 1, pp. 82–91, 2012.

[91] M. Boyce, K. F. Bryant, C. Jousse et al., "A selective inhibitor of elF2α dephosphorylation protects cells from ER stress," *Science*, vol. 307, no. 5711, pp. 935–939, 2005.

[92] P. Tsaytler, H. P. Harding, D. Ron, and A. Bertolotti, "Selective inhibition of a regulatory subunit of protein phosphatase 1 restores proteostasis," *Science*, vol. 332, no. 6025, pp. 91–94, 2011.

[93] K. Volkmann, J. L. Lucas, D. Vuga et al., "Potent and selective inhibitors of the inositol-requiring enzyme 1 endoribonuclease," *The Journal of Biological Chemistry*, vol. 286, no. 14, pp. 12743–12755, 2011.

[94] I. Papandreou, N. C. Denko, M. Olson et al., "Identification of an Ire1alpha endonuclease specific inhibitor with cytotoxic activity against human multiple myeloma," *Blood*, vol. 117, no. 4, pp. 1311–1314, 2011.

[95] N. Mimura, M. Fulciniti, G. Gorgun et al., "Blockade of XBP1 splicing by inhibition of IRE1α is a promising therapeutic option in multiple myeloma," *Blood*, vol. 119, no. 24, pp. 5772–5781, 2012.

[96] B. C. S. Cross, P. J. Bond, P. G. Sadowski et al., "The molecular basis for selective inhibition of unconventional mRNA splicing by an IRE1-binding small molecule," *Proceedings of the National Academy of Sciences of the United States of America*, vol. 109, no. 15, pp. E869–E878, 2012.

[97] R. Ghosh, L. Wang, E. S. Wang et al., "Allosteric inhibition of the IRE1α RNase preserves cell viability and function during endoplasmic reticulum stress," *Cell*, vol. 158, no. 3, pp. 534–548, 2014.

[98] R. Ringseis, J. Keller, and K. Eder, "Role of carnitine in the regulation of glucose homeostasis and insulin sensitivity: evidence from in vivo and in vitro studies with carnitine supplementation and carnitine deficiency," *European Journal of Nutrition*, vol. 51, no. 1, pp. 1–18, 2012.

[99] J. C. Bae, W. Y. Lee, K. H. Yoon et al., "Improvement of nonalcoholic fatty liver disease with carnitine-orotate complex in type 2 diabetes (CORONA): a randomized controlled trial," *Diabetes Care*, vol. 38, no. 7, pp. 1245–1252, 2015.

[100] N. Suksomboon, N. Poolsup, and N. Juanak, "Effects of coenzyme Q_{10} supplementation on metabolic profile in diabetes: a systematic review and meta-analysis," *Journal of Clinical Pharmacy and Therapeutics*, vol. 40, no. 4, pp. 413–418, 2015.

[101] J. C. Ratliff, L. B. Palmese, E. L. Reutenauer, and C. Tek, "An open-label pilot trial of alpha-lipoic acid for weight loss in patients with schizophrenia without diabetes," *Clinical Schizophrenia and Related Psychoses*, vol. 8, no. 4, pp. 196–200, 2015.

[102] S. Porasuphatana, S. Suddee, A. Nartnampong, J. Konsil, B. H. B.Pharm, and A. Santaweesuk, "Glycemic and oxidative status of patients with type 2 diabetes mellitus following oral administration of alphalipoic acid: a randomized double-blinded placebocontrolled study," *Asia Pacific Journal of Clinical Nutrition*, vol. 21, no. 1, pp. 12–21, 2012.

[103] A. E. Huerta, S. Navas-Carretero, P. L. Prieto-Hontoria, J. A. Martínez, and M. J. Moreno-Aliaga, "Effects of α-lipoic acid and eicosapentaenoic acid in overweight and obese women during weight loss," *Obesity*, vol. 23, no. 2, pp. 313–321, 2015.

[104] E. H. Koh, W. J. Lee, S. A. Lee et al., "Effects of alpha-lipoic acid on body weight in obese subjects," *The American Journal of Medicine*, vol. 124, no. 1, pp. 85.e1–85.e8, 2011.

[105] Y. Zhang, P. Han, N. Wu et al., "Amelioration of lipid abnormalities by α-lipoic acid through antioxidative and anti-inflammatory effects," *Obesity*, vol. 19, no. 8, pp. 1647–1653, 2011.

[106] P. L. Prieto-Hontoria, P. Pérez-Matute, M. Fernández-Galilea, J. Alfredo Martinez, and M. J. Moreno-Aliaga, "Effects of lipoic acid on AMPK and adiponectin in adipose tissue of low- and high-fat-fed rats," *European Journal of Nutrition*, vol. 52, no. 2, pp. 779–787, 2013.

[107] W. L. Chen, C. H. Kang, S. G. Wang, and H. M. Lee, "alpha-Lipoic acid regulates lipid metabolism through induction of sirtuin 1 (SIRT1) and activation of AMP-activated protein kinase," *Diabetologia*, vol. 55, no. 6, pp. 1824–1835, 2012.

[108] Y. Wang, X. Li, Y. Guo, L. Chan, and X. Guan, "Alpha-lipoic acid increases energy expenditure by enhancing adenosine monophosphate-activated protein kinase-peroxisome proliferator-activated receptor-gamma coactivator-1alpha signaling in the skeletal muscle of aged mice," *Metabolism*, vol. 59, no. 7, pp. 967–976, 2010.

[109] M.-S. Kim, J.-Y. Park, C. Namkoong et al., "Anti-obesity effects of α-lipoic acid mediated by suppression of hypothalamic AMP-activated protein kinase," *Nature Medicine*, vol. 10, no. 7, pp. 727–733, 2004.

[110] M. C. Castro, F. Francini, J. J. Gagliardino, and M. L. Massa, "Lipoic acid prevents fructose-induced changes in liver carbohydrate metabolism: role of oxidative stress," *Biochimica et Biophysica Acta*, vol. 1840, no. 3, pp. 1145–1151, 2014.

[111] S. K. Jain, R. McVie, J. J. Jaramillo, M. Palmer, and T. Smith, "Effect of modest vitamin E supplementation on blood glycated hemoglobin and triglyceride levels and red cell indices in type I diabetic patients," *Journal of the American College of Nutrition*, vol. 15, no. 5, pp. 458–461, 1996.

[112] A. Ceriello, D. Giugliano, A. Quatraro, C. Donzella, G. Dipalo, and P. J. Lefebvre, "Vitamin E reduction of protein glycosylation in diabetes: new prospect for prevention of diabetic complications?" *Diabetes Care*, vol. 14, no. 1, pp. 68–72, 1991.

[113] S. Shab-Bidar, Z. Mazloum, and Z. Mousavi-Shirazifard, "Daily vitamin E supplementation does not improve metabolic and glycemic control in type 2 diabetic patients: a double blinded randomized controlled trial," *Journal of Diabetes*, vol. 5, no. 1, pp. 57–58, 2013.

[114] P. A. Economides, L. Khaodhiar, A. Caselli et al., "The effect of vitamin E on endothelial function of micro- and macrocirculation and left ventricular function in type 1 and type 2 diabetic patients," *Diabetes*, vol. 54, no. 1, pp. 204–211, 2005.

[115] F. J. Gómez-Pérez, V. E. Valles-Sánchez, J. C. López-Alvarenga et al., "Vitamin E modifies neither fructosamine nor HbA1c levels in poorly controlled diabetes," *Revista de Investigación Clínica*, vol. 48, no. 6, pp. 421–424, 1996.

[116] Y.-C. Chang, Y.-H. Yu, J.-Y. Shew et al., "Deficiency of NPGPx, an oxidative stress sensor, leads to obesity in mice and human," *The EMBO Molecular Medicine*, vol. 5, no. 8, pp. 1165–1179, 2013.

[117] J.-R. Kim, H.-H. Ryu, H. J. Chung et al., "Association of anti-obesity activity of N-acetylcysteine with metallothionein-II down-regulation," *Experimental and Molecular Medicine*, vol. 38, no. 2, pp. 162–172, 2006.

[118] E. L. B. Novelli, P. P. Santos, H. B. Assalin et al., "N-acetylcysteine in high-sucrose diet-induced obesity: energy expenditure and metabolic shifting for cardiac health," *Pharmacological Research*, vol. 59, no. 1, pp. 74–79, 2009.

[119] J. R. Mercer, E. Yu, N. Figg et al., "The mitochondria-targeted antioxidant MitoQ decreases features of the metabolic syndrome in $ATM^{+/-}/ApoE^{-/-}$ mice," *Free Radical Biology and Medicine*, vol. 52, no. 5, pp. 841–849, 2012.

[120] K. Liu, R. Zhou, B. Wang, and M.-T. Mi, "Effect of resveratrol on glucose control and insulin sensitivity: a meta-analysis of 11 randomized controlled trials," *American Journal of Clinical Nutrition*, vol. 99, no. 6, pp. 1510–1519, 2014.

[121] D.-K. Kim, D. Ryu, M. Koh et al., "Orphan nuclear receptor estrogen-related receptor γ (ERRγ) is key regulator of hepatic gluconeogenesis," *Journal of Biological Chemistry*, vol. 287, no. 26, pp. 21628–21639, 2012.

[122] A. J. Sanyal, N. Chalasani, K. V. Kowdley et al., "Pioglitazone, vitamin E, or placebo for nonalcoholic steatohepatitis," *The New England Journal of Medicine*, vol. 362, no. 18, pp. 1675–1685, 2010.

[123] W. Li, W. Wu, H. Song et al., "Targeting Nrf2 by dihydro-CDDO-trifluoroethyl amide enhances autophagic clearance and viability of β-cells in a setting of oxidative stress," *FEBS Letters*, vol. 588, no. 12, pp. 2115–2124, 2014.

[124] R. Baerga, Y. Zhang, P.-H. Chen, S. Goldman, and S. Jin, "Targeted deletion of autophagy-related 5 (atg5) impairs adipogenesis in a cellular model and in mice," *Autophagy*, vol. 5, no. 8, pp. 1118–1130, 2009.

[125] J.-O. Pyo, S.-M. Yoo, H.-H. Ahn et al., "Overexpression of Atg5 in mice activates autophagy and extends lifespan," *Nature Communications*, vol. 4, article 2300, 2013.

[126] S. Kaushik, J. A. Rodriguez-Navarro, E. Arias et al., "Autophagy in hypothalamic agrp neurons regulates food intake and energy balance," *Cell Metabolism*, vol. 14, no. 2, pp. 173–183, 2011.

[127] S. Kaushik, E. Arias, H. Kwon et al., "Loss of autophagy in hypothalamic POMC neurons impairs lipolysis," *EMBO Reports*, vol. 13, no. 3, pp. 258–265, 2012.

[128] B. Coupé, Y. Ishii, M. O. Dietrich, M. Komatsu, T. L. Horvath, and S. G. Bouret, "Loss of autophagy in pro-opiomelanocortin neurons perturbs axon growth and causes metabolic dysregulation," *Cell Metabolism*, vol. 15, no. 2, pp. 247–255, 2012.

[129] N. Martinez-Lopez, D. Athonvarangkul, S. Sahu et al., "Autophagy in Myf5+ progenitors regulates energy and glucose homeostasis through control of brown fat and skeletal muscle development," *EMBO Reports*, vol. 14, no. 9, pp. 795–803, 2013.

[130] R. Malhotra, J. P. Warne, E. Salas, A. W. Xu, and J. Debnath, "Loss of Atg12, but not Atg5, in pro-opiomelanocortin neurons exacerbates diet-induced obesity," *Autophagy*, vol. 11, no. 1, pp. 145–154, 2015.

[131] S. G. Fonseca, S. Ishigaki, C. M. Oslowski et al., "Wolfram syndrome 1 gene negatively regulates ER stress signaling in rodent and human cells," *The Journal of Clinical Investigation*, vol. 120, no. 3, pp. 744–755, 2010.

6

Diphenyl Ditelluride Intoxication Triggers Histological Changes in Liver, Kidney, and Lung of Mice

Sônia Cristina Almeida da Luz,[1] Melissa Falster Daubermann,[2] Gustavo Roberto Thomé,[3] Matheus Mülling dos Santos,[3] Angelica Ramos,[3] Gerson Torres Salazar,[3] João Batista Teixeira da Rocha,[3] and Nilda Vargas Barbosa[3]

[1]*Departamento de Patologia, Universidade Federal de Santa Maria (UFSM), Campus Universitário, Camobi, 97105-900 Santa Maria, RS, Brazil*
[2]*Serviço de Patologia, Hospital Universitário de Santa Maria (UFSM), Campus Universitário, Camobi, 97105-900 Santa Maria, RS, Brazil*
[3]*Departamento de Bioquímica e Biologia Molecular, Universidade Federal de Santa Maria (UFSM), Campus Universitário, Camobi, 97105-900 Santa Maria, RS, Brazil*

Correspondence should be addressed to Nilda Vargas Barbosa; nvbarbosa@yahoo.com.br

Academic Editor: Andrea Stringer

Tellurium compounds may be cytotoxic to different cells types. Thus, this work evaluated the effect of diphenyl ditelluride ($(PhTe)_2$), an organotellurium commonly used in organic synthesis, on the morphology of liver, kidney, and lung. Adult mice were acutely (a subcutaneous single dose: 250 μmol/kg) or subchronically (one daily subcutaneous dose: 10 or 50 μmol/kg for 7 and 14 days) exposed to $(PhTe)_2$. Afterwards, the histological analyses of liver, kidney, and lungs were performed. Liver histology revealed that the hepatocytes of mice subchronically exposed to $(PhTe)_2$ presented cytoplasmic vacuolization, hydropic degeneration, and hyperchromatic nuclei. Subchronic exposure to 50 μmol/kg $(PhTe)_2$ also caused hepatic necrosis. Microvesicular and macrovesicular steatosis were identified in liver of mice acutely exposed to $(PhTe)_2$. Acute and subchronic intoxication with $(PhTe)_2$ induced changes on epithelial cells of renal tubules, namely, loss of brush border and cytoplasmatic vacuolization. Atrophy and hypertrophy, cast proteinaceous formation, and acute tubular necrosis were also identified in renal tissue. Mice subchronically exposed to 50 μmol/kg $(PhTe)_2$ developed intra-alveolar edema and alveolar wall congestion in some areas of lungs. Acute exposure to $(PhTe)_2$ did not cause histological changes in lungs. Our data show that $(PhTe)_2$ may be considered a histotoxic agent for liver, kidney, and lung.

1. Introduction

Tellurium (Te) is a rare metalloid, which has been regarded as a toxic and nonessential trace element. It can be found in the environment as elemental and ionic inorganic forms [1, 2]. Methylation of Te inorganic forms can produce and release volatile organic forms of tellurium in the environment. Industrially, Te is obtained as by-product of copper refinement [2, 3]. Te has important applications in several industrial processes, and currently many inorganic Te compounds are used in rubber production, in metallurgy, and in the industry of nanoparticulate semiconductors [4–6]. Concerning organic Te compounds, it is important to highlight their role as reagent in organic synthesis [7]. Although Te has been known to be present in plants and microorganisms as bacteria, and fungi, there is no evidence that Te has biological functions [8]. The investigations regarding the toxicology/pharmacology of Te are still limited in literature; however, the therapeutic and toxic role of Te compounds has received more attention in the last decades. With emphasis on toxicological properties, experimental studies have highlighted the detrimental effects of different Te compounds in several tissues including liver, kidney, and blood [9–11]. Te compounds can induce severe neurodegeneration, which

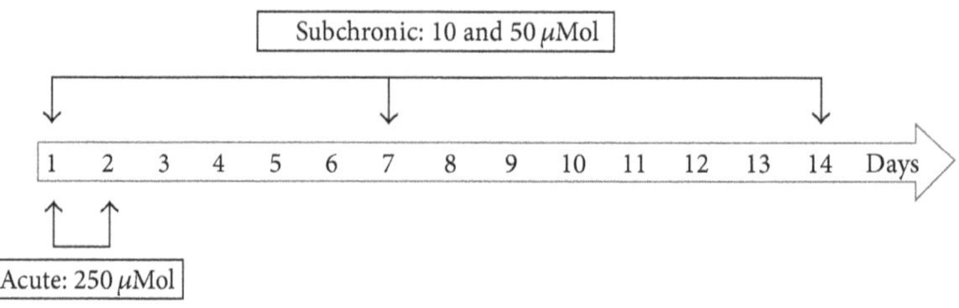

SCHEME 1

is strongly associated with the demyelination processes via inhibition of enzyme squalene epoxidase [1, 12, 13]. With regard to mechanisms, it has been postulated that the toxic action of Te forms (organic and inorganic) involves their prooxidant potential towards thiol groups from biologically active molecules [10, 14–19]. In a similar way, accumulating evidence has showed that the compound diphenyl ditelluride ($(PhTe)_2$), an organotellurium used commonly as intermediate in organic synthesis [9], is toxic to different tissues [20–29] and inhibits sulfhydryl containing enzymes *in vitro* and *in vivo* [9, 16, 19]. Moreover, $(PhTe)_2$ exposure has been associated with teratogenic, mutagenic, and genotoxic events [28–30]. Although a growing body of biochemical evidence shows the close relationship between diphenyl ditelluride intoxication and oxidative damage, there are few experimental works characterizing the putative histological changes triggered by the compound in specific mammalian organs. Only few studies have demonstrated that the exposure to certain Te compounds may induce morphological alterations in tissues such as liver, thymus, bone marrow, heart, retina, and kidney [31–33]. Specifically about $(PhTe)_2$, literature data show that rats exposed to compound develop an accentuated cerebral vacuolization [1, 20]. However, the effects of $(PhTe)_2$ intoxication on other target organs are still unknown morphologically. Thus, keeping in mind the $(PhTe)_2$ toxicity and the scarcity of data on its action on the morphology of targets tissues such as liver, kidney and lung, the present study aimed to assess the histology of liver, kidney and lungs of mice exposed acute and subchronically to $(PhTe)_2$ in order to extend, characterize and confirm morphologically the biochemical toxicity of $(PhTe)_2$.

2. Materials and Methods

2.1. Materials. Hematoxylin and eosin (H&E) and Periodic Acid-Schiff (PAS) staining were purchased from and acquired from Renylab. Diphenyl ditelluride was synthesized according to the literature method [34] (Paulmier, 1986). Analysis of ^{1}H NMR and ^{13}C NMR spectra showed that diphenyl ditelluride presented analytical and spectroscopic data in full agreement with their assigned structures. The chemical purity of the compounds (99.9%) was determined by CGMS.

2.2. Animals. Adult male Swiss albino mice (25–35 g) from our own breeding colony were used. Animals were kept on a 12 h light/dark cycle, at a room maintained at constant temperature (22 ± 2°C), with free access to food and water and housed in solid plastic-bottomed cages. The animals were used according to the guidelines of the Committee on Care and Use of Experimental Animal Resources, from the Federal University of Santa Maria, Brazil.

2.3. Experimental Protocol

2.3.1. Treatments. The mice were treated for different times and with doses of $(PhTe)_2$ according to Scheme 1. The animals were randomly divided into control ($n = 5$) and $(PhTe)_2$ ($n = 5$) groups; and the experiments were carried out 3 times. Mice in the $(PhTe)_2$ groups were administered (s.c) once a day with 10 or 50 μmol/kg (for 7 or 14 days) or with a single dose of 250 μmol/kg of $(PhTe)_2$. The compound was dissolved in DMSO and the control group was treated with the vehicle (DMSO 1 mL/Kg). The choice of $(PhTe)_2$ doses used in this experimental protocol was based on a previous study [6].

2.3.2. Tissue Preparation. Twenty-four hours after the end of each experimental period, the animals were euthanized by cervical dislocation. The organs designed for morphological analysis (liver, kidney, and lungs) were quickly removed, rinsed with saline solution (0.9%), and fixed in formalin 10%. The diagonal section of the liver and lung as well as the longitudinal section of the kidney was obtained and processed (Pathology laboratory, Pathology Department of Federal University of Santa Maria). The processed tissues were embedded in paraffin, sectioned at 4 μm thickness, and placed on frosted glass slides for further evaluation. The tissue macroscopic alterations were also analyzed.

The samples were stained using hematoxylin and eosin (H&E) stains [35], which can detect changes in the nucleus and cytoplasm; for instance, degenerative lesions and necrosis. The slides were assessed using a light microscopy coupled to the photomicrographic camera, both adapted to a microcomputer with *software* Honestech for image capture.

3. Results

3.1. Macroscopic Analysis. In macroscopic examination, we observed that the organs of mice exposed to $(PhTe)_2$ (independently of dose and period) had a gray-black coloration. This effect was more marked in kidneys, lungs, muscles, and abdominal cavity (Figures 1(a), 1(b), and 1(c)).

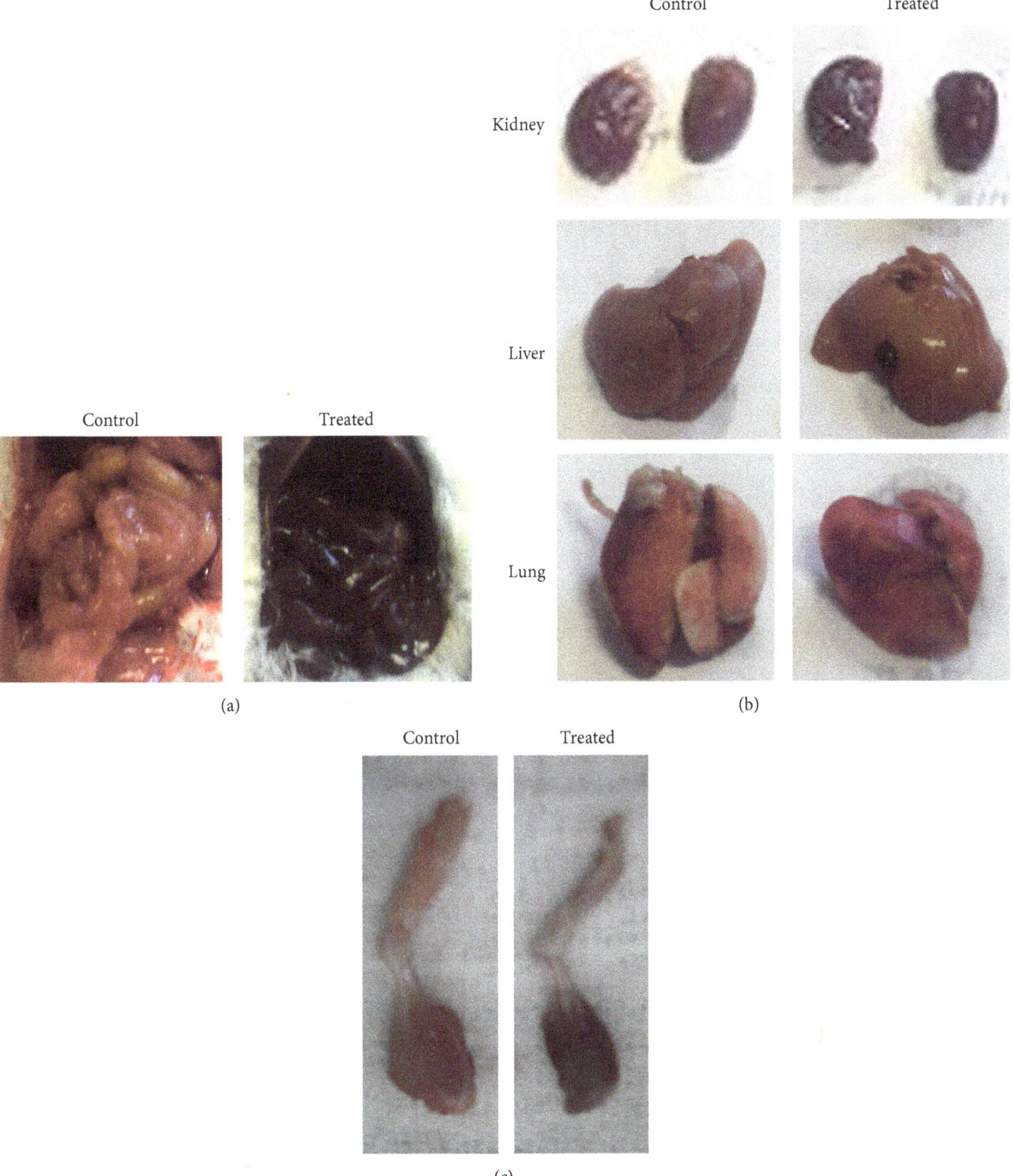

FIGURE 1: Abdominal cavity and organs of mice acutely or subchronically exposed to different diphenyl ditelluride treatments: (a) abdominal cavity of control (left) and diphenyl ditelluride (right) treated mice; (b) kidneys, liver, and lungs of control (left) and diphenyl ditelluride (right) treated mice; (c) muscles of lower limbs of control (left) and diphenyl ditelluride (right) treated mice. The picture is a representation of three independent experiments in all doses tested.

3.2. Microscopic Analysis

3.2.1. Hepatic Tissue

$(PhTe)_2$-10 μmol/kg. Liver histopathological analysis showed that the hepatocytes of mice exposed to $(PhTe)_2$ (10 μmol/kg for 7 days) presented marked cytoplasmic vacuolation (vacuoles of different sizes), hydropic degeneration (intracellular edema), and hyperchromatic nuclei when compared to the control mice (Figure 2). The same kind of morphological changes was found in the liver of mice exposed for 14 days to $(PhTe)_2$ (data not shown).

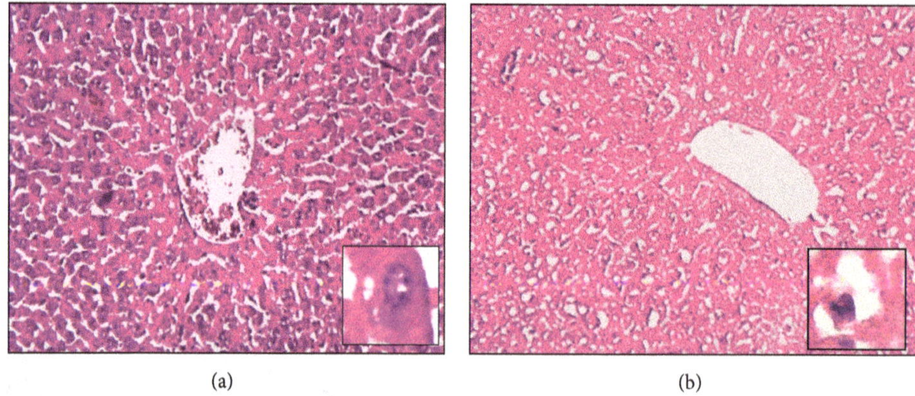

FIGURE 2: Liver histological analysis of mice exposed to diphenyl ditelluride 10 μmol/kg for 7 days. (a) Hepatocytes of mice control: cells with normal nuclei, dispersed chromatin and nucleolus arranged towards hepatic central vein (detail in 40x); (b) liver section of mice treated with diphenyl ditelluride showing cytoplasmic vacuolation, edema, and hyperchromatic nuclei (detail in 40x) (H&E 10x). The picture is a representation of three independent experiments.

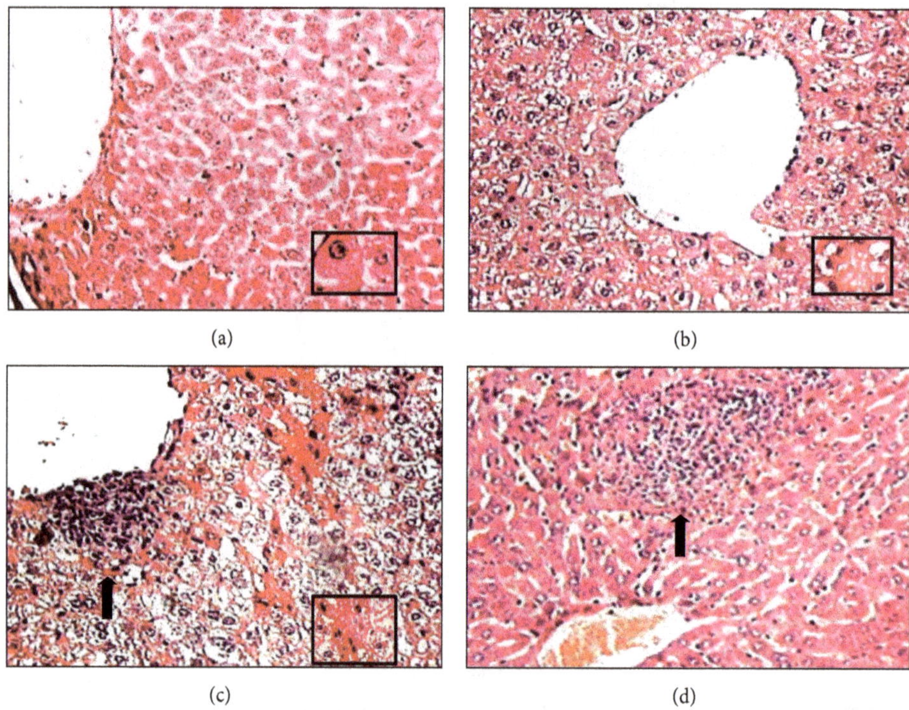

FIGURE 3: Liver histological analysis of mice exposed to diphenyl ditelluride 50 μmol/kg for 7 days. (a) Liver section of control group showing polygonal hepatocytes with oval shaped nuclei, dispersed chromatin, and prominent nucleolus cordially arranged towards hepatic central vein (detail in 40x); (b) liver section of diphenyl ditelluride treated mice showing hepatocytes with manifestation of hydropic degeneration (detail in 40x); (c) pyknotic nuclei and eosinophilic cytoplasm (arrow) (detail in 40x) and (d) mononuclear infiltrate in centrilobular (zone 3) and mediolobular (zone 2) (arrow) areas (H&E 10x). The picture is a representation of three independent experiments.

$(PhTe)_2$-50 μmol/kg. In addition to hydropic degeneration, exposure to 50 μmol/kg $(PhTe)_2$ for 7 days caused hepatic necrosis (Figure 3). The signs of necrosis were evidenced by presence of hepatocytes with pyknotic nuclei and eosinophilic cytoplasm (Figure 3(c)). Aggregation of mononuclear cells in centrilobular (zone 3) and mediolobular areas (zone 2) was also found in the hepatic parenchyma (Figure 3(d)). Similar histological changes were identified in the livers of mice intoxicated with 50 μmol/kg of $(PhTe)_2$ for 14 days (data not shown).

$(PhTe)_2$-250 μmol/kg. Histopathologic analysis revealed that the liver of mice exposed to a single dose of $(PhTe)_2$ (250 μmol/kg) developed microvesicular and macrovesicular steatosis (Figure 4). Microvesicular steatosis was characterized by presence of small vesicles filling the cytoplasm of the hepatocytes (foamy hepatocytes) and nucleus localized on the cell center. Macrovesicular steatosis was characterized by large vacuoles, apparently "without filling" and rounded by a clear outline (Figure 4(b)). The acute intoxication was also associated with a marked and focal dilatation of sinusoids,

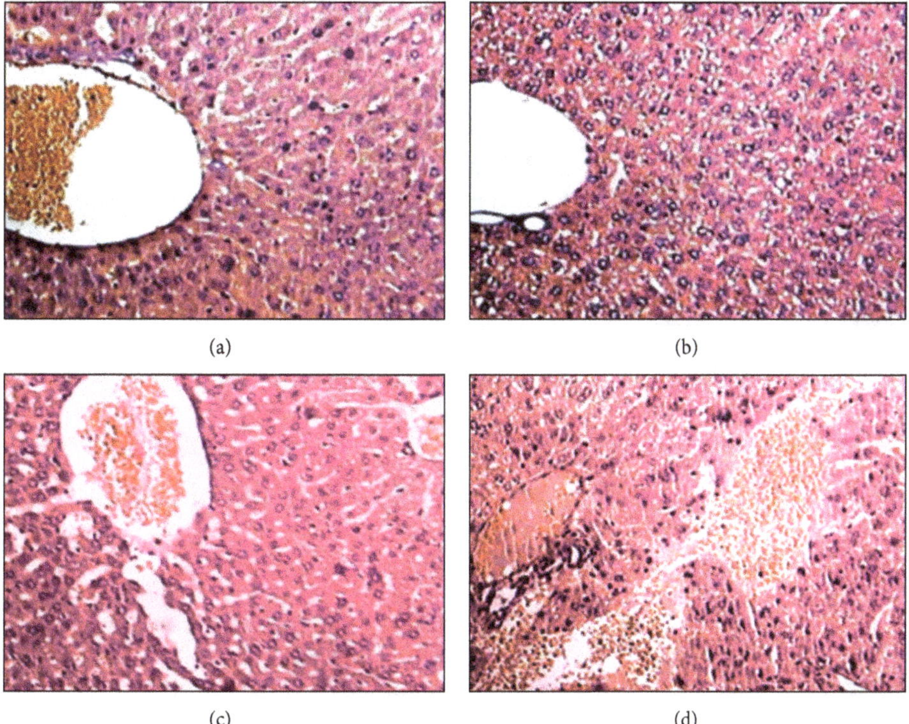

(a) (b) (c) (d)

FIGURE 4: Liver histological analysis of mice acutely exposed to diphenyl ditelluride 250 μmol/kg. (a) Liver section of control group showing preserved polygonal hepatocytes with oval-shaped nuclei, dispersed chromatin, and prominent nucleolus cordially arranged towards hepatic central vein; (b) liver section of diphenyl ditelluride treated mice showing microvesicular steatosis and macrovesicular steatosis; (c) presence of sinusoidal dilatation mainly in centrilobular and mediolobular areas; (d) hepatocytes with pyknotic nuclei surrounded area with vascular congestion and hepatic laminae disorganized (H&E 10x). The picture is a representation of three independent experiments.

which was more prominent in the centrilobular (Zone 3) and mediolobular (Zone 2) areas of the hepatic parenchyma (Figure 4(c)). In some areas a mild venous congestion and hepatocytes with pyknotic nucleus surrounding the congested area were observed (Figure 4(d)). A disorganization of hepatic laminae was also observed in this group when compared to control.

3.2.2. Renal Tissue

$(PhTe)_2$-10 μmol/kg. Exposure to $(PhTe)_2$ (10 μmol/kg for 7 days) caused a prominent degeneration of epithelial cells lining the renal tubules (Figure 5). Degenerative processes were evidenced by presence of edema and epithelial cells with large vacuoles (Figures 5(b) and 5(c)). In several tubules signals of acute tubular necrosis were observed, for instance, an apparent loss of tubular epithelial cells specialization (brush border) and presence of necrotic debris and necrotic epithelial cells in the lumen (Figure 5(c)). Indeed, various renal tubules were filled with eosinophilic homogenous material (cast proteinaceous) and had a marked tubular hypertrophy (Figures 5(c) and 5(d)). The same kind of morphological changes were found in mice treated for 14 days (data not shown).

$(PhTe)_2$-50 μmol/kg. The exposure to $(PhTe)_2$ (50 μmol for 7 days) induced degenerative changes in the lining epithelium of renal tubules, which had cytoplasmatic vacuoles and loss of brush border (Figure 6(b)). Some tubules also presented lumen filled with eosinophilic homogenous material, characterizing the cast proteinaceous formation (Figure 6(c)). Indeed, vascular congestion in cortical and medullar areas was identified (Figure 6(d)). No additional alteration was observed in the kidney of mice exposed to $(PhTe)_2$ 50 μmol/kg for 14 days (data not shown).

$(PhTe)_2$-250 μmol/kg. The histological analysis revealed that the renal tubules of mice exposed to a single dose of $(PhTe)_2$ (250 μmol/kg) contained epithelial cells in the lumen and presented different stages of compression (Figure 7(c)). Also the presence of hypertrophic tubules filled with cast proteinaceous and tubules containing a single layer of epithelial cells and small vacuoles was observed (Figures 7(c) and 7(d)). The occurrence of casts within the hypertrophic tubules was confirmed by PAS staining (Figure 7(e)).

3.2.3. Pulmonary Tissue

$(PhTe)_2$-10 μmol/kg. No morphological alteration was observed in the pulmonary tissue of mice exposed to 10 μmol/kg of $(PhTe)_2$, for 7 or 14 days, when compared with the control group (data not shown).

$(PhTe)_2$-50 μmol/kg. Lung histopathology revealed that the exposure to 50 μmol/kg of $(PhTe)_2$ for 7 days was accomplished by development of edema intra-alveolar and alveolar

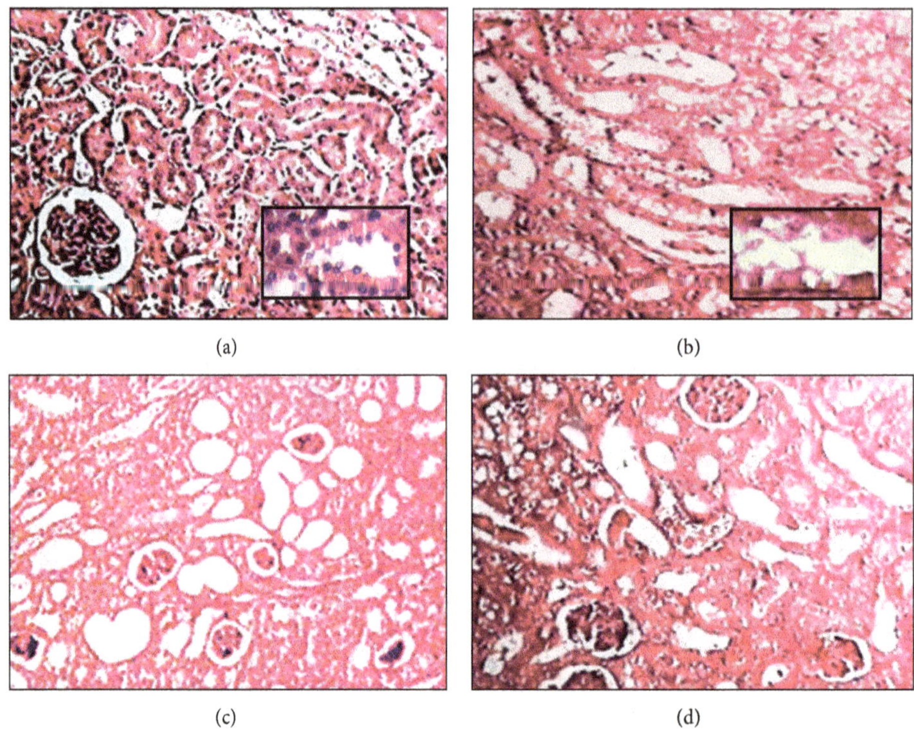

FIGURE 5: Kidney histological analysis of mice exposed to diphenyl ditelluride 10 μmol/kg for 7 days. (a) Kidney section of control group showing conserved architecture of cortex with convoluted tubules outlined for a single layer of cuboidal cells and preserved glomeruli (detail 40x). Kidney section of diphenyl ditelluride treated mice showing (b) vacuolar degeneration represented for marked epithelial cells swelling of renal tubules (detail 40x); (c) dilated distal tubules and proximal tubules in different stages of compression; loss of brush border and some tubular cells free in lumen; (d) hypertrophic tubules filled with eosinophilic homogeneous substance (cast proteinaceous) (H&E 10x). The picture is a representation of three independent experiments.

wall congestion in some areas (Figure 8(b)). Similar tissue changes were observed in the lung of mice exposed to $(PhTe)_2$ 50 μmol/kg for 14 days (data not shown).

$(PhTe)_2$-250 μmol/kg. The pulmonary analysis showed that the acute exposure to $(PhTe)_2$ at 250 μmol did not cause changes in alveolar morphology when compared to the control (data not shown).

4. Discussion

Our present work provided evidence that $(PhTe)_2$ can elicit several histological abnormalities in liver, kidney, and lung of adult mice. In general, $(PhTe)_2$ exposure caused degenerative lesions of reversible and irreversible character, principally in liver and kidney. In contrast, lung was little affected by $(PhTe)_2$ intoxication. The macroscopic findings showed that the kidneys, lungs, muscles, and abdominal cavity of mice intoxicated with $(PhTe)_2$ developed a gray-black coloration. In analogy, a blackened appearance has already been observed in the mucosa of the bladder and ureter during the necropsies analysis of a human fatally poisoned with sodium telluride [36]. In this case report, it was also emphasized that the individual intoxicated by sodium telluride presented a peculiar garlic odor in the breath and severe cyanosis [36]. Although the tissue metabolism of $(PhTe)_2$ is not well studied, other studies have suggested that the black color of some tissues observed in Te intoxication fatalities possibly reflects the deposition of reduced tellurium or elemental tellurium forms [4, 36].

Currently, the toxicological properties of $(PhTe)_2$ have been investigated in *in vivo* and *in vitro* experimental models. Especially in liver, acute and/or chronic intoxication have been reported to increase the organ-to-body weight ratio, inhibit δ-ALA-D enzyme, increase thiobarbituric acid reactive substances, decrease nonprotein SH levels, and modify antioxidant enzymes activities in rodents [17, 19, 29, 37]. In morphological terms, herein we observed that the liver of animals exposed to $(PhTe)_2$ (10 and 50 μmol/kg), for few days, contained hepatocytes with extensive cytoplasmic vacuolization, hydropic degeneration (edema), and hyperchromatic nuclei. The excessive accumulation of water associated with cytoplasmatic vacuolization and hydropic degeneration usually results from increased permeability of cell membranes [38]. Indeed, exposure to 50 μmol/kg of $(PhTe)_2$ induced a focal or nonspecific hepatitis and a focus of necrosis with dispersed cells followed by lymphocytic infiltration. Acute hepatitis with or without cholestasis is the most common histological pattern of drug-induced liver injury (DILI). It is widely recognized that DILI can be mediated by two main mechanisms: intrinsic and idiosyncratic hepatotoxicity. Commonly, intrinsic DILI is accompanied by hepatocellular

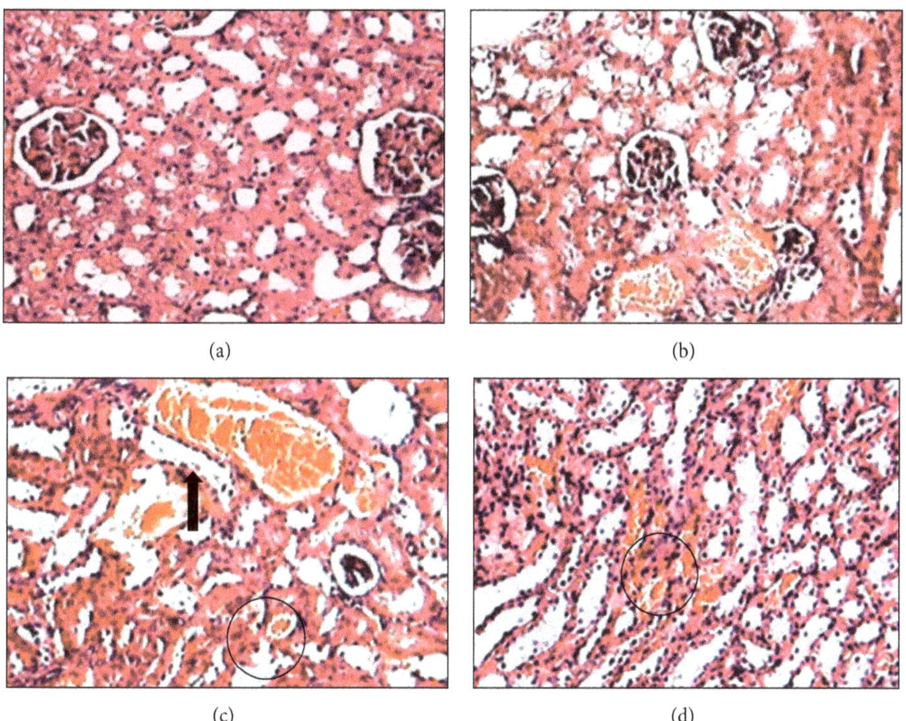

FIGURE 6: Kidney histological analysis of mice exposed to diphenyl ditelluride 50 μmol/kg for 7 days. (a) Kidney section of control group showing conserved architecture of cortex with convoluted tubules outlined for a single layer of cuboidal cells and preserved glomeruli; kidney section of diphenyl ditelluride treated mice revealing (b) vacuolar degeneration represented for marked epithelial cells swelling of renal tubules; (c) hypertrophic tubules filled with eosinophilic homogeneous substance (cast proteinaceous) (arrow); and (d) presence of vascular congestion in cortical and medullar areas (circle) (H&E 10x). The picture is a representation of three independent experiments.

necrosis and little inflammation, while the idiosyncratic DILI often with inflammation-dominant hepatic injury [39]. The liver of mice exposed acutely to $(PhTe)_2$ developed marked steatosis and changes consistent with cellular necrosis such as nuclear pyknosis and dense eosinophilic bodies unaccompanied by inflammation. Acute hepatocellular injury may result in necrosis affecting a single (spotty necrosis) or groups of hepatocytes (confluent necrosis). The necrosis signals associated with $(PhTe)_2$ intoxication were characterized by a confluent necrosis in centrilobular zone (zone 3), that is commonly caused by other drugs such as acetaminophen, halothane, and/or toxins like carbon tetrachloride. Frequently necrosis is accompanied by steatosis, which is characterized by presence of small fatty vesicles filling the cytoplasm of the hepatocyte (foamy hepatocyte) [40]. Here, the macrovesicular steatosis was represented by presence of single, large fat droplets in hepatocytes pushing the nucleus to the periphery of the cell. This change may be derived from the impaired egress of lipid from hepatocyte. Taken together, these sets of results indicate that $(PhTe)_2$ is a xenobiotic that induces acute hepatitis and cellular death. Although there are little data on the liver histology in models of intoxication by Te compounds, our findings are in accordance with some studies that identified vacuolization and necrosis signals in hepatocytes of rats exposed to tellurium dioxide [41].

In vivo data on the renal deleterious action of $(PhTe)_2$ are scarce in the literature. Unlike liver and brain, some biochemical analysis show that acute and/or chronic exposure to $(PhTe)_2$ did not affect the activity of renal sulfhydryl enzyme δ-ALA-D, a marker of oxidative damage [17]. Herein, the intoxication with $(PhTe)_2$ provoked several renal damage including vacuolar degeneration, atrophy and hypertrophy of renal tubules, hyaline cast formation, and acute tubular necrosis. These events reflect the cytotoxic effect of compound on renal parenchyma, which could impair the process of glomerular filtration and tubular reabsorption. Usually the hydropic changes and vacuolar degeneration appear whenever the cells are incapable of maintaining the ionic and fluid homeostasis. These features are considered the first manifestations of almost all forms of cell injury and characterize a reversible injury type [42]. In renal analysis, the atrophic aspect of tubules was distinguished by a decrease of their size following wrinkling and thickening of basal membrane. Some of atrophic tubules were also filled by cast proteinaceous, a pink mass in the lumen that corresponds to proteins filtered in glomerulus. In addition, the renal tubules of mice exposed subchronically to $(PhTe)_2$ presented signals of acute tubular necrosis that was identified by presence of cytoplasm fragment projections towards tubular lumen and loosening of some of these microvesicles ("blebbing"), loss of the brush border and some free cells in the lumen. Based on these observations, it is plausible to suppose that $(PhTe)_2$ exposure induced injuries on the basal membrane, the principal filtration structure, making the glomerulus abnormally

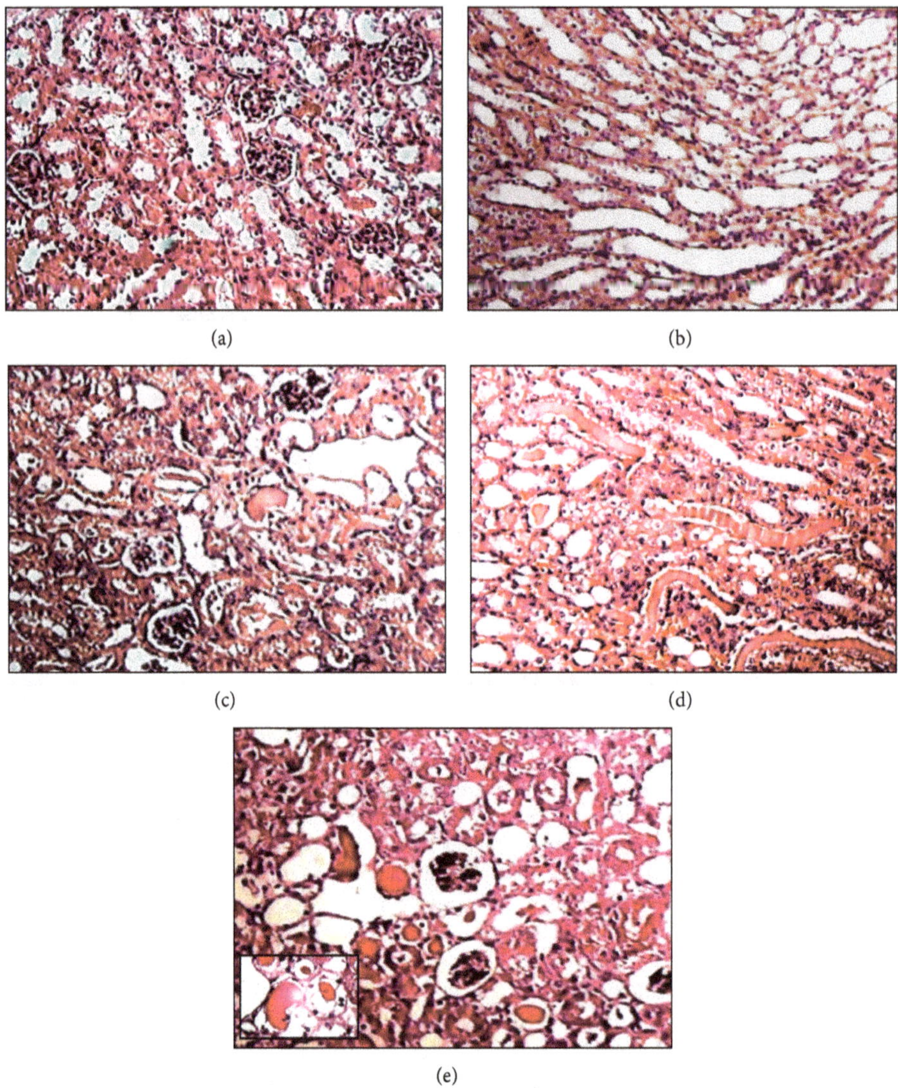

FIGURE 7: Kidney histological analysis of mice exposed acutely to diphenyl ditelluride 250 μmol/kg. Kidney section of control group showing (a) conserved architecture of renal cortex with convoluted tubules outlined for a single layer of cuboidal cells and preserved glomeruli and (b) renal medullar area with collecting tubule of normal morphology. Kidney of diphenyl ditelluride treated mice showing (c) tubules in different stages of compression (arrows), epithelial cells free in tubular lumen; presence of hypertrophic tubules filled with eosinophilic homogeneous substance (cast proteinaceous); (d) presence of tubules containing a single layer of epithelial cells and small vacuoles, presence of tubules filled with eosinophilic homogeneous substance (cast proteinaceous); (e) Kidney section with PAS stain, confirming the presence of cast proteinaceous in hypertrophic tubules (positive PAS stain/detail in 40x) (H&E 10x). The picture is a representation of three independent experiments.

permeable. In this way, there is evidence that inorganic Te compounds cause histological changes in the kidneys, ranging from cellular swelling to necrosis [31, 41]. For example, rats intoxicated with tellurium dioxide developed vacuolization of tubular cells and glomerular hemorrhage, followed by albuminuria and hematuria [31].

Regarding $(PhTe)_2$ exposure and its impact in humans, it is important to consider the growing use of this organochalcogen in the workplace and consequently the increased human exposure risk [9, 34]. In this context, the knowledge about the toxicological role of compound in the lungs is extremely important, since the inhalation is the major route of intoxication in the workplace. Although this route of exposure has not been used in this work and this fact may limit our findings, the results showed here are the first pathological data reporting the effects of $(PhTe)_2$ on the histology of lungs. Of toxicological importance, a recent study showed that acute exposure to $(PhTe)_2$ (via s.c, 0.3, 0.6, and 0.9 μmol/kg) caused oxidative damage in rat lungs, which was associated with increase in the levels of lipid peroxidation, reactive species, and nonprotein thiol as well as alterations in antioxidant enzymes activities [43]. In the histology analysis, we verified that, differing from the liver and kidney, the lung of mice intoxicated with $(PhTe)_2$ by

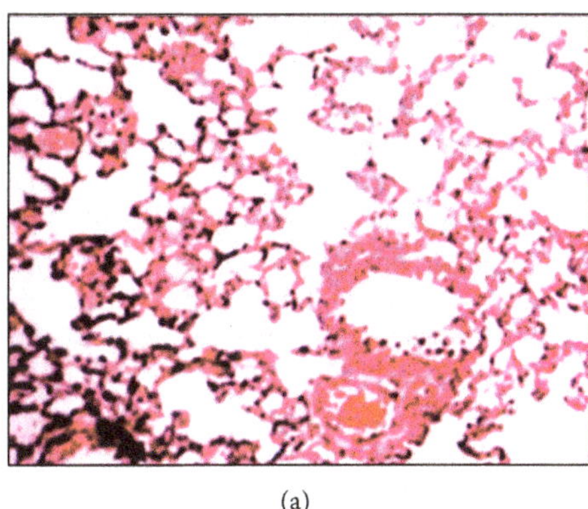

(a)

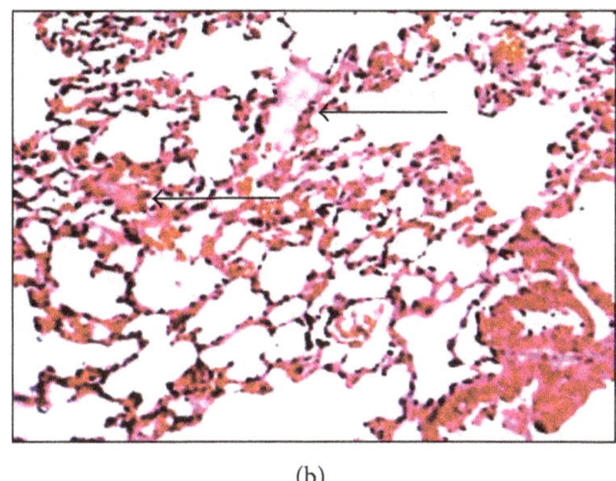

(b)

FIGURE 8: Lung histological analysis of mice exposed to diphenyl ditelluride 50 μmol/kg. (a) Lung section of control group showing bronchioles, blood vessels, and adjacent alveoli with normal morphology. (b) Lung section of diphenyl ditelluride treated mice showing the presence of some isolated areas with intra-alveolar edema (arrows) (H&E 10x). The picture represents the sum of three independent experiments.

s.c route did not present signals of severe lesions. However, it was possible to observe that $(PhTe)_2$ exposure induced edema and pulmonary congestion on some areas in the dose of 50 μmol/kg. It has been reported that other Te forms such as cadmium telluride (via intratracheal) and tellurium hexafluoride (via inhalation) cause significant lung changes, including parenchymal inflammation, lung fibrosis, necrosis of bronchiolar epithelium, inflammation of alveolar epithelium, and lung edema [44, 45]. The differences can be explained by the route and type of compounds administered.

In conclusion, our results indicate that $(PhTe)_2$ exposure provokes important morphological changes in liver, kidney, and lungs and, consequently, it represents a potential risk to human health in the work place. Although the mechanisms involved in $(PhTe)_2$ responses are still under debate, our data certainly will contribute to extending the knowledge on the toxicology of $(PhTe)_2$, since it is the first work that evaluates the histology of important organs after intoxication with the compound.

Conflict of Interests

The authors declare that there is no conflict of interests regarding the publication of this paper.

Acknowledgments

The financial support by FAPERGS/PRONEX/PRONEM, CAPES/SAUX, and CNPq is gratefully acknowledged. João Batista Teixeira da Rocha and Nilda Vargas Barbosa are the recipients of CNPq fellowships.

References

[1] L. Heimfarth, S. O. Loureiro, M. F. Dutra et al., "Disrupted cytoskeletal homeostasis, astrogliosis and apoptotic cell death in the cerebellum of preweaning rats injected with diphenyl ditelluride," *NeuroToxicology*, vol. 34, no. 1, pp. 175–188, 2013.

[2] W. C. Cooper, *Tellurium*, Van Nostrand Reinhod, New York, NY, USA, 1971.

[3] D. C. Dittmer, "Tellurium," *Chemical and Engineering News*, vol. 81, no. 36, p. 128, 2003.

[4] S. Duckett and K. A. O. Ellem, "Localization of tellurium in fetal tissues, particularly brain," *Experimental Neurology*, vol. 32, no. 1, pp. 49–57, 1971.

[5] M. C. Yarema and S. C. Curry, "Acute tellurium toxicity from ingestion of metal-oxidizing solutions," *Pediatrics*, vol. 116, no. 2, pp. 319–321, 2005.

[6] M. Green, H. Harwood, C. Barrowman et al., "A facile route to CdTe nanoparticles and their use in bio-labelling," *Journal of Materials Chemistry*, vol. 17, no. 19, pp. 1989–1994, 2007.

[7] N. Petragnani and H. A. Stefani, *Tellurium in Organic Synthesis*, 2nd edition, 2007.

[8] L. Gerhardsson, J. R. Glover, G. F. Nordberg, and V. Vouk, "Tellurium," in *Handbook on the Toxicology of Metals*, L. Friberg, G. F. Nordberg, and V. B. Vouk, Eds., vol. 2, pp. 532–548, Elsevier, Amsterdam, The Netherlands, 2nd edition, 1986.

[9] C. W. Nogueira, G. Zeni, and J. B. T. Rocha, "Organoselenium and organotellurium compounds: toxicology and pharmacology," *Chemical Reviews*, vol. 104, no. 12, pp. 6255–6285, 2004.

[10] C. A. S. Carvalho, T. Gemelli, R. B. Guerra et al., "Effect of in vitro exposure of human serum to 3-butyl-1-phenyl-2-(phenyltelluro)oct-en-1-one on oxidative stress," *Molecular and Cellular Biochemistry*, vol. 9, pp. 182–188, 2009.

[11] D. F. Meinerz, J. Allebrandt, D. O. C. Mariano et al., "Differential genotoxicity of diphenyl diselenide $(PhSe)_2$ and diphenyl ditelluride $(PhTe)_2$," *PeerJ*, vol. 2, article e290, 2014.

[12] M. Wagner, A. D. Toews, and P. Morell, "Tellurite specifically affects squalene epoxidase: investigations examining the mechanism of tellurium-induced neuropathy," *Journal of Neurochemistry*, vol. 64, no. 5, pp. 2169–2176, 1995.

[13] J. F. Goodrum, "Role of organotellurium species in tellurium neuropathy," *Neurochemical Research*, vol. 23, no. 10, pp. 1313–1319, 1998.

[14] F. X. Blais, R. T. Onischuk, and R. H. De Meio, "Hemolysis by tellurite. I. The tellurite test for hemolysis," *The Journal of the American Osteopathic Association*, vol. 72, no. 2, pp. 207–210, 1972.

[15] B. Deuticke, P. Lütkemeier, and B. Poser, "Tellurite-induced damage of the erythrocyte membrane. Manifestations and mechanisms," *Biochimica et Biophysica Acta (BBA)—Biomembranes*, vol. 1109, no. 1, pp. 97–107, 1992.

[16] N. V. Barbosa, J. B. T. Rocha, G. Zeni, T. Emanuelli, M. C. Beque, and A. L. Braga, "Effect of organic forms of selenium on δ-aminolevulinate dehydratase from liver, kidney, and brain of adult rats," *Toxicology and Applied Pharmacology*, vol. 149, no. 2, pp. 243–253, 1998.

[17] E. N. Maciel, E. M. M. Flores, J. B. T. Rocha, and V. Folmer, "Comparative deposition of diphenyl diselenide in liver, kidney, and brain of mice," *Bulletin of Environmental Contamination and Toxicology*, vol. 70, no. 3, pp. 470–476, 2003.

[18] V. C. Borges, J. B. T. Rocha, and C. W. Nogueira, "Effect of diphenyl diselenide, diphenyl ditelluride and ebselen on cerebral Na(+), K(+)-ATPase activity in rats," *Toxicology*, vol. 215, no. 3, pp. 191–197, 2005.

[19] J. B. T. Rocha, R. A. Saraiva, S. C. Garcia, F. S. Gravina, and C. W. Nogueira, "Aminolevulinate dehydratase (δ-ALA-D) as marker protein of intoxication with metals and other pro-oxidant situations," *Toxicology Research*, vol. 1, no. 2, pp. 85–102, 2012.

[20] C. W. Nogueira, L. N. Rotta, M. L. Perry, D. O. Souza, and J. B. Teixeira da Rocha, "Diphenyl diselenide and diphenyl ditelluride affect the rat glutamatergic system in vitro and in vivo," *Brain Research*, vol. 906, no. 1-2, pp. 157–163, 2001.

[21] B. L. Sailer, N. Liles, S. Dickerson, and T. G. Chasteen, "Cytometric determination of novel organotellurium compound toxicity in a promyelocytic (HL-60) cell line," *Archives of Toxicology*, vol. 77, no. 1, pp. 30–36, 2003.

[22] M. B. Moretto, C. Funchal, G. Zeni, J. B. T. Rocha, and R. Pessoa-Pureur, "Organoselenium compounds prevent hyperphosphorylation of cytoskeletal proteins induced by the neurotoxic agent diphenyl ditelluride in cerebral cortex of young rats," *Toxicology*, vol. 210, no. 2-3, pp. 213–222, 2005.

[23] E. C. Stangherlin, A. M. Favero, G. Zeni, J. B. T. Rocha, and C. W. Nogueira, "Teratogenic vulnerability of Wistar rats to diphenyl ditelluride," *Toxicology*, vol. 207, no. 2, pp. 231–239, 2005.

[24] V. C. Borges, J. B. T. Rocha, L. Savegnago, and C. W. Nogueira, "Repeated administration of diphenyl ditelluride induces hematological disorders in rats," *Food and Chemical Toxicology*, vol. 45, no. 8, pp. 1453–1458, 2007.

[25] V. P. P. Schiar, D. B. dos Santos, M. W. Paixão, C. W. Nogueira, J. B. T. Rocha, and G. Zeni, "Human erythrocyte hemolysis induced by selenium and tellurium compounds increased by GSH or glucose: a possible involvement of reactive oxygen species," *Chemico-Biological Interactions*, vol. 177, no. 1, pp. 28–33, 2009.

[26] S. Pinton, C. Luchese, E. C. Stangherlin, S. S. Roman, and C. W. Nogueira, "Diphenyl ditelluride induces neurotoxicity and impairment of developmental behavioral in rat pups," *Journal of the Brazilian Chemical Society*, vol. 21, no. 11, pp. 2130–2137, 2010.

[27] B. Comparsi, D. F. Meinerz, J. L. Franco et al., "Diphenyl ditelluride targets brain selenoproteins *in vivo*: inhibition of cerebral thioredoxin reductase and glutathione peroxidase in mice after acute exposure," *Molecular and Cellular Biochemistry*, vol. 370, no. 1-2, pp. 173–182, 2012.

[28] D. Caeran Bueno, D. F. Meinerz, J. Allebrandt et al., "Cytotoxicity and genotoxicity evaluation of organochalcogens in human leucocytes: a comparative study between ebselen, diphenyl diselenide, and diphenyl ditelluride," *BioMed Research International*, vol. 2013, Article ID 537279, 6 pages, 2013.

[29] R. Pessoa-Pureur, L. Heimfarth, and J. B. Rocha, "Signaling mechanisms and disrupted cytoskeleton in the diphenyl ditelluride neurotoxicity," *Oxidative Medicine and Cellular Longevity*, vol. 2014, Article ID 458601, 21 pages, 2014.

[30] T. H. Degrandi, I. M. de Oliveira, G. S. D'Almeida et al., "Evaluation of the cytotoxicity, genotoxicity and mutagenicity of diphenyl ditelluride in several biological models," *Mutagenesis*, vol. 25, no. 3, pp. 257–269, 2010.

[31] S. E. Sandrackaja, *Experimental Studies of the Characteristics of Telluriumas an Industrial Poison*, First Moscow Medical Institute, Moscow, Russia, 1962.

[32] W. W. Carlton and W. A. Kelly, "Tellurium toxicosis in Pekin ducks," *Toxicology and Applied Pharmacology*, vol. 11, no. 2, pp. 203–214, 1967.

[33] A. Nyska, T. Waner, M. Pirak, M. Albeck, and B. Sredni, "Toxicity study in rats of a tellurium based immunomodulating drug, AS-101: a potential drug for AIDS and cancer patients," *Archives of Toxicology*, vol. 63, no. 5, pp. 386–393, 1989.

[34] C. Paulmier, "Selenorganic functional groups," in *Selenium Reagents and Intermediates in Organic Synthesis*, C. Paulmier, Ed., pp. 25–51, Pergamon Press, Oxford, UK, 1st edition, 1986.

[35] L. P. Gartner and J. L. Hiatt, *Tratado de Histologia*, Guanabara Koogan, Rio de Janeiro, Brazil, 1999.

[36] J. H. Keall, N. H. Martin, and R. E. Tunbridge, "A report of three cases of accidental poisoning by sodium tellurite," *British Journal of Industrial Medicine*, vol. 3, pp. 175–176, 1946.

[37] F. C. Meotti, V. C. Borges, G. Zeni, J. B. T. Rocha, and C. W. Nogueira, "Potential renal and hepatic toxicity of diphenyl diselenide, diphenyl ditelluride and ebselen for rats and mice," *Toxicology Letters*, vol. 143, no. 1, pp. 9–16, 2003.

[38] T. S. Davies and A. Monro, "Marketed human pharmaceuticals reported to be tumorigenic in rodents," *Journal of the American College of Toxicology*, vol. 14, no. 2, pp. 90–107, 1995.

[39] R. Ramachandran and S. Kakar, "Histological patterns in drug-induced liver disease," *Journal of Clinical Pathology*, vol. 62, no. 6, pp. 481–492, 2009.

[40] N. F. Chevile, "Interpretation of acute cell injury: degeneration," in *Ultraestructural Pathology: An Introduction to Interpretation*, N. Cheville, Ed., chapter 2, pp. 51–79, Iowa State University Press, Ames, Iowa, USA, 1st edition, 1994.

[41] R. H. De Meio and W. W. Jetter, "Tellurium: the toxicity of ingested tellurium dioxide for rats," *The Journal of Industrial Hygiene and Toxicology*, vol. 30, no. 1, pp. 53–58, 1948.

[42] S. L. Robbins, V. Kumar, and R. S. Cotran, *Robbins and Cotran Pathologic Basis of Disease*, Saunders/Elsevier, Philadelphia, Pa, USA, 8th edition, 2010.

[43] S. Pinton, C. Luchese, E. C. Stangherlin, and C. W. Nogueira, "Acute exposure to diphenyl ditelluride causes oxidative damage in rat lungs," *Ecotoxicology and Environmental Safety*, vol. 74, no. 3, pp. 521–526, 2011.

[44] D. L. Morgan, C. J. Shines, S. P. Jeter et al., "Comparative pulmonary absorption, distribution, and toxicity of copper gallium diselenide, copper indium diselenide, and cadmium telluride in sprague–dawley rats," *Toxicology and Applied Pharmacology*, vol. 147, no. 2, pp. 399–410, 1997.

[45] G. Kimmerle, "Comparative studies on the inhalation toxicity of selenium sulfide and tellurium hexafluoride," *Archives of Toxicology*, vol. 18, pp. 140–144, 1960.

7

Stabilizing versus Destabilizing the Microtubules: A Double-Edge Sword for an Effective Cancer Treatment Option?

Daniele Fanale,[1] Giuseppe Bronte,[1] Francesco Passiglia,[1] Valentina Calò,[1] Marta Castiglia,[1] Florinda Di Piazza,[1] Nadia Barraco,[1] Antonina Cangemi,[1] Maria Teresa Catarella,[1] Lavinia Insalaco,[1] Angela Listì,[1] Rossella Maragliano,[1] Daniela Massihnia,[1] Alessandro Perez,[1] Francesca Toia,[2] Giuseppe Cicero,[1] and Viviana Bazan[1]

[1]*Department of Surgical, Oncological and Oral Sciences, Section of Medical Oncology, University of Palermo, 90127 Palermo, Italy*
[2]*Department of Surgical, Oncological and Oral Sciences, Section of Plastic Surgery, University of Palermo, 90127 Palermo, Italy*

Correspondence should be addressed to Daniele Fanale; fandan@libero.it

Academic Editor: Jérome Devy

Microtubules are dynamic and structural cellular components involved in several cell functions, including cell shape, motility, and intracellular trafficking. In proliferating cells, they are essential components in the division process through the formation of the mitotic spindle. As a result of these functions, tubulin and microtubules are targets for anticancer agents. Microtubule-targeting agents can be divided into two groups: microtubule-stabilizing, and microtubule-destabilizing agents. The former bind to the tubulin polymer and stabilize microtubules, while the latter bind to the tubulin dimers and destabilize microtubules. Alteration of tubulin-microtubule equilibrium determines the disruption of the mitotic spindle, halting the cell cycle at the metaphase-anaphase transition and, eventually, resulting in cell death. Clinical application of earlier microtubule inhibitors, however, unfortunately showed several limits, such as neurological and bone marrow toxicity and the emergence of drug-resistant tumor cells. Here we review several natural and synthetic microtubule-targeting agents, which showed antitumor activity and increased efficacy in comparison to traditional drugs in various preclinical and clinical studies. Cryptophycins, combretastatins, ombrabulin, soblidotin, D-24851, epothilones and discodermolide were used in clinical trials. Some of them showed antiangiogenic and antivascular activity and others showed the ability to overcome multidrug resistance, supporting their possible use in chemotherapy.

1. Introduction

Microtubules are dynamic and structural cellular components, typically formed by 13 protofilaments, which constitute the wall of a tube; each of the protofilaments consists of a head-to-tail arrangement of α/β tubulin heterodimers [1]. They are involved in several cell functions, including cell shape, motility, and intracellular trafficking. In proliferating cells, they are one of the essential components in the division process through the formation of the mitotic spindle. This event can take place because of the dynamic nature of microtubules through polymerization and depolymerization cycles [2]. As a result of these functions, tubulin and microtubules are targets for anticancer agents [3, 4]. Microtubule-targeting agents can be divided into two groups: microtubule-stabilizing and microtubule-destabilizing agents. The former bind to the tubulin polymer and stabilize microtubules, while the latter bind to the tubulin dimers and destabilize microtubules [5, 6].

Despite these differences, alteration of tubulin-microtubule equilibrium leads to the same final result: it disrupts the mitotic spindle, halting the cell cycle at the metaphase-anaphase transition and eventually resulting in cell death [7] (Figure 1).

Clinical application, however, has unfortunately shown several limits, such as a high level of neurological and bone marrow toxicity and the emergence of drug-resistant tumor cells due to the overproduction of P-glycoprotein (Pgp),

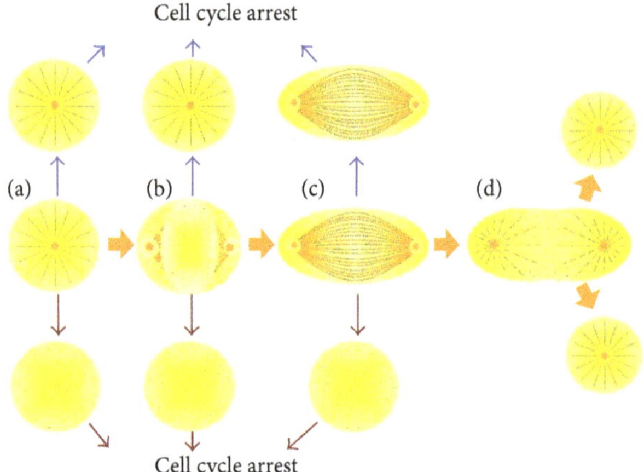

FIGURE 1: The dynamic nature of cytoskeleton is due to cycles of microtubule catastrophes. (a) Model structure of assembled cytoskeleton. The variety of shapes and sizes of the microtubule cytoskeleton is as great as the number of different cell types. In interphase, microtubules are long and stable because there are almost no catastrophes. (b) In mitosis, catastrophes are relatively frequent, resulting in highly dynamic microtubules that reach a steady-state length after a few minutes of growth (c). (d) After the segregation of chromatids, a new cycle of depolymerization and polymerization begins, resulting in a new stable microtubule cytoskeleton in daughter's cells (d). Blue and red arrows indicate effects of stabilizing and destabilizing agents, all resulting in cell cycle arrest.

an ATP-binding cassette (ABC) transmembrane transporter [8], the overexpression of different beta-tubulin isotypes, including βIII-tubulin [9, 10], or tubulin mutations [11].

Several natural and synthetic microtubule-targeting agents, exhibiting antitumor activity and increased efficacy in comparison to traditional drugs in various preclinical and clinical studies, have been discovered and their mechanisms have been elucidated [12, 13]. Apart from the well-known antimitotic function, for some of these drugs antiangiogenic and antivascular activity were demonstrated; for others the ability to overcome multidrug resistance was found. Many of these new generation microtubule-targeting agents are still under evaluation for clinical use. Some of them showed good tolerability and antitumor activity in particular cancers.

This review provides an overview of those microtubule-targeting drugs which are to date under clinical evaluation. A particular attention will be paid to the translation of preclinical data into the design of clinical trials.

2. Microtubule-Destabilizing Agents

Colchicine and Vinca alkaloids are two of the first microtubule-destabilizing agents to be discovered. These two compounds depolymerize microtubules by interacting with various β-tubulin sites. In particular, Vinca alkaloids interact with tubulin at specific binding sites which differ from those of other agents, including colchicine or taxanes, interfering with microtubule dynamics, blocking polymerization at the end of the mitotic spindle, and leading to metaphase arrest. Thanks to their peculiar mechanism of action, Vinca alkaloids have been widely used in anticancer therapy, usually in combination with other chemotherapeutic agents which do not have cross-resistance with them. First-generation Vinca alkaloids such as vinblastine have been included in the treatment protocol of both Hodgkin and non-Hodgkin lymphomas and testicular carcinoma, while vincristine has been approved for several years in the treatment of hematological tumors such as acute leukemia and multiple myeloma but also of rare tumors such as rhabdomyosarcoma and neuroblastoma. However, vincristine treatment was associated with a severe neurotoxicity, while the suppression of the bone marrow was more frequently reported during vinblastine therapy [14]. Second-generation semisynthetic Vinca alkaloids, vinorelbine and vindesine, have shown a broader spectrum of antitumor activity *in vitro*, along with a decreased neurotoxicity. Vinorelbine was approved as single agent and in combination therapy for the treatment of both hematological and solid tumors, including lung cancer, breast cancer, and gynecological tumors [15]. Recently, another synthetic Vinca alkaloid, vinflunine, has been approved in Europe for the second-line treatment of metastatic urothelial carcinoma. It is the first fluorinated microtubule inhibitor, which was associated with a higher antitumor activity than other Vinca alkaloids, showing also an excellent safety profile [16].

In order to overcome the clinical limits of these agents, in the last years attention has been focused on natural and synthetic compounds with a different structure but which act in a similar way [7, 17] (Table 1).

2.1. Cryptophycins. Cryptophycins are synthetic derivatives of macrocyclic depsipeptides, isolated by *Nostoc sp.* [18]. They block cell division and prevent the correct formation of the mitotic spindle, by inhibiting tubulin polymerization, probably at the binding site of the *Vinca alkaloids* [19]. In particular, C-52 and C-55 induce apoptosis by means of Bcl-2 hyperphosphorylation and inactivation [20–22] (Figure 2). These compounds are able to induce this phosphorylation at a greater extent than other microtubule inhibitors [23]. The first form discovered was epoxide cryptophycin 1, which showed antitumoral activity both in preclinical *in vitro* (colon, breast, ovarian, lung, and nasopharyngeal carcinomas) and *in vivo* (lung, breast, and prostate tumors) models. This has led to isolation and synthesis of cryptophycin analogs, divided into epoxides, chlorohydrins, and glycinate chlorohydrins [24] (Figure 3).

Cryptophycin 8 is the first C-1 analog synthesized in order to improve its antitumoral efficacy by means of conversion of the epoxide group into chlorohydrin. Its activity has been shown both in murine and human tumors. Although it is not as powerful as C-1, it is more soluble in water and has a stronger therapeutic effect. Nevertheless, it is still too unstable in solution to be considered clinically relevant [25].

TABLE 1: Microtubule-destabilizing agents.

Chemical lead	Properties and effects	Clinical trial/status	References
Cryptophycins	Apoptosis induction. Synergistic with chemotherapy and radiation.	Phase II clinical trials in platinum-resistant ovarian cancer and in NSCLC (C-52) but withdrawn due to peripheral neuropathy.	[26, 28, 31, 32, 36]
Combretastatin A-4-P	Antivascular and antiangiogenic activity. Synergistic with radiation, hyperthermia, chemotherapy, and immunoradiotherapy.	Phases II and III clinical trials in advanced solid tumors (lung and thyroid cancer) and in combination with carboplatin.	[63, 64, 66–70, 72, 73]
Combretastatin A-1-P	Antivascular and antitumoral activity superior to CA-4-P. Synergistic with chemotherapy.	Phase I clinical trials in solid tumors and in acute myelogenous leukaemia and myelodysplastic syndromes.	[78, 79]
Ombrabulin	Antivascular and antitumoral activity superior to CA-4-P. Synergistic with chemotherapy.	Phase I clinical trials as a single agent or in combination; phase III clinical trial in advanced soft-tissue sarcoma.	[86]
Soblidotin	Apoptosis induction. Antivascular activity. Antitumoral activity in tumors resistant to vincristine, docetaxel, and paclitaxel.	Phase II clinical trials in advanced solid tumors (soft-tissue sarcoma, NSCLC).	[99–105]
D-24851	Curative at nontoxic doses in rat tumor. No neurotoxic effects. Oral applicability. Activity versus MDR cell lines.	Phase I/II clinical trials in advanced solid tumors.	[140, 141]
Pseudolaric acid B	Antiangiogenic activity. No neurotoxic effects in tested animal. Activity versus MDR cell lines.	Preclinical phase.	[148, 149]
Embellistatin	Antiangiogenic activity.	Preclinical phase.	[150]

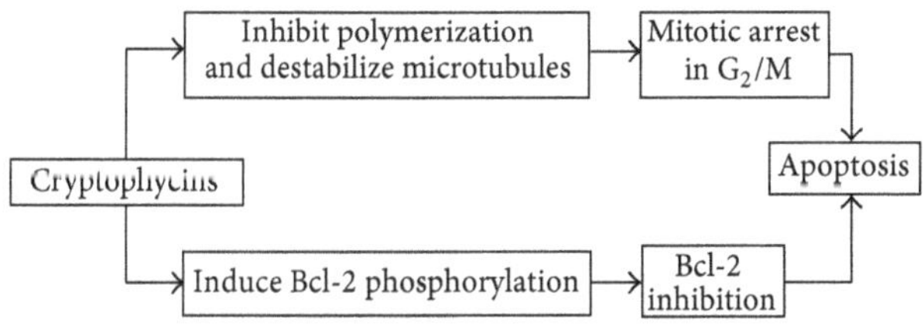

FIGURE 2: Mechanism of action of cryptophycins.

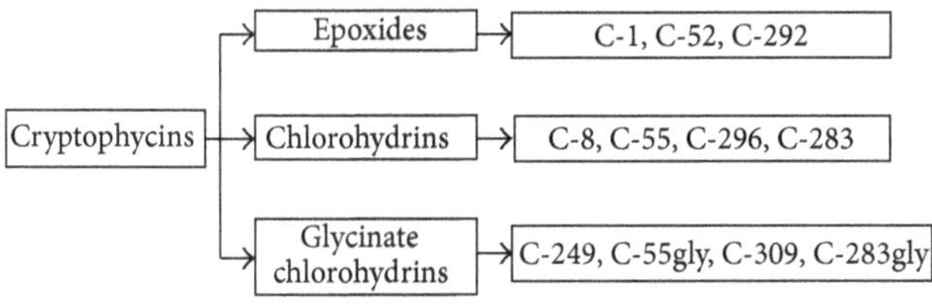

FIGURE 3: Classification of cryptophycins.

2.1.1. Cryptophycins 52 and 55. Cryptophycin 52 (LY355703) is a synthetic epoxide, used in phase II clinical trials, which presents a cytotoxic effect 400 times stronger than paclitaxel and *Vinca* alkaloids [26, 27]. It shows *in vitro* antitubulin, antimitotic, and cytotoxic activity which is dose-dependent against tumor cells. Furthermore, its activity has been evaluated both in murine tumor models and in human tumor xenografts [23]. C-52 resulted to be also effective against multidrug-resistant tumors [26, 28, 29].

Paclitaxel and the Vinca alkaloids are sensitive to the multidrug resistance (MDR) transporters P-glycoprotein (P-gp, MDR-1) and/or MDR-associated protein (MRP-1). Cryptophycin 52 was tested for its sensitivity to multidrug resistance in several paired cell lines in which a sensitive parental line was matched with a multidrug-resistant derivative line. Compared to other antimitotic agents (paclitaxel, vinblastine, and vincristine), the potency of cryptophycin 52 was shown to be minimally affected in multidrug-resistant cells compared to their sensitive parental lines [30]. Cryptophycin 52 fragment A analogues was synthesized to improve the potency and the aqueous solubility of the molecule allowing for the modification of its formulation. However, the same functional groups that rendered these analogues more potent and more water soluble also contributed to making them better substrates of the Pgp efflux pump. It is an unacceptable feature in the development of a clinically relevant antitumor agent [29].

Preclinical toxicological studies on animals (rats and dogs) have shown that above a certain concentration level C-52 causes secondary effects such as neutropenia and gastrointestinal problems but not neurotoxicity. These studies have allowed evaluating the optimum phase II dosage and tracing the plasma pharmacokinetic profile [26]. Furthermore, phase I clinical trials identified 1.5 mg/m^2 as a well-tolerated dose level of C-52. It was delivered as a 2-hour i.v. infusion on day 1 and day 8 repeated every 3 weeks [31]. This schedule was employed in a phase II study to determine the activity of C-52 in non-small cell lung cancer (NSCLC) patients previously treated with platinum-based chemotherapy and to characterize its toxicity profile. A good rate of disease stabilization and an unacceptable toxicity was found in this setting [32]. Also, a multicenter trial was performed to evaluate the same schedule of the drug in patients with platinum-resistant advanced ovarian cancer. A considerable clinical benefit without serious adverse events was achieved [28]. Afterwards, these phase II clinical trials were terminated due to significant neurological toxicity [12].

Cryptophycin 55, a C-52 chlorohydrin, shows higher cytotoxic activity and therapeutic efficacy than its epoxide precursor, but its low stability in solution has delayed its clinical application [33]. This problem has been overcome, however, by means of the synthesis of glycinate esters (C-55gly, C-283gly, and C-309) which show not only an *in vivo* activity similar to their precursors but also a high level of stability [34].

Treatment with C-52 and C-55 combined with other chemotherapy agents has produced synergic effects without increased toxicity, bringing about a greater survival rate in ovarian carcinoma murine models [23, 28]. The use of human tumor xenografts has made it possible to evaluate C-52 and C-55 activity combined with cisplatin, carboplatin, and oxaliplatin in different tumors. C-52 showed a synergic effect only when associated with cisplatin, whereas C-55 showed increased activity with all the platinum compounds [35]. *In vivo* antitumoral activity of C-52 and C-55 has been assessed in combination with radiotherapy (2γ) or with 5-FU in tumor xenografts, showing an increased effect. Pharmacokinetic analyses performed in murine models have demonstrated that C-52 concentration in the tumor increased after administration and remained high for 24 hours. The mean life of C-55 was the longest in the liver, intermediate in tumor tissue, and less in plasma. After C-55 administration, the mean life of C-52 was the longest in tumor tissue, less in plasma, and even less in the liver, suggesting almost total conversion of C-55 into C-52 in the tumor. The greater C-52 accumulation in tumor tissue depends on the bioconversion of C-55 in C-52 and different binding affinities towards different tissue proteins. The use of C-55 to deliver C-52 increased the retention of C-52 in tumor tissue and reduced its presence in all studied normal tissues. Furthermore, extracellular acid pH of the tumor increased C-55 stability, whereas intracellular basic pH encouraged bioconversion by stimulating its pharmacological activity [36].

The obtained results indicated that C-52 and C-55 fulfilled all the criteria required by ideal chemotherapy agents, since they showed an action mechanism against a specific target and considerable activity against drug-resistant cells. However, the lack of response observed in some tumors and peripheral neuropathy have been limiting factors in the development of these agents leading to termination of their study.

2.1.2. Second-Generation Cryptophycins. C-309, C-249, and C-283 are second-generation candidates for clinical use. The first two are glycinate esters, synthesized in order to provide a higher chemical stability and more solubility in water. C-309 is a derivative of C-296 which has proved to have more therapeutic activity than C-55, C-283, C-249, and C-296; it is able to bring about a complete or partial regression of murine tumors at lower doses than those of other glycinate analogs. C-249 derives from C-8 and is active against MDR tumors. Moreover, it has the advantage of being easier to synthesize.

These second-generation analogs have proved to be up to 1000 times as active as those of the first clinical candidates (C-52) but with the same or even less toxicity [34].

2.2. Combretastatins. The combretastatins, isolated from *Combretum caffrum*, are molecules structurally related to colchicine which have been extensively developed since the late 1990s as vascular-disrupting agents (VDAs) [37]. The vascular-disrupting effect of these compounds is present well below the maximum tolerated dose, with a wide therapeutic window [38]. A number of combretastatins are currently in clinical trials: combretastatins A4- and A1-phosphate, verubulin, crolibulin, plinabulin, and ombrabulin [12].

2.2.1. CA-4-P. Combretastatin A-4 interacts with tubulin at the colchicine binding site but not in the same pseudoirreversible manner. It is used as a combretastatin A-4 3-O-phosphate (CA-4-P), a prodrug which is soluble in water and transformed into its active form by endogenous phosphatases [39]. It showed cytotoxicity in tumor cell lines and in human endothelial cells, HUVEC, which are sensitive to the drug only if they are actively proliferating, suggesting a potential use as an antiangiogenic agent [38]. By interfering with microtubule polymerization and with mitotic spindle assembly, CA-4-P induces G2/M arrest, thus bringing about cell death by either mitotic catastrophe or apoptosis [38, 40, 41].

Recent computational studies, using fluorescence spectroscopy, identified a potential binding site on γ-tubulin for both CA-4-P and colchicines [42]. Since high levels of γ-tubulin have been reported in poorly differentiated and aggressive brain tumors, such as human glioblastoma and medulloblastoma [43, 44] and lung [45] and breast cancer [46], the discovery of a potential site interaction on this molecule would offer the possibility of targeting inhibition with a new class of chemotherapeutic agents. However, the experimental validation of such interesting observation is underway.

CA-4-P (also known as Zybrestat or fosbretabulin) shows a potent *in vivo* antivascular activity since it causes a rapid and widespread reduction of the tumoral blood flow and an increased vascular resistance, effects which are extremely reduced in the normal tissues [47]. At a dose of 1/5–1/10 of the maximum tolerated dose (MTD), the central area of the tumor undergoes hemorrhagic necrosis, while a thin peripheral ring of live cells remains [38, 48, 49]. On the contrary, colchicine and other drugs act only at approximately MTD [50]. This constitutes an important advantage for the therapeutic application of CA-4-P. An immediate effect of CA-4-P treatment is an increased vascular permeability, which is important for the reduction of blood flow through vascular collapse, and an increased viscosity consequent to fluid loss from the vasculature. However, endothelial barrier function alterations and increased vascular permeability might contribute to hastening tumor cell extravasation, causing progression to stages of greater malignancy, with heightened invasiveness and, in some cases, increased distant metastasis. It is no coincidence that susceptibility of tumors to CA-4-P showed a positive correlation with tumor vascular permeability [51]. Experiments conducted on HUVEC cells have shown that the CA-4-P-inducted microtubule depolymerization triggers off the actin reorganization through Rho activation and MLC (Myosin Light Chain) phosphorylation, thus causing rounding and retraction of cells and membrane blebbing. These events are associated with increased permeability, while the morphological cell change might contribute to determining the effects observed *in vivo* by means of vascular constriction [52, 53]. Furthermore, since CA-4-P interferes with the formation of stress fibers, it inhibits the VE-cadherin/β-catenin complex, thus leading to the destabilization of cell-cell junctions and increasing endothelial permeability [54].

The *ex vivo* perfusion of animal tumors highlights a lower increase in vascular resistance to that found *in vivo*, suggesting that the blood might also contribute towards the antivascular action of the drug [48]. It has been demonstrated that CA-4-P induces increased expression of endothelial CAM, responsible for the observed neutrophil recruitment which *in vivo* probably contributes both to vascular damage and to tumor cell death [55].

Apart from being an antivascular agent, CA-4-P inhibits the formation of new blood vessels, both *in vitro* and *in vivo*, presumably through inactivation of the VE-cadherin/β-catenin complex and Akt, all proteins required for cell adhesion, survival, and proliferation during neoangiogenesis. The same study has shown that smooth muscle cells, which are resistant to the drug, interfere with its antiangiogenic activity *in vitro*, suggesting that they may confer resistance to the endothelium by stabilizing cell-cell junctions [54]. CA-4-P selectivity towards the neoplastic tissue might therefore depend on the immaturity of tumor vessels, together with the proliferative status of tumor endothelial cells. Moreover, CA-4-P reduces *in vitro* HIF-1 expression (Hypoxia Inducible Factor-1) under hypoxia mainly in endothelial cells compared to that in cancer cell lines, suggesting a further possible mechanism of action for the drug [56] (Figure 4).

However, the effects of CA-4-P on tumor growth are not particularly significant, probably because of the persistent presence of vital peripheral cells [50], although the administration of several doses compared to the same total dose of the drug does increase its antitumoral effect [57, 58]. Furthermore, CA-4-P activity is directly proportional to tumor size [49]. This aspect, together with its capacity to act on the tumor core, differentiates this drug from more common therapeutic approaches, which target the peripheral tumor area. These complementary properties, together with the limited action of CA-4-P as a single agent, have led to experimentation involving combined treatments. It has been demonstrated that CA-4-P increases the response to radiotherapy and hyperthermia in treated tumors [57, 59] and, what is more, leads to a 90% increase in the retention of the anti-CEA antibody marked with I^{131} in the tumor, which is eradicated in 83% of the cases [60]. Similarly, CA-4-P increases the effect of chemotherapy drugs such as cisplatin, vinblastine, 5-fluorouracil, and irinotecan [57, 61].

The overall *in vivo* results obtained with CA-4-P have led to its introduction in phase I clinical trials [12, 62–66]. A phase I trial was performed to determine the MTD, safety, and pharmacokinetic profile of CA-4-P. This study showed absence of traditional cytotoxic side effects, with a toxicity profile which seems consistent with a "vascularly active" drug [67, 68]. The effects on tumor blood flow were assessed using dynamic contrast-enhanced magnetic resonance imaging (DCE-MRI) techniques. Dosages < or = 60 mg/m^2, as a 10 min infusion at 3-week intervals, define the upper boundary of the MTD. Similar effects were seen in other phase I clinical trials using a weekly and daily schedule [69, 70]. Afterwards, a further phase I trial investigated the combination of CA-4-P with carboplatin. A greater thrombocytopenia was observed as a consequence of altered carboplatin pharmacokinetics [63].

In order to improve its efficiency and reduce its side effects, a specific therapeutic system has been realized, based on the use of liposomes containing CA-4-P, carrying superficial RGD-peptides able to bind with the $\alpha_v\beta3$ integrins overexpressed on proliferating tumor endothelium. *In vitro* tests have demonstrated the specificity and stability of the system, essential properties for its *in vivo* application [71]. To date, phase II/III clinical trials in lung and thyroid cancer are currently being evaluated [12]. These studies showed that CA-4-P with or without carboplatin and paclitaxel combination therapy was well tolerated in thyroid cancer patients, although it did not meet statistical significance in OS improvement [72]. Instead, preliminary data suggests survival benefits and increased responses without significant additional toxicity in NSCLC patients treated with CA-4-P in combination with carboplatin, paclitaxel, and bevacizumab compared to patients treated with carboplatin, paclitaxel, and bevacizumab only [73].

2.2.2. CA-1-P. Combretastatin A1 phosphate (also known as Oxi4503), a CA-1 water-soluble prodrug, shows a powerful antivascular activity. When used in murine and human tumor xenografts at much lower doses than those required by CA-4-P, CA-1-P brings about a drastic reduction of blood flow, with resulting necrosis [74]. CA-1-P causes an increase in vessel permeability, in VEGF production and apoptosis induction in endothelial cells [75]. At high doses it is more easily tolerated than CA-4-P and shows a much higher antitumoral activity, leading to complete regression of human tumors even at extremely low doses [74]. Excellent results have been obtained with combined treatments involving several chemotherapy agents [76].

In vitro pharmacokinetic studies have suggested that CA-1-P is transformed into a more reactive metabolite than CA-4-P, which is responsible for most of the antitumoral activity; this has formed the basis for further clinical developments of the drug as an antivascular and antitumor agent [77]. The drug has completed the phase I evaluation as a potential anticancer drug at three different centres in the United Kingdom, and it was studied in other phase I clinical trials [78, 79].

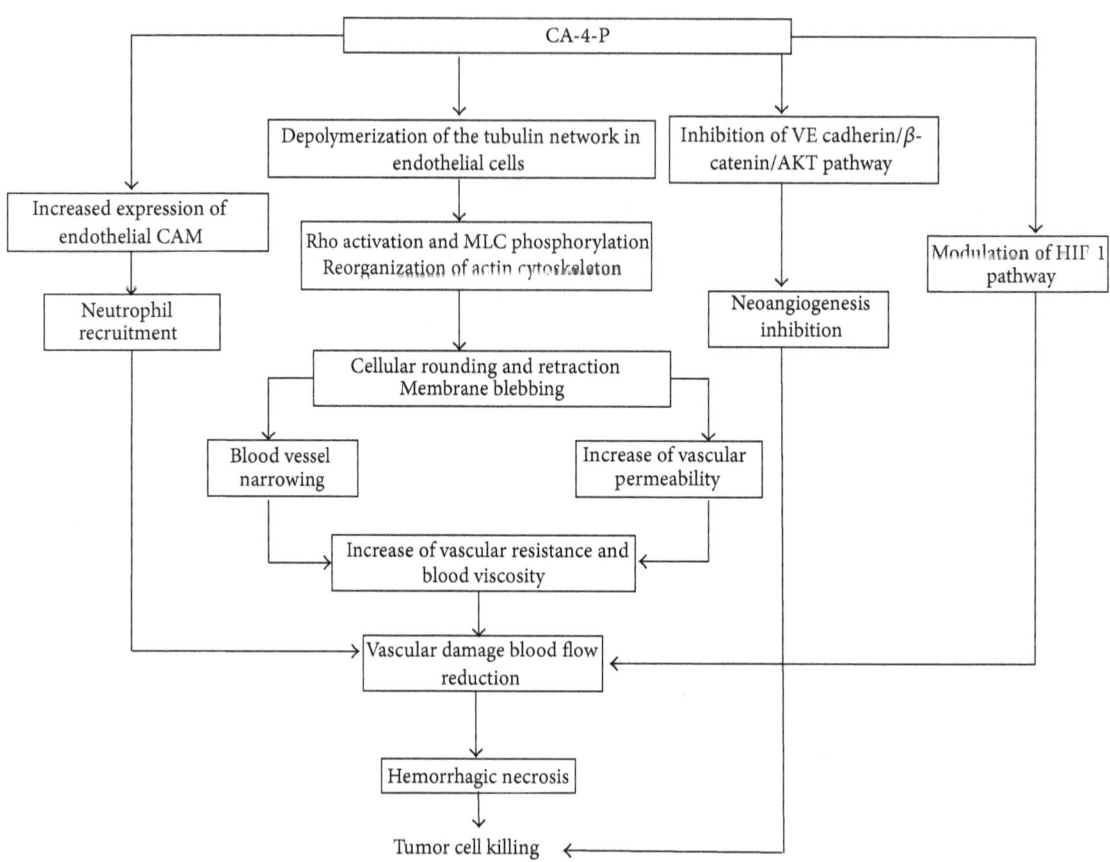

FIGURE 4: Combretastatin A-4-P: mechanisms of action at tumor level.

Recently, a new series of combretastatin derivatives have been synthesized and evaluated in seven cancer cell lines, exhibiting good anticancer activity [80, 81].

2.2.3. Ombrabulin. Ombrabulin (also known as AC-7700) is a serinamide hydrochloride, synthetic derivative of CA-4-P, which inhibits growth in a large number of drug-resistant animal tumors and carcinogen-induced tumors [39, 82]. Differently from CA-4-P, it does not act directly on the tumor vessels but instead causes constriction of the arterioles, resulting in complete downstream arrest of the blood flow and tumor growth [83]. These effects are obtained at doses half of MTD and 100 times less than that of CA-4-P [84]. Finally, the combination of AC-770 with cisplatin increases the effect of both drugs in murine tumors, with curative effects, and in human tumor xenografts [85]. In 2002, AC-7700 was introduced into phase I clinical trials in the United States and in Europe (AVE8062, *Aventis Pharma*). Recently, ombrabulin in combination with cisplatin was used in a phase III clinical trial for patients with advanced soft-tissue sarcomas after failure of anthracycline and ifosfamide chemotherapy, significantly improving progression-free survival. However, this improvement was not clinically relevant, despite being statistically significant [86].

2.3. Dolastatins. Dolastatins are pseudopeptides isolated from the sea hare *Dolabella auricularia* [50]. Dolastatins 10 and 15 showed antiproliferative activity. These agents induce apoptosis through interaction with tubulin [87]. Dolastatin 10 is a natural peptide able to interfere in microtubule assembly by means of the noncompetitive binding to the Vinca alkaloid site [88]. A phase II trial investigated dolastatin 10 in NSCLC patients. A low response rate was observed, even though a good tolerability was achieved. Myelosuppression was confirmed as the only noteworthy toxicity [89].

Other phase II clinical trials of dolastatin 10 were carried out in patients with metastatic melanoma, advanced colorectal and breast cancers, recurrent platinum-sensitive ovarian carcinoma, and hormone-refractory metastatic prostate adenocarcinoma [90–94]. These studies confirmed the same results previously obtained in terms of tumor response and toxicity. No activity was found in advanced pancreaticobiliary cancers and metastatic soft-tissue sarcomas [95, 96]. For this reason, it was suggested to not pursue the clinical development of this drug in further studies, not only because of its side effects [97] but also because of the low mean survival rate of the treated patients [95].

2.3.1. Soblidotin. Soblidotin (TZT-1027) is a synthetic analog of dolastatin 10 which inhibits the growth of several tumoral cell lines and induces caspase-3-dependent apoptosis. It shows *in vivo* antivascular effects in tumoral models overexpressing VEGF and in murine colon tumors, with an increase in vascular permeability, vessel closure, and widespread hemorrhage. Soblidotin also shows antitumoral activity in vincristine-, docetaxel-, and paclitaxel-resistant tumors, which makes it a potential chemotherapy drug for use in tumors which do not respond to other microtubule inhibitors [98].

The first two European phase I clinical trials identified a recommended dose of soblidotin between 2.4 and 2.7 mg/m^2 for a 3-weekly administration with neutropenia, fatigue, and a reversible peripheral neuropathy as the DLT. Moreover neurological side effects seemed to correlate with previous exposure to other neurotoxic agents such as platinum compounds. No correlation was found with body surface area suggesting possible use of flat dose regimen for next trials [99, 100]. In a Japanese phase I clinical trial MTD of 1.5 mg/m^2 administered on days 1 and 8 in 3-week courses was found [101]. A combination of this drug with carboplatin was also tested. The recommended dose was 1.5 mg/m^2 for soblidotin and AUC 5 for carboplatin and no pharmacokinetics interaction was observed [102]. In NSCLC patients a phase I trial indicated a recommended dose of 4.8 mg/m^2, administered every 3-4 weeks as recommended dose [103].

Phase II clinical investigations suggested activity in advanced or metastatic soft-tissue sarcomas with prior treatment with anthracycline-based chemotherapy. This study confirmed tolerability profile, but objective response was demonstrated in none of the patients [104]. Another phase II trial showed no anticancer activity for soblidotin in NSCLC patients previously treated with platinum-based chemotherapy [105].

2.3.2. Dolastatin 15. Dolastatin 15 is very similar to dolastatin 10. It was demonstrated by chromatography that the binding domain is the same as Vinca alkaloids and antimicrotubule peptides. The site of the binding is not a well-defined locus but a series of overlapping domains [106]. This drug showed an effect on growth and differentiation in leukaemia cell lines [107], induction of apoptosis through Bcl-2 phosphorylation in small cell lung cancer cell lines [108], and G2/M cell cycle arrest in human myeloma cell lines [109]. Romidepsin (Istodax), a dolastatin 15 analog, which also possesses activity as a histone deacetylase inhibitor, was found to be active in cutaneous T-cell lymphoma with a 34% objective response rate and for this it was approved in 2009 [110, 111]. Other two analogues of dolastatin 15 are used in clinical trials: cemadotin and tasidotin.

2.3.3. Cemadotin. Cemadotin (LU103793) exerts its effect by inhibition of microtubule polymerization [112]. This drug is not able to inhibit the binding of vinblastine to tubulin and it can suppress microtubule growth without a significant microtubule depolymerization [113]. This agent was first evaluated in three phase I clinical trials for advanced refractory solid tumors with different schedules. Daily 5-day every 3 weeks schedule identified a recommended dose of 2.5 mg/m^2 per day. It was associated with neutropenia, peripheral edema, and liver function test abnormalities as DLTs. This dose showed lack of prohibitive cardiovascular effects. Acceptable general toxicity profile has allowed prompting phase II trials [114]. Meanwhile, cemadotin was studied for 24-hour intravenous (i.v.) continuous infusion every three weeks. 15 mg/m^2 was the recommended dose for this schedule. Hypertension was highlighted as the DLT, even if its nature remained unclear [115]. Even 5-day continuous intravenous (CIV) infusion was investigated. MTD was 12.5 mg/m^2. There were moderate nonhematologic toxicities and no evidence of the cardiovascular toxicity [116]. Pharmacokinetic analysis in these phase I trials suggested that cardiovascular toxicity may be associated with the magnitude of the peak blood levels of cemadotin or its metabolites, whereas myelotoxicity depends on the duration of time that blood levels exceed a threshold concentration.

The first phase II clinical trial which used this drug at 2.5 mg/m^2 daily 5-day schedule repeated every three weeks obtained clinical activity with durable response in chemotherapy-naïve patients with metastatic melanoma. Toxicity profile previously determined for this schedule was confirmed [117]. In contrast, no activity was observed with the same schedule in metastatic breast cancer patients previously treated with two lines of chemotherapy and in untreated non-small cell cancer patients [118, 119].

2.3.4. Tasidotin. Tasidotin (ILX651) is a third-generation dolastatin 15 analogue that is metabolically stable through its resistance to hydrolysis [120]. It demonstrated *in vitro* cell cycle arrest in the G2 and M phases and inhibition of tubulin polymerization similar to cemadotin and the Vinca alkaloids. It can inhibit the extent of microtubule assembly even at low concentrations [121]. *In vitro* study with MCF7/GFP breast cancer cells and *in vivo* pharmacokinetic analysis through LOX tumors xenografts proposed that tasidotin is converted in tasidotin C-carboxylate, a functionally active intracellular metabolite, 10 to 30 times more potent [122]. Capability of inducing apoptosis was observed in Ewing's sarcoma, rhabdomyosarcoma, synovial sarcoma, and osteosarcoma cell lines. Preclinical xenograft models of pediatric sarcomas showed antitumor activity [123].

Like cemadotin the schedule indicated for clinical use is daily administration for 5 days every 3 weeks. The recommended dose for investigation in phase II trial was 27.3 mg/m^2/day. The toxicity profile was favourable and antitumor activity was found in melanoma patients [124]. The other two schedules were evaluated in phase I trial: 34.4 mg/m^2 d1,3,5 q3 wk and 46.8 mg/m^2 d1,8,15 q4 wk [125, 126]. Tolerability was similar with these schedules.

2.4. Rhizoxin. Rhizoxin (NSC 332598) is a macrolide antitumor antibiotic extracted from a pathogenic fungus, *Rhizopus chinensis*. It is known for its antifungal activity, but it is also studied for cytotoxic activity in a variety of human tumor cell lines, including melanoma, leukaemia, sarcoma, and some human tumor xenografts of melanoma, lung, and breast cancer [127]. The drug can bind to tubulin and inhibits microtubule assembly, blocking the cell cycle at the G2-M phase [128]. It is a more potent cytotoxic compound than vincristine *in vitro*, and, in addition, it showed activity in vincristine-resistant cells [129].

A recommended dose of 2.0 mg/m^2 administered by i.v. bolus injection at 3-week intervals was identified through phase I trial because of its good tolerability with mucositis and neutropenia as the main toxicities [130]. Minimal or absent antitumor activity was found in phase II studies for patients with various advanced solid tumors [131–134]. A pharmacological study demonstrated the rapid and variable elimination of rhizoxin. These data could explain the low levels of systemic toxicity and the little response rates [135]. For this reason, alternative dosage and schedule were studied in phase I trial. A 72-hour continuous i.v. infusion indicated the dose of 1.2 mg/m^2/72 hours as the MTD. The toxicity profile was similar to that obtained with brief infusion, but yet no antitumor responses were found [136].

2.5. D-24851. D-24851 (N-(pyridin-4-yl)-[1-(4-chlorbenzyl)-indol-3-yl]-glyoxyl-amid) is a synthetic compound which has been selected by a cell-based screening assay by ASTA Medica AG, Germany. This drug destabilizes microtubules by interacting with a binding site that does not overlap with those of known microtubule-destabilizing agents like vincristine or colchicine [137, 138].

D-24851 (also known as indibulin) induces Bcl-2 and Bax-mediated apoptosis in both p53^{wt} and p53$^{-/-}$ cell lines [137, 139]. It produces *in vivo* curative effects in rat sarcomas at nontoxic doses, is suitable for oral use, does not give rise to neurotoxic effects at curative doses, unlike vincristine and paclitaxel, and is effective in MDR tumor cells, so that it is an excellent candidate as a chemotherapy agent [137]. In 2004, an LC/MS/MS (liquid chromatography/tandem mass spectrometry) system was proposed for quantitative analysis of D-24851 in human plasma and urine in phase I clinical trials. Indibulin was used in phase I/II clinical trials of patients with advanced solid tumors (metastatic breast cancer) [27, 140, 141]. In a phase I clinical trial indibulin was studied for oral administration once daily for 14 days every 3 weeks in patients with various solid tumors. Pharmacokinetic analysis showed a better tolerability under feeding condition. The recommended dose identified for further studies was 60 mg daily for 14 days. Dose-limiting toxicities were nausea and vomiting, which seemed to be related to solvent lactic acid [141].

Furthermore, the effects of two N-heterocyclic indolyl glyoxylamides derivatives of D-24851, BPR0C259, and BPR0C123 were investigated in NSCLC cells. The obtained results showed that these compounds can suppress the cell proliferation, by inducing p53-independent apoptosis and G2/M phase arrest, and potentially increase radiosensitivity of human lung cancer cells in a p53-independent manner [142].

2.6. Pseudolaric Acid B. Pseudolaric acid B (PAB) is a diterpene isolated from *Pseudolarix kaempferi Gordon* which is able to selectively inhibit the growth of actively proliferating cancer cells. It induces apoptosis through the intrinsic pathway, involving JNK/SAPK and p53. Nevertheless, its cytotoxic effects were found also in p53$^{-/-}$ cell lines, which is interesting for its therapeutic use [143, 144].

It interacts with a different binding site on tubulin compared with those of colchicine and vinblastine [143] and, both *in vitro* and *in vivo*, inhibits endothelial cells proliferation and VEGF-dependent formation of blood vessels. In fact, PAB antagonizes VEGF-mediated antiapoptotic activity by inhibiting the phosphorylation/activation of KDR, the VEGF receptor implicated in mediating this effect [145]. Furthermore, at nontoxic doses, PAB inhibits VEGF secretion from tumor cells by reducing its HIF-1-dependent transcription. PAB, in fact, acts by accelerating the proteasome-mediated degradation of HIF-1α, by means of a mechanism so far unknown [146]. PAB also induces endothelial cell retraction, intercellular gap formation, and actin stress fiber formation, effects which can be attributed to disruption of tubulin cytoskeleton and which contribute to its antiangiogenic action [147]. Moreover, PAB circumvents P-glycoprotein overexpression-induced drug resistance and the doses used are well tolerated and nontoxic and have not proved lethal on tested animals [143]. PAB showed significant inhibitory effect and an additive inhibitory effect in combination with adriamycin on the growth of gastric cancer *in vivo* [148, 149].

2.7. Embellistatin. Embellistatin is a ketone isolated from *Embellisia chlamydospora* which inhibits microtubule polymerization and shows a strong antiangiogenic activity. It inhibits *in vitro* bovine endothelial cells (BAEC) proliferation through p53 and p21 activation, thus inhibiting bFGF-induced formation of vessels. This antiangiogenic activity has been confirmed *in vivo* on murine models. Similar effects have been found in human tumor cell lines, suggesting that it could be suitable for use in the development of new anticancer drugs [150].

2.8. CI-980. CI-980 (mivobulin) acts at the colchicine binding site and it appears to have significantly less vesicant activity than vinblastine [151]. It is a mitotic inhibitor with *in vivo* and *in vitro* activity against murine multidrug-resistant sublines. Its interactions with microtubules *in vitro* are similar to other drugs, but cellular microtubule and mitotic inhibition is more potent [152]. The uptake of CI-980 is not temperature or energy dependent, and its passive diffusion is followed by a significant but largely reversible binding to intracellular or membrane components [153].

Mivobulin was tested in a phase I trial using 24-hour infusion repeated every 3 weeks. MTD was 14.4 mg/m^2. The main toxicities were neutropenia, dose-dependent but not dose-limiting, and early and reversible neurotoxicity characterized by dizziness, headache, loss of coordination, loss of consciousness, nervousness, and other symptoms. Tumor responses and tumor marker reductions were observed in a colon cancer patient and two ovarian cancer patients, respectively [154]. The same toxicity profile was confirmed in other studies [155, 156]. A continuous 72-hour infusion of MTD 4.5 mg/m^2/day every 21 days was associated with reduced neurotoxicity but dose-limiting neutropenia [157]. For this reason, it was used in phase II clinical trials. A similar tolerability profile was found. CI-980 seems inactive in metastatic colorectal carcinoma, advanced soft-tissue sarcomas, treated and untreated melanoma, hormone-refractory prostate cancer, and malignant gliomas [158, 159]. Minimal activity was observed in platinum-refractory advanced epithelial ovarian carcinoma [160].

2.9. T138067. T138067 is a synthetic compound which irreversibly disrupts microtubule assembly by a selective and covalent binding to beta1, beta2, and beta4 isotypes of beta-tubulin at a conserved cysteine residue (Cys-239). Its action results in cell cycle arrest at G2/M and induction of apoptosis. It exhibits cytotoxic activity in tumor cell lines resistant to various antimicrotubule agents (vinblastine, paclitaxel, etc.) and in multidrug-resistant human tumor xenografts [161]. The covalent interaction of T138067 with β-tubulin may be proposed as a new way to overcome MDR. *In vivo* studies showed that this drug can cross the blood-brain barrier in mice, suggesting a possible use for brain tumors [162].

Phase I trials of T138067 were conducted by using a 3-hour infusion of drug given weekly or every 21 days with a recommended dose of 330 mg/m^2 per week. DLTs were neutropenia and neurological effects, consisting of encephalopathy, headache, hearing loss, and ataxia [163, 164]. This weekly dosage was used in two phase II clinical trials for patients with malignant glioma and metastatic colorectal cancer previously treated with irinotecan and 5-fluorouracil, respectively. The good toxicity profile was confirmed in both studies. No clinical activity in terms of antitumor responses was observed in both cases [165, 166].

2.9.1. T900607. T900607 is similar to T138067 for the kind of binding to tubulin in Cys-239 residue, but it is distinguished for a reduced ability to cross the blood-brain barrier.

A phase I trial indicated a recommended dose of 130 mg/m^2 delivered in i.v. infusion over 60 minutes on a 21-day cycle. No objective responses were observed but stable disease was reported in 7/20. Cardiac toxicity is the main drug-related side effect with this schedule. A different schedule consisting of weekly administration of T900607 identified MTD of 100 mg/m^2. This schedule was used in a phase II clinical trial for untreated patients with unresectable hepatocellular carcinoma. It showed good tolerability and moderate activity in some of these patients [167].

2.10. ABT-751. ABT-751, also known as E7010, is a sulfonamide able to impair microtubule formation and inhibit cell growth. Its binding characteristics seem to be different from that of colchicine and Vinca alkaloids. This agent has antiproliferative effects in many tumor cell lines which are drug-resistant due to the P-glycoprotein overexpression [168]. It showed a broad spectrum of activity against a variety of tumors in mice and human tumor xenografts, when administered orally [169]. Beta3 isotype is the preferential binding target. ABT-751-resistant cells were characterized by decreased expression of this tubulin isotype [170]. A warning derived from an *in vivo* study, which shed light on a possible testicular toxicity related to this drug administration in mice. It consisted of loss of seminiferous epithelial cells due to apoptosis of meiotic spermatocytes [171]. This drug selectively reduces tumor blood flow through tumor necrosis, regardless of a direct cytotoxic effect on tumor cells. Negligible is the effect on normal vascular function [172].

In a phase I clinical trial ABT-751 was administered as oral single or 5-day doses. The recommended dose for phase II trials is identified at 320 mg/m^2 for single dose and 200 mg/m^2/day for 5-day repeated dose. Peripheral neuropathy and intestinal paralysis were the DLTs. Gastrointestinal toxicity was dose-dependent but hematological toxicity was not dose-dependent [173]. Pharmacokinetic analysis of this study suggested that activity of ABT-751 may be time-dependent. For this reason a new schedule using a divided dose in order to maintain the blood level of ABT-751 has been formulated. The recommended dose in hematologic malignancies is 175 mg/m^2/day orally for 21 days every 4 weeks [174]. In a phase I trial for a pediatric population of patients with solid tumors ABT-751 was administered orally once daily for 21 days, repeated every 28 days. The MTD obtained for this schedule was 100 mg/m^2/day. DLTs included fatigue, sensory neuropathy, transient hypertension, neutropenia, thrombocytopenia, nausea, vomiting, dehydration, abdominal pain, and constipation [175]. In a phase II clinical trial, 21-day every 28 days schedule at the dose of 200 mg daily was studied in taxane-refractory NSCLC patients. Toxicity was acceptable. Median time to tumor progression and overall survival was 2.1 and 8.4 months, respectively. The objective response rate was 2.9% [176]. The combination of this agent with other cytotoxic drugs was proposed for future clinical studies. A phase IB study investigated clinical antitumor activity of ABT-751 in combination with docetaxel in patients with castration-resistant prostate cancer. Based on the cumulative safety analysis, the recommended phase II dose of ABT-751 is 200 mg daily with docetaxel 60 mg/m^2 for this patient population [177]. Further phases I and II clinical trials were carried out to evaluate activity of ABT-751 in combination with other drugs in advanced or metastatic NSCLC patients [178, 179]. ABT-751 showed adverse effects, although it has the advantage of being orally bioavailable.

3. Microtubule-Stabilizing Agents

Unlike the microtubule-destabilizing agents, there are other compounds that enhance microtubule polymerization. One of the most important classes of microtubule-stabilizing chemotherapy agents is that of taxanes, which target the cytoskeleton and spindle apparatus of tumor cells by binding to the microtubules, thereby disrupting key cellular mechanisms, including mitosis. The first microtubule-stabilizing agent used in anticancer chemotherapy [180] was paclitaxel. Thanks to their peculiar mechanism of action, taxanes are among the most effective chemotherapeutic agents used in the treatment of multiple solid tumors, such as breast, ovarian, lung, and prostate cancers. However, the occurrence of resistance limits treatment options and creates a major challenge for clinicians. Several potential mechanisms of resistance to these drugs have been identified, occurring at different pharmacodynamics levels. Besides the well-known overexpression of Pgp, an ABC transmembrane transporter

TABLE 2: Microtube-stabilizing agents.

Chemical lead	Properties and effects	Clinical trial/status	References
Epothilones	Elevated water solubility, activity versus MDR cell lines, and chemical malleability.	Phase II/III clinical trials in taxane-sensitive solid tumors (breast, lung, and prostate).	[195, 196]
Ixabepilone	Epothilone B analog, superior metabolic stability, and activity versus MDR cell lines.	Approved in 2007 for metastatic breast cancer; several ongoing trials in solid tumors.	[194, 197]
Laulimalide	Activity versus MDR cell lines and angiogenic activity, synergistic with docetaxel.	Preclinical phase.	[199, 201]
Dictyostatin	Activity against MDR cell lines, synergistic with taxol.	Preclinical phase.	[205, 206]

which pumps the drugs out of the tumor cells [8], the altered expression of specific beta-tubulin isotypes, seems to play an important role. Most notably, the increased expression of βIII-tubulin isotype has been associated with resistance to taxanes in several cancers, including ovarian, breast, and lung cancer [9, 181, 182]. It was originally correlated to the qualitative or quantitative modifications of the microtubule complex, which represents the target of such agents, definitively reducing the drug binding affinity [27]. However, the aberrant expression of βIII-tubulin can also interfere with microtubule dynamics, increasing the dynamic instability and counteracting the stabilizing effect of taxanes, with consequences for drug sensitivity/resistance [183]. Recent studies have suggested βIII-tubulin as a prosurvival factor adaptively expressed by cancer cells exposed to microenvironmental stressors, such as hypoxia or deficient nutrient supply [184, 185]. The activation of the βIII-tubulin-dependent pathway in partnership with GTPases, such as guanylate-binding protein 1 (GBP1), is associated with the incorporation of PIM1 into the cytoskeleton of tumor cells, conferring a survival advantage in a hostile microenvironment and ultimately leading to the development of drug resistance [186]. Finally, a multitude of alterations involving the apoptotic signaling pathways downstream the microtubule complex, as well as aberrant expression of microRNA, have been also found in resistant tumors. A better understanding of the mechanism underlying the occurrence of acquired resistance has led to the development of a new class of microtubule-stabilizing agents, including epothilones, discodermolide, sarcodictyins, eleutherobin, and laulimalide, which are more readily modifiable, with different structures but a similar mechanism of action [187] (Table 2). Epothilones, discodermolide, eleutherobins, and sarcodictyins compete with paclitaxel for binding to microtubules and bind at or near the taxane site, whereas laulimalide seems to bind to unique sites on microtubules (Figure 5). Recently, a novel generation of paclitaxel derivatives have been designed, targeting a specific intermediate binding site in the microtubule with differential affinity, depending on the β-tubulin isotype expressed in the tumor. Since βIII-tubulin is overexpressed in the majority of aggressive, resistant tumors, the design of a βIII-tubulin targeted agent was expected to enhance the drug activity, reducing common toxicities. However, none of the new molecules tested in breast cancer cell lines was superior to the currently used taxanes [188].

3.1. Epothilones. Among several classes of microtubule-targeting chemotherapy agents that may maintain activity despite clinical resistance to taxanes, there are the epothilones which have been isolated from the soil bacterium *Solangium cellulosum* and have been studied most extensively in the clinical setting [189]. They induce the formation of an aberrant mitotic spindle, mitotic arrest, and apoptosis [190]. Their greater solubility in water and their activity in MDR cells have made them an alternative to paclitaxel in anticancer treatment [191, 192]. Moreover, their simple structure makes it easy to produce synthetic analogs during the clinical experimentation phase [190]. There are 4 classes of natural epothilones (A, B, C, and D). By means of the selection of resistant or taxane-dependent cells, it has been observed that tubulin β1 plays an important role in epothilone B functionality [193].

Ixabepilone (Ixempra) is a semisynthetic analog of epothilone B, selected because of its greater metabolic stability and its simple preparation. It is more powerful *in vitro* than paclitaxel and also presents cytotoxicity against MDR cells. It causes regression of MDR tumors and is more effective than paclitaxel in a wide spectrum of pediatric tumors [194]. Ixabepilone is currently the only approved epothilone derivative and the most clinically advanced (phases II and III clinical trials), showing efficacy in several patient subgroups and in various stages of breast cancer. This analog is used for the treatment of locally advanced or metastatic breast cancer as monotherapy after failure of a taxane, an anthracycline, and capecitabine, or in combination with capecitabine after failure of a taxane and an anthracycline [195].

A great number of phase II clinical studies of epothilones in cancer treatment have been reported, and significant activity in taxane-sensitive tumor types (such as breast, lung, and prostate cancers) has been observed [12, 17]. Response rates in taxane-refractory metastatic breast cancer are relatively modest, but ixabepilone and patupilone have shown promising efficacy in hormone-refractory metastatic prostate cancer and in taxane-refractory ovarian cancer [196, 197].

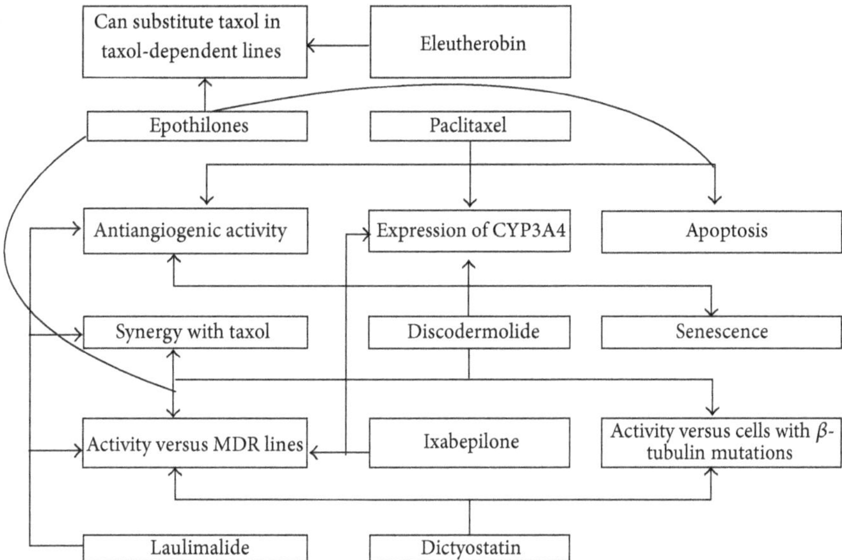

FIGURE 5: Similarities and differences between mechanisms of action and activity of microtubule-stabilizing agents.

3.2. Laulimalide. Laulimalide is a macrolide isolated from marine sponge (*Cacospongia mycofijiensis*) which inhibits cell proliferation, promoting assembly of the microtubules and stabilizing them in a taxol-like way, but at a different binding site located on two adjacent β-tubulin units between tubulin protofilaments of a microtubule [198–200]. This agent is also active in MDR cells which overexpress glycoprotein-P. When administered below cytotoxic doses, the drug prevents blood vessel formation and the VEGF-induced endothelial cell migration [201]. Docetaxel and laulimalide possess a synergic effect in these two processes, whereas they have antagonistic effects towards cell proliferation.

Used at low doses, laulimalide inhibits events downstream of VEGFR-2 activation, such as FAK and paxillin phosphorylation, VEGFR-2/FAK/Hsp90 interaction, and integrin activation. Compared with docetaxel, laulimalide has less effect on the VEGF-induced VEGFR-2/integrin $\alpha5\beta1$ interaction and is more effective with regard to phosphorylated paxillin levels. Furthermore, it inhibits RhoA/integrin $\alpha5\beta1$ association, suggesting that synergic effects of the two drugs might be explained by two different modalities of action.

The low quantities of the drug found in nature, together with its instability caused by its transformation into isolaulimalide, have led to the synthesis of the drug itself and of several analogs. The removal of a electrophilic and/or nucleophilic group, which prevents the substitution process, leads to major functional stability of the drug [202]. In preclinical phase, laulimalide so far showed poor efficacy and systematic toxicity [12]. The macrolide peloruside A shared many of the same properties of laulimalide, including its binding site and synergistic effects with the taxanes [203].

3.3. Dictyostatin. Dictyostatin is a macrolactone produced from sponges which induces *in vitro* tubulin assembly in the same way of paclitaxel but more rapidly. Like discodermolide, this drug possesses an antiproliferative action against paclitaxel-resistant human tumor cells as a result of β-tubulin mutations [204]. Dictyostatin inhibits the binding of discodermolide with microtubules and both drugs are able to inhibit the binding of epothilone B and paclitaxel with microtubules [204]. Several discodermolide/dictyostatin hybrids have been designed and have been found to maintain antiproliferative activities against several taxane-resistant cell lines [205, 206].

3.4. Eleutherobin. Eleutherobin is a glycosylate diterpene isolated from *Eleutherobia sp.* [207], which inhibits cell proliferation stabilizing microtubules. It binds at a site overlapping that of paclitaxel [208]. There is another group of cytotoxic agents, called sarcodictyins, which are structurally and functionally correlated to eleutherobins but not so toxic [209]. A form of cytotoxic diterpene, known as (Z)-sarcodictyine A, has been isolated from *Bellonia albiflora*; this exhibits a high level of toxicity towards human HeLa cells of the cervix [210]. Eleutherobin and the sarcodictyins have not been pursued clinically likely due to their susceptibility to Pgp-mediated transport [211].

4. Clinical Implications

In the last few years, a great amount of efforts has been put into the identification of new microtubule-targeting agents for use in anticancer therapy [212]. These last generation agents are also active in MDR tumors, which are resistant to the traditional antitubulin drugs used in chemotherapy, such as Vinca alkaloids and taxanes. Furthermore, these compounds have shown significant antivascular and antiangiogenic activity, leading to the possibility of using them both as alternatives to or in combination with preexistent drugs, as already indicated in several published studies [213]. A lot of clinical trials were conducted to study microtubule-targeting agents. In particular, epothilones are in advanced phases of clinical development [214, 215]. In cancer therapy, microtubule-targeting agents can target angiogenesis, cell migration, and intracellular trafficking to prevent tumor growth and induce cancer cell apoptosis. These new agents, which impair or enhance tubulin polymerization, can be classified in two groups: natural and synthetic drugs. The natural compounds are derived from different species of uni- and multicellular organisms. To improve their pharmacodynamic and pharmacokinetic features some of these compounds are transformed in semisynthetic molecules. Other agents are produced by a totally synthetic procedure. The great diversity of natural and synthetic compounds capable of interacting with microtubules represents an important source for developing of novel potential anticancer agents. However, the effectiveness of these agents in cancer therapy has been impaired by various side effects and drug resistance. Phase I trials have allowed identifying more tolerable schedules with the most frequent toxicities represented by neutropenia and neurological, cardiovascular, and gastrointestinal effects. The main way of delivery is the i.v. infusion. Oral assumption was studied for the synthetic compounds D-24851 and ABT-751. The most evident efficacy was observed for rhizoxin, above all in NSCLC. For the other agents only minor or no responses were obtained. The identification of new schedules or the transformation in more potent analogues should allow overcoming these hurdles in their clinical advancement.

5. Conclusions

Data obtained up till now have allowed introducing some of these microtubule-targeting drugs into the clinical experimentation phase, whereas others, still in their preclinical phase, represent excellent candidates for a future use in cancer treatment, thus opening new roads towards the development of new, individual, and efficient therapeutic approaches.

Conflict of Interests

The authors declare no conflict of interests.

References

[1] L. G. Wang, X. M. Liu, W. Kreis, and D. R. Budman, "The effect of antimicrotubule agents on signal transduction pathways of apoptosis: a review," *Cancer Chemotherapy and Pharmacology*, vol. 44, no. 5, pp. 355–361, 1999.

[2] J. J. Vicente and L. Wordeman, "Mitosis, microtubule dynamics and the evolution of kinesins," *Experimental Cell Research*, vol. 334, no. 1, pp. 61–69, 2015.

[3] A. Desai and T. J. Mitchison, "Microtubule polymerization dynamics," *Annual Review of Cell and Developmental Biology*, vol. 13, pp. 83–117, 1997.

[4] H. Bringmann, G. Skiniotis, A. Spilker, S. Kandels-Lewis, I. Vernos, and T. Surrey, "A kinesin-like motor inhibits microtubule dynamic instability," *Science*, vol. 303, no. 5663, pp. 1519–1522, 2004.

[5] H. H. Loong and W. Yeo, "Microtubule-targeting agents in oncology and therapeutic potential in hepatocellular carcinoma," *OncoTargets and Therapy*, vol. 7, pp. 575–585, 2014.

[6] K. Klute, E. Nackos, S. Tasaki, D. P. Nguyen, N. H. Bander, and S. T. Tagawa, "Microtubule inhibitor-based antibody-drug conjugates for cancer therapy," *OncoTargets and Therapy*, vol. 7, pp. 2227–2236, 2014.

[7] M. Kavallaris, N. M. Verrills, and B. T. Hill, "Anticancer therapy with novel tubulin-interacting drugs," *Drug Resistance Updates*, vol. 4, no. 6, pp. 392–401, 2001.

[8] K. Katayama, K. Noguchi, and Y. Sugimoto, "Regulations of P-Glycoprotein/ABCB1/MDR1 in human cancer cells," *New Journal of Science*, vol. 2014, Article ID 476974, 10 pages, 2014.

[9] M. Kavallaris, "Microtubules and resistance to tubulin-binding agents," *Nature Reviews Cancer*, vol. 10, no. 3, pp. 194–204, 2010.

[10] C. D. Katsetos, M. M. Herman, and S. J. Mörk, "Class III beta-tubulin in human development and cancer," *Cell Motility and the Cytoskeleton*, vol. 55, no. 2, pp. 77–96, 2003.

[11] M. Kavallaris, A. S. Tait, B. J. Walsh et al., "Multiple microtubule alterations are associated with Vinca alkaloid resistance in human leukemia cells," *Cancer Research*, vol. 61, no. 15, pp. 5803–5809, 2001.

[12] J. J. Field, A. Kanakkanthara, and J. H. Miller, "Microtubule-targeting agents are clinically successful due to both mitotic and interphase impairment of microtubule function," *Bioorganic and Medicinal Chemistry*, vol. 22, no. 18, pp. 5050–5059, 2014.

[13] Y.-M. Liu, H.-L. Chen, H.-Y. Lee, and J.-P. Liou, "Tubulin inhibitors: a patent review," *Expert Opinion on Therapeutic Patents*, vol. 24, no. 1, pp. 69–88, 2014.

[14] M. Moudi, R. Go, C. Y. S. Yien, and M. Nazre, "Vinca alkaloids," *International Journal of Preventive Medicine*, vol. 4, no. 11, pp. 1231–1235, 2013.

[15] R. K. Gregory and I. E. Smith, "Vinorelbine—a clinical review," *British Journal of Cancer*, vol. 82, no. 12, pp. 1907–1913, 2000.

[16] S. Vallo, M. Michaelis, F. Rothweiler et al., "Drug-resistant urothelial cancer cell lines display diverse sensitivity profiles to potential second-line therapeutics," *Translational Oncology*, vol. 8, no. 3, pp. 210–216, 2015.

[17] E. Mukhtar, V. M. Adhami, and H. Mukhtar, "Targeting microtubules by natural agents for cancer therapy," *Molecular Cancer Therapeutics*, vol. 13, no. 2, pp. 275–284, 2014.

[18] G. V. Subbaraju, T. Golakoti, G. M. L. Patterson, and R. E. Moore, "Three new cryptophycins from *Nostoc* sp. GSV 224," *Journal of Natural Products*, vol. 60, no. 3, pp. 302–305, 1997.

[19] C. Weiss, B. Sammet, and N. Sewald, "Recent approaches for the synthesis of modified cryptophycins," *Natural Product Reports*, vol. 30, no. 7, pp. 924–940, 2013.

[20] C. D. Smith and X. Zhang, "Mechanism of action of cryptophycin. Interaction with the Vinca alkaloid domain of tubulin," *Journal of Biological Chemistry*, vol. 271, no. 11, pp. 6192–6198, 1996.

[21] S. L. Mooberry, L. Busquets, and G. Tien, "Induction of apoptosis by cryptophycin 1, a new antimicrotubule agent," *International Journal of Cancer*, vol. 73, no. 3, pp. 440–448, 1997.

[22] D. Panda, V. Ananthnarayan, G. Larson, C. Shih, M. A. Jordan, and L. Wilson, "Interaction of the antitumor compound cryptophycin-52 with tubulin," *Biochemistry*, vol. 39, no. 46, pp. 14121–14127, 2000.

[23] C. Shih and B. A. Teicher, "Cryptophycins: a novel class of potent antimitotic antitumor depsipeptides," *Current Pharmaceutical Design*, vol. 7, no. 13, pp. 1259–1276, 2001.

[24] K. L. Bolduc, S. D. Larsen, and D. H. Sherman, "Efficient, divergent synthesis of cryptophycin unit A analogues," *Chemical Communications*, vol. 48, no. 51, pp. 6414–6416, 2012.

[25] T. H. Corbett, F. A. Valeriote, L. Demchik et al., "Preclinical anticancer activity of cryptophycin-8," *Journal of Experimental Therapeutics and Oncology*, vol. 1, no. 2, pp. 95–108, 1996.

[26] C. Sessa, K. Weigang-Köhler, O. Pagani et al., "Phase I and pharmacological studies of the cryptophycin analogue LY355703 administered on a single intermittent or weekly schedule," *European Journal of Cancer*, vol. 38, no. 18, pp. 2388–2396, 2002.

[27] C. Dumontet and M. A. Jordan, "Microtubule-binding agents: a dynamic field of cancer therapeutics," *Nature Reviews Drug Discovery*, vol. 9, no. 10, pp. 790–803, 2010.

[28] G. D'Agostino, J. del Campo, B. Mellado et al., "A multicenter phase II study of the cryptophycin analog LY355703 in patients with platinum-resistant ovarian cancer," *International Journal of Gynecological Cancer*, vol. 16, no. 1, pp. 71–76, 2006.

[29] R. S. Al-Awar, T. H. Corbett, J. E. Ray et al., "Biological evaluation of cryptophycin 52 fragment A analogues: effect of the multidrug resistance ATP binding cassette transporters on antitumor activity," *Molecular Cancer Therapeutics*, vol. 3, no. 9, pp. 1061–1067, 2004.

[30] M. M. Wagner, D. C. Paul, C. Shih, M. A. Jordan, L. Wilson, and D. C. Williams, "In vitro pharmacology of cryptophycin 52 (LY355703) in human tumor cell lines," *Cancer Chemotherapy and Pharmacology*, vol. 43, no. 2, pp. 115–125, 1999.

[31] J. P. Stevenson, W. Sun, M. Gallagher et al., "Phase I trial of the cryptophycin analogue LY355703 administered as an intravenous infusion on a day 1 and 8 schedule every 21 days," *Clinical Cancer Research*, vol. 8, no. 8, pp. 2524–2529, 2002.

[32] M. J. Edelman, D. R. Gandara, P. Hausner et al., "Phase 2 study of cryptophycin 52 (LY355703) in patients previously treated with platinum based chemotherapy for advanced non-small cell lung cancer," *Lung Cancer*, vol. 39, no. 2, pp. 197–199, 2003.

[33] T. Corbett, L. Polin, P. LoRusso et al., "In Vivo methods for screening and preclinical testing," in *Anticancer Drug Development Guide: Preclinical Screening, Clinical Trials, and Approval*, pp. 99–123, Springer, Berlin, Germany, 2004.

[34] J. Liang, R. E. Moore, E. D. Moher et al., "Cryptophycins-309, 249 and other cryptophycin analogs: preclinical efficacy studies with mouse and human tumors," *Investigational New Drugs*, vol. 23, no. 3, pp. 213–224, 2005.

[35] K. Menon, E. Alvarez, P. Forler et al., "Antitumor activity of cryptophycins: effect of infusion time and combination studies," *Cancer Chemotherapy and Pharmacology*, vol. 46, no. 2, pp. 142–149, 2000.

[36] R. R. Boinpally, L. Polin, S.-L. Zhou et al., "Pharmacokinetics and tissue distribution of cryptophycin 52 (C-52) epoxide and cryptophycin 55 (C-55) chlorohydrin in mice with subcutaneous tumors," *Cancer Chemotherapy and Pharmacology*, vol. 52, no. 1, pp. 25–33, 2003.

[37] J. Griggs, J. C. Metcalfe, and R. Hesketh, "Targeting tumour vasculature: the development of combretastatin A4," *The Lancet Oncology*, vol. 2, no. 2, pp. 82–87, 2001.

[38] G. G. Dark, S. A. Hill, V. E. Prise, G. M. Tozer, G. R. Pettit, and D. J. Chaplin, "Combretastatin A-4, an agent that displays potent and selective toxicity toward tumor vasculature," *Cancer Research*, vol. 57, no. 10, pp. 1829–1834, 1997.

[39] G. M. Tozer, C. Kanthou, C. S. Parkins, and S. A. Hill, "The biology of the combretastatins as tumour vascular targeting agents," *International Journal of Experimental Pathology*, vol. 83, no. 1, pp. 21–38, 2002.

[40] S. M. Nabha, R. M. Mohammad, M. H. Dandashi et al., "Combretastatin-A4 prodrug induces mitotic catastrophe in chronic lymphocytic leukemia cell line independent of caspase activation and poly(ADP-ribose) polymerase cleavage," *Clinical Cancer Research*, vol. 8, no. 8, pp. 2735–2741, 2002.

[41] I. Vitale, A. Antoccia, C. Cenciarelli et al., "Combretastatin CA-4 and combretastatin derivative induce mitotic catastrophe dependent on spindle checkpoint and caspase-3 activation in non-small cell lung cancer cells," *Apoptosis*, vol. 12, no. 1, pp. 155–166, 2007.

[42] D. E. Friesen, K. H. Barakat, V. Semenchenko et al., "Discovery of small molecule inhibitors that interact with γ-tubulin," *Chemical Biology and Drug Design*, vol. 79, no. 5, pp. 639–652, 2012.

[43] C. D. Katsetos, G. Reddy, E. Dráberová et al., "Altered cellular distribution and subcellular sorting of γ-tubulin in diffuse astrocytic gliomas and human glioblastoma cell lines," *Journal of Neuropathology and Experimental Neurology*, vol. 65, no. 5, pp. 465–477, 2006.

[44] V. Caracciolo, L. D'Agostino, E. Dráberová et al., "Differential expression and cellular distribution of gamma-tubulin and betaIII-tubulin in medulloblastomas and human medulloblastoma cell lines," *Journal of Cellular Physiology*, vol. 223, no. 2, pp. 519–529, 2010.

[45] N. F. Maounis, E. Dráberová, E. Mahera et al., "Overexpression of γ-tubulin in non-small cell lung cancer," *Histology and Histopathology*, vol. 27, no. 9, pp. 1183–1194, 2012.

[46] T. Liu, Y. Niu, Y. Yu, Y. Liu, and F. Zhang, "Increased γ-tubulin expression and $P16^{INK4A}$ promoter methylation occur together in preinvasive lesions and carcinomas of the breast," *Annals of Oncology*, vol. 20, no. 3, pp. 441–448, 2009.

[47] M. M. Mita, L. Sargsyan, A. C. Mita, and M. Spear, "Vascular-disrupting agents in oncology," *Expert Opinion on Investigational Drugs*, vol. 22, no. 3, pp. 317–328, 2013.

[48] G. M. Tozer, V. E. Prise, J. Wilson et al., "Combretastatin A-4 phosphate as a tumor vascular-targeting agent: early effects in tumors and normal tissues," *Cancer Research*, vol. 59, no. 7, pp. 1626–1634, 1999.

[49] W. Landuyt, O. Verdoes, D. O. Darius et al., "Vascular targeting of solid tumoursa major 'inverse' volume-response relationship following combretastatin A-4 phosphate treatment of rat rhabdomyosarcomas," *European Journal of Cancer*, vol. 36, no. 14, pp. 1833–1843, 2000.

[50] D. J. Chaplin and S. A. Hill, "The development of combretastatin A4 phosphate as a vascular targeting agent," *International Journal of Radiation Oncology Biology Physics*, vol. 54, no. 5, pp. 1491–1496, 2002.

[51] D. A. Beauregard, S. A. Hill, D. J. Chaplin, and K. M. Brindle, "The susceptibility of tumors to the antivascular drug combretastatin A4 phosphate correlates with vascular permeability," *Cancer Research*, vol. 61, no. 18, pp. 6811–6815, 2001.

[52] C. Kanthou and G. M. Tozer, "The tumor vascular targeting agent combretastatin A-4-phosphate induces reorganization of the actin cytoskeleton and early membrane blebbing in human endothelial cells," *Blood*, vol. 99, no. 6, pp. 2060–2069, 2002.

[53] A. Hussain, M. Steimle, H. Hoppeler, O. Baum, and S. Egginton, "The vascular-disrupting agent combretastatin impairs splitting

and sprouting forms of physiological angiogenesis," *Microcirculation*, vol. 19, no. 4, pp. 296–305, 2012.

[54] L. Vincent, P. Kermani, L. M. Young et al., "Combretastatin A4 phosphate induces rapid regression of tumor neovessels and growth through interference with vascular endothelial-cadherin signaling," *Journal of Clinical Investigation*, vol. 115, no. 11, pp. 2992–3006, 2005.

[55] A. C. Brooks, C. Kanthou, I. H. Cook et al., "The vascular targeting agent combretastatin A-4-phosphate induces neutrophil recruitment to endothelial cells in vitro," *Anticancer Research*, vol. 23, no. 4, pp. 3199–3206, 2003.

[56] G. U. Dachs, A. J. Steele, C. Coralli et al., "Anti-vascular agent Combretastatin A-4-P modulates hypoxia inducible factor-1 and gene expression," *BMC Cancer*, vol. 6, article 280, 2006.

[57] L. Li, A. M. Rojiani, and D. W. Siemann, "Preclinical evaluations of therapies combining the vascular targeting agent combretastatin A-4 disodium phosphate and conventional anticancer therapies in the treatment of Kaposi's sarcoma," *Acta Oncologica*, vol. 41, no. 1, pp. 91–97, 2002.

[58] S. A. Hill, D. J. Chaplin, G. Lewis, and G. M. Tozer, "Schedule dependence of combretastatin A4 phosphate in transplanted and spontaneous tumour models," *International Journal of Cancer*, vol. 102, no. 1, pp. 70–74, 2002.

[59] M. R. Horsman and R. Murata, "Combination of vascular targeting agents with thermal or radiation therapy," *International Journal of Radiation Oncology Biology Physics*, vol. 54, no. 5, pp. 1518–1523, 2002.

[60] K. J. Lankester, R. J. Maxwell, R. B. Pedley et al., "Combretastatin A-4-phosphate effectively increases tumor retention of the therapeutic antibody, 131I-A5B7, even at doses that are sub-optimal for vascular shut-down," *International Journal of Oncology*, vol. 30, no. 2, pp. 453–460, 2007.

[61] H. Wildiers, B. Ahmed, G. Guetens et al., "Combretastatin A-4 phosphate enhances CPT-11 activity independently of the administration sequence," *European Journal of Cancer*, vol. 40, no. 2, pp. 284–290, 2004.

[62] S. L. Young and D. J. Chaplin, "Combretastatin A4 phosphate: Background and current clinical status," *Expert Opinion on Investigational Drugs*, vol. 13, no. 9, pp. 1171–1182, 2004.

[63] J. H. Bilenker, K. T. Flaherty, M. Rosen et al., "Phase I trial of combretastatin A-4 phosphate with carboplatin," *Clinical Cancer Research*, vol. 11, no. 4, pp. 1527–1533, 2005.

[64] M. M. Cooney, T. Radivoyevitch, A. Dowlati et al., "Cardiovascular safety profile of combretastatin a4 phosphate in a single-dose phase I study in patients with advanced cancer," *Clinical Cancer Research*, vol. 10, no. 1, part 1, pp. 96–100, 2004.

[65] D. W. Siemann, D. J. Chaplin, and P. A. Walicke, "A review and update of the current status of the vasculature-disabling agent combretastatin-A4 phosphate (CA4P)," *Expert Opinion on Investigational Drugs*, vol. 18, no. 2, pp. 189–197, 2009.

[66] R. Granata, L. D. Locati, and L. Licitra, "Fosbretabulin for the treatment of anaplastic thyroid cancer," *Future Oncology*, vol. 10, no. 13, pp. 2015–2021, 2014.

[67] A. Dowlati, K. Robertson, M. Cooney et al., "A phase I pharmacokinetic and translational study of the novel vascular targeting agent combretastatin A-4 phosphate on a single-dose intravenous schedule in patients with advanced cancer," *Cancer Research*, vol. 62, no. 12, pp. 3408–3416, 2002.

[68] H. L. Anderson, J. T. Yap, M. P. Miller, A. Robbins, T. Jones, and P. M. Price, "Assessment of pharmacodynamic vascular response in a phase I trial of combretastatin A4 phosphate," *Journal of Clinical Oncology*, vol. 21, no. 15, pp. 2823–2830, 2003.

[69] G. J. S. Rustin, S. M. Galbraith, H. Anderson et al., "Phase I clinical trial of weekly combretastatin A4 phosphate: clinical and pharmacokinetic results," *Journal of Clinical Oncology*, vol. 21, no. 15, pp. 2815–2822, 2003.

[70] J. P. Stevenson, M. Rosen, W. Sun et al., "Phase I trial of the antivascular agent combretastatin A4 phosphate on a 5-day schedule to patients with cancer: magnetic resonance imaging evidence for altered tumor blood flow," *Journal of Clinical Oncology*, vol. 21, no. 23, pp. 4428–4438, 2003.

[71] R. Nallamothu, G. C. Wood, M. F. Kiani, B. M. Moore, F. P. Horton, and L. A. Thoma, "A targeted liposome delivery system for combretastatin A4: formulation optimization through drug loading and in vitro release studies," *PDA Journal of Pharmaceutical Science and Technology*, vol. 60, no. 3, pp. 144–155, 2006.

[72] J. A. Sosa, R. Elisei, B. Jarzab et al., "Randomized safety and efficacy study of fosbretabulin with paclitaxel/carboplatin against anaplastic thyroid carcinoma," *Thyroid*, vol. 24, no. 2, pp. 232–240, 2014.

[73] G. Korpanty, E. Smyth, and D. N. Carney, "Update on anti-angiogenic therapy in non-small cell lung cancer: are we making progress?" *Journal of Thoracic Disease*, vol. 3, no. 1, pp. 19–29, 2011.

[74] J. Hua, Y. Sheng, K. G. Pinney et al., "Oxi4503, a novel vascular targeting agent: effects on blood flow and antitumor activity in comparison to combretastatin A-4 phosphate," *Anticancer Research*, vol. 23, no. 2, pp. 1433–1440, 2003.

[75] Y. Sheng, J. Hua, K. G. Pinney et al., "Combretastatin family member OXI4503 induces tumor vascular collapse through the induction of endothelial apoptosis," *International Journal of Cancer*, vol. 111, no. 4, pp. 604–610, 2004.

[76] K. Staflin, S. Järnum, J. Hua, G. Honeth, P. Kannisto, and M. Lindvall, "Combretastatin A-1 phosphate potentiates the antitumor activity of carboplatin and paclitaxel in a severe combined immunodeficiency disease (SCID) mouse model of human ovarian carcinoma," *International Journal of Gynecological Cancer*, vol. 16, no. 4, pp. 1557–1564, 2006.

[77] I. G. Kirwan, P. M. Loadman, D. J. Swaine et al., "Comparative preclinical pharmacokinetic and metabolic studies of the combretastatin prodrugs combretastatin A4 phosphate and A1 phosphate," *Clinical Cancer Research*, vol. 10, no. 4, pp. 1446–1453, 2004.

[78] D. M. Patterson, M. Zweifel, M. R. Middleton et al., "Phase I clinical and pharmacokinetic evaluation of the vascular-disrupting agent OXi4503 in patients with advanced solid tumors," *Clinical Cancer Research*, vol. 18, no. 5, pp. 1415–1425, 2012.

[79] J. Cummings, M. Zweifel, N. Smith et al., "Evaluation of cell death mechanisms induced by the vascular disrupting agent OXi4503 during a phase I clinical trial," *British Journal of Cancer*, vol. 106, no. 11, pp. 1766–1771, 2012.

[80] S. Kumar, S. Mehndiratta, K. Nepali et al., "Novel indole-bearing combretastatin analogues as tubulin polymerization inhibitors," *Organic and Medicinal Chemistry Letters*, vol. 3, no. 1, article 3, 2013.

[81] S. Zheng, Q. Zhong, M. Mottamal et al., "Design, synthesis, and biological evaluation of novel pyridine-bridged analogues of combretastatin-A4 as anticancer agents," *Journal of Medicinal Chemistry*, vol. 57, no. 8, pp. 3369–3381, 2014.

[82] K. Hori, S. Saito, Y. Sato, and K. Kubota, "Stoppage of blood flow in 3-methylcholanthrene-induced autochthonous primary tumor due to a novel combretastatin A-4 derivative, AC7700,

and its antitumor effect," *Medical Science Monitor*, vol. 7, no. 1, pp. 26–33, 2001.

[83] A. Delmonte and C. Sessa, "AVE8062: a new combretastatin derivative vascular disrupting agent," *Expert Opinion on Investigational Drugs*, vol. 18, no. 10, pp. 1541–1548, 2009.

[84] K. Hori and S. Saito, "Microvascular mechanisms by which the combretastatin A-4 derivative AC7700 (AVE8062) induces tumour blood flow stasis," *British Journal of Cancer*, vol. 89, no. 7, pp. 1334–1344, 2003.

[85] Y. Morinaga, Y. Suga, S. Ehara, K. Harada, Y. Nihei, and M. Suzuki, "Combination effect of AC-7700, a novel combretastatin A-4 derivative, and cisplatin against murine and human tumors in vivo," *Cancer Science*, vol. 94, no. 2, pp. 200–204, 2003.

[86] J. Y. Blay, Z. Pápai, A. W. Tolcher et al., "Ombrabulin plus cisplatin versus placebo plus cisplatin in patients with advanced soft-tissue sarcomas after failure of anthracycline and ifosfamide chemotherapy: a randomised, double-blind, placebo-controlled, phase 3 trial," *The Lancet Oncology*, vol. 16, no. 5, pp. 531–540, 2015.

[87] J. Poncet, "The dolastatins, a family of promising antineoplastic agents," *Current Pharmaceutical Design*, vol. 5, no. 3, pp. 139–162, 1999.

[88] F. Erik and S. Jayaram, "The dolastatins," in *Anticancer Agents from Natural Products*, pp. 263–290, CRC Press, 2nd edition, 2011.

[89] L. M. Krug, V. A. Miller, G. P. Kalemkerian et al., "Phase II study of dolastatin-10 in patients with advanced non-small-cell lung cancer," *Annals of Oncology*, vol. 11, no. 2, pp. 227–228, 2000.

[90] K. Margolin, J. Longmate, T. W. Synold et al., "Dolastatin-10 in metastatic melanoma: a phase II and pharmokinetic trial of the California Cancer Consortium," *Investigational New Drugs*, vol. 19, no. 4, pp. 335–340, 2001.

[91] E. D. Saad, E. H. Kraut, P. M. Hoff et al., "Phase II study of dolastatin-10 as first-line treatment for advanced colorectal cancer," *American Journal of Clinical Oncology: Cancer Clinical Trials*, vol. 25, no. 5, pp. 451–453, 2002.

[92] M. A. Hoffman, J. A. Blessing, and S. S. Lentz, "A phase II trial of dolastatin-10 in recurrent platinum-sensitive ovarian carcinoma: a Gynecologic Oncology Group Study," *Gynecologic Oncology*, vol. 89, no. 1, pp. 95–98, 2003.

[93] U. Vaishampayan, M. Glode, W. Du et al., "Phase II study of dolastatin-10 in patients with hormone-refractory metastatic prostate adenocarcinoma," *Clinical Cancer Research*, vol. 6, no. 11, pp. 4205–4208, 2000.

[94] E. A. Perez, D. W. Hillman, P. A. Fishkin et al., "Phase II trial of dolastatin-10 in patients with advanced breast cancer," *Investigational New Drugs*, vol. 23, no. 3, pp. 257–261, 2005.

[95] H. L. Kindler, P. K. Tothy, R. Wolff et al., "Phase II trials of dolastatin-10 in advanced pancreaticobiliary cancers," *Investigational New Drugs*, vol. 23, no. 5, pp. 489–493, 2005.

[96] M. von Mehren, S. P. Balcerzak, A. S. Kraft et al., "Phase II trial of dolastatin-10, a novel anti-tubulin agent, in metastatic soft tissue sarcomas," *Sarcoma*, vol. 8, no. 4, pp. 107–111, 2004.

[97] T. L. Simmons, E. Andrianasolo, K. McPhail, P. Flatt, and W. H. Gerwick, "Marine natural products as anticancer drugs," *Molecular Cancer Therapeutics*, vol. 4, no. 2, pp. 333–342, 2005.

[98] J. Watanabe, T. Natsume, N. Fujio, K. Miyasaka, and M. Kobayashi, "Induction of apoptosis in human cancer cells by TZT-1027, an antimicrotubule agent," *Apoptosis*, vol. 5, no. 4, pp. 345–353, 2000.

[99] P. Schöffski, B. Thate, G. Beutel et al., "Phase I and pharmacokinetic study of TZT-1027, a novel synthetic dolastatin 10 derivative, administered as a 1-hour intravenous infusion every 3 weeks in patients with advanced refractory cancer," *Annals of Oncology*, vol. 15, no. 4, pp. 671–679, 2004.

[100] M. J. A. de Jonge, A. van der Gaast, A. S. T. Planting et al., "Phase I and pharmacokinetic study of the dolastatin 10 analogue TZT-1027, given on days 1 and 8 of a 3-week cycle in patients with advanced solid tumors," *Clinical Cancer Research*, vol. 11, no. 10, pp. 3806–3813, 2005.

[101] K. Tamura, K. Nakagawa, T. Kurata et al., "Phase I study of TZT-1027, a novel synthetic dolastatin 10 derivative and inhibitor of tubulin polymerization, which was administered to patients with advanced solid tumors on days 1 and 8 in 3-week courses," *Cancer Chemotherapy and Pharmacology*, vol. 60, no. 2, pp. 285–293, 2007.

[102] A. Greystoke, S. Blagden, A. L. Thomas et al., "A phase I study of intravenous TZT-1027 administered on day 1 and day 8 of a three-weekly cycle in combination with carboplatin given on day 1 alone in patients with advanced solid tumours," *Annals of Oncology*, vol. 17, no. 8, pp. 1313–1319, 2006.

[103] J. Horti, E. Juhasz, Z. Monostori, K. Maeda, S. Eckhardt, and I. Bodrogi, "Phase I study of TZT-1027, a novel synthetic dolastatin 10 derivative, for the treatment of patients with non-small cell lung cancer," *Cancer Chemotherapy and Pharmacology*, vol. 62, no. 1, pp. 173–180, 2008.

[104] S. Patel, M. L. Keohan, M. W. Saif et al., "Phase II study of intravenous TZT-1027 in patients with advanced or metastatic soft-tissue sarcomas with prior exposure to anthracycline-based chemotherapy," *Cancer*, vol. 107, no. 12, pp. 2881–2887, 2006.

[105] G. J. Riely, S. Gadgeel, I. Rothman et al., "A phase 2 study of TZT-1027, administered weekly to patients with advanced non-small cell lung cancer following treatment with platinum-based chemotherapy," *Lung Cancer*, vol. 55, no. 2, pp. 181–185, 2007.

[106] Z. Cruz-Monserrate, J. T. Mullaney, P. G. Harran, G. R. Pettit, and E. Hamel, "Dolastatin 15 binds in the vinca domain of tubulin as demonstrated by Hummel-Dreyer chromatography," *European Journal of Biochemistry*, vol. 270, no. 18, pp. 3822–3828, 2003.

[107] K. G. Steube, D. Grunicke, T. Pietsch, S. M. Gignac, G. R. Pettit, and H. G. Drexler, "Dolastatin 10 and dolastatin 15: effects of two natural peptides on growth and differentiation of leukemia cells," *Leukemia*, vol. 6, no. 10, pp. 1048–1053, 1992.

[108] M. A. Ali, R. Rosati, G. R. Pettit, and G. P. Kalemkerian, "Dolastatin 15 induces apoptosis and BCL-2 phosphorylation in small cell lung cancer cell lines," *Anticancer Research*, vol. 18, no. 2, pp. 1021–1026, 1998.

[109] M. Sato, M. Sagawa, T. Nakazato, Y. Ikeda, and M. Kizaki, "A natural peptide, dolastatin 15, induces G2/M cell cycle arrest and apoptosis of human multiple myeloma cells," *International Journal of Oncology*, vol. 30, no. 6, pp. 1453–1459, 2007.

[110] R. L. Piekarz, R. Frye, M. Turner et al., "Phase II multi-institutional trial of the histone deacetylase inhibitor romidepsin as monotherapy for patients with cutaneous T-cell lymphoma," *Journal of Clinical Oncology*, vol. 27, no. 32, pp. 5410–5417, 2009.

[111] S. E. Bates, R. Eisch, A. Ling et al., "Romidepsin in peripheral and cutaneous T-cell lymphoma: mechanistic implications from clinical and correlative data," *British Journal of Haematology*, vol. 170, no. 1, pp. 96–109, 2015.

[112] M. de Arruda, C. A. Cocchiaro, C. M. Nelson et al., "LU103793 (NSC D-669356): a synthetic peptide that interacts with microtubules and inhibits mitosis," *Cancer Research*, vol. 55, no. 14, pp. 3085–3092, 1995.

[113] M. A. Jordan, D. Walker, M. de Arruda, T. Barlozzari, and D. Panda, "Suppression of microtubule dynamics by binding of cemadotin to tubulin: possible mechanism for its antitumor action," *Biochemistry*, vol. 37, no. 50, pp. 17571–17578, 1998.

[114] M. A. Villalona-Calero, S. D. Baker, L. Hammond et al., "Phase I and pharmacokinetic study of the water-soluble dolastatin 15 analog LU103793 in patients with advanced solid malignancies," *Journal of Clinical Oncology*, vol. 16, no. 8, pp. 2770–2779, 1998.

[115] K. Mross, W. E. Berdel, H. H. Fiebig, R. Velagapudi, I. M. von Broen, and C. Unger, "Clinical and pharmacologic phase I study of Cemadotin-HCl (LU103793), a novel antimitotic peptide, given as 24-hour infusion in patients with advanced cancer. A study of the Arbeitsgemeinschaft Internistische Onkologie (AIO) Phase I Group and Arbeitsgruppe Pharmakologie in der Onkologie und Haematologie (APOH) Group of the German Cancer Society," *Annals of Oncology*, vol. 9, no. 12, pp. 1323–1330, 1998.

[116] J. G. Supko, T. J. Lynch, J. W. Clark et al., "A phase I clinical and pharmacokinetic study of the dolastatin analogue cemadotin administered as a 5-day continuous intravenous infusion," *Cancer Chemotherapy and Pharmacology*, vol. 46, no. 4, pp. 319–328, 2000.

[117] J. Smyth, M. E. Boneterre, J. Schellens et al., "Activity of the dolastatin analogue, LU103793, in malignant melanoma," *Annals of Oncology*, vol. 12, no. 4, pp. 509–511, 2001.

[118] P. Kerbrat, V. Dieras, N. Pavlidis, A. Ravaud, J. Wanders, and P. Fumoleau, "Phase II study of LU 103793 (dolastatin analogue) in patients with metastatic breast cancer," *European Journal of Cancer*, vol. 39, no. 3, pp. 317–320, 2003.

[119] R. S. Marks, D. L. Graham, J. A. Sloan et al., "A phase II study of the dolastatin 15 analogue LU 103793 in the treatment of advanced non-small-cell lung cancer," *American Journal of Clinical Oncology*, vol. 26, no. 4, pp. 336–337, 2003.

[120] K. K. Rasila and C. Verschraegen, "Tasidotin HCI genzyme," *Current Opinion in Investigational Drugs*, vol. 6, no. 6, pp. 631–638, 2005.

[121] R. Bai, M. C. Edler, P. L. Bonate et al., "Intracellular activation and deactivation of tasidotin, an analog of dolastatin 15: correlation with cytotoxicity," *Molecular Pharmacology*, vol. 75, no. 1, pp. 218–226, 2009.

[122] A. Ray, T. Okouneva, T. Manna et al., "Mechanism of action of the microtubule-targeted antimitotic depsipeptide tasidotin (formerly ILX651) and its major metabolite tasidotin C-carboxylate," *Cancer Research*, vol. 67, no. 8, pp. 3767–3776, 2007.

[123] V. Garg, W. Zhang, P. Gidwani, M. Kim, and E. A. Kolb, "Preclinical analysis of tasidotin HCl in Ewing's sarcoma, rhabdomyosarcoma, synovial sarcoma, and osteosarcoma," *Clinical Cancer Research*, vol. 13, no. 18, part 1, pp. 5446–5454, 2007.

[124] S. Ebbinghaus, E. Rubin, E. Hersh et al., "A phase I study of the dolastatin-15 analogue tasidotin (ILX651) administered intravenously daily for 5 consecutive days every 3 weeks in patients with advanced solid tumors," *Clinical Cancer Research*, vol. 11, no. 21, pp. 7807–7816, 2005.

[125] C. Cunningham, L. J. Appleman, M. Kirvan-Visovatti et al., "Phase I and pharmacokinetic study of the dolastatin-15 analogue tasidotin (ILX651) administered intravenously on days 1, 3, and 5 every 3 weeks in patients with advanced solid tumors," *Clinical Cancer Research*, vol. 11, no. 21, pp. 7825–7833, 2005.

[126] A. C. Mita, L. A. Hammond, P. L. Bonate et al., "Phase I and pharmacokinetic study of tasidotin hydrochloride (ILX651), a third-generation dolastatin-15 analogue, administered weekly for 3 weeks every 28 days in patients with advanced solid tumors," *Clinical Cancer Research*, vol. 12, no. 17, pp. 5207–5215, 2006.

[127] H. R. Hendriks, J. Plowman, D. P. Berger et al., "Preclinical antitumour activity and animal toxicology studies of rhizoxin, a novel tubulin-interacting agent," *Annals of Oncology*, vol. 3, no. 9, pp. 755–763, 1992.

[128] A. E. Prota, K. Bargsten, J. F. Diaz et al., "A new tubulin-binding site and pharmacophore for microtubule-destabilizing anticancer drugs," *Proceedings of the National Academy of Sciences of the United States of America*, vol. 111, no. 38, pp. 13817–13821, 2014.

[129] T. Tsuruo, T. Oh-hara, H. Iida et al., "Rhizoxin, a macrocyclic lactone antibiotic, as a new antitumor agent against human and murine tumor cells and the vincristine-resistant sublines," *Cancer Research*, vol. 46, no. 1, pp. 381–385, 1986.

[130] D. Bissett, M. A. Graham, A. Setanoians et al., "Phase I and pharmacokinetic study of rhizoxin," *Cancer Research*, vol. 52, no. 10, pp. 2894–2898, 1992.

[131] D. J. Kerr, G. J. Rustin, S. B. Kaye et al., "Phase II trials of rhizoxin in advanced ovarian, colorectal and renal cancer," *British Journal of Cancer*, vol. 72, no. 5, pp. 1267–1269, 1995.

[132] A. R. Hanauske, G. Catimel, S. Aamdal et al., "Phase II clinical trials with rhizoxin in breast cancer and melanoma. The EORTC early clinical trials group," *British Journal of Cancer*, vol. 73, no. 3, pp. 397–399, 1996.

[133] J. Verweij, J. Wanders, T. Gil et al., "Phase II study of rhizoxin in squamous cell head and neck cancer," *British Journal of Cancer*, vol. 73, no. 3, pp. 400–402, 1996.

[134] S. Kaplan, A. R. Hanauske, N. Pavlidis et al., "Single agent activity of rhizoxin in non-small-cell lung cancer: a phase II trial of the EORTC early clinical trials group," *British Journal of Cancer*, vol. 73, no. 3, pp. 403–405, 1996.

[135] H. L. McLeod, L. S. Murray, J. Wanders et al., "Multicentre phase II pharmacological evaluation of rhizoxin. Eortc early clinical studies (ECSG)/pharmacology and molecular mechanisms (PAMM) groups," *British Journal of Cancer*, vol. 74, no. 12, pp. 1944–1948, 1996.

[136] A. W. Tolcher, C. Aylesworth, J. Rizzo et al., "A phase I study of rhizoxin (NSC 332598) by 72-hour continuous intravenous infusion in patients with advanced solid tumors," *Annals of Oncology*, vol. 11, no. 3, pp. 333–338, 2000.

[137] G. Bacher, B. Nickel, P. Emig et al., "D-24851, a novel synthetic microtubule inhibitor, exerts curative antitumoral activity *in vivo*, shows efficacy toward multidrug-resistant tumor cells, and lacks neurotoxicity," *Cancer Research*, vol. 61, no. 1, pp. 392–399, 2001.

[138] A. Wienecke and G. Bacher, "Indibulin, a novel microtubule inhibitor, discriminates between mature neuronal and nonneuronal tubulin," *Cancer Research*, vol. 69, no. 1, pp. 171–177, 2009.

[139] H. Ito, T. Kanzawa, S. Kondo, and Y. Kondo, "Microtubule inhibitor D-24851 induces p53-independent apoptotic cell death in malignant glioma cells through Bcl-2 phosphorylation and Bax translocation," *International Journal of Oncology*, vol. 26, no. 3, pp. 589–596, 2005.

[140] E. Stokvis, L. G. A. H. Nan-Offeringa, M. Ouwehand et al., "Quantitative analysis of D-24851, a novel anticancer agent, in human plasma and urine by liquid chromatography coupled

with tandem mass spectrometry," *Rapid Communications in Mass Spectrometry*, vol. 18, no. 13, pp. 1465–1471, 2004.

[141] I. E. L. M. Kuppens, P. O. Witteveen, M. Schot et al., "Phase I dose-finding and pharmacokinetic trial of orally administered indibulin (D-24851) to patients with solid tumors," *Investigational New Drugs*, vol. 25, no. 3, pp. 227–235, 2007.

[142] T.-H. Huang, S.-J. Chiu, P.-H. Chiang et al., "Antiproliferative effects of N-heterocyclic indolyl glyoxylamide derivatives on human lung cancer cells," *Anticancer Research*, vol. 31, no. 10, pp. 3407–3415, 2011.

[143] V. K. W. Wong, P. Chiu, S. S. M. Chung et al., "Pseudolaric acid B, a novel microtubule-destabilizing agent that circumvents multidrug resistance phenotype and exhibits antitumor activity *in vivo*," *Clinical Cancer Research*, vol. 11, no. 16, pp. 6002–6011, 2005.

[144] X. Gong, M. Wang, S.-I. Tashiro, S. Onodera, and T. Ikejima, "Involvement of JNK-initiated p53 accumulation and phosphorylation of p53 in pseudolaric acid B induced cell death," *Experimental and Molecular Medicine*, vol. 38, no. 4, pp. 428–434, 2006.

[145] W.-F. Tan, X.-W. Zhang, M.-H. Li et al., "Pseudolarix acid B inhibits angiogenesis by antagonizing the vascular endothelial growth factor-mediated anti-apoptotic effect," *European Journal of Pharmacology*, vol. 499, no. 3, pp. 219–228, 2004.

[146] M.-H. Li, Z.-H. Miao, W.-F. Tan et al., "Pseudolaric acid B inhibits angiogenesis and reduces hypoxia-inducible factor 1alpha by promoting proteasome-mediated degradation," *Clinical Cancer Research*, vol. 10, no. 24, pp. 8266–8274, 2004.

[147] Y.-G. Tong, X.-W. Zhang, M.-Y. Geng et al., "Pseudolarix acid B, a new tubulin-binding agent, inhibits angiogenesis by interacting with a novel binding site on tubulin," *Molecular Pharmacology*, vol. 69, no. 4, pp. 1226–1233, 2006.

[148] Q. Sun and Y. Li, "The inhibitory effect of pseudolaric acid B on gastric cancer and multidrug resistance via Cox-2/PKC-α/P-gp pathway," *PLoS ONE*, vol. 9, no. 9, Article ID e107830, 2014.

[149] F. Yu, K. Li, S. Chen, Y. Liu, and Y. Li, "Pseudolaric acid B circumvents multidrug resistance phenotype in human gastric cancer SGC7901/ADR cells by downregulating Cox-2 and P-gp expression," *Cell Biochemistry and Biophysics*, vol. 71, no. 1, pp. 119–126, 2015.

[150] H. J. Jung, J. S. Shim, H. B. Lee et al., "Embellistatin, a microtubule polymerization inhibitor, inhibits angiogenesis both in vitro and in vivo," *Biochemical and Biophysical Research Communications*, vol. 353, no. 2, pp. 376–380, 2007.

[151] A. Kiselyov, K. V. Balakin, S. E. Tkachenko, N. Savchuk, and A. V. Ivachtchenko, "Recent progress in discovery and development of antimitotic agents," *Anti-Cancer Agents in Medicinal Chemistry*, vol. 7, no. 2, pp. 189–208, 2007.

[152] C. de Ines, D. Leynadier, I. Barasoain et al., "Inhibition of microtubules and cell cycle arrest by a new 1-deaza-7,8- dihydropteridine antitumor drug, CI 980, and by its chiral isomer, NSC 613863 ," *Cancer Research*, vol. 54, no. 1, pp. 75–84, 1994.

[153] K. E. Hook, S. A. Przybranowski, and W. R. Leopold, "Cellular transport of CI-980," *Investigational New Drugs*, vol. 14, no. 4, pp. 341–347, 1996.

[154] N. T. Sklarin, C. D. Lathia, L. Benson et al., "A phase I trial and pharmacokinetic evaluation of CI-980 in patients with advanced solid tumors," *Investigational New Drugs*, vol. 15, no. 3, pp. 235–246, 1997.

[155] C. A. Meyers, A. P. Kudelka, C. A. Conrad, C. K. Gelke, W. Grove, and R. Pazdur, "Neurotoxicity of CI-980, a novel mitotic inhibitor," *Clinical Cancer Research*, vol. 3, no. 3, pp. 419–422, 1997.

[156] M. L. Bernstein, S. Baruchel, S. Devine et al., "Phase I and pharmacokinetic study of CI-980 in recurrent pediatric solid tumor cases: a Pediatric Oncology Group study," *Journal of Pediatric Hematology/Oncology*, vol. 21, no. 6, pp. 494–500, 1999.

[157] E. K. Rowinsky, G. S. Long, D. A. Noe et al., "Phase I and pharmacological study of CI-980, a novel synthetic antimicrotubule agent," *Clinical Cancer Research*, vol. 3, no. 3, pp. 401–407, 1997.

[158] R. Pazdur, C. Meyers, E. Diaz-Canton et al., "Phase II trial of intravenous CI-980 (NSC 370147) in patients with metastatic colorectal carcinoma. Model for prospective evaluation of neurotoxicity," *American Journal of Clinical Oncology: Cancer Clinical Trials*, vol. 20, no. 6, pp. 573–576, 1997.

[159] J. P. Thomas, T. Moore, E. H. Kraut, S. P. Balcerzak, S. Galloway, and D. D. Vandre, "A phase II study of CI-980 in previously untreated extensive small cell lung cancer: an Ohio State University phase II research consortium study," *Cancer Investigation*, vol. 20, no. 2, pp. 192–198, 2002.

[160] A. P. Kudelka, A. Hasenburg, C. F. Verschraegen et al., "Phase II study of i.v. CI-980 in patients with advanced platinum refractory epithelial ovarian carcinoma," *Anti-Cancer Drugs*, vol. 9, no. 5, pp. 405–409, 1998.

[161] B. Shan, J. C. Medina, E. Santha et al., "Selective, covalent modification of β-tubulin residue Cys-239 by T138067, an antitumor agent with in vivo efficacy against multidrug-resistant tumors," *Proceedings of the National Academy of Sciences of the United States of America*, vol. 96, no. 10, pp. 5686–5691, 1999.

[162] S. M. Rubenstein, V. Baichwal, H. Beckmann et al., "Hydrophilic, pro-drug analogues of T138067 are efficacious in controlling tumor growth in vivo and show a decreased ability to cross the blood brain barrier," *Journal of Medicinal Chemistry*, vol. 44, no. 22, pp. 3599–3605, 2001.

[163] R. C. Donehower, G. Schwartz, A. C. Wolf et al., "Phase I and pharmacokinetic study of T138067 administered as a weekly 3-hour infusion," *Clinical Cancer Research*, vol. 6, pp. 4578s–4579s, 2000.

[164] G. Schwartz, E. K. Rowinsky, P. O'Dwyer et al., "Phase I and pharmacokinetic study of T138067, a synthetic microtubule depolymerizing agent, administered as a 3-hour infusion daily x 5 every 3 weeks," *Clinical Cancer Research*, vol. 6, pp. 4579s–4579s, 2000.

[165] S. Kirby, S. Z. Gertler, W. Mason et al., "Phase 2 study of T138067-sodium in patients with malignant glioma: trial of the National Cancer Institute of Canada Clinical Trials Group," *Neuro-Oncology*, vol. 7, no. 2, pp. 183–188, 2005.

[166] J. D. Berlin, A. Venook, E. Bergsland, M. Rothenberg, A. C. Lockhart, and L. Rosen, "Phase II trial of T138067, a novel microtubule inhibitor, in patients with metastatic, refractory colorectal carcinoma," *Clinical Colorectal Cancer*, vol. 7, no. 1, pp. 44–47, 2008.

[167] K. A. Gelmon, K. Belanger, D. Soulieres et al., "A phase I study of T900607 given once every 3 weeks in patients with advanced refractory cancers; National Cancer Institute of Canada Clinical Trials Group (NCIC-CTG) IND 130," *Investigational New Drugs*, vol. 23, no. 5, pp. 445–453, 2005.

[168] K. Yoshimatsu, A. Yamaguchi, H. Yoshino, N. Koyanagi, and K. Kitoh, "Mechanism of action of E7010, an orally active sulfonamide antitumor agent: inhibition of mitosis by binding to the colchicine site of tubulin," *Cancer Research*, vol. 57, no. 15, pp. 3208–3213, 1997.

[169] Y. Funahashi, N. Koyanagi, and K. Kitoh, "Effect of E7010 on liver metastasis and life span of syngeneic C57BL/6 mice bearing orthotopically transplanted murine Colon 38 tumor," *Cancer Chemotherapy and Pharmacology*, vol. 47, no. 2, pp. 179–184, 2001.

[170] Y. Iwamoto, K. Nishio, H. Fukumoto, K. Yoshimatsu, M. Yamakido, and N. Saijo, "Preferential binding of E7010 to murine β3-tubulin and decreased β3-tubulin in E7010-resistant cell lines," *Japanese Journal of Cancer Research*, vol. 89, no. 9, pp. 954–962, 1998.

[171] K. Hayakawa, T. Tashiro, K. Sato et al., "Collaborative work to evaluate toxicity on male reproductive organs by repeated dose studies in rats: 17) testicular toxicity of e7010, a sulfonamide tubulin polymerization inhibitor," *Journal of Toxicological Sciences*, vol. 25, pp. 173–178, 2000.

[172] Y. Nihei, M. Suzuki, A. Okano et al., "Evaluation of antivascular and antimitotic effects of tubulin binding agents in solid tumor therapy," *Japanese Journal of Cancer Research*, vol. 90, no. 12, pp. 1387–1395, 1999.

[173] K. Yamamoto, K. Noda, A. Yoshimura, M. Fukuoka, K. Furuse, and H. Niitani, "Phase I study of E7010," *Cancer Chemotherapy and Pharmacology*, vol. 42, no. 2, pp. 127–134, 1998.

[174] K. W. L. Yee, A. Hagey, S. Verstovsek et al., "Phase 1 study of ABT-751, a novel microtubule inhibitor, in patients with refractory hematologic malignancies," *Clinical Cancer Research*, vol. 11, no. 18, pp. 6615–6624, 2005.

[175] E. Fox, J. M. Maris, B. C. Widemann et al., "A phase I study of ABT-751, an orally bioavailable tubulin inhibitor, administered daily for 21 days every 28 days in pediatric patients with solid tumors," *Clinical Cancer Research*, vol. 14, no. 4, pp. 1111–1115, 2008.

[176] A. M. Mauer, E. E. W. Cohen, P. C. Ma et al., "A phase II study of ABT-751 in patients with advanced non-small cell lung cancer," *Journal of Thoracic Oncology*, vol. 3, no. 6, pp. 631–636, 2008.

[177] J. Michels, S. L. Ellard, L. Le et al., "A phase IB study of ABT-751 in combination with docetaxel in patients with advanced castration-resistant prostate cancer," *Annals of Oncology*, vol. 21, no. 2, pp. 305–311, 2010.

[178] C. M. Rudin, A. Mauer, M. Smakal et al., "Phase I/II study of pemetrexed with or without ABT-751 in advanced or metastatic non-small-cell lung cancer," *Journal of Clinical Oncology*, vol. 29, no. 8, pp. 1075–1082, 2011.

[179] T. Ma, A. D. Fuld, J. R. Rigas et al., "A phase i trial and in vitro studies combining ABT-751 with carboplatin in previously treated non-small cell lung cancer patients," *Chemotherapy*, vol. 58, no. 4, pp. 321–329, 2012.

[180] M. C. Wani, H. L. Taylor, M. E. Wall, P. Coggon, and A. T. McPhail, "Plant antitumor agents. VI. The isolation and structure of taxol, a novel antileukemic and antitumor agent from Taxus brevifolia," *Journal of the American Chemical Society*, vol. 93, no. 9, pp. 2325–2327, 1971.

[181] M. Kavallaris, D. Y.-S. Kuo, C. A. Burkhart et al., "Taxol-resistant epithelial ovarian tumors are associated with altered expression of specific beta-tubulin isotypes," *The Journal of Clinical Investigation*, vol. 100, no. 5, pp. 1282–1293, 1997.

[182] J. A. McCarroll, P. P. Gan, M. Liu, and M. Kavallaris, "BetaIII-tubulin is a multifunctional protein involved in drug sensitivity and tumorigenesis in non-small cell lung cancer," *Cancer Research*, vol. 70, no. 12, pp. 4995–5003, 2010.

[183] P. P. Gan, J. A. McCarroll, S. T. Po'Uha, K. Kamath, M. A. Jordan, and M. Kavallaris, "Microtubule dynamics, mitotic arrest, and apoptosis: drug-induced differential effects of βIII-tubulin," *Molecular Cancer Therapeutics*, vol. 9, no. 5, pp. 1339–1348, 2010.

[184] A. L. Parker, M. Kavallaris, and J. A. McCarroll, "Microtubules and their role in cellular stress in cancer," *Frontiers in Oncology*, vol. 4, article 153, 2014.

[185] G. Raspaglio, F. Filippetti, S. Prislei et al., "Hypoxia induces class III beta-tubulin gene expression by HIF-1α binding to its 3' flanking region," *Gene*, vol. 409, no. 1-2, pp. 100–108, 2008.

[186] M. De Donato, M. Mariani, L. Petrella et al., "Class III beta-tubulin and the cytoskeletal gateway for drug resistance in ovarian cancer," *Journal of Cellular Physiology*, vol. 227, no. 3, pp. 1034–1041, 2012.

[187] I. Ojima, S. Chakravarty, T. Inoue et al., "A common pharmacophore for cytotoxic natural products that stabilize microtubules," *Proceedings of the National Academy of Sciences of the United States of America*, vol. 96, no. 8, pp. 4256–4261, 1999.

[188] M. St. George, A. T. Ayoub, A. Banerjee et al., "Designing and testing of novel taxanes to probe the highly complex mechanisms by which taxanes bind to microtubules and cause cytotoxicity to cancer cells," *PLoS ONE*, vol. 10, no. 6, Article ID e0129168, 2015.

[189] G. Höfle, N. Bedorf, H. Steinmetz, D. Schomburg, K. Gerth, and H. Reichenbach, "Epothilone A and B—novel 16-membered macrolides with cytotoxic activity: isolation, crystal structure, and conformation in solution," *Angewandte Chemie*, vol. 35, no. 13-14, pp. 1567–1569, 1996.

[190] M. Wartmann and K.-H. Altmann, "The biology and medicinal chemistry of epothilones," *Current Medicinal Chemistry: Anti-Cancer Agents*, vol. 2, no. 1, pp. 123–148, 2002.

[191] K.-H. Altmann, G. Bold, G. Caravatti, A. Flörsheimer, V. Guagnano, and M. Wartmann, "Synthesis and biological evaluation of highly potent analogues of epothilones B and D," *Bioorganic and Medicinal Chemistry Letters*, vol. 10, no. 24, pp. 2765–2768, 2000.

[192] D. M. Bollag, P. A. McQueney, J. Zhu et al., "Epothilones, a new class of microtubule-stabilizing agents with a taxol- like mechanism of action," *Cancer Research*, vol. 55, no. 11, pp. 2325–2333, 1995.

[193] C.-P. H. Yang, P. Verdier-Pinard, F. Wang et al., "A highly epothilone B-resistant A549 cell line with mutations in tubulin that confer drug dependence," *Molecular Cancer Therapeutics*, vol. 4, no. 6, pp. 987–995, 2005.

[194] J. K. Peterson, C. Tucker, E. Favours et al., "In vivo evaluation of ixabepilone (BMS247550), a novel epothilone B derivative, against pediatric cancer models," *Clinical Cancer Research*, vol. 11, part 1, no. 19, pp. 6950–6958, 2005.

[195] C. F. Brogdon, F. Y. Lee, and R. M. Canetta, "Development of other microtubule-stabilizer families: the epothilones and their derivatives," *Anticancer Drugs*, vol. 25, no. 5, pp. 599–609, 2014.

[196] J. M. G. Larkin and S. B. Kaye, "Epothilones in the treatment of cancer," *Expert Opinion on Investigational Drugs*, vol. 15, no. 6, pp. 691–702, 2006.

[197] K. De Geest, J. A. Blessing, R. T. Morris et al., "Phase II clinical trial of ixabepilone in patients with recurrent or persistent platinum- and taxane-resistant ovarian or primary peritoneal cancer: a gynecologic oncology group study," *Journal of Clinical Oncology*, vol. 28, no. 1, pp. 149–153, 2010.

[198] S. L. Mooberry, G. Tien, A. H. Hernandez, A. Plubrukarn, and B. S. Davidson, "Laulimalide and isolaulimalide, new paclitaxel-like microtubule-stabilizing agents," *Cancer Research*, vol. 59, no. 3, pp. 653–660, 1999.

[199] D. E. Pryor, A. O'Brate, G. Bilcer et al., "The microtubule stabilizing agent laulimalide does not bind in the taxoid site, kills cells resistant to paclitaxel and epothilones, and may not require its epoxide moiety for activity," *Biochemistry*, vol. 41, no. 29, pp. 9109–9115, 2002.

[200] C. D. Churchill, M. Klobukowski, and J. A. Tuszynski, "The unique binding mode of laulimalide to two tubulin protofilaments," *Chemical Biology & Drug Design*, vol. 86, no. 2, pp. 190–199, 2015.

[201] H. Lu, J. Murtagh, and E. L. Schwartz, "The microtubule binding drug laulimalide inhibits vascular endothelial growth factor-induced human endothelial cell migration and is synergistic when combined with docetaxel (taxotere)," *Molecular Pharmacology*, vol. 69, no. 4, pp. 1207–1215, 2006.

[202] P. A. Wender, M. K. Hilinski, N. Soldermann, and S. L. Mooberry, "Total synthesis and biological evaluation of 11-desmethyllaulimalide, a highly potent simplified laulimalide analogue," *Organic Letters*, vol. 8, no. 7, pp. 1507–1510, 2006.

[203] A. E. Prota, K. Bargsten, P. T. Northcote et al., "Structural basis of microtubule stabilization by laulimalide and peloruside A," *Angewandte Chemie*, vol. 53, no. 6, pp. 1621–1625, 2014.

[204] C. Madiraju, M. C. Edler, E. Hamel et al., "Tubulin assembly, taxoid site binding, and cellular effects of the microtubule-stabilizing agent dictyostatin," *Biochemistry*, vol. 44, no. 45, pp. 15053–15063, 2005.

[205] L. L. Vollmer, M. Jiménez, D. P. Camarco et al., "A simplified synthesis of novel dictyostatin analogues with *in vitro* activity against epothilone B-resistant cells and antiangiogenic activity in zebrafish embryos," *Molecular Cancer Therapeutics*, vol. 10, no. 6, pp. 994–1006, 2011.

[206] K. R. Brunden, N. M. Gardner, M. J. James et al., "MT-stabilizer, dictyostatin, exhibits prolonged brain retention and activity: potential therapeutic implications," *ACS Medicinal Chemistry Letters*, vol. 4, no. 9, pp. 886–889, 2013.

[207] T. Lindel, P. R. Jensen, W. Fenical et al., "ChemInform abstract: eleutherobin, a new cytotoxin that mimics paclitaxel (taxol) by stabilizing microtubules," *ChemInform*, vol. 28, no. 51, 2010.

[208] B. H. Long, J. M. Carboni, A. J. Wasserman et al., "Eleutherobin, a novel cytotoxic agent that induces tubulin polymerization, is similar to paclitaxel (Taxol)," *Cancer Research*, vol. 58, no. 6, pp. 1111–1115, 1998.

[209] E. Hamel, B. W. Day, J. H. Miller et al., "Synergistic effects of peloruside A and laulimalide with taxoid site drugs, but not with each other, on tubulin assembly," *Molecular Pharmacology*, vol. 70, no. 5, pp. 1555–1564, 2006.

[210] Y. Nakao, S. Yoshida, S. Matsunaga, and N. Fusetani, "(Z)-sarcodictyin A, a new highly cytotoxic diterpenoid from the soft coral *Bellonella albiflora*," *Journal of Natural Products*, vol. 66, no. 4, pp. 524–527, 2003.

[211] A. L. Risinger, F. J. Giles, and S. L. Mooberry, "Microtubule dynamics as a target in oncology," *Cancer Treatment Reviews*, vol. 35, no. 3, pp. 255–261, 2009.

[212] R. Kaur, G. Kaur, R. K. Gill, R. Soni, and J. Bariwal, "Recent developments in tubulin polymerization inhibitors: an overview," *European Journal of Medicinal Chemistry*, vol. 87, pp. 89–124, 2014.

[213] Z. Liu, P. Xu, T. Wu, and W. Zeng, "Microtubule-targeting anticancer agents from marine natural substance," *Anti-Cancer Agents in Medicinal Chemistry*, vol. 14, no. 3, pp. 409–417, 2014.

[214] J. Cortes and J. Baselga, "Targeting the microtubules in breast cancer beyond taxanes: the epothilones," *Oncologist*, vol. 12, no. 3, pp. 271–280, 2007.

[215] L. Vahdat, "Ixabepilone: a novel antineoplastic agent with low susceptibility to multiple tumor resistance mechanisms," *Oncologist*, vol. 13, no. 3, pp. 214–221, 2008.

8

Melatonin Modulates Endoplasmic Reticulum Stress and Akt/GSK3-Beta Signaling Pathway in a Rat Model of Renal Warm Ischemia Reperfusion

Kaouther Hadj Ayed Tka,[1] Asma Mahfoudh Boussaid,[1] Mohamed Amine Zaouali,[1] Rym Kammoun,[2] Mohamed Bejaoui,[3] Sonia Ghoul Mazgar,[2] Joan Rosello Catafau,[3] and Hassen Ben Abdennebi[1]

[1] *Unit of Molecular Biology and Anthropology Applied to Development and Health (UR12ES11), Faculty of Pharmacy, University of Monastir, rue Avicenne, 5000 Monastir, Tunisia*
[2] *Laboratory of Histology and Embryology, Faculty of Dental Medicine, University of Monastir, rue Avicenne, 5000 Monastir, Tunisia*
[3] *Unit of Experimental Hepatic Ischemia-Reperfusion, Institute of Biomedical Investigations, Higher Council of Scientific Investigations, 08036 Barcelona, Spain*

Correspondence should be addressed to Hassen Ben Abdennebi; hbenabdennebi@yahoo.fr

Academic Editor: Monica Cantile

Melatonin (Mel) is widely used to attenuate ischemia/reperfusion (I/R) injury in several organs. Nevertheless, the underlying mechanisms remain unclear. This study was conducted to explore the effect of Mel on endoplasmic reticulum (ER) stress, Akt and MAPK cascades after renal warm I/R. Eighteen Wistar rats were randomized into three groups: Sham, I/R, and Mel + I/R. The ischemia period was 60 min followed by 120 min of reperfusion. Mel (10 mg/kg) was administrated 30 min prior to ischemia. The creatinine clearance, MDA, LDH levels, and histopathological changes were evaluated. In addition, Western blot was performed to study ER stress and its downstream apoptosis as well as phosphorylation of Akt, GSK-3β, VDAC, ERK, and P38. Mel decreased cytolysis and lipid peroxidation and improved renal function and morphology compared to I/R group. Parallely, it significantly reduced the ER stress parameters including GRP 78, p-PERK, XBP 1, ATF 6, CHOP, and JNK. Simultaneously, p-Akt level was significantly enhanced and its target molecules GSK-3β and VDAC were inhibited. Furthermore, the ERK and P38 phosphorylation were evidently augmented after Mel administration in comparison to I/R group. In conclusion, Mel improves the recovery of renal function by decreasing ER stress and stimulating Akt pathway after renal I/R injury.

1. Introduction

Ischemia/reperfusion (I/R) injury remains a major problem encountered in vascular surgery, organ procurement, and transplantation and can lead to structural and functional cell damage [1]. In renal disease, I/R represents the most frequent cause of acute kidney injury [2]. The last years have witnessed a burgeoning development in our understanding of the molecular pathways involved in I/R and various mechanisms have been proposed to explain the origins of tissue injury. It is generally believed that reactive oxygen species (ROS) are key mediators of the I/R induced damage to the kidney. The excessive formation of ROS activates a host of signaling pathways including endoplasmic reticulum (ER) stress and cell death [3].

ER plays an important role in synthesis and maturation of proteins, biosynthesis of lipids, regulation of calcium, and maintenance of cell homeostasis [4]. Disturbances such as hypoxia, glucose starvation, and oxidative stress may lead to ER disorder which can provoke ER stress. Subsequently, a signal transduction cascade termed the unfolded protein response (UPR) is induced [3]. UPR is an adaptive response that aims to restore normal ER function. It comprises three branches: activating transcription factor (ATF) 6, inositol-requiring enzyme (IRE) 1, and RNA activated protein kinase-(PKR-) like ER kinase (PERK). These proteins are normally held in inactive states in ER membranes by binding to an intra-ER chaperone, the glucose regulated protein (GRP) 78. In response to stress, GRP78 dissociates from ER membrane to bind misfolding proteins freeing in this way, ATF6, IRE1, and PERK, which initiate signal transduction processes in order to reestablish ER homeostasis [5]. Though UPR normally helps in cell survival by removing misfolded proteins, an elevated and prolonged ER stress level can cause cell death [4]. Consequently, this can contribute to a diverse range of pathophysiological events including acute and chronic renal disease [3]. Hence, therapeutic strategies targeting ER stress and its downstream apoptosis might have the potential to provide a powerful tool in an attempt to reduce I/R injury.

Melatonin (N-acetyl-5-methoxytryptamine) (Mel) is a hormone secreted by pineal gland and is mainly responsible for controlling circadian cycle [6]. It is a highly lipophilic molecule that crosses cell membranes to easily reach subcellular compartments [7]. This small amphiphilic molecule and its metabolites are likewise potent scavengers of ROS [8]. Apart from this, Mel was shown to possess anti-inflammatory and antiapoptotic actions [9, 10] as well as other remarkable cell protective properties [11, 12]. The efficacy of Mel treatment to reduce renal I/R injury has been well-documented. However, experiments evaluating the underlying mechanisms of action, particularly its effect on ER stress and apoptosis, are lacking. Therefore, the present study was made to investigate whether Mel can influence the I/R induced ER stress in the kidney and whether its renoprotective effect implicates the activation of prosurival signaling cascades including Akt/GSK-3β pathway.

2. Materials and Methods

2.1. Animals and Experimental Groups. Male Wistar rats weighing 200–250 g were used in this study. Animals were maintained at constant temperature (23 ± 2°C) with a 12 h light-dark cycle and free access to water and food. All procedures were carried out in accordance with the European Union Regulations (Directive 86/609/CEE) for animal experiments. Animals were randomly assigned into the following experimental groups, each containing 6 rats.

I/R Group. Rats had been injected with a vehicle solution consisting of ethanol and NaCl 0.9% mixture (the final concentration of ethanol was 1%) intraperitoneally (i.p.) 30 min before they were subjected to bilateral renal ischemia. The renal pedicles were occluded for 60 min using nontraumatic vascular clips, followed by reperfusion for 120 min [13].

Mel + I/R Group. This group was the same as I/R group but animals were treated with Mel (10 mg/kg i.p.) 30 min before renal clamping [6, 14]. Mel (Sigma Chemical, St. Louis, MO, USA) was dissolved in the vehicle solution.

Sham Group. Animals were subjected to the same surgical procedure described above but were not subjected to renal I/R and did not receive any treatment.

2.2. Surgery and Experimental Protocols. As described previously by Mahfoudh-Boussaid et al. [13] rats were anesthetized through an intraperitoneal injection of ketamine hydrochloride (50 mg/kg) and xylazine (10 mg/kg) and placed onto a thermostatically controlled warm board to maintain body temperature at 37°C. After performing a midline laparotomy, the renal pedicles containing the renal artery, vein, and nerves supplying each kidney were carefully isolated and occluded. After clamps' removal, the bladder was cannulated for the collection of urine during the last 30 min of reperfusion and the abdomen was closed in layers. The mean arterial pressure was measured using a pressure transducer (Pression Monitor BP-1; Pression Instruments, Sarasota, FL) connected to the right carotid artery. The left jugular vein was cannulated for mannitol (10%) and heparin (50 U/mL) infusion (Minipuls 3 peristaltic pump, Gilson, France).

At the end of the reperfusion period, rats were euthanized and blood samples were collected via carotid artery. Simultaneously, both kidneys were harvested and weighed. Plasma, urine, and tissue samples were immediately kept at −80°C for biochemical and Western blot analyses.

2.3. Assessment of Renal Function. The renal function was evaluated during the last thirty minutes of reperfusion by calculating the creatinine clearance using the standard formula:

$$\text{Creatinine clearance } (\mu\text{L/min/g of weight}) = \frac{(\text{Creat U} * \text{V})}{\text{Creat P}}. \tag{1}$$

Creat U is the creatinine concentration in urine (μmol/L), V is urine flow rate (μL/min/g of weight), and Creat P is the creatinine concentration in plasma (μmol/L).

Serum and urine creatinine concentrations were measured spectrophotometrically at 490 nm by the Jaffé kinetic reaction (BioMerieux Kit, France).

2.4. LDH Assay. The activity of lactate dehydrogenase (LDH) in the plasma was quantified using LDH assay kit (Spinreact, Spain).

2.5. Lipid Peroxidation Assessment. Malondialdehyde (MDA) is an end product of peroxidation of cell membrane lipids caused by oxygen derived free radicals. It was measured in renal tissue using the thiobarbiturate reaction at 530 nm [15].

2.6. Renal Histology. Samples from all kidneys were fixed in 10% formalin solution and processed for histology by hematoxylin and eosin (H&E) staining. Histological evaluations were performed using light microscopy at a magnification of 40–400 by an experienced renal pathologist without having knowledge about the treatment groups. Morphological changes from the whole cross-sectional area of the kidneys were assessed and a semiquantitative analysis of histological

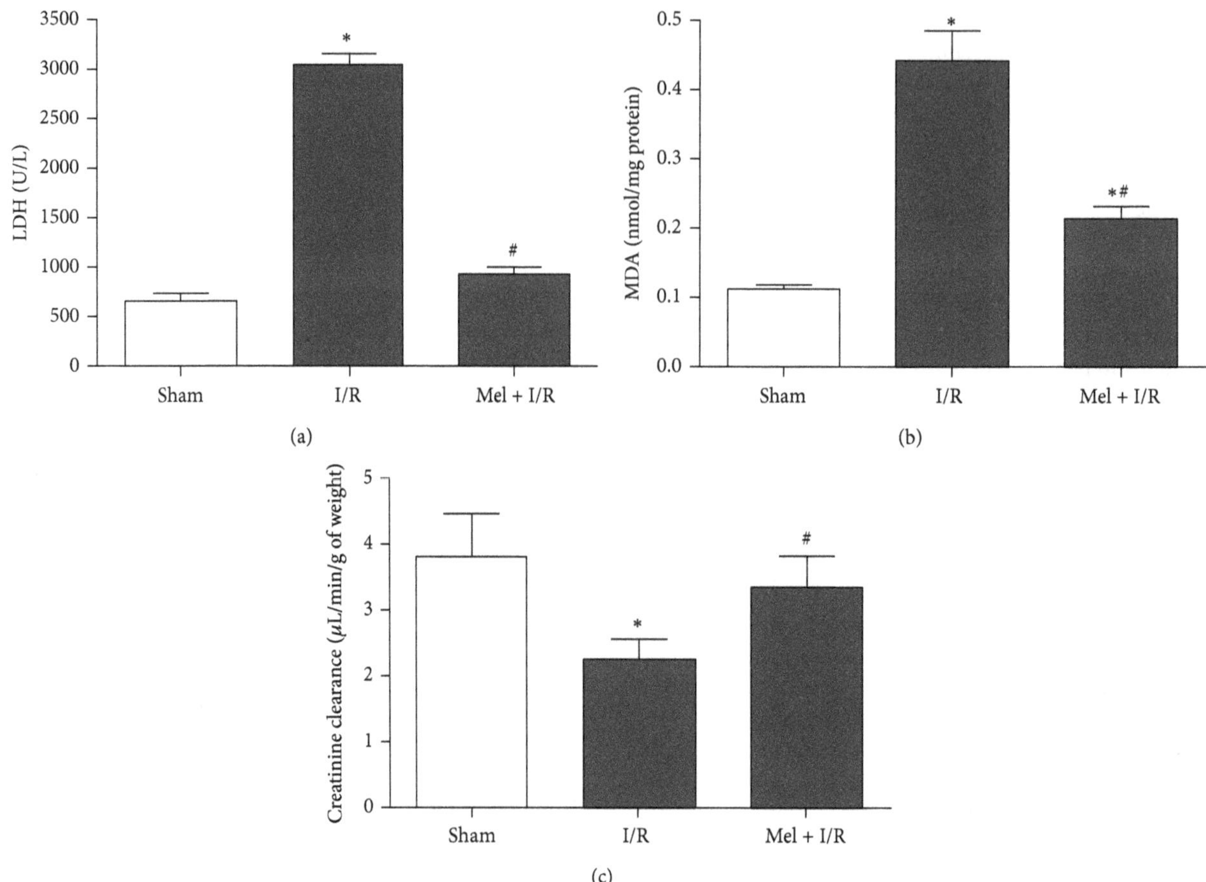

FIGURE 1: Evaluation of lactate dehydrogenase activity in plasma (a), malondialdehyde concentration in tissue (b), and creatinine clearance (c). Results are expressed as mean ± SEM ($n = 6$ for each group). $^*p < 0.05$ versus Sham. $^\# p < 0.05$ versus I/R.

damage was conducted. A score from 0 to 4 was given to assess necrosis according to the method of Jablonski et al. [16] as the following: 0, normal; 1, necrosis of individual cells; 2, necrosis of all cells in adjacent proximal convoluted tubule (PCT), with survival of surrounding tubules; 3, necrosis confined to distal third PCT with bands of necrosis extending across inner cortex; 4, necrosis of all three segments of PCT.

2.7. Western Blot Analysis. Western blot analysis was performed as previously described by Mahfoudh-Boussaid et al. [13]. Briefly, tissue samples from the kidneys were prepared with lysis buffer (150 mM NaCl, 50 mM Tris HCl, 1 mM DTT, 50 mM NaF, 1 mM PMSF, 1 mM EDTA, 1 mM EGTA, 0.1 mM orthovanadate, 0.05% Triton X-100, and 2% protease inhibitor cocktails). Protein concentrations were determined according to the Bradford method. Protein extracts (50 μg/lane) were then separated by SDS-PAGE electrophoresis and transferred to polyvinylidene fluoride membranes. Membranes were immunoblotted with antibodies directed against GRP78, total and p-PERK, XBP-1, ATF6α and CHOP (Santa Cruz Biotechnology, Santa Cruz, CA, USA), β-actin (Sigma chemical, St. Louis, MO), total and p-JNK, total and p-Akt, total and p-GSK-3β, total and p-ERK, total and p-P38 (Cell Signalling Technology Inc., Beverly, MA, USA), and total and p-VDAC. The bands were visualized using an enhanced chemiluminescence kit (Bio Rad Laboratories, Hercules, CA, USA). The values were obtained by densitometric scanning and the Quantity One software program (Bio Rad Laboratories, Hercules, CA, USA).

2.8. Statistical Analysis. The data are presented as means ± SEM. Statistical analysis was performed using one-way ANOVA, followed by Newman-Keuls multiple comparisons. $p < 0.05$ was considered statistically significant.

3. Results

Cytolysis was assessed by measuring the activity of LDH in the plasma (Figure 1(a)). Level of LDH increased from baseline values of 654 ± 81 U/L in Sham to 3044 ± 109 U/L in the I/R group ($p < 0.05$). This rise was significantly lower after Mel treatment with values of 930 ± 69 U/L compared to I/R group ($p < 0.05$).

Then, we examined the protective effect of Mel on lipid peroxidation (Figure 1(b)). Renal I/R significantly increased MDA level to 0.44 ± 0.04 nmol/mg protein compared with nontreated group where MDA concentration was 0.11 ± 0.01 nmol/mg protein ($p < 0.05$). After the administration

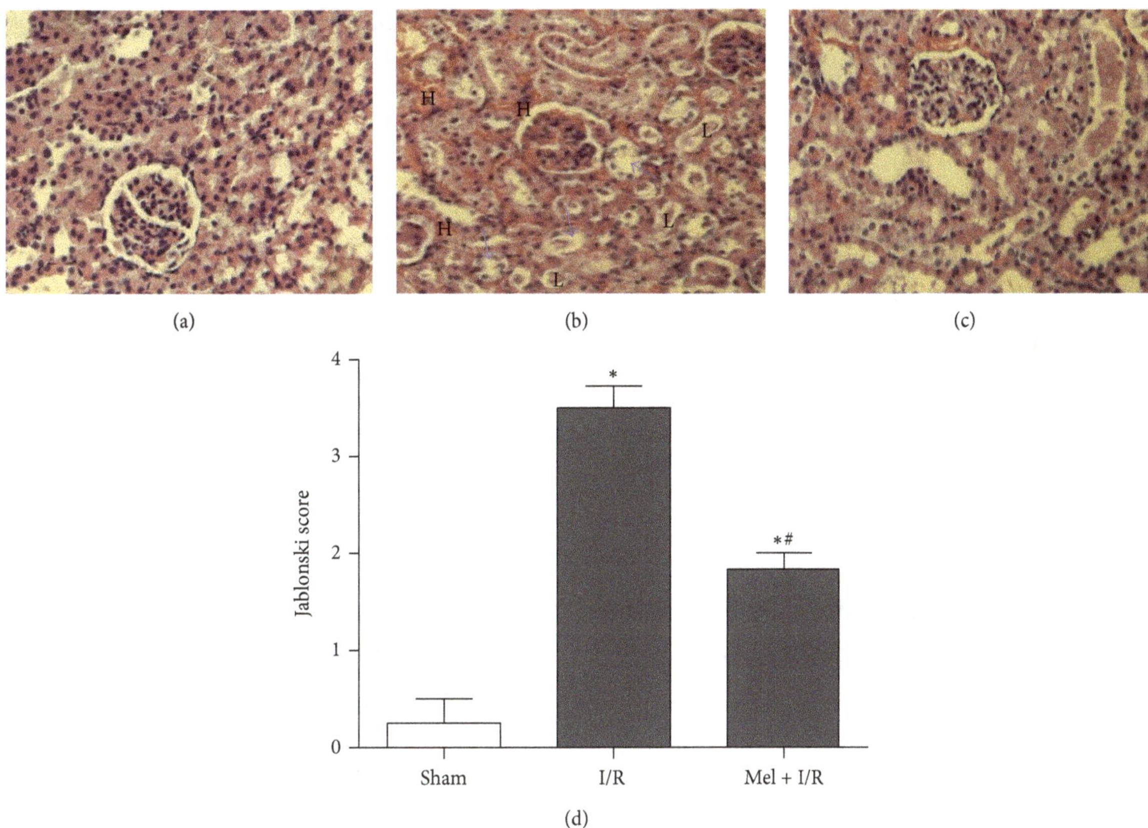

FIGURE 2: Representative histological photographs of kidney tissues from Sham (a), I/R (b), and Mel + I/R (c) groups (H&E) ×400. Semiquantitative assessment of renal necrosis among the different experimental groups using the Jablonski score (d). The arrows denote brush border loss, "H" denotes hemorrhage, and "L" denotes nuclei loss. Results are expressed as mean ± SEM ($n = 6$ for each group). $^{*}p < 0.05$ versus Sham. $^{\#}p < 0.05$ versus I/R.

of Mel, we observed a significant drop in this parameter reaching 0.21 ± 0.02 nmol/mg protein regarding I/R group ($p < 0.05$).

Renal function was evaluated comparing the variation of creatinine clearance among the three groups (Figure 1(c)). Kidneys from I/R group revealed a dramatic decrease in creatinine clearance with values of 2.3 ± 0.2 μL/min/g of weight compared to those of Sham group with values of 3.8 ± 0.4 μL/min/g of weight ($p < 0.05$). An important functional recovery was observed subsequently to Mel administration prior to renal I/R and the creatinine clearance was 3.36 ± 0.3 μL/min/g of weight ($p < 0.05$) in comparison to I/R group.

Histological changes were in keeping with biochemical parameters of renal injury. The morphological examination of all groups confirmed that there was renal impairment by severe tubular damage after I/R (Figure 2(b)) compared to Sham group (Figure 2(a)). These features included brush border loss, nuclear condensation, cell swelling, a consistent loss of nuclei, and hemorrhage. Renal sections obtained from rats pretreated with Mel demonstrated a marked reduction of the histological features of renal injury (Figure 2(c)). The Jablonski score (Figure 2(d)) in the I/R rat kidney was 3.5 ± 0.2 versus 0.33 ± 0.33 in the Sham kidney ($p < 0.05$). In comparison to the I/R group, treatment with Mel significantly attenuated this score reaching 1.83 ± 0.2 ($p < 0.05$).

Afterwards, we examined the possible involvement of Mel in modulating ER stress induced by I/R injury. Different ER stress pathways were explored (Figure 3). Renal I/R significantly increased the relative amounts of GRP78, p-PERK, XBP-1, and ATF6α from Sham values of 98 ± 23, 56 ± 20, 62 ± 4, and 73 ± 61, respectively, to 391 ± 8, 205 ± 24, 305 ± 51, and 160 ± 21, respectively ($p < 0.05$). Interestingly, rats undergoing Mel treatment demonstrated a lower level activation of these ER stress parameters in the kidney compared with their respective I/R groups with values of 227 ± 2, 105 ± 13, 102 ± 22, and 66 ± 5, respectively ($p < 0.05$).

In line with this, we studied the ER stress induced apoptosis by focusing on two proapoptotic parameters. As indicated in Figure 4, renal I/R markedly enhanced the activation of CHOP as well as JNK and the respective values were 228 ± 33 and 307 ± 1 versus 161 ± 5 and 203 ± 17 for Sham ($p < 0.05$). In contrast, this effect was significantly attenuated by preischemic Mel administration and values dropped to 123 ± 13 and 267 ± 4, respectively, in comparison to I/R solely.

Furthermore, we evaluated the influence of Mel on some targets of the Akt signaling pathway. We found that Akt

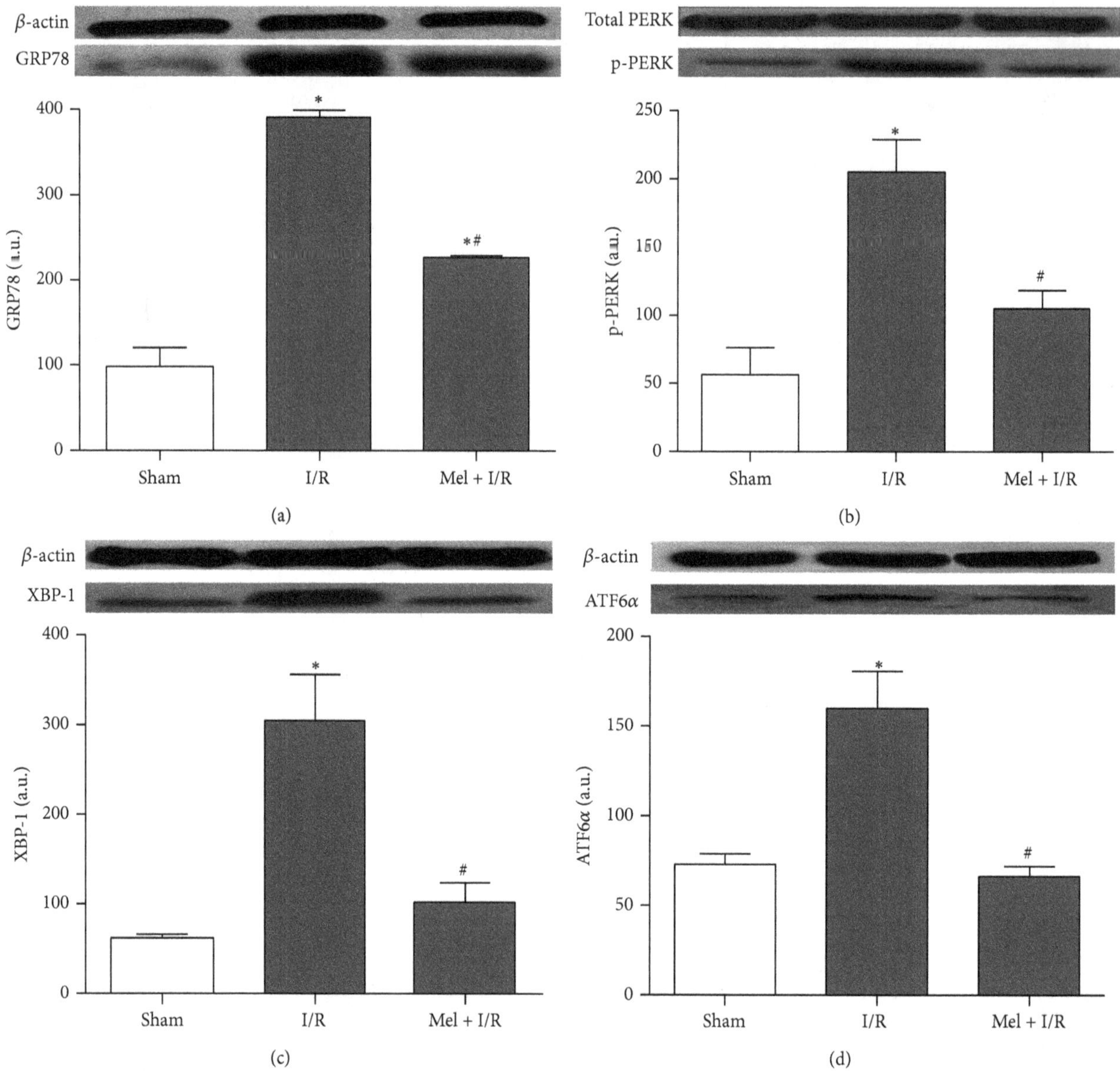

FIGURE 3: Western blot of GRP 78 (a), total and phosphorylated PERK (b), XBP-1 (c), and ATF6α (d). β-actin was used as a loading control. One representative blot of six independent experiments is shown at the top whereas densitometric analysis is shown at the bottom. Results are expressed as mean ± SEM. $^{*}p < 0.05$ versus Sham. $^{\#}p < 0.05$ versus I/R.

phosphorylation was notably decreased after I/R to values of 93 ± 4 when compared to Sham where p-Akt level was 141 ± 18 ($p < 0.05$) (Figure 5(a)). This was concomitant with a significant increase in phosphorylated VDAC amount with values of 486 ± 31 as compared to Sham with values of 366 ± 35 ($p < 0.05$) (Figure 5(c)). However, there was no obvious difference between I/R and sham groups regarding GSK-3β phosphorylation (Figure 5(b)). The administration of Mel was found to reverse the effect of I/R on Akt and VDAC phosphorylation and thus p-Akt level rose noticeably reaching 145 ± 8 whereas p-VDAC amount dropped until 375 ± 9 ($p < 0.05$). Moreover, GSK-3β phosphorylation was significantly enhanced after Mel treatment to 354 ± 36 in comparison to both other groups.

To finally explore the relevance of Mel treatment on some MAPK features after exposure to renal I/R, immunoblot analyses of ERK and P38 in kidneys from all groups were performed. As shown in Figure 6, our results reveal no significant differences between Sham and I/R groups regarding phosphorylated ERK and P38 levels. However, Mel treatment resulted in a significant enhancement in these two parameters with values of 123 ± 14 and 314 ± 18, respectively ($p < 0.05$), in comparison to both other groups.

The effect of Mel without I/R (Sham + Mel group) was assessed regarding the parameters used in the present study (data not shown) and no significant differences were recorded in comparison with Sham group. Therefore, only the data obtained in Sham group were mentioned in this study and

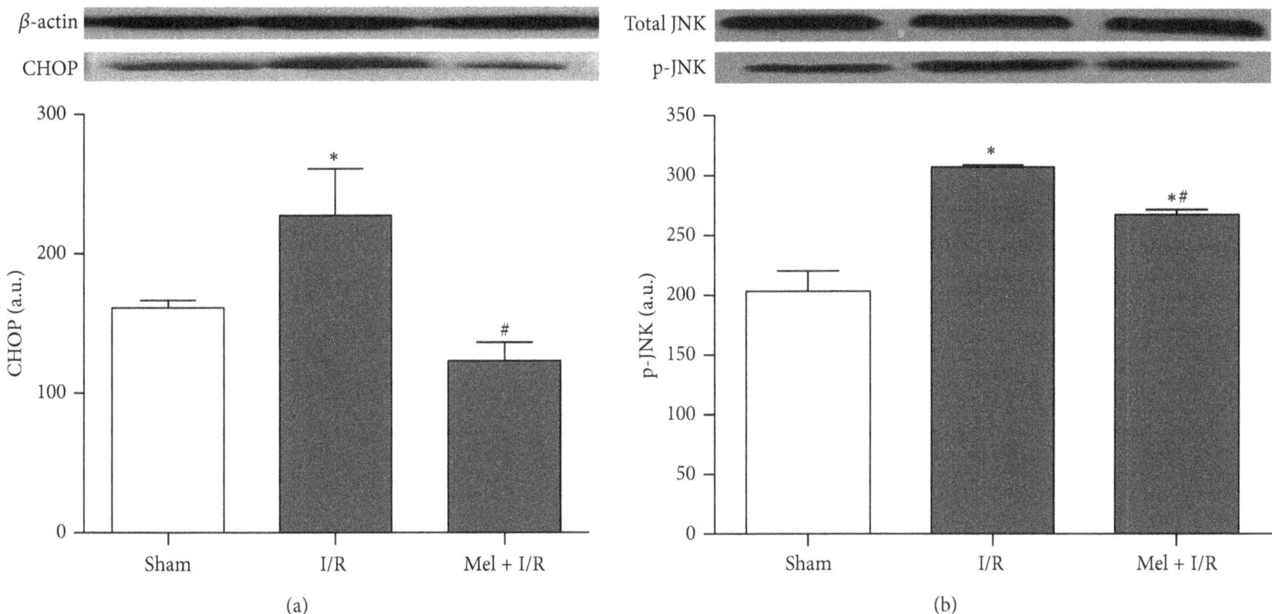

FIGURE 4: Western blot of CHOP (a) and total and phosphorylated JNK (b). The β-actin was used as a loading control. One representative blot of six independent experiments is shown at the top whereas densitometric analysis is shown at the bottom. Results are expressed as mean ± SEM. $^{*}p < 0.05$ versus Sham. $^{\#}p < 0.05$ versus I/R.

were used for further statistical analysis with I/R and Mel + I/R groups.

4. Discussion

Renal I/R injury remains an unresolved problem that has immediate and deleterious effects in both native and transplanted kidneys [17]. The pathogenesis underlying I/R injury is complex involving different molecular pathways which are not fully understood [18]. The present study investigated the effects of Mel on renal I/R injury. We showed that preischemic treatment with Mel significantly reduced I/R induced injury in the rat kidney. The current data are in agreement with previous results demonstrating that Mel pretreatment protects against warm I/R injury in a variety of tissues and organs, including the heart [19], liver [20], brain [21], and kidney [22, 23].

In addition to the decrease of I/R induced elevation in lipid peroxidation, our findings revealed that Mel reduced LDH release and improved the creatinine clearance of ischemic kidneys. It has been suggested that lipid peroxidation is closely related to I/R induced tissue damage and that MDA is an indicator of lipid peroxidation rate [24]. The peroxidation of membrane lipids can disrupt membrane fluidity and cell compartmentalization which may result in cell lysis [25] and thus LDH release. It is well-recognized that Mel has antioxidant effects and its role in lipid peroxidation inhibition has been well-established [26, 27]. Besides, the effect of Mel on LDH leakage suggests that it appears to preserve the integrity of cell membranes and renal architecture as well. This may, in part, explain the important function recovery observed after Mel administration.

The next finding of this study shows that Mel significantly attenuated the level of several ER stress parameters induced by renal I/R. It is well-documented that ER stress plays a significant role in the pathogenesis of renal I/R injury [28, 29]. In line with this, Mahfoudh-Boussaid et al. [13] have described that renal I/R is concomitant with amplified levels of GRP 78, p-PERK, ATF4, and XBP-1. These data are in agreement with the present investigation showing that renal I/R induced elevations in GRP78, XBP-1, p-PERK, CHOP, and ATF6. Interestingly, Mel treatment was found to counteract these elevations. Our results are in keeping with recent findings demonstrating that melatonin reduces ER stress in different models of cell injury. For instance, Mel represses the UPR in rabbits with lethal fulminant hepatitis [30]. Similar effects were also observed in the steatotic liver [31]. Furthermore, a marked reduction of ER stress after Mel treatment was also observed in brain of rats subjected to arsenite-induced neurotoxic conditions [32]. However, whether Mel is involved in protection against ER stress in warm renal I/R injury is unclear. In this report, we demonstrate for the first time the reduction of ER stress after melatonin treatment in this experimental model of renal I/R. The effectiveness of Mel in reducing ER stress was also associated with attenuation of cell death as evidenced by lower levels of CHOP and p-JNK. CHOP and JNK activation has been correlated with apoptosis as an ER stress downstream event [33, 34]. Increasing evidence has shown that induction of CHOP is an important element of switch from prosurvival to proapoptotic signaling cascades [35, 36]. In this same context, activation of JNK was correlated with triggering apoptotic signaling mechanisms following I/R injury in various organs [37, 38]. In light of the findings that Mel reduced ER stress induced apoptosis,

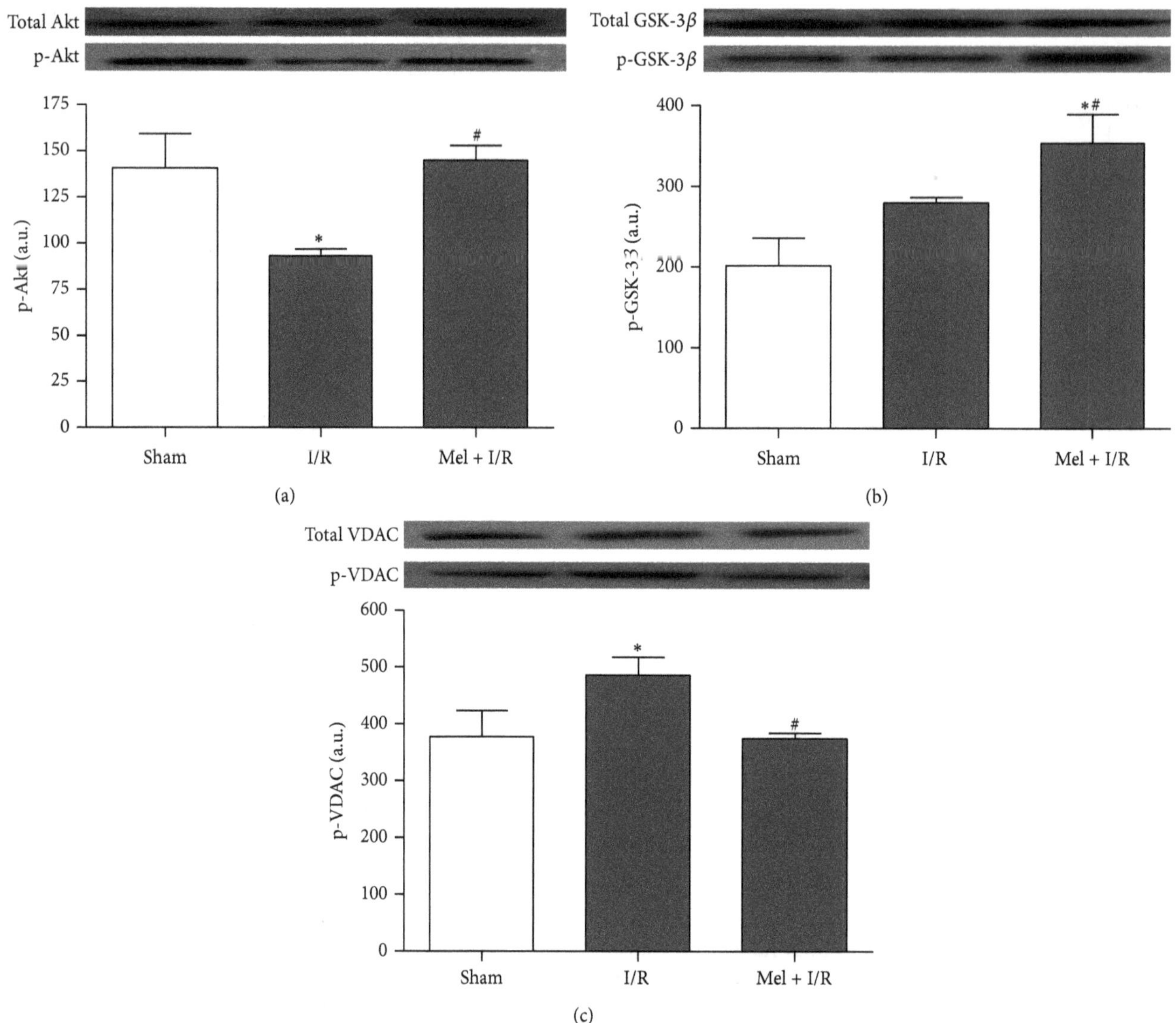

FIGURE 5: Western blot of total and phosphorylated Akt (a), total and phosphorylated GSK-3β (b), and total and phosphorylated VDAC (c). One representative blot of six independent experiments is shown at the top whereas densitometric analysis is shown at the bottom. Results are expressed as mean ± SEM. $^{*}p < 0.05$ versus Sham. $^{\#}p < 0.05$ versus I/R.

we hypothesized that this cell death attenuation would be in favor of survival enhancement.

To further elucidate the mechanisms by which Mel modulates cell survival during renal I/R, we evaluated its effects on Akt and its downstream targets, GSK-3β and VDAC. Results of the current study showed that p-Akt decreased in the case of I/R injury and that Mel prevented this downregulation. Many researchers have demonstrated that Akt plays a crucial role in the protection of liver [39], heart [40] and kidney [41] against I/R injury. One of the proposed mechanisms is that Akt phosphorylates GSK-3β which decreases the level of phosphorylated VDAC, the most abundant protein in mitochondrial outer membrane, leading to inhibition of the apoptotic process [13, 42]. The capability of Mel to enhance Akt activation in the setting of I/R has been documented in several organs including brain [43] and liver [44] but is not yet proven in kidney. Our data suggest that antiapoptotic effect of Mel is mediated, in part, by Akt signaling axis activation during renal I/R.

There are likely many other mechanisms by which Mel can promote cell survival. In order to explore other possible pathways, we examined the phosphorylation levels of ERK and P38 which are serine/threonine kinases belonging to the MAPK family. ERK activation is commonly considered as protective in the setting of renal I/R [45]. Besides, some studies report that p-ERK could be responsible, at least partially, for the inhibition of GSK-3β activity [46] thus contributing to apoptosis decrease. Our results indicated that preconditioning with Mel induced a significant increase in p-ERK level regarding kidneys undergoing I/R injury. This is in keeping with a previous report demonstrating that Mel effectively promotes ERK phosphorylation in case of cerebral I/R [47]. P38 is a crucial signaling protein that is involved in cellular proliferation, differentiation, inflammation, and

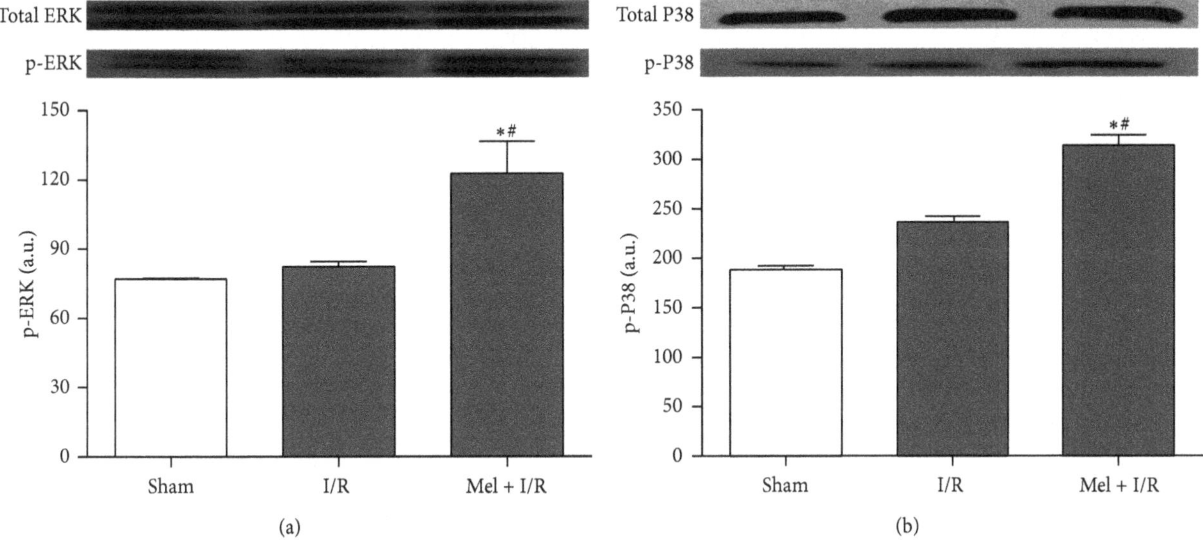

FIGURE 6: Western blot of total and phosphorylated ERK (a) and total and phosphorylated P38 (b). One representative blot of six independent experiments is shown at the top whereas densitometric analysis is shown at the bottom. Results are expressed as mean ± SEM. $^{*}p < 0.05$ versus Sham. $^{\#}p < 0.05$ versus I/R.

apoptosis [48]. According to our findings, Mel administration results in a significant activation of P38. While the evidence is mounting that P38 inhibition might be beneficial in reducing inflammation and I/R injury [49]. Other reports suggest that P38 activation may confer protection [50]. Importantly, some of the downstream targets of P38 are protective, while others are inducers of cell death, and the overall result of P38 activation may depend on the balance between them [51]. Hernendez and coworkers identified a beneficial role for P38 in the setting of cardiac I/R [52]. It is obviously critical to be certain that P38 inhibition will not exacerbate I/R injury. Unfortunately, there is no clear answer to this question. Nevertheless, given that Mel is shown to reduce molecular damage and cellular loss, our hypothesis would be in favor of beneficial role of P38 signaling cascade regarding our renal I/R model. However, how Mel activates the protective aspects of P38 pathway will be a major issue to be addressed in the future.

5. Conclusion

On the basis of the previous findings, we conclude that Mel could ameliorate renal damage related to I/R. The underlying mechanisms of this protection essentially involve the modulation of ER stress, Akt and MAPK pathways.

Conflict of Interests

The authors declare that there is no conflict of interests regarding the publication of this paper.

Acknowledgments

This work was supported by the Tunisian Ministry of Higher Education and Scientific Research. The authors thank Mr. Fraj Alaya at the language service of the Faculty of Pharmacy, University of Monastir, Tunisia, for revising the English text.

References

[1] S. Rodríguez-Reynoso, C. Leal, E. Portilla-De Buen, J. C. Castillo, and F. Ramos-Solano, "Melatonin ameliorates renal ischemia/reperfusion injury," *Journal of Surgical Research*, vol. 116, no. 2, pp. 242–247, 2004.

[2] N. Arfian, N. Emoto, N. Vignon-Zellweger, K. Nakayama, K. Yagi, and K.-I. Hirata, "ET-1 deletion from endothelial cells protects the kidney during the extension phase of ischemia/reperfusion injury," *Biochemical and Biophysical Research Communications*, vol. 425, no. 2, pp. 443–449, 2012.

[3] R. Inagi, "Endoplasmic reticulum stress in the kidney as a novel mediator of kidney injury," *Nephron—Experimental Nephrology*, vol. 112, no. 1, pp. e1–e9, 2009.

[4] S. Sharma, J. Sarkar, C. Haldar, and S. Sinha, "Melatonin reverses fas, E2F-1 and endoplasmic reticulum stress mediated apoptosis and dysregulation of autophagy induced by the herbicide atrazine in murine splenocytes," *PLoS ONE*, vol. 9, no. 9, Article ID e108602, 2014.

[5] I. Ben Mosbah, I. Alfany-Fernández, C. Martel et al., "Endoplasmic reticulum stress inhibition protects steatotic and non-steatotic livers in partial hepatectomy under ischemia-reperfusion," *Cell Death and Disease*, vol. 1, no. 7, article e52, 2010.

[6] J. Sehajpal, T. Kaur, R. Bhatti, and A. P. Singh, "Role of progesterone in melatonin-mediated protection against acute kidney injury," *Journal of Surgical Research*, vol. 191, no. 2, pp. 441–447, 2014.

[7] R. J. Reiter, D.-X. Tan, L. C. Manchester, and W. Qi, "Biochemical reactivity of melatonin with reactive oxygen and nitrogen species: a review of the evidence," *Cell Biochemistry and Biophysics*, vol. 34, no. 2, pp. 237–256, 2001.

[8] W. Z. Wang, X.-H. Fang, L. L. Stephenson, X. Zhang, K. T. Khiabani, and W. A. Zamboni, "Melatonin attenuates I/R-induced mitochondrial dysfunction in skeletal muscle," *Journal of Surgical Research*, vol. 171, no. 1, pp. 108–113, 2011.

[9] A. Galano, D. X. Tan, and R. J. Reiter, "Melatonin as a natural ally against oxidative stress: a physicochemical examination," *Journal of Pineal Research*, vol. 51, no. 1, pp. 1–16, 2011.

[10] J. L. Mauriz, P. S. Collado, C. Veneroso, R. J. Reiter, and J. González-Gallego, "A review of the molecular aspects of melatonin's anti-inflammatory actions: recent insights and new perspectives," *Journal of Pineal Research*, vol. 54, no. 1, pp. 1–14, 2013.

[11] W. Balduini, S. Carloni, S. Perrone et al., "The use of melatonin in hypoxic-ischemic brain damage: an experimental study," *Journal of Maternal-Fetal and Neonatal Medicine*, vol. 25, no. 1, pp. 119–124, 2012.

[12] A. Lochner, B. Huisamen, and F. Nduhirabandi, "Cardioprotective effect of melatonin against ischaemia/reperfusion damage," *Frontiers in Bioscience*, vol. 5, no. 1, pp. 305–315, 2013.

[13] A. Mahfoudh-Boussaid, M. A. Zaouali, T. Hauet et al., "Attenuation of endoplasmic reticulum stress and mitochondrial injury in kidney with ischemic postconditioning application and trimetazidine treatment," *Journal of Biomedical Science*, vol. 19, pp. 71–84, 2012.

[14] Z. Kurcer, E. Oguz, H. Ozbilge et al., "Melatonin protects from ischemia/reperfusion-induced renal injury in rats: this effect is not mediated by proinflammatory cytokines," *Journal of Pineal Research*, vol. 43, no. 2, pp. 172–178, 2007.

[15] I. B. Mosbah, J. Roselló-Catafau, R. Franco-Gou et al., "Preservation of steatotic livers in IGL-1 solution," *Liver Transplantation*, vol. 12, no. 8, pp. 1215–1223, 2006.

[16] P. Jablonski, B. O. Howden, D. A. Rae, C. S. Birrell, V. C. Marshall, and J. Tange, "An experimental model for assessment of renal recovery from warm ischemia," *Transplantation*, vol. 35, no. 3, pp. 198–204, 1983.

[17] J. Chen, W. Wang, Q. Zhang et al., "Low molecular weight fucoidan against renal ischemia-reperfusion injury via inhibition of the MAPK signaling pathway," *PLoS ONE*, vol. 8, no. 2, Article ID e56224, 2013.

[18] L.-T. Wang, B.-L. Chen, C.-T. Wu, K.-H. Huang, C.-K. Chiang, and S. H. Liu, "Protective role of AMP-activated protein kinase-evoked autophagy on an *in vitro* model of ischemia/reperfusion-induced renal tubular cell injury," *PLoS ONE*, vol. 8, no. 11, Article ID e79814, 2013.

[19] Z. Chen, C. C. Chua, J. Gao et al., "Prevention of ischemia/reperfusion-induced cardiac apoptosis and injury by melatonin is independent of glutathione peroxdiase 1," *Journal of Pineal Research*, vol. 46, no. 2, pp. 235–241, 2009.

[20] Y. Okatani, A. Wakatsuki, R. J. Reiter, H. Enzan, and Y. Miyahara, "Protective effect of melatonin against mitochondrial injury induced by ischemia and reperfusion of rat liver," *European Journal of Pharmacology*, vol. 469, no. 1–3, pp. 145–152, 2003.

[21] P.-O. Koh, "Melatonin attenuates the focal cerebral ischemic injury by inhibiting the dissociation of pBad from 14-3-3," *Journal of Pineal Research*, vol. 44, no. 1, pp. 101–106, 2008.

[22] O. R. Kunduzova, G. Escourrou, M.-H. Seguelas et al., "Prevention of apoptotic and necrotic cell death, caspase-3 activation, and renal dysfunction by melatonin after ischemia/reperfusion," *The FASEB Journal*, vol. 17, no. 8, pp. 872–874, 2003.

[23] Z. Li, A. Nickkholgh, X. Yi et al., "Melatonin protects kidney grafts from ischemia/reperfusion injury through inhibition of NF-kB and apoptosis after experimental kidney transplantation," *Journal of Pineal Research*, vol. 46, no. 4, pp. 365–372, 2009.

[24] T. Aktoz, N. Aydogdu, B. Alagol, O. Yalcin, G. Huseyinova, and I. H. Atakan, "The protective effects of melatonin and vitamin E against renal ischemia-reperfusion injury in rats," *Renal Failure*, vol. 29, no. 5, pp. 535–542, 2007.

[25] A. D. Yalcin, A. Bisgin, R. H. Erbay et al., "Trimetazidine effect on burn-induced intestinal mucosal injury and kidney damage in rats," *International Journal of Burns and Trauma*, vol. 2, pp. 110–117, 2012.

[26] D. Y. Yoo, W. Kim, C. H. Lee et al., "Melatonin improves D-galactose-induced aging effects on behavior, neurogenesis, and lipid peroxidation in the mouse dentate gyrus via increasing pCREB expression," *Journal of Pineal Research*, vol. 52, no. 1, pp. 21–28, 2012.

[27] N. Ersoz, A. Guven, T. Cayci et al., "Comparison of the efficacy of melatonin and 1400w on renal ischemia/reperfusion injury: a role for inhibiting iNOS," *Renal Failure*, vol. 31, no. 8, pp. 704–710, 2009.

[28] B. Bailly-Maitre, C. Fondevila, F. Kaldas et al., "Cytoprotective gene bi-1 is required for intrinsic protection from endoplasmic reticulum stress and ischemia-reperfusion injury," *Proceedings of the National Academy of Sciences of the United States of America*, vol. 103, no. 8, pp. 2809–2814, 2006.

[29] G. Kuznetsov, K. T. Bush, P. L. Zhang, and S. K. Nigam, "Perturbations in maturation of secretory proteins and their association with endoplasmic reticulum chaperones in a cell culture model for epithelial ischemia," *Proceedings of the National Academy of Sciences of the United States of America*, vol. 93, no. 16, pp. 8584–8589, 1996.

[30] M. J. Tuñõn, B. San-Miguel, I. Crespo et al., "Melatonin treatment reduces endoplasmic reticulum stress and modulates the unfolded protein response in rabbits with lethal fulminant hepatitis of viral origin," *Journal of Pineal Research*, vol. 55, no. 3, pp. 221–228, 2013.

[31] M. A. Zaouali, E. Boncompagni, R. J. Reiter et al., "AMPK involment in endoplasmic reticulum stress and autophagy modulation after fatty liver graft preservation: a role for melatonin and trimetazidine cocktail," *Journal of Pineal Research*, vol. 55, pp. 65–78, 2013.

[32] A. M. Y. Lin, S. F. Fang, P. L. Chao, and C. H. Yang, "Melatonin attenuates arsenite-induced apoptosis in rat brain: involvement of mitochondrial and endoplasmic reticulum pathways and aggregation of α-synuclein," *Journal of Pineal Research*, vol. 43, no. 2, pp. 163–171, 2007.

[33] L. Yu, M. Lu, P. Wang, and X. Chen, "Trichostatin A ameliorates myocardial ischemia/reperfusion injury through inhibition of endoplasmic reticulum stress-induced apoptosis," *Archives of Medical Research*, vol. 43, no. 3, pp. 190–196, 2012.

[34] M. Kitamura, "Endoplasmic reticulum stress and unfolded protein response in renal pathophysiology: janus faces," *American Journal of Physiology: Renal Physiology*, vol. 295, no. 2, pp. F323–F334, 2008.

[35] K. Zhang and R. J. Kaufman, "From endoplasmic-reticulum stress to the inflammatory response," *Nature*, vol. 454, no. 7203, pp. 455–462, 2008.

[36] C. Xu, B. Bailly-Maitre, and J. C. Reed, "Endoplasmic reticulum stress: cell life and death decisions," *Journal of Clinical Investigation*, vol. 115, no. 10, pp. 2656–2664, 2005.

[37] E. L. Marderstein, B. Bucher, Z. Guo, X. Feng, K. Reid, and D. A. Geller, "Protection of rat hepatocytes from apoptosis by inhibition of c-Jun N-terminal kinase," *Surgery*, vol. 134, no. 2, pp. 280–284, 2003.

[38] T. Yin, G. Sandhu, C. D. Wolfgang et al., "Tissue-specific pattern of stress kinase activation in ischemic/reperfused heart and kidney," *The Journal of Biological Chemistry*, vol. 272, no. 32, pp. 19943–19950, 1997.

[39] X. Yang, L. Qin, J. Liu, L. Tian, and H. Qian, "17β-Estradiol protects the liver against cold ischemia/reperfusion injury through the Akt kinase pathway," *Journal of Surgical Research*, vol. 178, no. 2, pp. 996–1002, 2012.

[40] S.-J. Fang, X.-S. Wu, Z.-H. Han et al., "Neuregulin-1 preconditioning protects the heart against ischemia/reperfusion injury through a PI3K/Akt-dependent mechanism," *Chinese Medical Journal*, vol. 123, no. 24, pp. 3597–3604, 2010.

[41] A. Satake, M. Takaoka, M. Nishikawa et al., "Protective effect of 17β estradiol on ischemic acute renal failure through the PI3K/Akt/eNOS pathway," *Kidney International*, vol. 73, no. 3, pp. 308–317, 2008.

[42] M. A. Zaouali, S. Padrissa-Altés, I. B. Mosbah et al., "Improved rat steatotic and nonsteatotic liver preservation by the addition of epidermal growth factor and insulin-like growth factor-I to University of Wisconsin solution," *Liver Transplantation*, vol. 16, no. 9, pp. 1098–1111, 2010.

[43] J. Song, S. M. Kang, W. T. Lee, K. A. Park, K. M. Lee, and J. E. Lee, "The benefecial effect of melatonin in brain endothelial cells against oxygen-glucose deprivation followed by reperfusion induced injury," *Oxidative Medicine and Cellular Longevity*, vol. 2014, Article ID 639531, 14 pages, 2014.

[44] P. O. Koh, "Melatonin prevents hepatic injury-induced decrease in Akt downstream targets phosphorylations," *Journal of Pineal Research*, vol. 51, no. 2, pp. 214–219, 2011.

[45] I. Kyriazis, G. C. Kagadis, P. Kallidonis et al., "PDE5 inhibition against acute renal ischemia reperfusion injury in rats: does vardenafil offer protection?" *World Journal of Urology*, vol. 31, no. 3, pp. 597–602, 2013.

[46] T. Miura, M. Nishihara, and T. Miki, "Drug development targeting the glycogen synthase kinase-3beta (GSK-3beta) mediated signal transduction pathway: role of GSK-3beta in myocardial protection against ischemia reperfusion injury," *Journal of Pharmacological Sciences*, vol. 109, no. 2, pp. 162–167, 2009.

[47] P.-O. Koh, "Melatonin attenuates the cerebral ischemic injury via the MEK/ERK/p90RSK/Bad signaling cascade," *Journal of Veterinary Medical Science*, vol. 70, no. 11, pp. 1219–1223, 2008.

[48] X. Lv, J. Tan, D. Liu, P. Wu, and X. Cui, "Intratracheal administration of p38α short-hairpin RNA plasmid ameliorates lung ischemia-reperfusion injury in rats," *Journal of Heart and Lung Transplantation*, vol. 31, no. 6, pp. 655–662, 2012.

[49] Y. Wang, "Mitogen-activated protein kinases in heart development and diseases," *Circulation*, vol. 116, no. 12, pp. 1413–1423, 2007.

[50] J. E. Clark, N. Sarafraz, and M. S. Marber, "Potential of p38-MAPK inhibitors in the treatment of ischaemic heart disease," *Pharmacology and Therapeutics*, vol. 116, no. 2, pp. 192–206, 2007.

[51] B. A. Rose, T. Force, and Y. Wang, "Mitogen-activated protein kinase signaling in the heart: angels versus demons in a heart-breaking tale," *Physiological Reviews*, vol. 90, no. 4, pp. 1507–1546, 2010.

[52] G. Hernández, H. Lal, M. Fidalgo et al., "A novel cardioprotective p38-MAPK/mTOR pathway," *Experimental Cell Research*, vol. 317, no. 20, pp. 2938–2949, 2011.

9

Transcription Factor HBP1 Enhances Radiosensitivity by Inducing Apoptosis in Prostate Cancer Cell Lines

Yicheng Chen,[1] Yueping Wang,[2] Yanlan Yu,[1] Liwei Xu,[1] Youyun Zhang,[1] Shicheng Yu,[1] Gonghui Li,[1] and Zhigeng Zhang[1]

[1]*Department of Urology, Sir Run-Run Shaw Hospital, College of Medicine, Zhejiang University, Hangzhou 310016, China*
[2]*Department of Urology, Wuyi First People's Hospital, Zhejiang 321200, China*

Correspondence should be addressed to Zhigeng Zhang; zhangzhigeng2015@sina.com

Academic Editor: Giovanni L. Gravina

Radiotherapy for prostate cancer has been gradually carried out in recent years; however, acquired radioresistance often occurred in some patients after radiotherapy. HBP1 (HMG-box transcription factor 1) is a transcriptional inhibitor which could inhibit the expression of dozens of oncogenes. In our previous study, we showed that the expression level of HBP1 was closely related to prostate cancer metastasis and prognosis, but the relationship between HBP1 and radioresistance for prostate cancer is largely unknown. In this study, the clinical data of patients with prostate cancer was compared, and the positive correlation was revealed between prostate cancer brachytherapy efficacy and the expression level of HBP1 gene. Through research on prostate cancer cells in vitro, we found that HBP1 expression levels were negatively correlated with oncogene expression levels. Furthermore, HBP1 overexpression could sensitize prostate cancer cells to radiation and increase apoptosis in prostate cancer cells. In addition, animal model was employed to analyze the relationship between HBP1 gene and prostate cancer radiosensitivity in vivo; the result showed that knockdown of HBP1 gene could decrease the sensitivity to radiation of xenograft. These studies identified a specific molecular mechanism underlying prostate cancer radiosensitivity, which suggested HBP1 as a novel target in prostate cancer radiotherapy.

1. Introduction

Prostate cancer is very common in western countries, the incidence of which ranks first in male cancers [1]. With increased life expectancy and the change of diet and lifestyle, the incidence and mortality rate of prostate cancer are rising in China, which is particularly prominent in some economically developed regions [2, 3]. As such, studies on prostate cancer pathogenesis and therapy are prevalent.

In the past, radical prostatectomy was preferred clinically for localized prostate cancer of early stage and low-risk patients [4], while for late stage, intermediate- and high-risk patients, androgen deprivation therapy has been used [5]. In the last 20 years in western countries, radiotherapy (including EBRT and permanent radioactive seed implantation) for the treatment of prostate cancer has gradually replaced the radical prostatectomy and androgen deprivation therapy and has become one of the main methods for the treatment of prostate cancer [6, 7]. Radiotherapy for prostate cancer has been gradually carried out in China in recent years with good effect. However, biochemical recurrence or clinical relapse occurred in some patients after radiotherapy, potentially due to acquired radioresistance [8, 9]. While the mechanism of radioresistance for prostate cancer is unclear, the methodology into the research and treatment for prostate cancer radioresistance is lacking. Studies that focus on the reduction of prostate cancer cell resistance and promote increased tumor cell sensitivity to radiotherapy treatment are predominant in prostate cancer.

HBP1 (HMG-box transcription factor 1) is a transcriptional inhibitor belonging to HMG-box transcription factor family and could inhibit the expression of a number of growth regulatory genes and oncogenes [10]. Our recently published study showed that the expression level of HBP1 in prostate cancer cells and prostate cancer tissues was significantly lower than the normal cells and normal adjacent matched tissues, respectively. Lower expression level of HBP1 resulted in the increased expression level of MIF gene (macrophage migration inhibitory factor) and promoted the ability of colony formation and invasion of prostate cancer cells. Though the expression level of HBP1 in prostate cancer is closely related to metastasis and prognosis [3], the relationship between HBP1 and prostate cancer radiotherapy is unknown.

Therefore, we hypothesized that decreased expression of HBP1 in prostate cancer leads to radioresistance. In this study, we combined clinical data of patients with prostate cancer, prostate cancer cells, and animal models to analyze the relationship between HBP1 gene and prostate cancer radiosensitivity. Furthermore, we determined the relationship between HBP1 and apoptosis during prostate cancer radiotherapy. These studies clarify the role of HBP1 in prostate cancer radiotherapy and identify HBP1 as a new biomarker in prostate cancer radiotherapy as well as a novel target for radiosensitization.

2. Materials and Methods

2.1. Patient Information. Sample collection was in accordance with the terms of the Medical Ethical Committee of the Zhejiang University and followed the guidelines of the Declaration of Helsinki. Blood samples from 66 patients with low-risk and intermediate-risk prostate cancer treated with brachytherapy were obtained from the Department of Urology, Sir Run-Run Shaw Hospital (Zhejiang University, China) from February 2009 to February 2011. The inclusion criteria are National Comprehensive Cancer Network (NCCN) risk grouping criteria, which are low-risk patients, defined as Gleason score < 6, prostate-specific antigen (PSA) < 10 ng/mL, and T1c-T2a, and intermediate-risk patients, defined as Gleason score = 7, PSA 10–20 ng/mL, and T2b-T2c. The age of patients was ranged from 69 to 87; the median age was 78 years. All patients were diagnosed by prostate needle biopsy, according to the Gleason score system: the lowest score is 3 + 3 = 6, and the highest is 4 + 3 = 7; the lowest serum PSA before treatment was 2.86 ng/dL, and the highest was 19.3 ng/dL. All patients underwent prostate magnetic resonance imaging and the whole body bone PET/CT examination, and no bone metastases were found in any patient. All patients underwent the implantation of ^{125}iodine (^{125}I) particles according to the guidelines of American Society for Radiation Oncology (ASTRO) and American College of Radiology (ACR). The three-dimensional image is reconstructed of the prostate; Brachy probpsstep V3.02 planning software was applied to develop treatment plans and the expected target dose is 144 Gy. The median number of particles was 64, with a minimum of 54 and a maximum of 91. The implantation condition was checked via pelvic CT scan on the first day after operation, calculating the value of D90. In 66 patients, the median D90 value was 142 Gy, with a minimum of 122 Gy and a maximum of 151 Gy. Patients were discharged after three days and the catheter was removed after one week. The blood samples were collected from patients before and after radiation therapy. Full ethical consent was obtained from all patients.

2.2. Cell Culture. DU-145 cell lines (prostate carcinoma cell lines) were purchased from the American Type Culture Collection (ATCC; Manassas, VA, USA). All cells were cultured in Dulbecco's modified Eagle's medium (DMEM; Gibco, Grand Island, NY) containing 10% fetal bovine serum (Hyclone, Logan, UT), supplemented with 50 units of penicillin/streptomycin.

Irradiation was carried out using 6 MV X-rays generated by a linear accelerator (PRIMUS-M, Siemens) at a dose rate of 2 Gy/min. During irradiation, cells were put at room temperature with 2 cm thick tissue glue placed on the culture dish and irradiated by X-rays at a source distance of 100 mm.

2.3. Plasmid Construction. The pBaBE-HBP1 expression vectors were a kind gift from Dr. Amy S. Yee [11]; pBabe Vector was used as the control. Retroviral gene transduction was carried out using Phoenix packaging cells. RNAi-mediated HBP1 knockdown was accomplished by shRNA produced by the DNA-based shRNA-expressing retroviral vector (pSuper-Retro). The vectors were a kind gift from Dr. Amy S. Yee. The knockdown experiment was performed as described previously [3]. The HBP1 shRNA target sequence is ACTGT-GAGTGCCACTTCTC as the pGenesil-HBP1-shRNA plasmid and pGenesil-scramble plasmid were used as the control.

2.4. Real-Time PCR. Total RNA was isolated from tissues or cells using TRIzol reagent (Invitrogen, Carlsbad, USA) according to the manufacturer's instructions. Reverse transcription was performed with an iScript cDNA synthesis kit (Bio-Rad) in 20 μL reaction volume containing 1 μg of total RNA. Real-time PCR was performed with Power SYBR Green PCR Master Mix (Applied Biosystems) using a 7500 real-time PCR System (Applied Biosystems). The primers for cyclin D (CCND) (sense: 5′-TGGAGCCCG-TGAAAAAGAGC-3′; anti-sense: 5′-TCTCCTTCATCT-TAGAGGCCAC-3′), MIF (sense: 5′-GCGGGTCTCCTG-GTCCTTCTG-3′; anti-sense: 5′-GTGGGTCCCTGCGG-CTCTTA-3′), N-Myc (sense: 5′-ACTTCTACTTCGGCGG-3′; anti-sense: 5′-TCTCCGTAGCCCAAT-3′), and GAPDH (sense: 5′-CACCAGGGCTGCTTTTAACTC-3′; anti-sense: 5′-GAAGATGGTGATGGGATTTC-3′) were designed with Primer Premier Version 5.0 software and their efficiency was confirmed by sequencing their conventional PCR products.

2.5. Western Blots. Proteins extracted from cells were quantified by the modified Lowry method. Discontinuous sodium dodecyl sulphate-polyacrylamide gel electrophoresis (SDS-PAGE) was performed using Bio-Rad mini-protein II electrophoresis and transferred into polyvinylidenedifluoride membrane (PVDF, Amersham Pharmacia Biotech, Piscataway, NJ). Protein extract was electrophoresed and electroblotted onto supported nitrocellulose membranes. Blots were blocked for 2 h with 5% nonfat dry milk in Tris-buffered saline (TBS) at room temperature for 1 h and then incubated with anti-HBP1 and anti-GAPDH (cat. sc-8488 and sc-32233, Santa Cruz Biotechnology, Santa Cruz, CA, USA) specific primary antibodies (1 : 1000 dilution) at room temperature for 2 h. Blots were incubated with HRP-conjugated secondary anti-rabbit antiserum (Santa Cruz, CA, USA, 1 : 5000 dilution in TBS) for 1 h. After several washes with 0.1% TBS-Tween 20, immunoreactive proteins were visualized with enhanced chemiluminescence (ECL) and captured on an X-ray film. Protein levels were quantified using Biosense 300 software (Oberhaching, Germany). Relative protein expression level was calculated by comparing with the expression of controls.

2.6. MTT Analysis. Chondrocytes were seeded in a 96-well culture plate. After 12 h, cells were treated with diosgenin (0, 10, 50, and 100 μM) for 24 h. The cells were incubated with MTT solution (5 mg/mL) at 37°C for 4 h and then with dimethylsulfoxide (DMSO) by shaking at room temperature for 10 min. The spectrophotometric absorbance was measured at 570 nm on a multifunctional microplate reader (Tecan, Durham, NC, USA).

2.7. Flow Cytometry Analysis for Apoptosis. The percentage of apoptotic cells was assayed by the Annexin-V-FLUOS Staining Kit (Roche). Briefly, 1×10^5 cells were seeded in six-well plates and cultured for 24 hours. The cells were collected and resuspended in 100 μL binding buffer. Then, the cells were incubated with 5 μL FITC-Annexin-V in the dark for 15 minutes at room temperature. Subsequently, 5 μL PI was added and incubated with the cells for 20 minutes at room temperature in the dark. Finally, the cell samples were examined in the flow cytometer. Each assessment of proliferation and apoptosis was repeated three times.

2.8. Xenograft Model. All animal care and experimental protocols in this study were approved by the animal ethics committee of Zhejiang University, China. Male BALB/c nude mice (4~6 weeks old) were purchased from Weitong Lihua Experimental Animal Technical Company (Beijing, China). Approximately 5×10^7 cells in 0.1 mL of PBS were subcutaneously injected in the right thigh of nude mice and treatment was started when the tumors reached an average volume of 50 mm^3. Mice bearing similar tumor volumes were chosen and randomly divided into 2 groups for irradiation with 3 mice in each group: Con shRNA group and HBP1 shRNA group. Mice were checked daily for mortality relevant to treatment. Body weight and tumor size were measured every 3 days. Mice were sacrificed three weeks after treatment and tumor volumes were calculated using the formula: tumor volume (mm^3) = [length (mm) × width (mm)^2]/2.

2.9. Statistical Analysis. All experiments were repeated three times with independent cultures and similar results were obtained. Data are presented as the mean and 95% confidence interval (CI). Statistical significance was determined by the two-tailed unpaired Student's t-test. P values less than 0.05 were considered significant.

3. Results

3.1. Positive Correlation between Prostate Cancer Brachytherapy Efficacy and the Expression Level of HBP1 Gene. The expression level of HBP1 gene in blood samples was detected via RT-PCR in 66 patients who received radiotherapy and compared to preradiation control samples. As shown in Figure 1(a), we found that HBP1 expression level increased in the blood samples of brachytherapy-treated patients compared with pretreatment blood samples. For these patients, PSA levels were as the main criteria to judge the efficacy of brachytherapy; we found that PSA was significantly downregulated in irradiated patient samples (Figure 1(b)). Furthermore, the relationship between the expression level of HBP1 and serum PSA was analyzed, and the statistical results suggested that the expression level of HBP1 was positively correlated with serum PSA; the prognosis of patients with low expression level of HBP1 is poor (Figure 1(c)).

3.2. HBP1 Expression Levels Are Negatively Correlated with Oncogene Expression Levels. To examine the function of HBP1 in prostate cancer in response to brachytherapy, monoclonal cell lines stably transfected by pBaBE-vector and pBaBE-HBP1 plasmid were selected with puromycin in DU-145 cells. Western blot assay was employed to detect the expression level, and the result showed that HBP1 was significantly upregulated in pBaBE-HBP1 group (HBP1 OE) compared with pBaBE-vector (Vector) group (Figure 2(a)). Furthermore, the mRNA levels of the HBP1 downstream effector genes were detected; we found that HBP1 overexpression could upregulate the expression of these genes, such as CCND, MIF, and N-Myc (Figure 2(b)). Similarly, monoclonal cell lines stably transfected with pGenesil-scramble and pGenesil-HBP1-shRNA plasmid were selected with G418 in DU-145 cells; the expression level of HBP1 was also verified by western blot, and the result showed that pGenesil-HBP1-shRNA (HBP1 shRNA) could markedly reduce the endogenous expression of HBP1 compared with cells transfected with pGenesil-scramble (Con shRNA) (Figure 2(c)). In addition, the knockdown of HBP1 results in an increase in the mRNA levels of CCND, MIF, and N-Myc (Figure 2(d)).

3.3. HBP1 Overexpression Sensitizes DU-145 Cells to Radiation. The four established clonal groups (HBP1 OE, Vector, HBP1 shRNA, and Con shRNA) were irradiated using a dose gradient (from 2 to 6 Gy). At 24 h and 48 h after irradiation, MTT assay was used to assess cell growth. Upon optimization of the experimental conditions, we irradiated cells with 4 Gy for subsequent experiments. The survival rates of all four different groups progressively declined following irradiation; the HBP1 OE cells which experienced an approximate 30% reduction in viability compared with the other three groups (Table 1) were especially affected. However, there was no significant difference observed between the Vector group and HBP1 shRNA group (Table 2). The results suggest that upregulation of HBP1 expression could enhance the short-term apoptotic effects of radiation or reduce radiation-resistant prostate cancer.

3.4. Overexpression of HBP1 Increases Apoptosis in DU-145 Cells. The amount of apoptotic cells of the four monoclonal cell lines was measured 48 h after irradiation with 4 Gy by flow cytometry. HBP1 overexpression increased the apoptosis rate compared to the other three groups (Figure 3(a)). Additionally, the activity of proapoptotic protein caspase-3 was detected by western blot in the four different irradiated cell

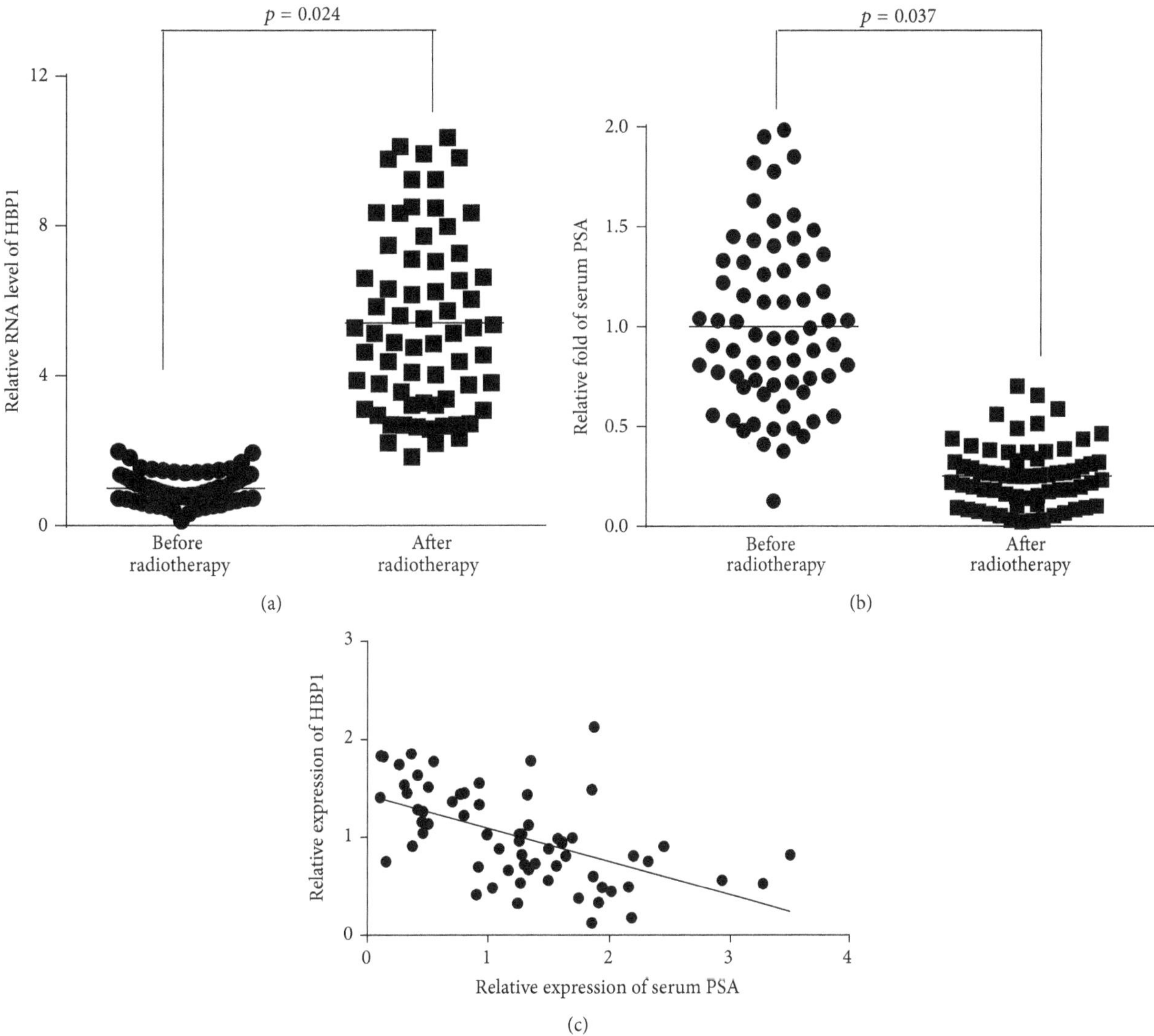

FIGURE 1: The relationship between prostate cancer brachytherapy efficacy and the expression level of HBP1 gene. (a) RT-PCR assay was used to detect the expression level of HBP1 gene in 66 pairs of blood samples of prostate cancer patients before or after brachytherapy. (b) The serum PSA level from patients was detected in 66 pairs of blood samples of prostate cancer patients before or after brachytherapy. (c) The relationship between the expression level of HBP1 and PSA was analyzed in 66 prostate patients who received brachytherapy.

TABLE 1: Comparison of cell viability of Vector group and HBP1 OE group at 48 h after different dose gradient radiation.

Dose	Vector group	HBP1 OE group	p value
2 Gy	0.590 ± 0.019	0.640 ± 0.014	0.003
4 Gy	0.614 ± 0.015	0.322 ± 0.014	0.001
6 Gy	0.565 ± 0.015	0.292 ± 0.015	0.0002

TABLE 2: Comparison of cell viability of Con shRNA group and HBP1 shRNA group at 48 h after different dose gradient radiation.

Dose	Con shRNA group	HBP1 shRNA group	p value
2 Gy	0.530 ± 0.019	0.588 ± 0.023	0.1
4 Gy	0.608 ± 0.006	0.628 ± 0.017	0.08
6 Gy	0.618 ± 0.018	0.595 ± 0.007	0.1

groups. We observed increased caspase-3 levels in HBP1 OE cells, which was consistent with the flow cytometry results (Figure 3(b)).

3.5. Sensitivity to Radiation of Xenograft with Different Expression Levels of HBP1 Gene. DU-145 cells from the four stable cell lines were digested to form cell suspensions, which were subcutaneously injected into the right thigh of 6-week-old Balb/c male mice. Tumor formation was observed and measured. Among the nude mice stably inoculated with HBP1 OE cells, viability was severely impaired and these mice were euthanized. Mice bearing tumors derived from the empty vector cells survived, while the specific reasons were not clear (data not shown). When the diameter of tumor reached 0.5 cm, we conducted irradiation sensitivity tests. Among the nude mice stably transfected with Con shRNA cells and HBP1

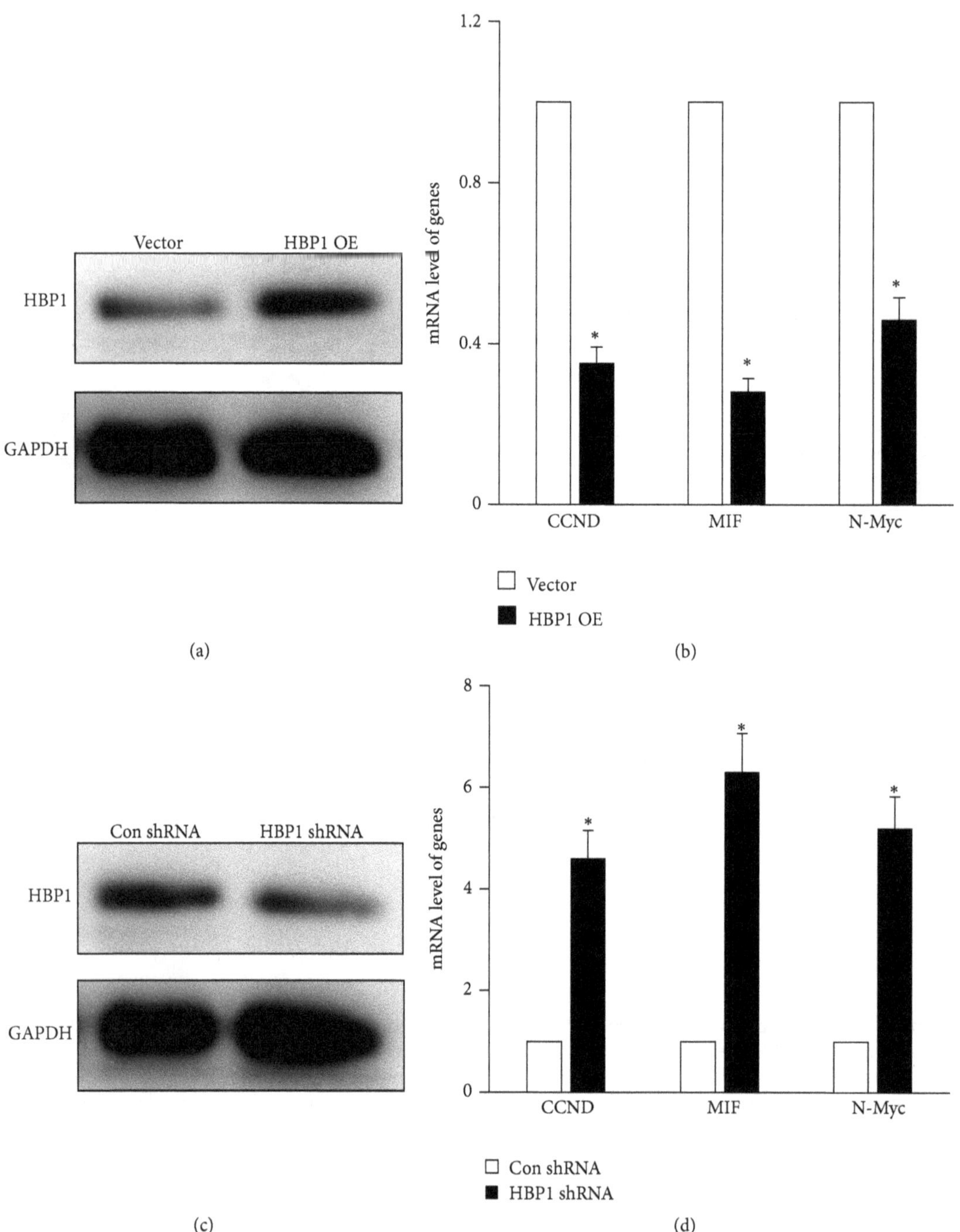

FIGURE 2: The establishment of prostate cancer cell lines with different expression levels of HBP1 gene. (a) Western blot assay was used to detect the protein level of HBP1 in monoclonal cell lines stably transfected by pBaBE-vector (Vector) and pBaBE-HBP1 (HBP1 OE) plasmid in DU-145 cells. (b) The mRNA level of the HBP1 downstream genes was detected via RT-qPCR including CCND, MIF, and N-Myc in Vector and HBP1 OE group. $^*p < 0.05$ versus control. (c) Western blot assay was used to detect the protein level of HBP1 in monoclonal cell lines stably transfected by pGenesil-scramble (Con shRNA) and pGenesil-HBP1-shRNA (HBP1 shRNA) plasmid in DU-145 cells. (d) The mRNA level of the HBP1 downstream genes was detected via RT-qPCR including CCND, MIF, and N-Myc in Con shRNA and HBP1 shRNA groups. $^*p < 0.05$ versus control.

shRNA cells, the knockdown of endogenous HBP1 could effectively promote the tumor size compared with the Con shRNA cells (Figure 4(a)). When the mice were sacrificed, the tumor was removed and measured; the tumor in HBP1 shRNA group was significantly bigger than Con shRNA group (Figure 4(b)). Furthermore, the expression of HBP1 in tumor was detected via western blot; we found that HBP1 expression was greatly decreased in HBP1 shRNA group (Figure 4(c)). All data suggested that HBP1 had an important role in the development of tumors.

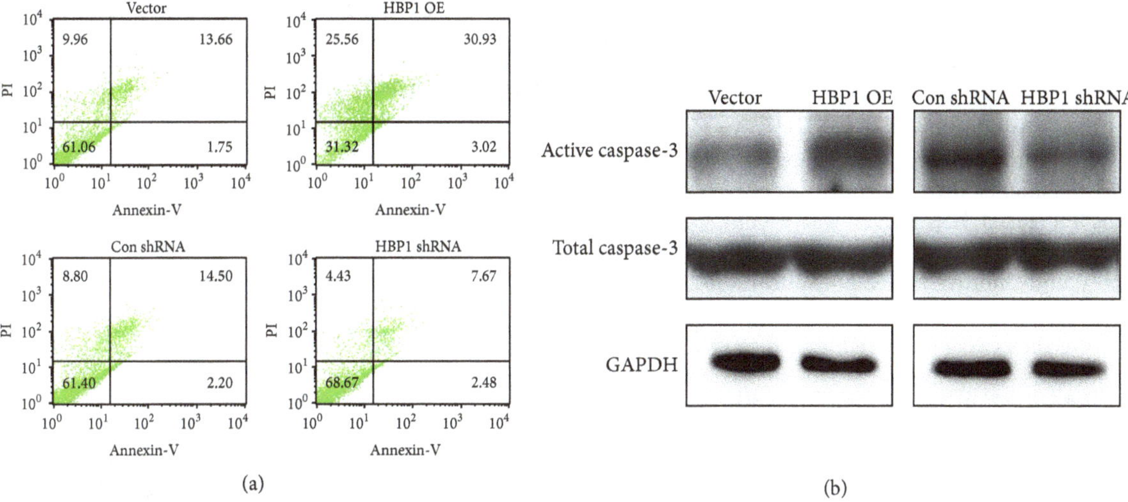

FIGURE 3: Apoptosis of DU-145 cells with different expression levels of HBP1 gene. (a) Flow cytometry assay was used to detect the apoptosis in Vector, HBP1 OE, Con shRNA, and HBP1 shRNA groups 48 h after irradiation with 4 Gy. (b) Western blot assay was used to detect the activity of proapoptotic protein caspase-3.

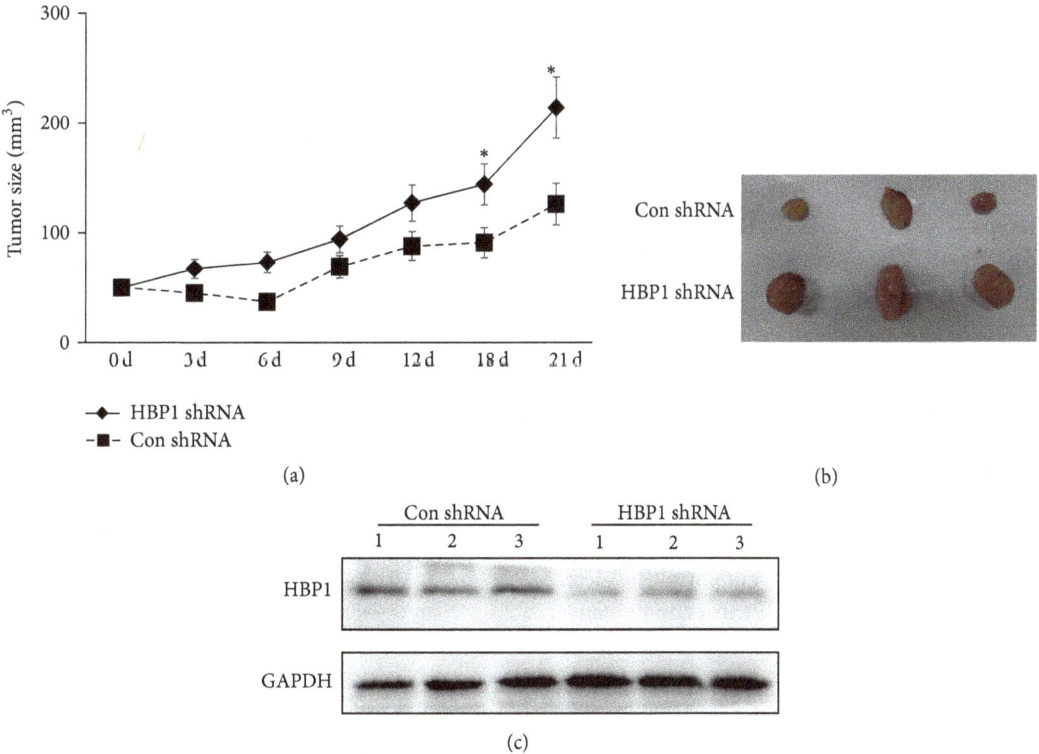

FIGURE 4: Sensitivity to radiation of xenograft with different expression levels of HBP1 gene. (a) The tumor size was measured in 6-week-old Balb/c male mice in Con shRNA and HBP1 shRNA groups after irradiation. $^*p < 0.05$ versus control. (b) The tumor was removed and observed in Con shRNA and HBP1 shRNA groups after irradiation. (c) The expression of HBP1 was detected via western blot in these tumors from Con shRNA and HBP1 shRNA groups after irradiation.

4. Discussion

Our preliminary results showed that DU-145 prostate cancer cell lines with high expression level of HBP1 were more sensitive to radiation. According to these results, it can be envisaged that increased expression of HBP1 can enhance the radiosensitivity of prostate cancer cells, whereas reduced expression level of HBP1 in prostate cancer cells is likely to be an important cause of prostate cancer radioresistance. However, additional research is required to support the hypothesis. Furthermore, the mechanism of HBP1 activity is needed to understand its role.

Many studies in cell and animal models have confirmed that HBP1 plays an important role in cell cycle arrest and apoptosis in the regulation of the cell cycle [12, 13]. Apoptosis, as a unique cell death process, plays an important role in irradiation-induced cell death [14]. Apoptosis and overall survival and local recurrence rates are significantly correlated. In patients with advanced cancer, apoptosis of tumor cells increased [15], which was accompanied with increased aneuploid cells [16, 17] and p53 overexpression [18], which could improve the response to radiotherapy of the tumor cells. The local control rate of patients with a high apoptotic index was improved, and distant metastasis was reduced; thus, the prognosis was better. Antiapoptotic mechanism of tumor cells and tumor cell radioresistance are closely linked [14]. Thus, HBP1, which regulates cell cycle progression, likely modulates radiation-induced apoptosis in prostate cancer cells, therefore affecting the efficiency of radiotherapy in prostate cancer cells. At present, there are two main caspase-dependent apoptotic pathways: one is activated by extracellular signals, which triggers intracellular cell death signaling by extracellular death ligand binding to the corresponding death receptor on the membrane and recruiting and activating caspase-2, caspase-8, and caspase-10; the second pathway is activated by intracellular stress signals, primarily mediated by the mitochondria cytochrome C activation that leads to caspase-9 activation [19, 20]. However, the regulation of apoptosis includes a complex series of cascades, involving p53 [21], RB [22], E2F [23], and other factors. The mechanisms of apoptosis vary as greatly as the different tissues themselves. Further study is required to determine if HBP1 is associated with apoptosis and if the interaction is mediated by irradiation.

Presently, while much is known about the upstream regulation of HBP1, little is known about its downstream targets and their roles in radiotherapy in the treatment of prostate cancer. HBP1, as an important transcriptional repressor, may regulate many target genes and signaling pathways. Future experiments to determine the role of HBP1 in apoptosis are worthwhile. New technologies, such as gene chips, could be employed to determine the downstream effectors of HBP1 in prostate cancer radiotherapy.

5. Conclusion

Taken together, our data demonstrated that suppression of HBP1 expression not only sensitized prostate cancer cells to radiation but also increased apoptosis in prostate cancer cells. Furthermore, xenograft model was carried on and the result showed that suppression of HBP1 attenuated the sensitivity to radiation in vivo. In addition, the results implied that HBP1 might exert its function via regulating the expression of CCND, MIF, and N-Myc. All these findings have essential implications for the treatment of prostate cancer by radiotherapy and further prospective investigations in a larger patient population might be needed.

Conflict of Interests

The authors declare that there is no conflict of interests regarding the publication of this paper.

Acknowledgments

This work was supported by the National Natural Science Foundation of China (no. 81101929 and no. 81101930) and Zhejiang Province Medical science and technology project of China (no. 2015RCA014).

References

[1] M. A. Bjurlin, A. B. Rosenkrantz, L. S. Beltran, R. A. Raad, and S. S. Taneja, "Imaging and evaluation of patients with high-risk prostate cancer," *Nature Reviews Urology*, vol. 12, no. 11, pp. 617–628, 2015.

[2] J. H. Lei, L. R. Liu, Q. Wei, S. B. Yan, T. R. Song et al., "Systematic review and meta-analysis of the survival outcomes of first-line treatment options in high-risk prostate cancer," *Scientific Reports*, vol. 5, article 7713, 2015.

[3] Y. C. Chen, X. W. Zhang, X. H. Niu et al., "Macrophage migration inhibitory factor is a direct target of HBP1-mediated transcriptional repression that is overexpressed in prostate cancer," *Oncogene*, vol. 29, no. 21, pp. 3067–3078, 2010.

[4] N. M. Fried and A. L. Burnett, "Novel methods for mapping the cavernous nerves during radical prostatectomy," *Nature Reviews Urology*, vol. 12, no. 8, pp. 451–460, 2015.

[5] A. Katzenwadel and P. Wolf, "Androgen deprivation of prostate cancer: leading to a therapeutic dead end," *Cancer Letters*, vol. 367, no. 1, pp. 12–17, 2015.

[6] R. G. Stock and N. N. Stone, "Permanent radioactive seed implantation in the treatment of prostate cancer," *Hematology/Oncology Clinics of North America*, vol. 13, no. 3, pp. 489–501, 1999.

[7] M. Albert, J. S. Song, D. Schultz et al., "Defining the rectal dose constraint for permanent radioactive seed implantation of the prostate," *Urologic Oncology*, vol. 26, no. 2, pp. 147–152, 2008.

[8] L. Chang, P. H. Graham, J. Ni et al., "Targeting PI3K/Akt/mTOR signaling pathway in the treatment of prostate cancer radioresistance," *Critical Reviews in Oncology/Hematology*, vol. 96, no. 3, pp. 507–517, 2015.

[9] J. L. Torrecilla, A. Hervas, A. Zapatero et al., "Uroncor consensus statement: management of biochemical recurrence after radical radiotherapy for prostate cancer: from biochemical failure to castration resistance," *Reports of Practical Oncology and Radiotherapy*, vol. 20, no. 4, pp. 259–272, 2015.

[10] X. Sun, X. Geng, J. Zhang, H. Zhao, and Y. Liu, "miR-155 promotes the growth of osteosarcoma in a HBP1-dependent mechanism," *Molecular and Cellular Biochemistry*, vol. 403, no. 1, pp. 139–147, 2015.

[11] S. P. Berasi, M. Xiu, A. S. Yee, and K. E. Paulson, "HBP1 repression of the p47phox gene: cell cycle regulation via the NADPH oxidase," *Molecular and Cellular Biology*, vol. 24, no. 7, pp. 3011–3024, 2004.

[12] A. S. Yee, E. K. Paulson, M. A. McDevitt et al., "The HBP1 transcriptional repressor and the p38 MAP kinase: unlikely partners in G1 regulation and tumor suppression," *Gene*, vol. 336, no. 1, pp. 1–13, 2004.

[13] N. Watanabe, R. Kageyama, and T. Ohtsuka, "Hbp1 regulates the timing of neuronal differentiation during cortical development by controlling cell cycle progression," *Development*, vol. 142, no. 13, pp. 2278–2290, 2015.

[14] M. Hassan, A. El Khattouti, A. Ejaeidi et al., "Elevated expression of hepatoma up-regulated protein inhibits γ-irradiation-induced apoptosis of prostate cancer cells," *Journal of Cellular Biochemistry*, 2015.

[15] X. Zhu, H. Zhao, Z. Lin, and G. Zhang, "Functional studies of miR-130a on the inhibitory pathways of apoptosis in patients with chronic myeloid leukemia," *Cancer Gene Therapy*, vol. 22, no. 12, pp. 573–580, 2015.

[16] A. Ohashi, M. Ohori, K. Iwai et al., "Aneuploidy generates proteotoxic stress and DNA damage concurrently with p53-mediated post-mitotic apoptosis in SAC-impaired cells," *Nature Communications*, vol. 6, article 7668, 2015.

[17] R. Wiedemuth, B. Klink, K. Töpfer, E. Schröck, G. Schackert, and M. Tatsuka, "Survivin safeguards chromosome numbers and protects from aneuploidy independently from p53," *Molecular Cancer*, vol. 13, article 107, 2014.

[18] A. A. Alshatwi, P. Subash-Babu, and P. Antonisamy, "Violacein induces apoptosis in human breast cancer cells through up regulation of BAX, p53 and down regulation of MDM2," *Experimental and Toxicologic Pathology*, vol. 68, no. 1, pp. 89–97, 2016.

[19] J. L. Koff, S. Ramachandiran, and L. Bernal-Mizrachi, "A time to kill: targeting apoptosis in cancer," *International Journal of Molecular Sciences*, vol. 16, no. 2, pp. 2942–2955, 2015.

[20] S. Shalini, L. Dorstyn, S. Dawar, and S. Kumar, "Old, new and emerging functions of caspases," *Cell Death & Differentiation*, vol. 22, pp. 526–539, 2015.

[21] S. Goldar, M. S. Khaniani, S. M. Derakhshan, and B. Baradaran, "Molecular mechanisms of apoptosis and roles in cancer development and treatment," *Asian Pacific Journal of Cancer Prevention*, vol. 16, no. 6, pp. 2129–2144, 2015.

[22] P. Indovina, F. Pentimalli, N. Casini, I. Vocca, and A. Giordano, "RB1 dual role in proliferation and apoptosis: cell fate control and implications for cancer therapy," *Oncotarget*, vol. 6, no. 20, pp. 17873–17890, 2015.

[23] M. Hazar-Rethinam, L. Endo-Munoz, O. Gannon, and N. Saunders, "The role of the E2F transcription factor family in UV-induced apoptosis," *International Journal of Molecular Sciences*, vol. 12, no. 12, pp. 8947–8960, 2011.

10

The Prognostic Role and Relationship between E2F1 and SV40 in Diffuse Large B-Cell Lymphoma of Egyptian Patients

Rehab M. Samaka, Hayam A. Aiad, Mona A. Kandil, Nancy Y. Asaad, and Nanes S. Holah

Pathology Department, Faculty of Medicine, Menoufia University, Shebin El-Kom, Egypt

Correspondence should be addressed to Rehab M. Samaka; rehabsamaka@yahoo.com

Academic Editor: Ekaterina S. Jordanova

Diffuse large B-cell lymphoma (DLBCL) is the most common type of lymphomas worldwide. The pathogenesis of lymphomas is not yet well understood. SV40 induces malignant transformation by the large T-antigen (L-TAG) and promotes transformation by binding and inactivating p53 and pRb. L-TAG can bind pRb promoting the activation of the E2F1 transcription factor, thus inducing the expression of genes required for the entry to the S phase and leading to cell transformation. This immunohistochemical study was conducted to assess the prognostic role and relationship of SV40 L-TAG and E2F1 in diffuse large B-cell lymphoma (DLBCL) of Egyptian patients. This retrospective study was conducted on 105 tissue specimens including 20 follicular hyperplasia and 85 DLBCL cases. SV40 L-TAG was identified in 3/85 (4%) of DLBCL. High Ki-67 labeling index (Ki-67 LI) and apoptotic count were associated with high E2F1 expression ($p < 0.001$ for all). No significant association was reached between E2F1 and SV40. E2F1 expression proved to be the most and first independent prognostic factor on overall survival of DLBCL patients (HR = 5.79, 95% CI= 2.3–14.6, and $p < 0.001$). Upregulation of E2F1 has been implicated in oncogenesis, prognosis, and prediction of therapeutic response but is not seemingly to have a relationship with the accused SV40.

1. Introduction

Non-Hodgkin's lymphoma (NHL) is the third common malignancy out of all malignances of Egyptian patients; it is of high rank among cancers in each sex, where it accounts for 8.4% of estimated incidence with 8.7 age standardized rate (ASR) per 100.000 [1]. In Egypt, NHL represents a major health problem as its rates are one of the highest in the world [2]. Diffuse large B-cell lymphoma (DLBCL) is the most common lymphoma worldwide [1].

Alarmingly, Simian virus (SV40) induces malignant transformation in rodents and human cells. This transformation is induced by the large T-antigen (L-TAG), known to promote transformation by binding and inactivating tumor suppressor genes, such as p53 and pRb [3]. Over the years, an increasing number of reports have suggested that SV40 causes specific tumor types, such as mesothelioma, brain, and bone tumors [4]. L-TAG can bind pRb promoting the activation of the E2F1 transcription factor, thus inducing the expression of genes required for the entry to the S phase [3]. Few studies have shown the presence of SV40 in lymphomas [4]. Nevertheless, SV40 could be taken into consideration for a putative role in human lymphomagenesis, alone or in combination with additional events, such as a transcription factor E2F1.

E2F is a family of transcription factors that regulate the expression of genes involved in a wide range of cellular processes, including cell-cycle progression, DNA repair, differentiation, and apoptosis [5]. E2F1, the founding member of the family, induces proliferation; both Rb-deficiency and ectopic expression of E2F1 in normal cells lead to high level of apoptosis owing to its ability to activate a large number of proapoptotic genes through a plethora of distinct apoptotic mechanisms [6]. However, the information about the role of E2F1 in human malignancy as depicted from its expression in relationship to tumor kinetic parameters and clinicopathological features is limited and incomplete.

The present immunohistochemical (IHC) study was conducted to assess the role and relationship of SV40 L-TAG and E2F1 in DLBCL of Egyptian patients, get a hint of whether

SV40 and E2F1 are coplayers in this malignancy or not, and correlate the results with the standard clinicopathological and survival data.

2. Materials and Methods

2.1. Studied Population. This retrospective case control study was conducted on 105 archival cases, including 85 DLBCL cases and 20 reactive follicular hyperplasia cases that were used as a control group. They were diagnosed in Pathology Department, Faculty of Medicine, Menoufia University, between January 2003 and December 2007. Written consent forms approved by The Committee of Human Rights in Research in Menoufia University were obtained from studied cases and control subjects before study initiation. Cases were newly diagnosed with no previous treatment taken.

2.2. Clinical Features. Staging was evaluated according to Ann-Arbor staging system and then the cases were divided into an early stage, by lumping stages I and II of the tumor, and an advanced stage, by lumping stages III and IV of the tumor. Revised international prognostic index (R-IPI) was calculated and the final scores stratified the DLBCL patients into 3 distinct prognostic groups [7]. For statistical purpose this score was simplified as 0–2 indicating good R-IPI and 3–5 indicating poor R-IPI. Age adjusted IPI (AAIPI) was applied separately in patients younger than or equal to 60 years (AAIPI < 60) and those older than 60 years (AAIPI > 60) to identify 3 risk groups for each category [8].

2.3. Histopathological Features. The hematoxylin and eosin (H&E) stained sections were evaluated for the presence and percentage of spontaneous coagulative tumor necrosis. Mitotic and apoptotic figures were counted in 10 randomly selected cellular fields under high power magnification (×400) and they were used as dichotomous covariant in the statistical analysis according to the median value for apoptosis and 25 for mitotic count [9]. The Ki-67 labeling index (Ki-67 LI) was determined using a semiquantitative visual approach and expressed as the percentage of Ki-67 positive malignant cells among a total number of 1000 malignant cells, at high power magnification [10]. Fifty percent cutoff point was applied to discriminate between low and high Ki-67 LI [11]. Scoring was carried out using an Olympus CH2 light microscope (Tokyo, Japan) with a wide angle (field size of 0.274 mm^2 and field diameter of 0.59 mm^2).

2.4. SV40 L-TAG and E2F1 Immunostaining Procedure. Five-micrometer-thick sections were cut from the paraffin-embedded blocks, deparaffinized in xylene, and rehydrated in a graded alcohol series. Epitope retrieval: the preferred method for SV40 is the use of Heat Induced Epitope Retrieval (HIER) techniques using Cell Marque's Trilogy (Cat. number 920P-04, Cell Marque, 6600 Sierra College Boulevard, Rocklin, CA 95677, USA) and followed by cooling at room temperature. For E2F1 epitope retrieval the tissue sections are boiled in 1 mM EDTA, pH 8.0. The slides were incubated overnight at 4°C with mouse monoclonal SV40 L-TAG Ab-2 with 1:100 as optimal dilution (Cat. number 351-14, Cell Marque, 6600 Sierra College Boulevard, Rocklin, CA 95677, USA). Positive control slides of SV40 infected renal tissues were used (Cat. number 351S, Thermo Scientific, Lab Vision Corporation, 46360 Fremont Boulevard, Fremont, CA 94538-6406, USA). The slides were incubated over night at 4°C with mouse monoclonal E2F1 with 1:200 as optimal dilution (Cat. number MS-879-P0Ab-2, Thermo Scientific, Lab Vision Corporation, 46360 Fremont Boulevard, Fremont, CA 94538-6406, USA). Breast carcinoma was used as a positive control. The detection kit used was ultravision detection system antipolyvalent HRP/DAB (ready to use) (Cat. number TP-015-HD, Thermo Scientific, Lab Vision Corporation, 46360 Fremont Boulevard, Fremont, CA 94538-6406, USA). The reaction was visualized by an appropriate substrate/chromogen (Diaminobenzidine, DAB) reagent with Mayer haematoxylin as a counterstain.

2.5. Assessment of SV40 and E2F1 Immunostained Slides. Positive SV40 expression is assigned when any number of cells shows true nuclear staining regardless of absence or presence of concomitant cytoplasmic staining while only cytoplasmic staining does not assign any positivity [12]. Evaluation of E2F-1 expression is based on the proportion of labeled nuclei either low E2F1 expression (≤10%) or high expression (>10%) [13]. Unintentional bias was prevented by coding patient tissue samples so that IHC analysis was done without knowledge of the patients' outcome and tumor characteristics. Assessment of slides was done by two of the authors (Rehab M. Samaka and Nanes S. Holah) separately.

2.6. Statistical Analysis. Statistical analysis was performed using SPSS "Statistical Package for the Social Science" program for windows, version 17, SPSS, Inc., Chicago, Illinois, USA. All factors were used as dichotomous covariates in the statistical analysis. To test whether these variables differed according to clinicopathological parameters and biological markers, the Fisher exact (FE), χ^2 test, Mann-Whitney test, and Student's t-test were used. Log-rank and Cox regression analysis were used for life-table assessment. All p values were two-sided; p values of <0.05 were considered statistically significant. Kaplan-Meier plots and hazard function curves were used to visualize the survival distribution.

3. Results

(i) Clinicopathological data of DLBCL cases studied are shown in Table 1.

(ii) SV40 expression in reactive lymphoid hyperplasia and DLBCL cases is as follows.

  (a) Negative expression of SV40 was noted in all reactive lymphoid hyperplasias (Figure 1(a)). Nuclear positivity for SV40 was identified in only 4% of DLBCL cases (3/85) (Figure 2).

  (b) The profiles of SV40 positive and negative DLBCL cases are shown in Table 2.

Table 1: Clinicopathological characteristics of DLBCL cases studied.

Variables	DLBCL (n = 85) No (%)
Age	
$\overline{x} \pm$ SD	54.31 ± 16.07
Median	56.0
Range	2.0–87.0
<60	49 (58)
≥60	36 (42)
Gender	
Male	42 (49)
Female	43 (51)
Primary site of involvement	
Nodal	56 (66)
Extranodal	29 (34)
Number of involved extranodal sites	
0	47 (55)
1-2	32 (38)
>2	6 (7)
Status	
Generalized	16 (29)
Localized	40 (71)
Size (cm)	
≤10	74 (87)
>10	11 (13)
Stage grouping	
Early	48 (56)
Advanced	37 (44)
PS	
<2	14 (16)
≥2	71 (84)
B symptoms	
Present	51 (60)
Absent	34 (40)
LDH	
Normal	11 (13)
Elevated	74 (87)
Prognostic group of R-IPI	
Good	29 (34)
Poor	56 (66)
Risk groups of AAIPI ≥60	
Low	6 (7)
Intermediate	16 (19)
High	17 (20)
Risk groups of AAIPI <60	
Low	17 (20)
Intermediate	11 (13)
High	18 (21)
Type of DLBCL	
Germinal	49 (57.6)
Nongerminal	36 (42.4)
Necrosis	
Present	14 (16)
Absent	71 (84)
$\overline{x} \pm$ SD	34.3 ± 22.4
Range	10.0–0.80
Mitosis	
$\overline{x} \pm$ SD	22.5 ± 9.5
Range	6.0–46.0
Media	21.0
Ki-67 LI	
<50	50 (59)
≥50	35 (41)
Apoptosis	
$\overline{x} \pm$ SD	13.5 ± 6.4
Range	3.0–31.0
Median	13.0

R-IPI: revised international prognostic index; AAIPI: age adjusted international prognostic index.
PS: performance status; LDH: lactate dehydrogenase; Ki-67 LI: Ki-67 labeling index.
DLBCL: diffuse large B-cell lymphoma.

(iii) E2F1 expression in reactive follicular hyperplasia and DLBCL cases is as follows.

(a) All reactive follicular hyperplasia cases showed nuclear E2F1 staining with variable percentages of positivity. The topography of positive lymphocytes was distributed in the germinal centers and in the interfollicular areas with complete negativity in the mantle zone lymphocytes (Figure 3). Low E2F1 expression (≤10%) was detected in 15/20 cases (75%), while high E2F1 expression (>10%) was detected in 5/20 (25%) of them.

(b) All DLBCL cases studied showed positive E2F1 expression. Regarding DLBCL cases, high E2F1 expression (>10%) (Figure 4(a)) presented in 44/85 of cases (52%), while low E2F1 expression (≤10%) (Figure 4(b)) presented in 41/85 of cases (48%).

(iv) Relationship of E2F1 expression in DLBCL cases studied with the clinicopathological features and presence of SV40 is shown in Table 3.

There was a highly significant difference between low and high E2F1 expression in DLBCL cases regarding the age and age grouping as the lower numerical values of age had associated with high E2F1 expression (p = 0.001 and p = 0.02, resp.). Numerous mitoses, high Ki-67 LI, and an abundant number of apoptotic counts were significantly associated with DLBCL cases with high E2F1 expression ($p < 0.001$ for all). There was a significant difference between low and high E2F1 expression in DLBCL cases regarding the risk groups of AAIPI < 60, as

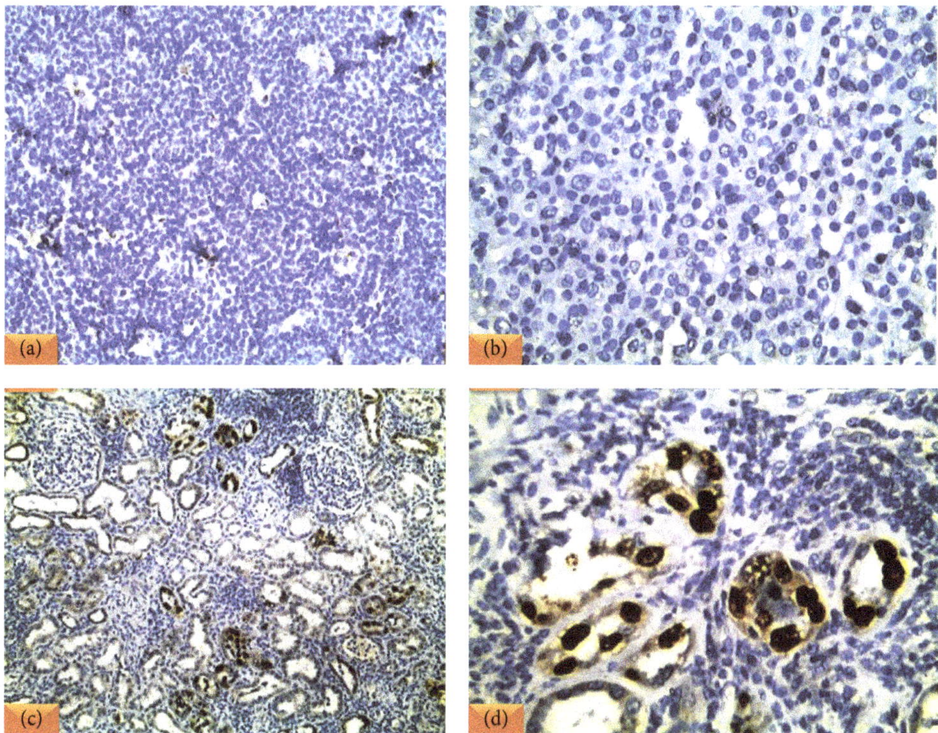

FIGURE 1: (a) Reactive follicular hyperplasia with prominent tangible body macrophages showed SV40 negativity. (b) Diffuse large B-cell lymphoma (DLBCL) displayed SV40 negativity. (c) SV40 infected renal tissue was the positive control. (d) High power view demonstrating the nuclear SV40 positivity in the tubular cells (IHC ×200 for (a) and (c) and ×400 for (b) and (d)).

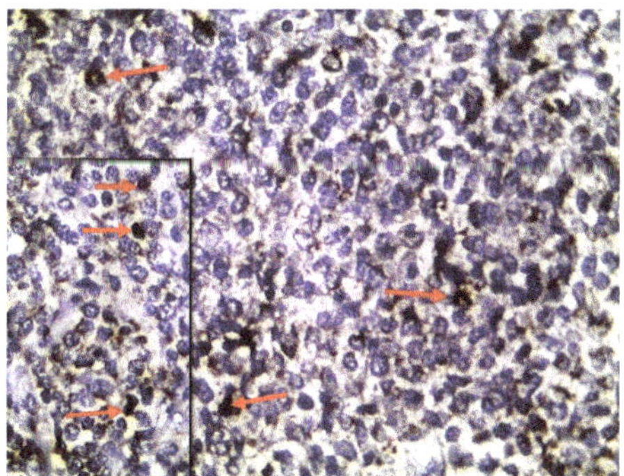

FIGURE 2: The malignant lymphocytes showed positive nuclear staining (arrows) of SV40 in a case of DLBCL. Inset closer view of nuclear staining of SV40 (arrows) (IHC ×400).

71% of cases with high risk group had high E2F1 expression ($p = 0.049$). There was no significant association between E2F1 expression and presence of SV40 in DLBCL cases.

(v) Survival analysis of DLBCL cases showed the following.

By univariate survival analysis, ≥60 years age group (log-rank (LR) test = 4.21, $p = 0.04$), worse PS (LR test = 34.94, $p < 0.001$) (Figure 5), elevated LDH (LR test = 4.15, $p = 0.042$), presence of B symptoms (LR test = 4.9, $p = 0.027$), advanced stage (LR = 12.19, $p < 0.001$), poor prognostic group of R-IPI (LR test = 19.95, $p < 0.001$) (Figure 6), high risk group of AAIPI < 60 (LR test = 15.01, $p < 0.001$), high Ki-67 LI and apoptotic counts (LR test = 16.93 and LR test = 12.66, resp., $p < 0.001$ for both), and high E2F1 expression (LR test = 14.99, $p < 0.001$) (Figure 7) had shorter survival time of DLBCL cases. By multivariate survival analysis, E2F1 expression proved to be the most and first independent prognostic factor on overall survival of DLBCL patients (HR = 5.79, 95% CI = 2.3–14.6, and $p < 0.001$).

4. Discussion

In Egypt, the high incidence of NHL is possibly related to the exposure of population, at a young age, to various bacterial, parasitic, and viral infections which result in a sustained stimulation of the lymphoid system [1, 14]. In view of limited and controversial data about SV40 in NHL, we decide to explore the prevalence of SV40 in DLBCL tissue specimens of Egyptian patients. In the current IHC study, 3/85 (4%) of DLBCL cases were positive for SV40 L-TAG. It was reported that there is no role of SV40 L-TAG in human lymphomas in patients at risk of having received SV40-contaminated poliomyelitis virus vaccines in Italian, Swiss, and Austrian patients [12]. Also, L-TAG was not detected in a lymphoma series of French and Canadian cases as well as in Spanish

Table 2: Descriptive data for SV40 expression in DLBCL.

Variables	Positive SV40 (n = 3) No (%)	Negative SV40 (n = 82) No (%)
Age		
$\overline{x} \pm$ SD	31.0 ± 19.5	55.2 ± 15.4
Median	30.0	56.0
Range	12–51	2–87
<60	1 (2)	48 (98)
≥60	2 (6)	34 (94)
Gender		
Male	1 (2)	41 (98)
Female	2 (5)	41 (95)
Primary site of involvement		
Nodal	2 (4)	54 (96)
Extranodal	1 (3)	28 (97)
Number of involved extranodal sites		
0	1 (2)	46 (98)
1-2	0 (0)	32 (100)
>2	2 (33)	4 (67)
Status		
Generalized	2 (12)	14 (88)
Localized	1 (2)	39 (98)
Size (cm)		
≤10	2 (3)	72 (97)
>10	1 (9)	10 (91)
Stage grouping		
Early	0 (0)	48 (100)
Advanced	3 (8)	34 (92)
PS		
<2	0 (0)	14 (100)
≥2	3 (4.2)	68 (95.8)
B symptoms		
Present	2 (4)	49 (96)
Absent	1 (3)	33 (97)
LDH		
Normal	0 (0)	11 (100)
Elevated	3 (4)	71 (96)
Prognostic group of R-IPI		
Good	0 (0)	29 (100)
Poor	3 (5)	53 (95)
Risk groups of AAIPI ≥60		
Low	0 (0)	0 (0)
Intermediate	0 (0)	0 (0)
High	2 (14)	0 (0)
Risk groups of AAIPI <60		
Low	0 (0)	0 (0)
Intermediate	0 (0)	0 (0)
High	1 (100)	0 (0)
Type of DLBCL		
Germinal	2 (4)	47 (96)
Nongerminal	1 (2.8)	35 (97.2)
Necrosis		
Present	0 (0)	14 (100)
Absent	3 (14)	68 (96)
$\overline{x} \pm$ SD	—	34.29 ± 22.43
Range	—	10.0–80.0

Table 2: Continued.

Variables	Positive SV40 (n = 3) No (%)	Negative SV40 (n = 82) No (%)
Mitosis		
$\overline{x} \pm$ SD	21.3 ± 1.5	22.5 ± 9.7
Range	20–23	6–46
Media	21.0	21.5
Ki-67 LI		
<50	3 (4)	74 (96)
≥50	0 (0)	8 (100)
Apoptosis		
$\overline{x} \pm$ SD	12.7 ± 3.1	13.5 ± 6.5
Range	10–16	3–31
Median	12	13

R-IPI: revised international prognostic index; AAIPI: age adjusted international prognostic index.
PS: performance status; LDH: lactate dehydrogenase; Ki-67 LI: Ki-67 labeling index.
DLBCL: diffuse large B-cell lymphoma.

patients [15, 16]. Similarly, SV40 L-TAG was detected in 1/25 posttransplant lymphoproliferative disorders and 1/5 AIDS lymphoma in USA [17]. Moreover, weak signals of SV40 L-TAG expression were detected in 12/55 HIV-associated lymphomas in USA and in 4% of Swiss mesothelioma patients [18, 19].

SV40 L-TAG expression in few numbers of DLBCL cases studied might be interpreted by one of the following attributions and theories: (a) absence of the integrated SV40 genome in the host cell and thus absence of permanent expression of the oncoprotein L-TAG [12, 15, 16], (b) the short half-life of the L-TAG [19], (c) the difference in geographic distribution and incidence of SV40 virus strains [17], (d) an underestimation of viral content as the DNAs recovered from paraffin-embedded tissues are highly fragmented [20], and (e) on the other hand the capability of adopting the "hit and run model" for L-TAG induced transformation claiming that viruses can mediate cellular transformations through an initial "hit" while maintenance of the transformed state is compatible with the loss "run" of viral molecules [21, 22].

Moreover, few polymerase chain reaction (PCR) studies have shown the presence of SV40 in lymphomas with contradicting results. Two Egyptian studies using multiplex nested PCR have shown that SV40 DNA sequences were found in 53.8% of NHL patients in both series [23, 24]. Other studies found 13, 10, 14, 42, and 43% incidence of SV40 in NHL, respectively [17, 25, 26]. However, other studies have not supported these findings [27, 28]. Despite these contradicting results, a recent report concluded that SV40 should be added to the list of factors playing a role in the pathogenesis of B-cell lymphoma, acting together with mutated p53 in the multistep tumorigenesis of lymphoproliferative disorders [4].

The reasons for the discrepant findings are not clear. You and colleagues assumed that a fascinating possibility of

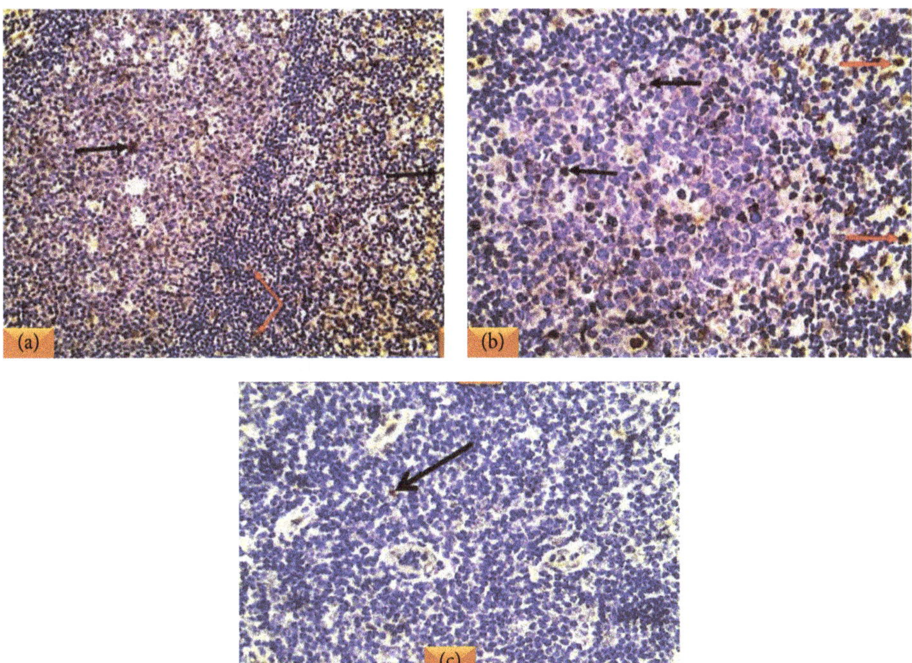

FIGURE 3: (a) A case of reactive follicular hyperplasia showed positive nuclear staining of E2F1 in the lymphocytes in the germinal center (black arrows) and in the interfollicular area (red arrows). (b) High power view of lymphocytes with nuclear positivity in the germinal center (black arrows) and in the interfollicular area (red arrows) together with negative mantle zone lymphocytes. (c) A germinal center exhibited single lymphocyte with nuclear E2F1 positivity (arrow) (IHC ×200 for (a) and ×400 (b) and (c)).

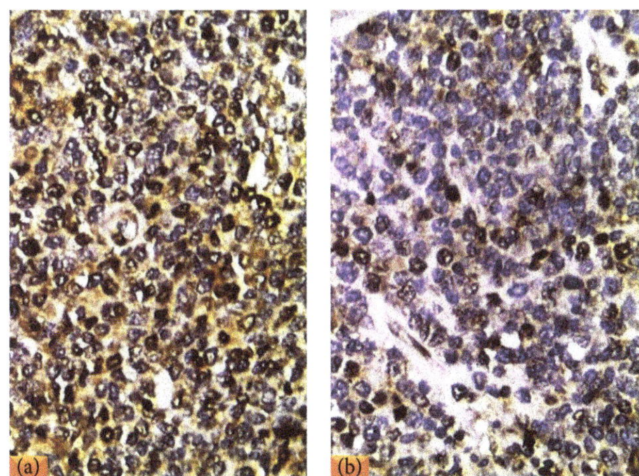

FIGURE 4: (a) A case of DLBCL showed high nuclear E2F1 expression. (b) A case of DLBCL displayed low nuclear E2F1 expression (IHC ×400 for (a) and (b)).

some viral microRNAs (miRNAs) may function as orthologs of cellular miRNAs, but the function of most of them is unknown [29, 30]. SV40-encoded miR-S1-5p was reported to downregulate the expression of viral T-antigen without reducing the yield of infectious virus, thus reducing host cytotoxic T lymphocyte (CTL) susceptibility and local cytokine release. This dispensable downregulation appears to be very helpful in maintaining the long-term relationship between the virus and the host during latent viral infection or virus-mediated tumorigenesis [34]. Nevertheless, the orthologous role of SV40-miR-S1-5p with cellular miR423-5p also implied that SV40-encoded miRNA not only autoregulates its viral gene expression but also may regulate cellular gene expression [29].

The functions and expression of SV40 are a complex process that depends on numerous factors depending on the cellular context, virus host interaction, and accuracy and sufficiency of detection techniques. E2F is a family of transcription factors that regulate the expression of genes involved in a wide range of cellular processes [5]. In the present study, E2F1 was expressed in 5/20 (25%) of reactive follicular hyperplasia cases mainly localized to the proliferating germinal center and few in the interfollicular areas with complete negativity in the mantle zone lymphocytes. Our results agreed with other reports that stated that E2F1 is a transcription factor that mediates cell-cycle progression from the G1 to S phase and is normally regulated by a group of proteins, including cyclin D1, mainly in the germinal center [31, 32].

In the current study all DLBCL cases with high mitosis (high Ki-67 LI) had high E2F1 expression that was consistent with other studies [31, 32]. They stated that E2F1 regulates the transcription of many genes necessary for G1/S and G2/M phase transitions, DNA replication, synthesis, and mitosis [6, 31, 33].

E2F1 modulates cell death via activation of proapoptotic genes and by inactivation of antiapoptotic survival factors through p53-dependent or p53-independent pathways [34]

TABLE 3: Relationship of E2F1 expression with the clinicopathological data and expression of SV40 in DLBCL cases.

Variables	E2F1 among DLBCL ≤10 ($n = 41$) No (%)	E2F1 among DLBCL >10 ($n = 44$) No (%)	Test of significance and p value
Age			
($\overline{x} \pm$ SD)	58.5 ± 6.8	50.4 ± 14.5	**t = 2.36** **0.020***
Median	69.0	56	
Range	32–75	41–70	
Age			
<60	16 (33)	33 (67)	**χ^2 = 11.25** **0.001****
≥60	25 (69)	11 (31)	
Gender			
Male	21 (50)	21 (50)	χ^2 = 0.10 0.748
Female	20 (47)	23 (53)	
Primary site of involvement			
Nodal	29 (52)	27 (48)	χ^2 = 0.83 0.363
Extranodal	12 (41)	17 (59)	
Number of involved extranodal sites			
0	25 (3)	22 (47)	FE = 1.21 0.553
1-2	13 (41)	19 (59)	
>2	3 (50)	3 (50)	
Status (nodal = 56)			
Generalized	9 (40)	9 (60)	FE = 0.809 0.779
Localized	17 (53)	21 (47)	
Size (cm)			
≤10	36 (49)	6 (51)	χ^2 = 0.04 0.843
>10	5 (45)	38 (55)	
Stage grouping			
Early	25 (52)	23 (48)	χ^2 = 0.65 0.419
Advanced	16 (43)	21 (57)	
PS			
<2	7 (50)	7 (50)	FE = 1.088 1.000
≥2	34 (48)	37 (52)	
B symptoms			
Present	23 (45)	28 (55)	χ^2 = 0.50 0.478
Absent	18 (53)	16 (47)	
LDH			
Normal	3 (27)	8 (73)	χ^2 = 2.22 0.136
Elevated	38 (51)	36 (49)	
Prognostic group of R-IPI			
Good	14 (48)	15 (52)	χ^2 = 0.00 0.996
Poor	27 (48)	29 (52)	
Risk groups of AAIPI ≥60			
Low	12 (86)	2 (14)	FE = 3.09 0.233
Intermediate	5 (63)	3 (37)	
High	6 (55)	5 (45)	

TABLE 3: Continued.

Variables	E2F1 among DLBCL ≤10 ($n = 41$) No (%)	E2F1 among DLBCL >10 ($n = 44$) No (%)	Test of significance and p value
Risk groups of AAIPI <60			
Low	2 (15)	11 (85)	**FE = 5.85 0.049***
Intermediate	10 (66)	8 (44)	
High	6 (29)	15 (71)	
Type of DLBCL			
Germinal	22 (45)	27 (55)	FE = 1.34
Nongerminal	18 (50)	18 (50)	0.80
Necrosis			
Present	5 (36)	9 (64)	$\chi^2 = 1.05$
Absent	36 (51)	35 (49)	0.305
Necrosis (%)			
$\bar{x} \pm$ SD	44.0 ± 23.0	28.9 ± 21.5	$U = 1.15$ 0.249
Median	60	20	
Range	10–60	10–80	
Mitosis			
$\bar{x} \pm$ SD	14.5 ± 4.4	29.9 ± 6.3	**U = 12.98 <0.001****
Median	13	34	
Range	12–14	24–43	
Ki-67 LI			
<50	41 (82)	9 (18)	**$\chi^2 = 55.44$**
≥50	0 (0)	35 (100)	**<0.001****
Apoptosis			
$\bar{x} \pm$ SD	10.5 ± 4.9	16.3 ± 6.4	**U = 4.29 <0.001****
Median	11	17	
Range	4–26	5–25	
SV40			
Positive	1 (33)	2 (67)	FE = 0.28
Negative	40 (49)	42 (51)	1.00

R-IPI: revised international prognostic index; AAIPI: age adjusted international prognostic index; PS: performance status; LDH: lactate dehydrogenase; *significant; **highly significant; t-test: Student's t-test; U: Mann-Whitney test; FE: Fisher's exact test; χ^2: Chi-square test; Ki-67 LI: Ki-67 labeling index; DLBCL: diffuse large B-cell lymphoma.

that is consistent with the current results as DLBCL cases with numerous apoptosis belonged to high E2F1 expression.

E2F1 can stabilize p53 via transcriptional induction of p14ARF, which binds directly to mouse double minutes (MDM2) and inhibits its ability to target p53 for subsequent degradation resulting in p53 accumulation and subsequent activation of its downstream target genes required for apoptosis [6]. A second major mechanism by which E2F1 sensitizes cells to apoptosis is mediated in a p53-independent manner through antiapoptotic signaling mediated by NFκB and Bcl-2 [35].

Viral T-antigens can bind all members of the pRb family promoting the activation of the E2F family, thus inducing the expression of genes required for the entry to the S phase [36]. However, the current study revealed no association between E2F1 expression and presence of SV40 was observed in DLBCL cases. This study offers novel insights into the assumed E2F1 activity that is not seemingly to have a relationship with the accused SV40 in DLBCL of the Egyptian patients.

According to the survival analysis multivariate Cox regression hazard analysis revealed that overexpression of E2F1 is independent prognostic factor for DLBCL cases studied and associated with dismal outcome.

Several reports were concordant with our findings on breast carcinoma, esophageal squamous cell carcinoma, pancreatic ductal carcinoma, non-small-cell lung cancer, and glioblastoma [37–41]. Few reports were in contrast with our findings; low E2F-1 was associated with shortened survival of DLBCL and bladder carcinoma patients [13, 42]. However, squamous cell lung carcinoma cases have no prognostic impact of E2F1 [43].

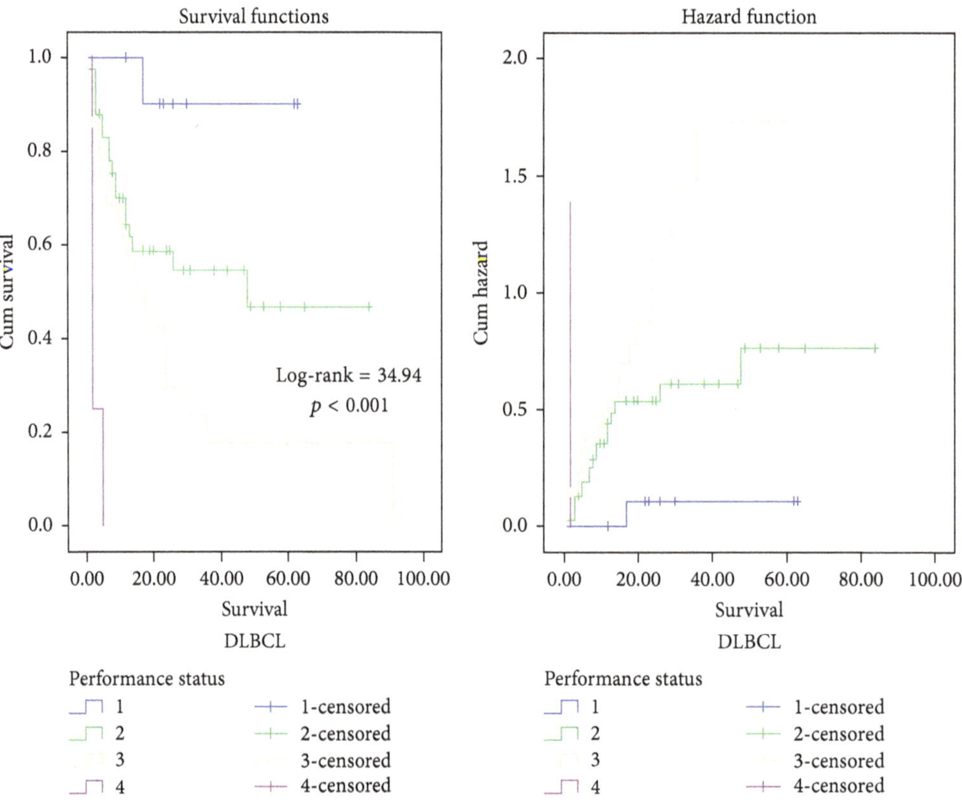

FIGURE 5: Kaplan-Meier and hazard function curve of overall survival (OS) for DLBCL patients with different categories of performance status (PS) indicating that patients with PS = 4 were more hazardous.

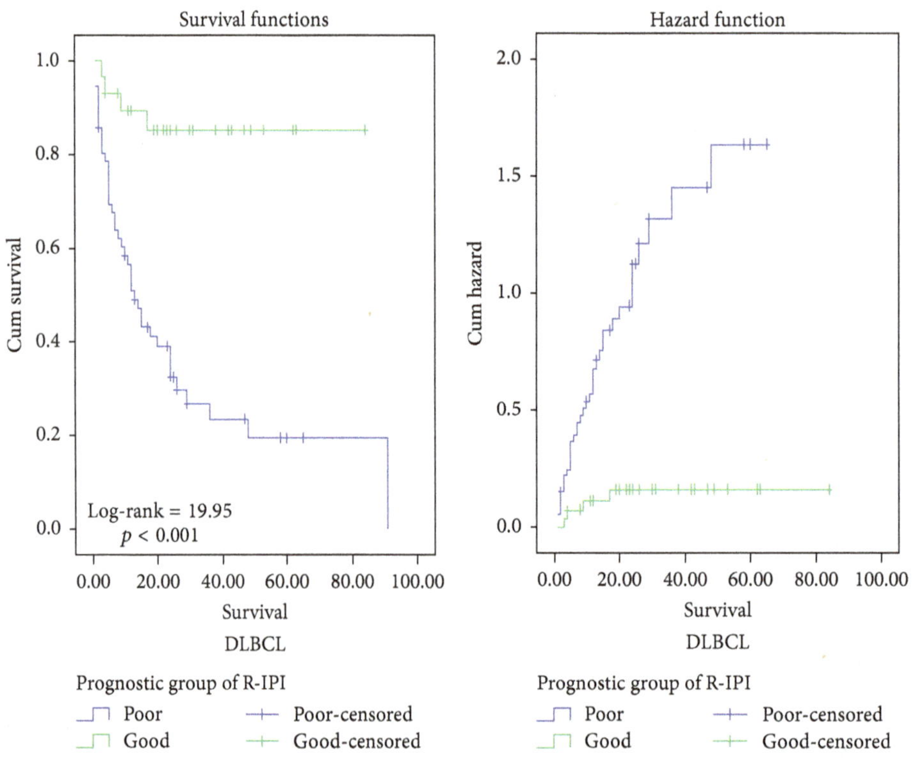

FIGURE 6: Kaplan-Meier and hazard function curve of OS for DLBCL patients with different categories of prognostic group of R-IPI indicating that poor prognostic group was more hazardous.

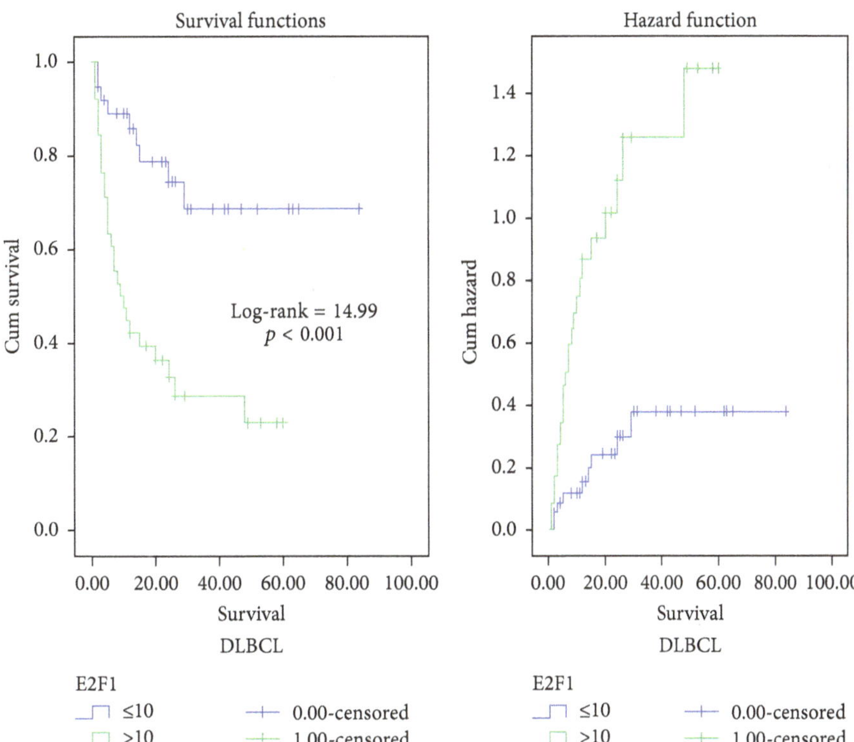

Figure 7: Kaplan-Meier and hazard function curve of OS for DLBCL patients with low and high E2F1 expression indicating that high E2F1 expression was more hazardous.

This dual role of E2F1 in cell-cycle progression and apoptosis gave it the property to be used as a target therapy. Currently, it is hypothesized that the evidence is inadequate to accept or to reject a causal relationship between SV40 and DLBCL in Egyptian patients. E2F1 has a putative oncogenic signaling in DLBCL in the current series by orchestrating and engaging cell death pathways either alone or in cooperation with cellular proliferation pathways. Overexpression of E2F1 is an indicator for short overall survival in DLBCL patients. It is therefore assumed that upregulation of E2F1 has been implicated in oncogenesis, prognosis, and prediction of therapeutic response together with development of novel target therapy. In DLBCL, the assumed E2F1 activity is not seemingly to have a relationship with the accused SV40.

Disclosure

This paper is original. The requirements for authorship have been met, and each author believes that the paper represents honest work. The paper is not currently under consideration for publication in another journal. This paper has not been published elsewhere and it has not been submitted simultaneously for publication elsewhere.

Disclaimer

The authors alone are responsible for the content and writing of the paper.

Conflict of Interests

The authors report no conflict of interests to declare pertaining to this paper.

Authors' Contribution

All the authors were active participants. This paper has been read and approved by all the authors.

References

[1] "Epidemiology of cancer," in *Pathology of Cancer*, M. N. El Bolkainy, M. A. Nouh, I. G. Farahat et al., Eds., chapter 2, pp. 15–31, Cairo Press, Cairo, Egypt, 4th edition, 2013.

[2] A. S. Soliman and P. Boffetta, "Lymphoma and leukemia," in *Cancer Incidence in Four Member Countries (Cyprus, Egypt, Israel, and Jordan) of the Middle East Cancer Consortium (MECC) Compared with US SEER*, L. S. Freedman, B. K. Edwards, L. A. G. Ries, and J. L. Young, Eds., chapter 14, pp. 131–140, National Cancer Institute, 1st edition, 2006.

[3] G. Barbanti-Brodano, F. Martini, A. Corallini et al., "Reactivation of infectious simian virus 40 from normal human tissues," *Journal of NeuroVirology*, vol. 10, no. 3, pp. 199–205, 2004.

[4] S. Heinsohn, R. Scholz, and H. Kabisch, "SV40 and p53 as team players in childhood lymphoproliferative disorders," *International Journal of Oncology*, vol. 38, no. 5, pp. 1307–1317, 2011.

[5] A. K. Biswas and D. G. Johnson, "Transcriptional and non-transcriptional functions of E2F1 in response to DNA damage," *Cancer Research*, vol. 72, no. 1, pp. 13–17, 2012.

[6] Z. Wu, S. Zheng, and Q. Yu, "The E2F family and the role of E2F1 in apoptosis," *International Journal of Biochemistry and Cell Biology*, vol. 41, no. 12, pp. 2389–2397, 2009.

[7] L. H. Sehn, B. Berry, M. Chhanabhai et al., "The revised International Prognostic Index (R-IPI) is a better predictor of outcome than the standard IPI for patients with diffuse large B-cell lymphoma treated with R-CHOP," *Blood*, vol. 109, no. 5, pp. 1857–1861, 2007.

[8] P. A. Hamlin, A. D. Zelenetz, T. Kewalramani et al., "Age-adjusted International Prognostic Index predicts autologous stem cell transplantation outcome for patients with relapsed or primary refractory diffuse large B-cell lymphoma," *Blood*, vol. 102, no. 6, pp. 1989–1996, 2003.

[9] A. López-Guillermo, L. Colomo, M. Jiménez et al., "Diffuse large B-cell lymphoma: clinical and biological characterization and outcome according to the nodal or extranodal primary origin," *Journal of Clinical Oncology*, vol. 23, no. 12, pp. 2797–2804, 2005.

[10] M. A. Aleskandarany, E. A. Rakha, R. D. MacMillan, D. G. Powe, I. O. Ellis, and A. R. Green, "MIB1/Ki-67 labelling index can classify grade 2 breast cancer into two clinically distinct subgroups," *Breast Cancer Research and Treatment*, vol. 127, no. 3, pp. 591–599, 2011.

[11] S. Uddin, A. Hussain, M. Ahmed et al., "S-phase kinase protein 2 is an attractive therapeutic target in a subset of diffuse large B-cell lymphoma," *The Journal of Pathology*, vol. 216, no. 4, pp. 483–494, 2008.

[12] P. Went, C. A. Seemayer, S. Pileri, R. Maurer, A. Tzankov, and S. Dirnhofer, "Lack of protein expression of the simian virus 40 large T antigen in human lymphomas," *Journal of Medical Virology*, vol. 80, no. 6, pp. 1112–1115, 2008.

[13] M. B. Møller, P. W. Kania, Y. Ino et al., "Frequent disruption of the RB1 pathway in diffuse large B cell lymphoma: prognostic significance of E2F-1 and $p16^{INK4A}$," *Leukemia*, vol. 14, no. 5, pp. 898–904, 2000.

[14] "Haematologic malignancy," in *Pathology of Cancer*, M. N. El Bolkainy, M. A. Nouh, I. G. Farahat et al., Eds., chapter 25, pp. 406–450, Cairo Press, Cairo, Egypt, 4th edition, 2013.

[15] P. Brousset, V. de Araujo, and R. D. Gascoyne, "Immunohistochemical investigation of SV40 large T antigen in Hodgkin and non-Hodgkin's lymphoma," *International Journal of Cancer*, vol. 112, no. 3, pp. 533–535, 2004.

[16] J. Hernández-Losa, C. G. Fedele, F. Pozo et al., "Lack of association of polyomavirus and herpesvirus types 6 and 7 in human lymphomas," *Cancer*, vol. 103, no. 2, pp. 293–298, 2005.

[17] P. Rizzo, M. Carbone, S. G. Fisher et al., "Simian virus 40 is present in most United States human mesotheliomas, but it is rarely present in non-Hodgkin's lymphoma," *Chest*, vol. 116, supplement 6, pp. 470S–473S, 1999.

[18] R. A. Vilchez, D. Lopez-Terrada, J. R. Middleton et al., "Simian virus 40 tumor antigen expression and immunophenotypic profile of AIDS-related non-Hodgkin's lymphoma," *Virology*, vol. 342, no. 1, pp. 38–46, 2005.

[19] A. Ziegler, C. A. Seemayer, M. Hinterberger et al., "Low prevalence of SV40 in Swiss mesothelioma patients after elimination of false-positive PCR results," *Lung Cancer*, vol. 57, no. 3, pp. 282–291, 2007.

[20] S. Toracchio, C. A. Kozinetz, D. E. Killen et al., "Variable frequency of polyomavirus SV40 and herpesvirus EBV in lymphomas from two different urban population groups in Houston, TX," *Journal of Clinical Virology*, vol. 46, no. 2, pp. 154–160, 2009.

[21] K. Khalili, L. Del Valle, J. Otte, M. Weaver, and J. Gordon, "Human neurotropic polyomavirus, JCV, and its role in carcinogenesis," *Oncogene*, vol. 22, no. 33, pp. 5181–5191, 2003.

[22] L. Ricciardiello, M. Baglioni, and C. Giovannini, "Induction of chromosomal instability in colonic cells by the human polyomavirus JC virus," *Cancer Research*, vol. 63, no. 21, pp. 7256–7262, 2003.

[23] W. S. Mohamed, M. A. Samra, and M. A. Fawzy, "Presence of simian virus 40 DNA sequences in Egyptian patients with lymphoproliferative disorders," *International Journal of Health Sciences*, vol. 1, no. 1, pp. 11–16, 2007.

[24] A.-R. Zekri, W. Mohamed, A. Bahnassy et al., "Detection of simian virus 40 DNA sequences in Egyptian patients with different hematological malignancies," *Leukemia and Lymphoma*, vol. 48, no. 9, pp. 1828–1834, 2007.

[25] F. Martini, R. Dolcetti, A. Gloghini et al., "Simian-virus-40 footprints in human lymphoproliferative disorders of HIV^- and HIV^+ patients," *International Journal of Cancer*, vol. 78, no. 6, pp. 669–674, 1998.

[26] R. A. Vilchez, C. R. Madden, C. A. Kozinetz et al., "Association between simian virus 40 and non-Hodgkin lymphoma," *The Lancet*, vol. 359, no. 9309, pp. 817–823, 2002.

[27] S. de Sanjose, K. V. Shah, E. Domingo-Domenech et al., "Lack of serological evidence for an association between simian virus 40 and lymphoma," *International Journal of Cancer*, vol. 104, no. 4, pp. 522–524, 2003.

[28] J. MacKenzie, K. S. Wilson, J. Perry, A. Gallagher, and R. F. Jarrett, "Association between simian virus 40 DNA and lymphoma in the United Kingdom," *Journal of the National Cancer Institute*, vol. 95, no. 13, pp. 1001–1003, 2003.

[29] X. You, Z. Zhang, J. Fan, Z. Cui, and X.-E. Zhang, "Functionally orthologous viral and cellular microRNAs studied by a novel dual-fluorescent reporter system," *PLoS ONE*, vol. 7, no. 4, Article ID e36157, 2012.

[30] C. S. Sullivan, A. T. Grundhoff, S. Tevethia, J. M. Pipas, and D. Ganem, "SV40-encoded microRNAs regulate viral gene expression and reduce susceptibility to cytotoxic T cells," *Nature*, vol. 435, no. 7042, pp. 682–686, 2005.

[31] J. A. Chan, M. Olvera, R. Lai, W. Naing, S. A. Rezk, and R. K. Brynes, "Immunohistochemical expression of the transcription factor DP-1 and its heterodimeric partner E2F-1 in non-Hodgkin lymphoma," *Applied Immunohistochemistry and Molecular Morphology*, vol. 10, no. 4, pp. 322–326, 2002.

[32] R. Lai, L. J. Medeiros, R. Coupland, A. McCourty, and R. K. Brynes, "Immunohistochemical detection of E2F-1 in non-Hodgkin's lymphomas: a survey of 124 cases," *Modern Pathology*, vol. 11, no. 5, pp. 457–463, 1998.

[33] A. Blais and B. D. Dynlacht, "Hitting their targets: an emerging picture of E2F and cell cycle control," *Current Opinion in Genetics and Development*, vol. 14, no. 5, pp. 527–532, 2004.

[34] S. Emmrich and B. M. Pützer, "Checks and balances: E2F-microRNA crosstalk in cancer control," *Cell Cycle*, vol. 9, no. 13, pp. 2555–2567, 2010.

[35] J. Stanelle and B. M. Pützer, "E2F1-induced apoptosis: turning killers into therapeutics," *Trends in Molecular Medicine*, vol. 12, no. 4, pp. 177–185, 2006.

[36] V. Caracciolo, K. Reiss, K. Khalili, G. De Falco, and A. Giordano, "Role of the interaction between large T antigen and Rb family members in the oncogenicity of JC virus," *Oncogene*, vol. 25, no. 38, pp. 5294–5301, 2006.

[37] V. Vuaroqueaux, P. Urban, M. Labuhn et al., "Low E2F1 transcript levels are a strong determinant of favorable breast cancer outcome," *Breast Cancer Research*, vol. 9, no. 3, article R33, 2007.

[38] Y. Ebihara, M. Miyamoto, T. Shichinohe et al., "Over-expression of E2F-1 in esophageal squamous cell carcinoma correlates with tumor progression," *Diseases of the Esophagus*, vol. 17, no. 2, pp. 150–154, 2004.

[39] K. Yamazaki, T. Yajima, T. Nagao et al., "Expression of transcription factor E2F-1 in pancreatic ductal carcinoma: an immunohistochemical study," *Pathology Research and Practice*, vol. 199, no. 1, pp. 23–28, 2003.

[40] C.-L. Huang, D. Liu, J. Nakano et al., "E2F1 overexpression correlates with thymidylate synthase and survivin gene expressions and tumor proliferation in non small-cell lung cancer," *Clinical Cancer Research*, vol. 13, no. 23, pp. 6938–6946, 2007.

[41] M. M. Alonso, J. Fueyo, J. W. Shay et al., "Expression of transcription factor E2F1 and telomerase in glioblastomas: mechanistic linkage and prognostic significance," *Journal of the National Cancer Institute*, vol. 97, no. 21, pp. 1589–1600, 2005.

[42] F. Rabbani, V. M. Richon, I. Orlow et al., "Prognostic significance of transcription factor E2F-1 in bladder cancer: genotypic and phenotypic characterization," *Journal of the National Cancer Institute*, vol. 91, no. 10, pp. 874–881, 1999.

[43] M. Volm, R. Koomägi, and W. Rittgen, "Clinical implications of cyclins, cyclin-dependent kinases, RB and E2F1 in squamous-cell lung carcinoma," *International Journal of Cancer*, vol. 79, no. 3, pp. 294–299, 1998.

11

FoxO Proteins in the Nervous System

Kenneth Maiese

Cellular and Molecular Signaling, Newark, NJ 07101, USA

Correspondence should be addressed to Kenneth Maiese; wntin75@yahoo.com

Academic Editor: Nady Braidy

Acute as well as chronic disorders of the nervous system lead to significant morbidity and mortality for millions of individuals globally. Given the ability to govern stem cell proliferation and differentiated cell survival, mammalian forkhead transcription factors of the forkhead box class O (FoxO) are increasingly being identified as potential targets for disorders of the nervous system, such as Alzheimer's disease, Parkinson's disease, Huntington's disease, amyotrophic lateral sclerosis, and auditory neuronal disease. FoxO proteins are present throughout the body, but they are selectively expressed in the nervous system and have diverse biological functions. The forkhead O class transcription factors interface with an array of signal transduction pathways that include protein kinase B (Akt), serum- and glucocorticoid-inducible protein kinase (SgK), IκB kinase (IKK), silent mating type information regulation 2 homolog 1 (*S. cerevisiae*) (SIRT1), growth factors, and Wnt signaling that can determine the activity and integrity of FoxO proteins. Ultimately, there exists a complex interplay between FoxO proteins and their signal transduction pathways that can significantly impact programmed cell death pathways of apoptosis and autophagy as well as the development of clinical strategies for the treatment of neurodegenerative disorders.

1. Clinical Significance of Nervous System Disorders

Nervous system disorders lead to disability and death in a significant proportion of the world's population. For example, almost ten percent of the global population suffers from the sporadic form of Alzheimer's disease (AD) while familial cases of AD account for less than 2% of all presentation [1, 2]. In the United States alone, greater than 5 million individuals have AD and another 3.5 million individuals are under treatment at an annual cost of almost 4 billion US dollars. In regards to cerebrovascular disease, stroke is presently ranked as the fourth leading cause of death and can also affect the lives of millions of individuals [3]. A number of factors are responsible for stroke no longer being ranked higher as a cause of death. These factors include improved management of hypertension and diabetes, reduction in tobacco consumption, heightened public awareness for seeking rapid care [3, 4], treatment with recombinant tissue plasminogen activator [5], and novel new strategies that focus on trophic factors, improved biomarkers, and cellular pathways of oxidative stress [3, 6–10].

Yet, the availability of treatments that can prevent the initiation of acute or chronic neurodegenerative disorders or block the progression of these diseases is scarce. Therapeutic strategies that can aggressively treat AD and stroke continue to remain limited for most individuals. Furthermore, multiple other neurodegenerative disorders also greatly impact the global population with treatments that are not always optimal. By the year 2030, epilepsy is predicted to affect over 50 million people, neuropathies are estimated to afflict almost 300 million individuals, and neurological injuries may alter the lives of 243 million individuals [11].

2. Targeting Forkhead Transcription Factors

Given the need for novel directions that can potentially diminish or resolve the onset and progression of neurological disorders, mammalian forkhead transcription factors are surfacing as potential effective targets that can offer new developments for drug discovery. Since the documentation of the *Drosophila melanogaster gene forkhead*, greater than 100 forkhead genes, and 19 human subgroups that range from *FOXA* to *FOXS* is now known to exist [12]. Prior terminology for forkhead proteins included forkhead in rhabdomyosarcoma (FKHR) (FOXO1), FKHRL1 (forkhead in rhabdomyosarcoma like protein 1) (FOXO3a), the *Drosophila*

TABLE 1: Forkhead box class O (FoxO) in the nervous system.

Pathway	Function
Tissue expression	FoxO proteins are expressed in all tissues of the body FoxO proteins appear to have selective expression in the nervous system that may offer insight into the biology of specific FoxO proteins FoxO proteins may be applicable for multiple neurodegenerative disorders that include Alzheimer's disease, Parkinson's disease, Huntington's disease, amyotrophic lateral sclerosis, and auditory neuronal disease
Epigenetic and posttranslational modification	FoxO proteins are controlled by posttranslation protein modifications that involve phosphorylation, acetylation, and ubiquitylation that involve Akt, SgK, MST1, IKK, SIRT1, and Wnt signaling with WISP1
Oxidative stress	FoxO proteins may be required for oxidative stress to result in apoptosis and can disrupt proliferative pathways of Wnt signaling FoxO proteins have been linked to disease progression and oxidative stress can modify FoxO interactions with other proteins that can ultimately influence cell neuronal survival
Autophagy and apoptosis	During oxidative stress, FoxO proteins can lead to the induction of autophagy and promote cell survival to clear the presence of toxic proteins such as mHtt, α-synuclein, and Aβ Under some circumstances with autophagy, a reduction in autophagy is required for protection indicating that FoxO cytoprotection may not always be directly tied to the induction of autophagy Protection against apoptosis usually requires inhibition or gene knockdown of FoxO proteins to protect against injuries such as cerebral ischemia, microglial and inflammatory cell demise, and Aβ exposure. Protection with metabotropic glutamate receptors, NAD^+ precursors, and trophic factors such as EPO requires inhibition and nuclear export of FoxO proteins
Stem cells	Activity of FoxO proteins can be necessary for the development of hematopoietic stem cells, dopaminergic cells, muscle regeneration, and oligodendrocyte progenitor development and myelination At times, reduction in FoxO protein activity is required for cell development and differentiation such as with pancreatic beta cell survival, osteoblast precursors, embryonic stem cells, and enteric nervous system precursors

Akt: protein kinase B; Aβ: beta-amyloid; EPO: erythropoietin; IKK: IκB kinase; MST1: mammalian sterile 20-like kinase-1; mHtt: mutant Huntingtin; SgK: NAD^+: nicotinamide adenine dinucleotide; serum- and glucocorticoid-inducible protein kinase; SIRT1: silent mating type information regulation 2 homolog 1 (*S. cerevisiae*); WISP1: wnt1 inducible signaling pathway protein 1.

gene fork head (*fkh*), Forkhead Related Activator- (FREAC-) 1 and FREAC-2, and the acute leukemia fusion gene located in chromosome X (*AFX*) (*FOXO4*) [13, 14]. For the current nomenclature, an Arabic number is provided with the designation of "Fox," and then a subclass or subgroup letter is provided, and finally the member number is listed within the subclasses of the Fox proteins [15]. All letters are capitalized for human Fox proteins. For the mouse, only the initial letter is listed as uppercase and for all other chordates the initial and subclass letters are uppercased [16–19].

Mammalian FOXO proteins are assigned to the O class of the forkhead box class transcription factors and consist of FOXO1, FOXO3, FOXO4, and FOXO6 [20]. With a butterfly-like appearance on X-ray crystallography [21] and nuclear magnetic resonance [22], the forkhead box (FOX) family of genes has a conserved forkhead domain (the "forkhead box") described as a "winged helix." The forkhead domain in FoxO proteins has three α-helices, three β-sheets, and two loops that compose the "wings" of the domain [23] which is specific for the forkhead proteins, since not all winged helix domains are considered to be Fox proteins [24]. The α-helices and β-sheets have high sequence homology with variations in either absent β-sheets and loops or additional α-helices. As transcription factors, FoxO proteins bind DNA through the FoxO-recognized element in the C-terminal basic region of the forkhead DNA binding domain [25, 26]. Target gene expression is repressed or activated through fourteen protein-DNA contacts with the primary recognition site located at α-helix H3 [21]. Phosphorylation or acetylation that can block FoxO activity may alter the binding of the C-terminal basic region to DNA to prevent transcriptional activity [27]. However, multiple mechanisms may contribute to forkhead DNA binding that involve variations in the N-terminal region of the recognition helix, changes in electrostatic distribution, and nuclear translocation of FoxO proteins [28–31].

FoxO proteins are expressed in all tissues of the body (Table 1). In relation to metabolic signaling, function of FoxO proteins appears to be conserved among multiple species that include *Caenorhabditis elegans, Drosophila melanogaster,* and mammals. FoxO proteins are homologous to the transcription factor DAuer Formation-16 (DAF-16) in the worm *Caenorhabditis elegans* that can determine metabolic insulin signaling and lead to lifespan extension [32, 33]. Furthermore, individual FoxO proteins appear to have selective expression in the nervous system that may provide clues to the biology for specific FoxO proteins [26, 34]. FoxO6 may oversee memory consolidation and emotion [35], since it is present in several regions of the brain, such as the hippocampus, the amygdala, and the nucleus accumbens [36, 37]. FoxO1 may have a vital role in a number of functions given its broad expression that may relate to astrocyte survival [38], modulation of embryonic endothelial stem cell survival [39], regulation of ischemic brain injury [10], vascular disease [40], and motor and memory pathways in the striatum and subregions of the hippocampus [36]. FoxO3 may have a more critical role in auditory synaptic transmission [41], cerebral endothelial vascular cell survival [42, 43], oxidative stress injury in mouse cerebellar granule neurons [44], neonatal hypoxic-ischemic encephalopathy [45], erythroid cell growth [46], and hippocampal neuronal injury [47, 48].

3. Epigenetic and Posttranslation Modification of Forkhead Transcription Factors

Activity of FoxO proteins is controlled by epigenetic [44, 49] and posttranslation protein modifications that involve phosphorylation [28, 30, 46–48, 50–56], acetylation [44, 50, 57], and ubiquitylation [26, 58–60] of these proteins (Table 1). Phosphorylation of forkhead transcription factors can be mediated by the serine-threonine kinase protein kinase B (Akt) [2, 61–66]. In the nervous system, Akt can protect cells during ischemic preconditioning [67], beta-amyloid (Aβ) toxicity [68–70], oxidative stress injury in the retina [71], inflammatory vascular injury [72], cerebral ischemia [73], experimental subarachnoid hemorrhage [74], flavonoid-dependent neuroprotection [75], lipoic acid protection [76, 77], epidermal growth factor receptor transactivation [78], neuroinflammation [79], tau homeostasis [80], senile plaque memory impairment [81], and growth factor administration [28, 71, 82–89]. Akt phosphorylates FoxO proteins that will bind FoxOs to 14-3-3 proteins prevent nuclear translocation and block the transcription of target genes that promote apoptosis [47, 52, 90, 91]. Akt also may control FoxO proteins activity and subsequently block caspase cleavage to prevent the induction of apoptotic cell death. Akt suppresses caspase activity that ultimately leads to mitochondrial pore opening and cytochrome c release [42, 66, 92–101]. Enhanced activity of FoxO proteins such as FoxO3a also can lead to cytochrome c release and caspase-induced apoptotic death [28, 51, 57, 66, 102–104]. As a result, one mechanism by which Akt prevents apoptotic cell death is through the blockade of FoxO protein activity that would prevent caspase activation. In addition, pathways such as Akt that block caspase 3 activity appear to offer another unique regulatory mechanism. Caspase 3 cleavage of FoxO3a may result in "proapoptotic" amino-terminal (Nt) fragments that can lead to cell death [105]. However, during caspase 3 inhibition such as that by Akt, phosphorylated FoxO3a remains intact and does not lead to apoptotic cell injury during oxidative stress [53, 106].

In addition to Akt, other pathways can lead to the phosphorylation and inactivation of FoxO proteins. The serum- and glucocorticoid-inducible protein kinase (SgK), a member of a family of kinases termed AGC (protein kinase A/protein kinase G/protein kinase C) kinases that includes Akt and phosphorylates FoxO3a and maintains this protein in the cytoplasm [107]. Importantly, Akt and SgK can phosphorylate FoxO proteins at different sites, suggesting greater options to control FoxO protein activity. However, some protein kinases such as mammalian sterile 20-like kinase-1 (MST1) can phosphorylate FOXO proteins and disrupt the binding to 14-3-3 which then allows FOXO nuclear translocation and subsequent death in neurons [29], indicating that the phosphorylation site of FoxO proteins is crucial in determining the activity of forkhead transcription factors. The ability of MST1 to activate FoxO proteins may be linked to c-Jun N-terminal kinase (JNK), since MST1 can increase JNK activation [108] which phosphorylates 14-3-3 protein, blocks binding to FoxO, and results in the nuclear localization of FoxO proteins [109].

Pathways associated with ubiquitylation and acetylation also control posttranslational modification of FoxO proteins [110, 111]. For example, Akt also leads to the ubiquitination and degradation through the 26S proteasome of FoxO proteins [111, 112]. Agents that can prevent the ubiquitination and degradation of FoxO proteins may serve as important agents to induce apoptotic cell death in cancers that can be tied to silent mating type information regulation 2 homolog 1 (*S. cerevisiae*) (SIRT1) [50, 113]. In a similar vein, SIRT1 activity also can lead to enhanced cell survival such as in the nervous system through inhibition of FoxO activity [57, 114–117]. Mammalian forkhead transcription factors can bind to the SIRT1 promoter region that contains a cluster of five putative core binding repeat motifs (IRS-1) and a forkhead-like consensus-binding site (FKHD-L) to affect FoxO transcription [118]. FoxO proteins, such as FoxO1, can subsequently regulate SIRT1 transcription and increase SIRT1 expression [119]. In some cases, SIRT1 and FoxO proteins may function synergistically to promote cell survival. In differentiated chondrocytes exposed to oxidative stress, loss of the forkhead transcription factors FoxO1 and FoxO3 in combination with decreased SIRT1 activity lead to cell death with reduced production of autophagic related proteins, indicating that SIRT1 with FoxO proteins may be necessary for cellular survival [120]. IκB kinase (IKK) also can directly phosphorylate and block the activity of FoxO proteins that results in the proteolysis of FoxO3a via the Ub-dependent proteasome pathway [121]. Acetylation of FoxO proteins provides another avenue for the control of these proteins. FoxO proteins are acetylated by histone acetyltransferases that include p300, the CREB-binding protein (CBP), and the CBP-associated factor. Once acetylated such as CBP, FoxO proteins translocate to the cell nucleus but have diminished activity since acetylation of lysine residues on FoxO proteins has been shown to limit the ability of FoxO proteins to bind to DNA [122]. Furthermore, acetylation can increase phosphorylation of FoxO proteins through Akt [122]. FoxO proteins are deacetylated by histone deacetylases, such as SIRT1 [13, 112, 123, 124]. Histone deacetylase 2 (HDAC2) also forms a physical complex with FoxO3a. This complex can influence FoxO3a-dependent gene transcription and oxidative stress-induced mouse cerebellar granule neuron cell death [44].

4. Forkhead Transcription Factors, Oxidative Stress, Apoptosis, and Autophagy

FoxO proteins are important components in the control of cell survival and neurodegenerative disorders determined by apoptosis and autophagy in the presence of oxidative stress [7, 125–128]. During oxidative stress, reactive oxygen species (ROS) are generated that include nitric oxide, peroxynitrite, superoxide free radicals, hydrogen peroxide, and singlet oxygen [97, 129–135]. These ROS can lead to cellular organelle injury, protein misfolding, DNA destruction, and neuronal synaptic dysfunction [48, 132, 136–138]. Endogenous systems exist in the body to prevent cellular injury during oxidative stress, but these systems can become overwhelmed such as glutathione peroxidase [139, 140], superoxide dismutase [120, 132, 138, 141–148], and vitamins B, C, D, and K [59, 140, 149–151]. FoxO proteins have been linked to disease progression and oxidative stress such as that with vitiligo [134] (Table 1). In patients with polymorphism of the *FOXO3A* gene, FOXO3A levels and catalase enzyme activity in vitiligo patients were decreased compared with control groups, suggesting in this case that FoxO proteins may confer protection. In other systems such as the maternal decidua, FoxO proteins may function independently in regards to oxidative stress with FOXO1 preventing oxidative stress damage and FOXO3a promoting oxidative cell death [152]. In addition, oxidative stress can serve as an epigenetic modifier of FoxO interactions with other proteins that can influence neuronal cell survival [44].

Autophagy is a process that recycles cytoplasmic components while removing dysfunctional organelles for tissue remodeling [7, 153–156]. Macroautophagy is the most prevalent type of autophagy that sequesters cytoplasmic proteins and organelles into autophagosomes [6, 157–160] and plays a role with FoxO proteins [2, 49, 127]. Autophagosomes, once produced, combine with lysosomes for degradation and are recycled for future cellular processes [125, 159, 161–163]. Under conditions of oxidative stress, FoxO proteins can lead to the induction of autophagy and promote cell survival (Table 1). During exposure with the oxidant tert-butyl hydroperoxide, constitutive active form of FoxO3 increases human articular chondrocyte cell viability and the expression of autophagy related proteins [120]. SIRT1-mediated deacetylation of FoxO1 also appears to mediate starvation-induced increases in autophagic flux that can maintain left ventricular function during periods of starvation [164]. Cardiac expression of constitutively active FoxO3 results in reversible heart atrophy through the activation of autophagic pathways [165]. In experimental models of full-length mutant Huntingtin (mHtt) transgenic mice, ectopic expression of FoxO1 enhances autophagy and toxic mHtt protein clearance in neuronal cell cultures [160]. However, under some conditions, a reduction in autophagy has been reported in the presence of increased FoxO expression, suggesting that FoxO cytoprotection may not always be directly tied to the induction of autophagy. Upregulation of FoxO3 and SIRT1 with a reduction in autophagy occurs in human bronchial epithelial cells exposed to cigarette smoke condensates in the presence of Amurensis H (Vam3), a dimeric derivative of resveratrol that can reduce oxidative stress [166].

In regards to the programmed cell death pathway of apoptosis, a later phase that leads to genomic DNA degradation is preceded by an early phase with the loss of plasma membrane lipid phosphatidylserine (PS) asymmetry [156, 167, 168]. The later phase of apoptosis results in DNA destruction [8, 19, 169–171], but the early phase of apoptosis represents an important target to save injured cells. Prevention or reversal of membrane PS externalization [68, 172–177] can result in the salvage of neurons and prevent inflammatory cells such as microglia from removing otherwise functional neurons [174, 178, 179]. During oxidative stress, FoxO proteins can lead to initial membrane PS externalization and subsequent DNA degradation (Table 1). In the presence of high glucose exposure, the development of endothelial cell dysfunction occurs with a reduction in SIRT1 expression and an increase in FoxO1 expression [180]. It has been suggested that FoxO proteins, such as FoxO1 and FoxO3a, must be present for oxidative stress to result in apoptosis [181]. This observation is supported by cell culture and animal studies demonstrating that inhibition or gene knockdown of FoxO1 or FoxO3a results in stroke reduction by estradiol [91], protects against microglial cell demise during oxidative stress [106] and Aβ exposure [182], promotes the protective effects of metabotropic glutamate receptors [102], increases neuronal cell survival through nicotinamide adenine dinucleotide (NAD^+) precursors [51], and provides trophic factor protection with erythropoietin (EPO) [28, 42, 46, 52] and neurotrophins [183–185]. However, under some scenarios that may impact other cellular signal transduction pathways, the activation of FoxO proteins may prevent apoptotic cell injury during oxidative stress such as chondrocytes [120]. Other studies show that in some cellular populations such as mouse hematopoietic stem cells, the conditional deletion of FoxO1, FoxO3a, and FoxO4 can lead to an increase in ROS [186], suggesting that FoxO proteins may be beneficial in regulation ROS in some cellular environments.

FoxO proteins such as FoxO3a can lead to the induction of "proapoptotic genes" and disrupt proliferative pathways of Wnt signaling [50]. A converse relationship exists between Wnt signaling and FoxO proteins. For example, FoxO3a can block prostate cell malignant phenotypes through the downregulation of Wnt signaling and β-catenin [187]. Wnt signaling includes the family member Wnt1 that can oversee neuronal development, angiogenesis, immunity, tumorigenesis, and stem cell proliferation [188–192]. Wnt1 expression is increased during injury of endothelial cells [28], metabolic disturbance [28], nonneuronal cell activation [69, 104, 193–195], spinal cord injury [196], stroke [197], and oxidative stress [104, 179, 197]. This increased expression of Wnt1 appears to be protective since loss of Wnt1 translates into progressive spinal cord injury [198], impaired neurogenesis [199], and apoptosis [156, 193, 200]. Wnt1 signaling pathways can prevent cellular injury during experimental diabetes [28, 201], ischemic brain injury [197, 202], dopaminergic neuronal cell injury [179, 189, 195, 203], toxic environments for microglia and other inflammatory cells [69, 104, 191, 193], and neuronal synaptic dysfunction [204]. Wnt signaling can afford cellular protection against apoptotic cell death through the inactivation of FoxO proteins. Phosphorylation and inhibition of FoxO3a activity by β-catenin during oxidative stress can protect hepatocytes from apoptotic cell death [54]. Osteoblastic differentiation can be preserved in the presence of oxidative stress through the increased expression of Wnt signaling pathways and the inhibition of FoxO3a [205]. In microglial cells of the central nervous system, Wnt1 prevents apoptosis through the posttranslational phosphorylation and maintenance of FoxO3a in the cytoplasm to prevent the loss of mitochondrial membrane permeability, cytochrome c release, Bad phosphorylation, and activation of caspases [104]. Neuroprotective trophic factors and cytokines, such as EPO [83, 87, 206, 207], also use Wnt signaling to offer cellular protection through the inhibition of FoxO proteins. EPO protects cerebral endothelial cells during oxygen-glucose deprivation by phosphorylating FoxO3a and preventing its subcellular trafficking to the nucleus [42, 208]. During elevated glucose exposure, EPO relies upon Wnt1 to block FoxO3a activity and maintain cerebral endothelial survival [28]. Wnt1 inducible signaling pathway protein 1 (WISP1), also known as CCN4, is a target of Wnt1 and affects programmed cell death, cancer cell growth, extracellular matrix production, cellular migration, and mitosis [159, 209–213]. WISP1 also protects neurons through the posttranslational phosphorylation of FoxO3a, by sequestering FoxO3a in the cytoplasm with protein 14-3-3, and by limiting deacetylation of FoxO3a [47]. Overexpression of FoxO3a during oxidative stress results in caspase 1 and caspase 3 [58, 214]. Through an autoregulatory loop, WISP1 has been shown to increase neuronal survival by limiting FoxO3a deacytelation, blocking caspases 1 and 3 activation, and fostering SIRT1 nuclear trafficking [47]. It should be noted that, under some conditions, Wnt signaling through β-catenin may increase *FoxO* transcriptional activity and competitively limit β-catenin interaction with members of the lymphoid enhancer factor/T cell factor family [215].

5. Forkhead Transcription Factors, Development, Stem Cell Proliferation, and Neurodegeneration

FoxO proteins have a prominent role not only in new cell development and differentiation, but also in determining the survival of mature cells in the nervous system (Table 1). Each of forkhead transcription factors may have different biological effects during development. For example, *Foxo3a* −/− and *Foxo4* −/− mice can develop without incidence and have similar weight gain [216]. Yet, mice singly deficient in *Foxo1* die by embryonic day eleven and lack development of the vascular system [216]. Overexpression of FoxO1, such as in skeletal muscle in mice, can lead to weight loss, reduced skeletal muscle mass, and impaired glycemic control [217]. On further analysis, FoxO3a −/− null animals experience a number of developmental abnormalities that were not present in mice singly deficient for FoxO4. *Foxo3a* −/− mice are known to become infertile with ovarian follicles that are depleted of oocytes [218]. FoxO3a overexpression retards oocyte growth and follicular development and leads to anovulation and luteinization of unruptured follicles [219], indicating a specific function for FoxO3a in the development and maintenance of the reproductive system. This work may suggest a role for FoxO3a in relation to oocyte and follicular development [220]. Mutations in *FOXO3a* and *FOXO1a* have been reported in a small percentage of women who suffer from premature ovarian failure [221]. Deletion of *Foxo1*, *Foxo3a*, and *Foxo4* or a single deletion of *Foxo3a* also blocks the repopulation of hematopoietic stem cells in murine models [186, 222], illustrating the need for FoxO proteins to maintain hematopoietic stem cells. Other work suggests that FoxO3a alone may play a role in maintaining hematopoietic stem cells, since hematopoietic stem cells are decreased in aged FoxO3 −/− mice compared to the littermate controls [222]. FoxO3 in combination with type 2 deiodinase (D2) and circulation thyroid hormone also is necessary for normal mouse myogenesis and muscle regeneration [223]. Nuclear translocation of FoxO1 in cooperation with SMAD3/4 and Sp1 by transforming growth factor β (TGFβ) is required for oligodendrocyte progenitor development and myelination in the central nervous system [224].

In contrast, other studies suggest that inhibition of FoxO protein activity or prevention of Wnt pathway disruption may be necessary for stem cell survival. FoxO1 may negatively affect pancreatic beta cell survival [225]. Work that examines osteoblastogenesis demonstrates that FoxO proteins during oxidative stress and aging may antagonize Wnt signaling pathways and block the proliferation of osteoblast precursors [226]. SIRT1 deficiency in mouse embryonic stem cells has been shown to enhance the acetylation and phosphorylation FoxO1, block nuclear localization of FoxO1, and prevent apoptotic cell death that would otherwise ensue with FoxO1 activity [227]. SIRT1 is also necessary to promote cortical bone formation with osteoblast progenitors by deacetylating FoxOs and preventing FoxO protein binding to β-catenin and inhibiting Wnt signaling [228].

In the nervous system, FoxO proteins similarly determine the fate of neuronal precursors and the maintenance of neurons [137, 229]. Studies that employ genetic deletions of Foxa1 and Foxa2 in mice result in the decline of striatal dopamine metabolites, reduction in dopaminergic cells, and locomotor deficits [230]. Stem cell maintenance may also be governed by the interactions between WISP1 and FoxO proteins. WISP1 is upregulated during stem cell migration [231] and WISP1 may be one of several components that affect induced pluripotent stem cell reprogramming [232, 233]. WISP1 requires β-catenin for the differentiation of marrow derived mesenchymal stem cells [234]. During oxidative stress, FoxO may bind to β-catenin and prevent stem cell development similar to the previously described pathways with Wnt signaling [212, 235]. Cellular mechanisms that utilize Wnt signaling such as EPO also control FoxO protein activity for stem cell growth [236–241]. EPO promotes erythroid progenitor cell development that requires the modulation of FoxO3a activity [46, 172, 242, 243]. Other trophic factors, such as glial cell line-derived neurotrophic factor, require the inhibition of FoxO1 and FoxO3a to promote rat enteric nervous system precursor development [244].

In relation to neurodegenerative disorders and neuronal cell survival, activation of FoxO proteins under most conditions leads to cell death [13, 245]. Manganese toxicity that may be a factor in neurodegenerative disorders such as Parkinson's disease has been associated with the cell death of astrocytes through increased expression and activation of FoxO proteins [246]. Iron-induced oxidative stress that results in apoptotic death of hippocampal neurons can lead to a protective response that activates Akt and blocks FoxO protein translocation to the nucleus [55]. Protection of primary hippocampal neurons by group I metabotropic receptors during exposure to ROS requires the phosphorylation and inactivation of FoxO3a as well as the prevention of caspase cleavage of FoxO3a [102] to block the generation of potentially "proapoptotic" amino-terminal (Nt) fragments [105]. Antioxidant administration to protect cortical neurons and hippocampal neuronal cell lines during excitotoxicity [247] and in experimental models of AD with Aβ toxicity [48] employs FoxO3 inactivation and blocked translocation to the cell nucleus [247]. Independent of Wnt signaling, EPO has been shown to offer neuronal and vascular cell protection through pathways that inactivate FoxO proteins, such as FoxO3a [46, 52]. During cerebral ischemia, FoxO3a expression increases in the hippocampus [248] and FoxO3a interaction with cell cycle induction proteins may play a role in neuronal apoptotic cell death [44]. Toxin exposure in cortical neurons that fosters FoxO3a activation and p27 (kip1) transcription leads to apoptosis [249]. In microglial cells of the nervous system as well as neurons, knockdown of FoxO3a and prevention of nuclear shuttling lead to the increased survival during oxidative stress [47, 104]. During periods of elevated glucose, cortical neurons [250] and vascular cells [28, 42, 53, 58] are protected through inhibitory phosphorylation of FoxO3a and the nuclear export of this protein.

However, it is important to recognize the antiproliferative and anticancer effects of FoxO proteins that make these transcription factors attractive targets for the inhibition of tumor growth [14, 50]. Increased activity of FoxO3a with cyclin-dependent kinase inhibitor p27 in isolated human breast cancer cells can suppress breast cancer progression [251]. Colorectal cancer progression may be checked by the activation of FoxO1 [252] and angiogenesis that is necessary for tumor growth can be blocked by the activation of FoxO3a [253]. Through the disruption of proliferative pathways such as Wnt signaling, a number of cancers that include breast cancer, gastric cancer, central nervous system tumors, and lung carcinoma [190, 209, 212, 254–257] can be inhibited through FoxO protein activity [187] while loss of FoxO activity may signal an increased risk for cancer development [258]. As a result, pathways that inactivate FoxO proteins may have some potential risk for latent tumor growth.

In some experimental scenarios, FoxO protein activation may be required for neuronal protection. Blockade of neurodegenerative disease and adverse behavioral deficits during selenium exposure that may be linked to the development of amyotrophic lateral sclerosis occurs during increased FoxO protein expression [259]. FoxO3a also may be necessary for cochlear auditory activity and the maintenance of synaptic function [41]. In Drosophila models of Aβ toxicity, loss of FoxO results in decreased survival and locomotive activity [260]. FoxO proteins such as FoxO3 may also be important for the control of autophagic flux in Parkinson's disease [261]. In dopaminergic neurons, overexpressing human α-synuclein, inhibition of FoxO3 is protective. However, a small degree of FoxO3 activity prevents nigral neuron cell death in the presence of human α-synuclein accumulation by reducing the amount of α-synuclein and fostering the accumulation of autophagic vacuoles containing lipofuscin [261]. Interestingly, a controlled upregulation of FoxO3a and SIRT1 expression in cardiac tissue may be important during exercise [262]. Levels of SIRT1 that are less than 7.5-fold are associated with catalase expression that is also controlled by FoxO1a to possibly reduce cell injury during oxidative stress. Conversely, elevated levels of SIRT1 at 12.5-fold can result in cardiomyocyte apoptosis and decreased cardiac function [263]. Activation of FoxO proteins may also be protective during aging. Loss of FoxO3a activity leads to decreased manganese-superoxide dismutase and enhanced cell injury with aging [264]. This extension of cellular lifespan that may be provided by FoxO proteins can be dependent on the negative regulation of Akt to allow for the activation of FoxO3a [265].

6. Conclusions

Neurodegenerative disorders result in significant death and disability for millions of individuals throughout the world but remain for the most part with limited treatment options and palliative therapies. Forkhead transcription factors and especially those of the FoxO subgroup are increasingly being identified as potential targets for disorders of the nervous system. FoxO proteins are expressed throughout the body, but their varied expression in the nervous system suggests that specific FoxO proteins may be vital for selective cellular and biological function and may be applicable for Alzheimer's disease, Parkinson's disease, Huntington's disease, amyotrophic lateral sclerosis, and auditory neuronal disease. For example, FoxO3 may be important for auditory synaptic transmission, cerebral endothelial vascular cell survival, and erythroid cell growth. In contrast, FoxO6 may be critical for memory consolidation and emotion. FoxOs are regulated by epigenetic and posttranslational modifications that involve phosphorylation, ubiquitylation, and acetylation by cellular pathways that involve Akt, SgK, MST1, IKK, SIRT1, and Wnt signaling to control the activity and integrity of these proteins. The ability of FoxO proteins to ultimately determine cell development and survival in the nervous system during oxidative stress resides with FoxO control of the programmed cell death pathways of apoptosis and autophagy. During oxidative stress cell injury, activation of FoxO proteins often leads to apoptotic cell death that initially fosters membrane PS residue externalization and subsequent DNA degradation. FoxO activity also can disrupt proliferative pathways of Wnt signaling involving β-catenin to result in apoptotic cell death. Conversely, Wnt signaling that includes WISP1 can phosphorylate, limit deacetylation, and sequester FoxO proteins in the cytoplasm to block apoptotic pathways that include caspase activation. FoxO proteins can promote autophagy to preserve cell survival during oxidative stress and clear toxic proteins from the cell. Yet, under some conditions, FoxO proteins may be tied to enhanced cell survival that is independent of autophagy. These observations do not always provide crisp conclusions and suggest the presence of a complex interplay between FoxO proteins and multiple signal transduction pathways in the cell. Furthermore, the degree of FoxO activity as well as companion pathways that involve SIRT1 can significantly impact cell development and survival. Elevated FoxO or SIRT1 activity can be detrimental to cells, but a minimal level of activity that can shepherd autophagic accumulation of toxic proteins may be beneficial. Importantly, these considerations provide further insight for the targeting of FoxO in the nervous system that may involve Wnt signaling, SIRT1, and trophic factors such as EPO to block cellular injury during oxidative stress. In addition, one should be cognizant of the nonproliferative role FoxO proteins play in tumorigenesis. Inactivation of FoxO proteins could yield unexpected cell growth not only in the nervous system but also in other regions of the body. Focusing upon FoxO proteins for the consideration of new therapeutic strategies against neurodegenerative disorders that oversee early cell development as well as differentiated cellular function can offer potentially high returns for new drug development.

Conflict of Interests

The author declares no conflict of interests regarding the publication of this paper.

Acknowledgments

This research was supported by the following grants to Kenneth Maiese: American Diabetes Association, American Heart Association, NIH NIEHS, NIH NIA, NIH NINDS, and NIH ARRA.

References

[1] C. M. Filley, Y. D. Rollins, C. Alan Anderson et al., "The genetics of very early onset Alzheimer disease," *Cognitive and Behavioral Neurology*, vol. 20, no. 3, pp. 149–156, 2007.

[2] K. Maiese, "Taking aim at Alzheimer's disease through the mammalian target of rapamycin," *Annals of Medicine*, vol. 46, no. 8, pp. 587–596, 2014.

[3] K. Maiese, "Cutting through the complexities of mTOR for the treatment of stroke," *Current Neurovascular Research*, vol. 11, no. 2, pp. 177–186, 2014.

[4] P. E. Pergola, C. L. White, J. M. Szychowski et al., "Achieved blood pressures in the secondary prevention of small subcortical strokes (SPS3) study: challenges and lessons learned," *American Journal of Hypertension*, vol. 27, no. 8, pp. 1052–1060, 2014.

[5] D. Pineda, C. Ampurdanés, M. G. Medina et al., "Tissue plasminogen activator induces microglial inflammation via a noncatalytic molecular mechanism involving activation of mitogen-activated protein kinases and Akt signaling pathways and AnnexinA2 and Galectin-1 receptors," *Glia*, vol. 60, no. 4, pp. 526–540, 2012.

[6] K. Maiese, "Driving neural regeneration through the mammalian target of rapamycin," *Neural Regeneration Research*, vol. 9, no. 15, pp. 1413–1417, 2014.

[7] V. P. Nakka, P. Prakash-babu, and R. Vemuganti, "Crosstalk between endoplasmic reticulum stress, oxidative stress, and autophagy: potential therapeutic targets for acute CNS injuries," *Molecular Neurobiology*, 2014.

[8] A. Q. Nguyen, B. H. Cherry, G. F. Scott, M. Ryou, and R. T. Mallet, "Erythropoietin: powerful protection of ischemic and post-ischemic brain," *Experimental Biology and Medicine*, vol. 239, no. 11, pp. 1461–1475, 2014.

[9] A. Selvamani, M. H. Williams, R. C. Miranda, and F. Sohrabji, "Circulating miRNA profiles provide a biomarker for severity of stroke outcomes associated with age and sex in a rat model," *Clinical Science*, vol. 127, no. 2, pp. 77–89, 2014.

[10] X. Xiong, R. Xie, H. Zhang et al., "PRAS40 plays a pivotal role in protecting against stroke by linking the Akt and mTOR pathways," *Neurobiology of Disease*, vol. 66, pp. 43–52, 2014.

[11] World Health Organization, *Neurological Disorders: Public Health Challenges*, WHO Library Cataloguing-in-Publication Data, 2006.

[12] D. Weigel, G. Jürgens, F. Küttner, E. Seifert, and H. Jäckle, "The homeotic gene *fork head* encodes a nuclear protein and is expressed in the terminal regions of the Drosophila embryo," *Cell*, vol. 57, no. 4, pp. 645–658, 1989.

[13] K. Maiese, Z. C. Zhao, and C. S. Yan, "'Sly as a FOXO': new paths with forkhead signaling in the brain," *Current Neurovascular Research*, vol. 4, no. 4, pp. 295–302, 2007.

[14] K. Maiese, Z. Z. Chong, Y. C. Shang, and J. Hou, "Clever cancer strategies with FoxO transcription factors," *Cell Cycle*, vol. 7, no. 24, pp. 3829–3839, 2008.

[15] K. Maiese, J. Hou, Z. Z. Chong, and Y. C. Shang, "A fork in the path: developing therapeutic inroads with foxO proteins," *Oxidative Medicine and Cellular Longevity*, vol. 2, no. 3, pp. 119–129, 2009.

[16] Z. Cheng and M. F. White, "Targeting forkhead Box O1 from the concept to metabolic diseases: Lessons from mouse models," *Antioxidants and Redox Signaling*, vol. 14, no. 4, pp. 649–661, 2011.

[17] K. H. Kaestner, W. Knöchel, and D. E. Martínez, "Unified nomenclature for the winged helix/forkhead transcription factors," *Genes and Development*, vol. 14, no. 2, pp. 142–146, 2000.

[18] K. Maiese, Z. Z. Chong, Y. C. Shang, and J. Hou, "FoxO proteins: cunning concepts and considerations for the cardiovascular system," *Clinical Science*, vol. 116, no. 3, pp. 191–203, 2009.

[19] S. Shao, Y. Yang, G. Yuan, M. Zhang, and X. Yu, "Signaling molecules involved in lipid-induced pancreatic beta-cell dysfunction," *DNA and Cell Biology*, vol. 32, no. 2, pp. 41–49, 2013.

[20] K. Maiese, *Forkhead Transcription Factors: Vital Elements in Biology and Medicine*, vol. 665 of *Advances in Experimental Medicine and Biology*, Springer Science+Business Media, 2010.

[21] K. L. Clark, E. D. Halay, E. Lai, and S. K. Burley, "Co-crystal structure of the HNF-3/fork head DNA-recognition motif resembles histone H5," *Nature*, vol. 364, no. 6436, pp. 412–420, 1993.

[22] C. Jin, I. Marsden, X. Chen, and X. Liao, "Sequence specific collective motions in a winged helix DNA binding domain detected by 15N relaxation NMR," *Biochemistry*, vol. 37, no. 17, pp. 6179–6187, 1998.

[23] K. Maiese, Z. Z. Chong, and Y. C. Shang, "OutFOXOing disease and disability: the therapeutic potential of targeting FoxO proteins," *Trends in Molecular Medicine*, vol. 14, no. 5, pp. 219–227, 2008.

[24] E. T. Larson, B. Eilers, S. Menon et al., "A winged-helix protein from sulfolobus turreted icosahedral virus points toward stabilizing disulfide bonds in the intracellular proteins of a hyperthermophilic virus," *Virology*, vol. 368, no. 2, pp. 249–261, 2007.

[25] W. H. Biggs III, W. K. Cavenee, and K. C. Arden, "Identification and characterization of members of the FKHR (FOX O) subclass of winged-helix transcription factors in the mouse," *Mammalian Genome*, vol. 12, no. 6, pp. 416–425, 2001.

[26] H. Huang and D. J. Tindall, "Dynamic FoxO transcription factors," *Journal of Cell Science*, vol. 120, no. 15, pp. 2479–2487, 2007.

[27] K. L. Tsai, Y. J. Sun, C. Y. Huang, J. Y. Yang, M. C. Hung, and C. D. Hsiao, "Crystal structure of the human FOXO3a-DBD/DNA complex suggests the effects of post-translational modification," *Nucleic Acids Research*, vol. 35, no. 20, pp. 6984–6994, 2007.

[28] Z. Z. Chong, J. Hou, Y. C. Shang, S. Wang, and K. Maiese, "EPO relies upon novel signaling of Wnt1 that requires Akt1, FoxO3a, GSK-3beta, and beta-catenin to foster vascular integrity during experimental diabetes," *Current Neurovascular Research*, vol. 8, no. 2, pp. 103–120, 2011.

[29] M. K. Lehtinen, Z. Yuan, P. R. Boag et al., "A conserved MST-FOXO signaling pathway mediates oxidative-stress responses and extends life span," *Cell*, vol. 125, no. 5, pp. 987–1001, 2006.

[30] P. Scodelaro Bilbao and R. Boland, "Extracellular ATP regulates FoxO family of transcription factors and cell cycle progression through PI3K/Akt in MCF-7 cells," *Biochimica et Biophysica Acta*, vol. 1830, no. 10, pp. 4456–4469, 2013.

[31] L. P. Van Der Heide, M. F. M. Hoekman, and M. P. Smidt, "The ins and outs of FoxO shuttling: mechanisms of FoxO translocation and transcriptional regulation," *Biochemical Journal*, vol. 380, no. 2, pp. 297–309, 2004.

[32] K. Lin, J. B. Dorman, A. Rodan, and C. Kenyon, "daf-16: an HNF-3/forkhead family member that can function to double the life-span of Caenorhabditis elegans," *Science*, vol. 278, no. 5341, pp. 1319–1322, 1997.

[33] S. Ogg, S. Paradis, S. Gottlieb et al., "The fork head transcription factor DAF-16 transduces insulin-like metabolic and longevity signals in *C. elegans*," *Nature*, vol. 389, no. 6654, pp. 994–999, 1997.

[34] K. Maiese, Z. Z. Chong, J. Hall, and Y. C. Shang, "The 'O' class: crafting clinical care with FoxO transcription factors," *Advances in Experimental Medicine and Biology*, vol. 665, pp. 242–260, 2009.

[35] D. A. M. Salih, A. J. Rashid, D. Colas et al., "FoxO6 regulates memory consolidation and synaptic function," *Genes and Development*, vol. 26, no. 24, pp. 2780–2801, 2012.

[36] M. F. M. Hoekman, F. M. J. Jacobs, M. P. Smidt, and J. P. H. Burbach, "Spatial and temporal expression of FoxO transcription factors in the developing and adult murine brain," *Gene Expression Patterns*, vol. 6, no. 2, pp. 134–140, 2006.

[37] L. P. van der Heide, F. M. J. Jacobs, J. P. H. Burbach, M. F. M. Hoekman, and M. P. Smidt, "FoxO6 transcriptional activity is regulated by Thr^{26} and Ser^{184}, independent of nucleo-cytoplasmic shuttling," *Biochemical Journal*, vol. 391, no. 3, pp. 623–629, 2005.

[38] S.-J. Lee, B.-R. Seo, E.-J. Choi, and J.-Y. Koh, "The role of reciprocal activation of cAbl and Mst1 in the Oxidative death of cultured astrocytes," *Glia*, vol. 62, no. 4, pp. 639–648, 2014.

[39] B. Merkely, E. Gara, Z. Lendvai et al., "Signaling via PI3K/FOXO1A pathway modulates formation and survival of human embryonic stem cell-derived endothelial cells," *Stem Cells and Development*, vol. 24, no. 7, pp. 869–878, 2015.

[40] Y. Zhao, Y. Yu, X. Tian et al., "Association study to evaluate FoxO1 and FoxO3 gene in CHD in Han Chinese," *PLoS ONE*, vol. 9, no. 1, Article ID e86252, 2014.

[41] F. Gilels, S. T. Paquette, J. Zhang, I. Rahman, and P. M. White, "Mutation of foxo3 causes adult onset auditory neuropathy and alters cochlear synapse architecture in mice," *Journal of Neuroscience*, vol. 33, no. 47, pp. 18409–18424, 2013.

[42] J. Hou, S. Wang, Y. C. Shang, Z. Z. Chong, and K. Maiese, "Erythropoietin employs cell longevity pathways of SIRT1 to foster endothelial vascular integrity during oxidant stress," *Current Neurovascular Research*, vol. 8, no. 3, pp. 220–235, 2011.

[43] K. Maiese, F. Li, and Z. Z. Chong, "Erythropoietin in the brain: can the promise to protect be fulfilled?" *Trends in Pharmacological Sciences*, vol. 25, no. 11, pp. 577–583, 2004.

[44] S. Peng, S. Zhao, F. Yan et al., "HDAC2 selectively regulates foxo3a-mediated gene transcription during oxidative stress-induced neuronal cell death," *Journal of Neuroscience*, vol. 35, no. 3, pp. 1250–1259, 2015.

[45] Z. Rong, R. Pan, Y. Xu, C. Zhang, Y. Cao, and D. Liu, "Hesperidin pretreatment protects hypoxia-ischemic brain injury in neonatal rat," *Neuroscience*, vol. 255, pp. 292–299, 2013.

[46] M. E. Chamorro, S. D. Wenker, D. M. Vota, D. C. Vittori, and A. B. Nesse, "Signaling pathways of cell proliferation are involved in the differential effect of erythropoietin and its carbamylated derivative," *Biochimica et Biophysica Acta*, vol. 1833, no. 8, pp. 1960–1968, 2013.

[47] S. Wang, Z. Z. Chong, Y. C. Shang, and K. Maiese, "WISP1 neuroprotection requires FoxO3a post-translational modulation with autoregulatory control of SIRT1," *Current Neurovascular Research*, vol. 10, no. 1, pp. 54–69, 2013.

[48] E. Zeldich, C. Chen, T. A. Colvin et al., "The neuroprotective effect of Klotho is mediated via regulation of members of the redox system," *The Journal of Biological Chemistry*, vol. 289, no. 35, pp. 24700–24715, 2014.

[49] A. Jenwitheesuk, C. Nopparat, S. Mukda, P. Wongchitrat, and P. Govitrapong, "Melatonin regulates aging and neurodegeneration through energy metabolism, epigenetics, autophagy and circadian rhythm pathways," *International Journal of Molecular Sciences*, vol. 15, no. 9, pp. 16848–16884, 2014.

[50] S. Carbajo-Pescador, J. L. Mauriz, A. García-Palomo, and J. González-Gallego, "FoxO proteins: regulation and molecular targets in liver cancer," *Current Medicinal Chemistry*, vol. 21, no. 10, pp. 1231–1246, 2014.

[51] Z. Z. Chong, S.-H. Lin, and K. Maiese, "The NAD^+ precursor nicotinamide governs neuronal survival during oxidative stress through protein kinase B coupled to FOXO3a and mitochondrial membrane potential," *Journal of Cerebral Blood Flow and Metabolism*, vol. 24, no. 7, pp. 728–743, 2004.

[52] Z. Z. Chong and K. Maiese, "Erythropoietin involves the phosphatidylinositol 3-kinase pathway, 14-3-3 protein and FOXO3a nuclear trafficking to preserve endothelial cell integrity," *British Journal of Pharmacology*, vol. 150, no. 7, pp. 839–850, 2007.

[53] J. Hou, Z. Z. Chong, Y. C. Shang, and K. Maiese, "Early apoptotic vascular signaling is determined by Sirt1 through nuclear shuttling, forkhead trafficking, bad, and mitochondrial caspase activation," *Current Neurovascular Research*, vol. 7, no. 2, pp. 95–112, 2010.

[54] G.-Z. Tao, N. Lehwald, K. Y. Jang et al., "Wnt/β-catenin signaling protects mouse liver against oxidative stress-induced apoptosis through the inhibition of forkhead transcription factor FoxO3," *Journal of Biological Chemistry*, vol. 288, no. 24, pp. 17214–17224, 2013.

[55] R. M. Uranga, S. Katz, and G. A. Salvador, "Enhanced phosphatidylinositol 3-kinase (PI3K)/Akt signaling has pleiotropic targets in hippocampal neurons exposed to iron-induced oxidative stress," *Journal of Biological Chemistry*, vol. 288, no. 27, pp. 19773–19784, 2013.

[56] C. P. Wong, T. Kaneda, A. H. A. Hadi, and H. Morita, "Ceramicine B, a limonoid with anti-lipid droplets accumulation activity from *Chisocheton ceramicus*," *Journal of Natural Medicines*, vol. 68, no. 1, pp. 22–30, 2014.

[57] W. Wang, C. Yan, J. Zhang et al., "SIRT1 inhibits TNF-alpha-induced apoptosis of vascular adventitial fibroblasts partly

through the deacetylation of FoxO1," *Apoptosis*, vol. 18, no. 6, pp. 689–701, 2013.

[58] J. Hou, Z. Z. Chong, Y. C. Shang, and K. Maiese, "FOXO3a governs early and late apoptotic endothelial programs during elevated glucose through mitochondrial and caspase signaling," *Molecular and Cellular Endocrinology*, vol. 321, no. 2, pp. 194–206, 2010.

[59] K. Maiese, Z. Z. Chong, J. Hou, and Y. C. Shang, "The vitamin nicotinamide: translating nutrition into clinical care," *Molecules*, vol. 14, no. 9, pp. 3446–3485, 2009.

[60] T. Tanaka and M. Iino, "Knockdown of Sec8 promotes cell-cycle arrest at G_1/S phase by inducing p21 via control of FOXO proteins," *The FEBS Journal*, vol. 281, no. 4, pp. 1068–1084, 2014.

[61] Z. Z. Chog, F. Li, and K. Maiese, "Activating Akt and the brain's resources to drive cellular survival and prevent inflammatory injury," *Histology and Histopathology*, vol. 20, no. 1, pp. 299–315, 2005.

[62] C.-Y. Huang, C.-Y. Chan, I.-T. Chou, C.-H. Lien, H.-C. Hung, and M.-F. Lee, "Quercetin induces growth arrest through activation of FOXO1 transcription factor in EGFR-overexpressing oral cancer cells," *Journal of Nutritional Biochemistry*, vol. 24, no. 9, pp. 1596–1603, 2013.

[63] K. Maiese, Z. Z. Chong, and Y. C. Shang, "Mechanistic insights into diabetes mellitus and oxidative stress," *Current Medicinal Chemistry*, vol. 14, no. 16, pp. 1729–1738, 2007.

[64] J. Park, Y. S. Ko, J. Yoon et al., "The forkhead transcription factor FOXO1 mediates cisplatin resistance in gastric cancer cells by activating phosphoinositide 3-kinase/Akt pathway," *Gastric Cancer*, vol. 17, no. 3, pp. 423–430, 2014.

[65] P. Puthanveetil, A. Wan, and B. Rodrigues, "FoxO1 is crucial for sustaining cardiomyocyte metabolism and cell survival," *Cardiovascular Research*, vol. 97, no. 3, pp. 393–403, 2013.

[66] X.-F. Qi, Y.-J. Li, Z.-Y. Chen, S.-K. Kim, K.-J. Lee, and D.-Q. Cai, "Involvement of the FoxO3a pathway in the ischemia/reperfusion injury of cardiac microvascular endothelial cells," *Experimental and Molecular Pathology*, vol. 95, no. 2, pp. 242–247, 2013.

[67] W. Balduini, S. Carloni, and G. Buonocore, "Autophagy in hypoxia-ischemia induced brain injury," *Journal of Maternal-Fetal and Neonatal Medicine*, vol. 25, supplement 1, pp. 30–34, 2012.

[68] L. Bing, J. Wu, J. Zhang, Y. Chen, Z. Hong, and H. Zu, "DHT inhibits the Aβ25-35-induced apoptosis by regulation of seladin-1, survivin, XIAP, bax, and bcl-xl expression through a rapid PI3-K/Akt signaling in C6 glial cell lines," *Neurochemical Research*, vol. 40, no. 1, pp. 41–48, 2015.

[69] Y. C. Shang, Z. Z. Chong, S. Wang, and K. Maiese, "Prevention of beta-amyloid degeneration of microglia by erythropoietin depends on Wnt1, the PI 3-K/mTOR pathway, Bad, and Bcl-xL," *Aging*, vol. 4, no. 3, pp. 187–201, 2012.

[70] Y. C. Shang, Z. Z. Chong, S. Wang, and K. Maiese, "Tuberous sclerosis protein 2 (TSC2) modulates CCN4 cytoprotection during apoptotic amyloid toxicity in microglia," *Current Neurovascular Research*, vol. 10, no. 1, pp. 29–38, 2013.

[71] Z.-Y. Chang, M.-K. Yeh, C.-H. Chiang, Y.-H. Chen, and D.-W. Lu, "Erythropoietin protects adult retinal ganglion cells against NMDA-, trophic factor withdrawal-, and TNF-alpha-induced damage," *PLoS ONE*, vol. 8, no. 1, Article ID e55291, 2013.

[72] Z. Z. Chong, J. Q. Kang, and K. Maiese, "AKT1 drives endothelial cell membrane asymmetry and microglial activation through Bcl-xL and caspase 1, 3, and 9," *Experimental Cell Research*, vol. 296, no. 2, pp. 196–207, 2004.

[73] C. Gubern, S. Camós, O. Hurtado et al., "Characterization of Gcf2/Lrrfip1 in experimental cerebral ischemia and its role as a modulator of Akt, mTOR and β-catenin signaling pathways," *Neuroscience*, vol. 268, pp. 48–65, 2014.

[74] Y. Hong, A. Shao, J. Wang et al., "Neuroprotective effect of hydrogen-rich saline against neurologic damage and apoptosis in early brain injury following subarachnoid hemorrhage: possible role of the Akt/GSK3β signaling pathway," *PLoS ONE*, vol. 9, no. 4, Article ID e96212, 2014.

[75] A. Jalsrai, T. Numakawa, Y. Ooshima, N. Adachi, and H. Kunugi, "Phosphatase-mediated intracellular signaling contributes to neuroprotection by flavonoids of *Iris tenuifolia*," *The American Journal of Chinese Medicine*, vol. 42, no. 1, pp. 119–130, 2014.

[76] M. N. A. Kamarudin, N. A. M. Raflee, S. S. S. Hussein, J. Y. Lo, H. Supriady, and H. Abdul Kadir, "(R)-(+)-α-Lipoic acid protected NG108-15 cells against H_2O_2-induced cell death through PI3K-Akt/GSK-3β pathway and suppression of NF-$\kappa\beta$-cytokines," *Drug Design Development and Therapy*, vol. 8, pp. 1765–1780, 2014.

[77] S. Zara, M. de Colli, M. Rapino et al., "Ibuprofen and lipoic acid conjugate neuroprotective activity is mediated by Ngb/Akt intracellular signaling pathway in alzheimer's disease rat model," *Gerontology*, vol. 59, no. 3, pp. 250–260, 2013.

[78] R. Kimura, M. Okouchi, T. Kato et al., "Epidermal growth factor receptor transactivation is necessary for glucagon-like peptide-1 to protect PC12 cells from apoptosis," *Neuroendocrinology*, vol. 97, no. 4, pp. 300–308, 2013.

[79] E. Russo, F. Andreozzi, R. Iuliano et al., "Early molecular and behavioral response to lipopolysaccharide in the WAG/Rij rat model of absence epilepsy and depressive-like behavior, involves interplay between AMPK, AKT/mTOR pathways and neuroinflammatory cytokine release," *Brain, Behavior, and Immunity*, vol. 42, pp. 157–168, 2014.

[80] Z. Tang, E. Bereczki, H. Zhang et al., "Mammalian target of rapamycin (mTor) mediates tau protein dyshomeostasis: implication for Alzheimer disease," *Journal of Biological Chemistry*, vol. 288, no. 22, pp. 15556–15570, 2013.

[81] Z. Zhu, J. Yan, W. Jiang et al., "Arctigenin effectively ameliorates memory impairment in Alzheimer's disease model mice targeting both β-amyloid production and clearance," *Journal of Neuroscience*, vol. 33, no. 32, pp. 13138–13149, 2013.

[82] S. Busch, A. Kannt, M. Kolibabka et al., "Systemic treatment with erythropoietin protects the neurovascular unit in a rat model of retinal neurodegeneration," *PLoS ONE*, vol. 9, no. 7, Article ID e102013, 2014.

[83] Z. Z. Chong, J. Q. Kang, and K. Maiese, "Erythropoietin is a novel vascular protectant through activation of AKt1 and mitochondrial modulation of cysteine proteases," *Circulation*, vol. 106, no. 23, pp. 2973–2979, 2002.

[84] Z. Z. Chong, Y. C. Shang, S. Wang, and K. Maiese, "PRAS40 is an integral regulatory component of erythropoietin mTOR signaling and cytoprotection," *PLoS ONE*, vol. 7, no. 9, Article ID e45456, 2012.

[85] M.-S. Kwon, M.-H. Kim, S.-H. Kim et al., "Erythropoietin exerts cell protective effect by activating PI3k/Akt and MAPK pathways in c6 cells," *Neurological Research*, vol. 36, no. 3, pp. 215–223, 2014.

[86] K. Maiese, Z. Z. Chong, Y. C. Shang, and S. Wang, "Erythropoietin: new directions for the nervous system," *International Journal of Molecular Sciences*, vol. 13, no. 9, pp. 11102–11129, 2012.

[87] K. Maiese, F. Li, and Z. Z. Chong, "New avenues of exploration for erythropoietin," *Journal of the American Medical Association*, vol. 293, no. 1, pp. 90–95, 2005.

[88] T. Maurice, M.-H. Mustafa, C. Desrumaux et al., "Intranasal formulation of erythropoietin (EPO) showed potent protective activity against amyloid toxicity in the $A\beta_{25-35}$ non-transgenic mouse model of Alzheimer's disease," *Journal of Psychopharmacology*, vol. 27, no. 11, pp. 1044–1057, 2013.

[89] G.-B. Wang, Y.-L. Ni, X.-P. Zhou, and W.-F. Zhang, "The AKT/mTOR pathway mediates neuronal protective effects of erythropoietin in sepsis," *Molecular and Cellular Biochemistry*, vol. 385, no. 1-2, pp. 125–132, 2014.

[90] E. Arimoto-Ishida, M. Ohmichi, S. Mabuchi et al., "Inhibition of phosphorylation of a Forkhead transcription factor sensitizes human ovarian cancer cells to cisplatin," *Endocrinology*, vol. 145, no. 4, pp. 2014–2022, 2004.

[91] C. K. Won, H. H. Ji, and P. O. Koh, "Estradiol prevents the focal cerebral ischemic injury-induced decrease of forkhead transcription factors phosphorylation," *Neuroscience Letters*, vol. 398, no. 1-2, pp. 39–43, 2006.

[92] C. Chen, Y. Xu, and Y. Song, "IGF-1 gene-modified muscle-derived stem cells are resistant to oxidative stress via enhanced activation of IGF-1R/PI3K/AKT signaling and secretion of VEGF," *Molecular and Cellular Biochemistry*, vol. 386, no. 1-2, pp. 167–175, 2014.

[93] Z. Z. Chong, J.-Q. Kang, and K. Maiese, "Erythropoietin fosters both intrinsic and extrinsic neuronal protection through modulation of microglia, Akt1, Bad, and caspase-mediated pathways," *British Journal of Pharmacology*, vol. 138, no. 6, pp. 1107–1118, 2003.

[94] Z. Z. Chong, S.-H. Lin, J.-Q. Kang, and K. Maiese, "Erythropoietin prevents early and late neuronal demise through modulation of akt1 and induction of caspase 1, 3, and 8," *Journal of Neuroscience Research*, vol. 71, no. 5, pp. 659–669, 2003.

[95] L. Dong, S. Zhou, X. Yang, Q. Chen, Y. He, and W. Huang, "Magnolol protects against oxidative stress-mediated neural cell damage by modulating mitochondrial dysfunction and PI3K/Akt signaling," *Journal of Molecular Neuroscience*, vol. 50, no. 3, pp. 469–481, 2013.

[96] Y. Jiang, L. Li, B. Liu et al., "Vagus nerve stimulation attenuates cerebral ischemia and reperfusion injury via endogenous cholinergic pathway in rat," *PLoS ONE*, vol. 9, no. 7, Article ID e102342, 2014.

[97] S. H. Kwon, S. I. Hong, S. X. Ma, S. Y. Lee, and C. G. Jang, "3′,4′,7-trihydroxyflavone prevents apoptotic cell death in neuronal cells from hydrogen peroxide-induced oxidative stress," *Food and Chemical Toxicology*, vol. 80, pp. 41–51, 2015.

[98] Y. Li, M. Zeng, W. Chen et al., "Dexmedetomidine reduces isoflurane-induced neuroapoptosis partly by preserving PI3K/Akt pathway in the hippocampus of neonatal rats," *PLoS ONE*, vol. 9, no. 4, Article ID e93639, 2014.

[99] Y. Nakazawa, T. Nishino, Y. Obata et al., "Recombinant human erythropoietin attenuates renal tubulointerstitial injury in murine adriamycin-induced nephropathy," *Journal of Nephrology*, vol. 26, no. 3, pp. 527–533, 2013.

[100] L.-L. Pan, X.-H. Liu, Y.-L. Jia et al., "A novel compound derived from danshensu inhibits apoptosis via upregulation of heme oxygenase-1 expression in SH-SY5Y cells," *Biochimica et Biophysica Acta*, vol. 1830, no. 4, pp. 2861–2871, 2013.

[101] Y. Zhu, G. Wu, G. Zhu, C. Ma, and H. Zhao, "Chronic sleep restriction induces changes in the mandibular condylar cartilage of rats: roles of Akt, Bad and Caspase-3," *International Journal of Clinical and Experimental Medicine*, vol. 7, no. 9, pp. 2585–2592, 2014.

[102] Z. Z. Chong, F. Li, and K. Maiese, "Group I metabotropic receptor neuroprotection requires Akt and its substrates that govern FOXO3a, bim, and β-catenin during oxidative stress," *Current Neurovascular Research*, vol. 3, no. 2, pp. 107–117, 2006.

[103] P. Obexer, K. Geiger, P. F. Ambros, B. Meister, and M. J. Ausserlechner, "FKHRL1-mediated expression of Noxa and Bim induces apoptosis via the mitochondria in neuroblastoma cells," *Cell Death and Differentiation*, vol. 14, no. 3, pp. 534–547, 2007.

[104] Y. C. Shang, Z. Z. Chong, J. Hou, and K. Maiese, "Wnt1, FoxO3a, and NF-kappaB oversee microglial integrity and activation during oxidant stress," *Cellular Signalling*, vol. 22, no. 9, pp. 1317–1329, 2010.

[105] C. Charvet, I. Alberti, F. Luciano et al., "Proteolytic regulation of Forkhead transcription factor FOXO3a by caspase-3-like proteases," *Oncogene*, vol. 22, no. 29, pp. 4557–4568, 2003.

[106] C. S. Yan, Z. C. Zhao, H. Jinling, and K. Maiese, "FoxO3a governs early microglial proliferation and employs mitochondrial depolarization with caspase 3, 8, and 9 cleavage during oxidant induced apoptosis," *Current Neurovascular Research*, vol. 6, no. 4, pp. 223–238, 2009.

[107] M. L. L. Leong, A. C. Maiyar, B. Kim, B. A. O'Keeffe, and G. L. Firestone, "Expression of the serum- and glucocorticoid-inducible protein kinase, Sgk, is a cell survival response to multiple types of environmental stress stimuli in mammary epithelial cells," *The Journal of Biological Chemistry*, vol. 278, no. 8, pp. 5871–5882, 2003.

[108] J. J. Song and Y. J. Lee, "Differential cleavage of Mst1 by caspase-7/-3 is responsible for TRAIL-induced activation of the MAPK superfamily," *Cellular Signalling*, vol. 20, no. 5, pp. 892–906, 2008.

[109] J. Sunayama, F. Tsuruta, N. Masuyama, and Y. Gotoh, "JNK antagonizes Akt-mediated survival signals by phosphorylating 14-3-3," *Journal of Cell Biology*, vol. 170, no. 2, pp. 295–304, 2005.

[110] H. Matsuzaki, H. Daitoku, M. Hatta, K. Tanaka, and A. Fukamizu, "Insulin-induced phosphorylation of FKHR (Foxo1) targets to proteasomal degradation," *Proceedings of the National Academy of Sciences of the United States of America*, vol. 100, no. 20, pp. 11285–11290, 2003.

[111] D. R. Plas and C. B. Thompson, "Akt activation promotes degradation of tuberin and FOXO3a via the proteasome," *Journal of Biological Chemistry*, vol. 278, no. 14, pp. 12361–12366, 2003.

[112] Z. Jagani, A. Singh, and R. Khosravi-Far, "FoxO tumor suppressors and BCR-ABL-induced leukemia: a matter of evasion of apoptosis," *Biochimica et Biophysica Acta—Reviews on Cancer*, vol. 1785, no. 1, pp. 63–84, 2008.

[113] F. Wang, C.-H. Chan, K. Chen, X. Guan, H.-K. Lin, and Q. Tong, "Deacetylation of FOXO3 by SIRT1 or SIRT2 leads to Skp2-mediated FOXO3 ubiquitination and degradation," *Oncogene*, vol. 31, no. 12, pp. 1546–1557, 2012.

[114] Z. Z. Chong, Y. C. Shang, S. Wang, and K. Maiese, "SIRT1: new avenues of discovery for disorders of oxidative stress," *Expert Opinion on Therapeutic Targets*, vol. 16, no. 2, pp. 167–178, 2012.

[115] Z. Z. Chong, S. Wang, Y. C. Shang, and K. Maiese, "Targeting cardiovascular disease with novel SIRT1 pathways," *Future Cardiology*, vol. 8, no. 1, pp. 89–100, 2012.

[116] K. Maiese, Z. Z. Chong, Y. C. Shang, and S. Wang, "Translating cell survival and cell longevity into treatment strategies with

SIRT1," *Romanian Journal of Morphology and Embryology*, vol. 52, no. 4, pp. 1173–1185, 2011.

[117] A. F. Paraíso, K. L. Mendes, and S. H. S. Santos, "Brain activation of SIRT1: role in neuropathology," *Molecular Neurobiology*, vol. 48, no. 3, pp. 681–689, 2013.

[118] Y. Kobayashi, Y. Furukawa-Hibi, C. Chen et al., "SIRT1 is critical regulator of FOXO-mediated transcription in response to oxidative stress," *International Journal of Molecular Medicine*, vol. 16, no. 2, pp. 237–243, 2005.

[119] S. Xiong, G. Salazar, N. Patrushev, and R. W. Alexander, "FoxO1 mediates an autofeedback loop regulating SIRT1 expression," *The Journal of Biological Chemistry*, vol. 286, no. 7, pp. 5289–5299, 2011.

[120] Y. Akasaki, O. Alvarez-Garcia, M. Saito, B. Caramés, Y. Iwamoto, and M. K. Lotz, "FOXO transcription factors support oxidative stress resistance in human chondrocytes," *Arthritis & Rheumatology*, vol. 66, no. 12, pp. 3349–3358, 2014.

[121] M. C.-T. Hu, D.-F. Lee, W. Xia et al., "IκB kinase promotes tumorigenesis through inhibition of forkhead FOXO3a," *Cell*, vol. 117, no. 2, pp. 225–237, 2004.

[122] H. Matsuzaki, H. Daitoku, M. Hatta, H. Aoyama, K. Yoshimochi, and A. Fukamizu, "Acetylation of Foxo1 alters its DNA-binding ability and sensitivity to phosphorylation," *Proceedings of the National Academy of Sciences of the United States of America*, vol. 102, no. 32, pp. 11278–11283, 2005.

[123] S. S. Myatt and E. W.-F. Lam, "The emerging roles of forkhead box (Fox) proteins in cancer," *Nature Reviews Cancer*, vol. 7, no. 11, pp. 847–859, 2007.

[124] A. van der Horst and B. M. T. Burgering, "Stressing the role of FoxO proteins in lifespan and disease," *Nature Reviews Molecular Cell Biology*, vol. 8, no. 6, pp. 440–450, 2007.

[125] K. A. Kim, Y. J. Shin, M. Akram et al., "High glucose condition induces autophagy in endothelial progenitor cells contributing to angiogenic impairment," *Biological and Pharmaceutical Bulletin*, vol. 37, no. 7, pp. 1248–1252, 2014.

[126] Y. Liu, S. Shi, Z. Gu et al., "Impaired autophagic function in rat islets with aging," *Age*, vol. 35, no. 5, pp. 1531–1544, 2013.

[127] K. Maiese, Z. Z. Chong, Y. C. Shang, and S. Wang, "Novel directions for diabetes mellitus drug discovery," *Expert Opinion on Drug Discovery*, vol. 8, no. 1, pp. 35–48, 2013.

[128] H. Zhang, C. Duan, and H. Yang, "Defective autophagy in Parkinson's disease: lessons from genetics," *Molecular Neurobiology*, vol. 51, no. 1, pp. 89–104, 2015.

[129] Z. C. Zhao, F. Li, and K. Maiese, "Stress in the brain: novel cellular mechanisms of injury linked to Alzheimer's disease," *Brain Research Reviews*, vol. 49, no. 1, pp. 1–21, 2005.

[130] Y. Liu, R. Palanivel, E. Rai et al., "Adiponectin stimulates autophagy and reduces oxidative stress to enhance insulin sensitivity during high fat diet feeding in mice," *Diabetes*, vol. 64, no. 1, pp. 36–48, 2014.

[131] K. Maiese, "mTOR: driving apoptosis and autophagy for neurocardiac complications of diabetes mellitus," *World Journal of Diabetes*, vol. 6, no. 2, pp. 217–224, 2015.

[132] K. Maiese, Z. Z. Chong, S. Wang, and Y. C. Shang, "Oxidant stress and signal transduction in the nervous system with the PI 3-K, Akt, and mTOR cascade," *International Journal of Molecular Sciences*, vol. 13, no. 11, pp. 13830–13866, 2012.

[133] E. Mhillaj, M. Morgese, and L. Trabace, "Early life and oxidative stress in psychiatric disorders: what can we learn from animal models?" *Current Pharmaceutical Design*, vol. 21, no. 11, pp. 1396–1403, 2015.

[134] U. Ozel Turkcu, N. Solak Tekin, T. Gokdogan Edgunlu, S. Karakas Celik, and S. Oner, "The association of FOXO3A gene polymorphisms with serum FOXO3A levels and oxidative stress markers in vitiligo patients," *Gene*, vol. 536, no. 1, pp. 129–134, 2014.

[135] P. Zolotukhin, Y. Kozlova, A. Dovzhik et al., "Oxidative status interactome map: towards novel approaches in experiment planning, data analysis, diagnostics and therapy," *Molecular BioSystems*, vol. 9, no. 8, pp. 2085–2096, 2013.

[136] G. Harish, A. Mahadevan, N. Pruthi et al., "Characterization of traumatic brain injury in human brains reveals distinct cellular and molecular changes in contusion and pericontusion," *Journal of Neurochemistry*, 2015.

[137] K. Maiese, "SIRT1 and stem cells: in the forefront with cardiovascular disease, neurodegeneration and cancer," *World Journal of Stem Cells*, vol. 7, no. 2, pp. 235–242, 2015.

[138] H. E. Palma, P. Wolkmer, M. Gallio et al., "Oxidative stress parameters in blood, liver, and kidney of diabetic rats treated with curcumin and/or insulin," *Molecular and Cellular Biochemistry*, vol. 386, no. 1-2, pp. 199–210, 2014.

[139] K. Rjiba-Touati, I. Ayed-Boussema, Y. Guedri, A. Achour, H. Bacha, and S. Abid-Essefi, "Effect of recombinant human erythropoietin on mitomycin C-induced oxidative stress and genotoxicity in rat kidney and heart tissues," *Human & Experimental Toxicology*, 2015.

[140] J. M. Yousef and A. M. Mohamed, "Prophylactic role of B vitamins against bulk and zinc oxide nano-particles toxicity induced oxidative DNA damage and apoptosis in rat livers," *Pakistan Journal of Pharmaceutical Sciences*, vol. 28, no. 1, pp. 175–184, 2015.

[141] S. Gezginci-Oktayoglu, O. Sacan, S. Bolkent et al., "Chard (*Beta vulgaris* L. var. cicla) extract ameliorates hyperglycemia by increasing GLUT2 through Akt2 and antioxidant defense in the liver of rats," *Acta Histochemica*, vol. 116, no. 1, pp. 32–39, 2014.

[142] R.-P. Li, Z.-Z. Wang, M.-X. Sun et al., "Polydatin protects learning and memory impairments in a rat model of vascular dementia," *Phytomedicine*, vol. 19, no. 8-9, pp. 677–681, 2012.

[143] X.-Y. Mao, D.-F. Cao, X. Li et al., "Huperzine A ameliorates cognitive deficits in streptozotocin-induced diabetic rats," *International Journal of Molecular Sciences*, vol. 15, no. 5, pp. 7667–7683, 2014.

[144] M. Moghaddasi, S. H. Javanmard, P. Reisi, M. Tajadini, and M. Taati, "The effect of regular exercise on antioxidant enzyme activities and lipid peroxidation levels in both hippocampi after occluding one carotid in rat," *The Journal of Physiological Sciences*, vol. 64, no. 5, pp. 325–332, 2014.

[145] M. M. Muley, V. N. Thakare, R. R. Patil, A. D. Kshirsagar, and S. R. Naik, "Silymarin improves the behavioural, biochemical and histoarchitecture alterations in focal ischemic rats: a comparative evaluation with piracetam and protocatachuic acid," *Pharmacology Biochemistry and Behavior*, vol. 102, no. 2, pp. 286–293, 2012.

[146] A. Srivastava and T. Shivanandappa, "Prevention of hexachlorocyclohexane-induced neuronal oxidative stress by natural antioxidants," *Nutritional Neuroscience*, vol. 17, no. 4, pp. 164–171, 2014.

[147] D. K. Vishwas, A. Mukherjee, C. Haldar, D. Dash, and M. K. Nayak, "Improvement of oxidative stress and immunity by melatonin: an age dependent study in golden hamster," *Experimental Gerontology*, vol. 48, no. 2, pp. 168–182, 2013.

[148] Q. Zhou, C. Liu, W. Liu et al., "Rotenone induction of hydrogen peroxide inhibits mTOR-mediated S6K and 4E-BP1/eIF4E

pathways, leading to neuronal apoptosis," *Toxicological Sciences*, vol. 143, no. 1, pp. 81–96, 2014.

[149] C. Bowes Rickman, S. Farsiu, C. A. Toth, and M. Klingeborn, "Dry age-related macular degeneration: mechanisms, therapeutic targets, and imaging," *Investigative Ophthalmology and Visual Science*, vol. 54, no. 14, pp. ORSF68–ORSF80, 2013.

[150] J. A. Miret and S. Munné-Bosch, "Plant amino acid-derived vitamins: biosynthesis and function," *Amino Acids*, vol. 46, no. 4, pp. 809–824, 2014.

[151] Y.-J. Xu, P. S. Tappia, N. S. Neki, and N. S. Dhalla, "Prevention of diabetes-induced cardiovascular complications upon treatment with antioxidants," *Heart Failure Reviews*, vol. 19, no. 1, pp. 113–121, 2014.

[152] T. Kajihara, M. Jones, L. Fusi et al., "Differential expression of FOXO1 and FOXO3a confers resistance to oxidative cell death upon endometrial decidualization," *Molecular Endocrinology*, vol. 20, no. 10, pp. 2444–2455, 2006.

[153] Z. Cai and L. J. Yan, "Rapamycin, autophagy, and Alzheimer's disease," *Journal of Biochemical and Pharmacological Research*, vol. 1, no. 2, pp. 84–90, 2013.

[154] W. Chen, Y. Sun, K. Liu, and X. Sun, "Autophagy: a double-edged sword for neuronal survival after cerebral ischemia," *Neural Regeneration Research*, vol. 9, no. 12, pp. 1210–1216, 2014.

[155] Y. Chen, X. Liu, Y. Yin et al., "Unravelling the multifaceted roles of Atg proteins to improve cancer therapy," *Cell Proliferation*, vol. 47, no. 2, pp. 105–112, 2014.

[156] K. Maiese, Z. Z. Chong, Y. C. Shang, and S. Wang, "Targeting disease through novel pathways of apoptosis and autophagy," *Expert Opinion on Therapeutic Targets*, vol. 16, no. 12, pp. 1203–1214, 2012.

[157] J. H. Fox, T. Connor, V. Chopra et al., "The mTOR kinase inhibitor Everolimus decreases S6 kinase phosphorylation but fails to reduce mutant huntingtin levels in brain and is not neuroprotective in the R6/2 mouse model of Huntington's disease," *Molecular Neurodegeneration*, vol. 5, no. 1, article 26, 2010.

[158] K. Maiese, "Novel applications of trophic factors, Wnt and WISP for neuronal repair and regeneration in metabolic disease," *Neural Regeneration Research*, vol. 10, no. 4, pp. 518–528, 2015.

[159] K. Maiese, "Programming apoptosis and autophagy with novel approaches for diabetes mellitus," *Current Neurovascular Research*, vol. 12, no. 2, pp. 173–188, 2015.

[160] R. L. Vidal, A. Figueroa, F. A. Court et al., "Targeting the UPR transcription factor XBP1 protects against Huntington's disease through the regulation of FoxO1 and autophagy," *Human Molecular Genetics*, vol. 21, no. 10, pp. 2245–2262, 2012.

[161] C. He, H. Zhu, H. Li, M.-H. Zou, and Z. Xie, "Dissociation of Bcl-2-Beclin1 complex by activated AMPK enhances cardiac autophagy and protects against cardiomyocyte apoptosis in diabetes," *Diabetes*, vol. 62, no. 4, pp. 1270–1281, 2013.

[162] Y. M. Lim, H. Lim, K. Y. Hur et al., "Systemic autophagy insufficiency compromises adaptation to metabolic stress and facilitates progression from obesity to diabetes," *Nature Communications*, vol. 5, article 4934, 2014.

[163] H. Vakifahmetoglu-Norberg, H. Xia, and J. Yuan, "Pharmacologic agents targeting autophagy," *Journal of Clinical Investigation*, vol. 125, no. 1, pp. 5–13, 2015.

[164] N. Hariharan, Y. Maejima, J. Nakae, J. Paik, R. A. Depinho, and J. Sadoshima, "Deacetylation of FoxO by Sirt1 plays an essential role in mediating starvation-induced autophagy in cardiac myocytes," *Circulation Research*, vol. 107, no. 12, pp. 1470–1482, 2010.

[165] T. G. Schips, A. Wietelmann, K. Höhn et al., "FoxO3 induces reversible cardiac atrophy and autophagy in a transgenic mouse model," *Cardiovascular Research*, vol. 91, no. 4, pp. 587–597, 2011.

[166] J. Shi, N. Yin, L. L. Xuan, C. S. Yao, A. M. Meng, and Q. Hou, "Vam3, a derivative of resveratrol, attenuates cigarette smoke-induced autophagy," *Acta Pharmacologica Sinica*, vol. 33, no. 7, pp. 888–896, 2012.

[167] Y. Fong, Y. Lin, C. Wu et al., "The antiproliferative and apoptotic effects of sirtinol, a sirtuin inhibitor on human lung cancer cells by modulating Akt/β-catenin-Foxo3a axis," *The Scientific World Journal*, vol. 2014, Article ID 937051, 8 pages, 2014.

[168] X. Guo, Y. Chen, Q. Liu et al., "Ac-cel, a novel antioxidant, protects against hydrogen peroxide-induced injury in PC12 cells via attenuation of mitochondrial dysfunction," *Journal of Molecular Neuroscience*, vol. 50, no. 3, pp. 453–461, 2013.

[169] Z. C. Zhao, F. Li, and K. Maiese, "Oxidative stress in the brain: novel cellular targets that govern survival during neurodegenerative disease," *Progress in Neurobiology*, vol. 75, no. 3, pp. 207–246, 2005.

[170] B. Favaloro, N. Allocati, V. Graziano, C. di Ilio, and V. de Laurenzi, "Role of apoptosis in disease," *Aging*, vol. 4, no. 5, pp. 330–349, 2012.

[171] J. Folch, F. Junyent, E. Verdaguer et al., "Role of cell cycle re-entry in neurons: a common apoptotic mechanism of neuronal cell death," *Neurotoxicity Research*, vol. 22, no. 3, pp. 195–207, 2012.

[172] K. Maiese, Z. Z. Chong, J. Hou, and Y. C. Shang, "Oxidative stress: biomarkers and novel therapeutic pathways," *Experimental Gerontology*, vol. 45, no. 3, pp. 217–234, 2010.

[173] K. Maiese, Z. Z. Chong, Y. C. Shang, and J. Hou, "Novel avenues of drug discovery and biomarkers for diabetes mellitus," *Journal of Clinical Pharmacology*, vol. 51, no. 2, pp. 128–152, 2011.

[174] K. Schutters and C. Reutelingsperger, "Phosphatidylserine targeting for diagnosis and treatment of human diseases," *Apoptosis*, vol. 15, no. 9, pp. 1072–1082, 2010.

[175] Z. Tang, A. T. Baykal, H. Gao et al., "MTor is a signaling hub in cell survival: a mass-spectrometry-based proteomics investigation," *Journal of Proteome Research*, vol. 13, no. 5, pp. 2433–2444, 2014.

[176] T. Wang, H. Cui, N. Ma, and Y. Jiang, "Nicotinamide-mediated inhibition of SIRT1 deacetylase is associated with the viability of cancer cells exposed to antitumor agents and apoptosis," *Oncology Letters*, vol. 6, no. 2, pp. 600–604, 2013.

[177] Y. Yang, H. Li, S. Hou, B. Hu, J. Liu, and J. Wang, "The noncoding RNA expression profile and the effect of lncRNA AK126698 on cisplatin resistance in non-small-cell lung cancer cell," *PLoS ONE*, vol. 8, no. 5, Article ID e65309, 2013.

[178] K. Maiese, "New insights for oxidative stress and diabetes mellitus," *Oxidative Medicine and Cellular Longevity*, vol. 2015, Article ID 875961, 17 pages, 2015.

[179] L. Wei, C. Sun, M. Lei et al., "Activation of Wnt/β-catenin pathway by exogenous Wnt1 protects SH-SY5Y cells against 6-hydroxydopamine toxicity," *Journal of Molecular Neuroscience*, vol. 49, no. 1, pp. 105–115, 2013.

[180] G. Arunachalam, S. M. Samuel, I. Marei, H. Ding, and C. R. Triggle, "Metformin modulates hyperglycaemia-induced endothelial senescence and apoptosis through SIRT1," *British Journal of Pharmacology*, vol. 171, no. 2, pp. 523–535, 2014.

[181] T. Nakamura and K. Sakamoto, "Forkhead transcription factor FOXO subfamily is essential for reactive oxygen species-induced apoptosis," *Molecular and Cellular Endocrinology*, vol. 281, no. 1-2, pp. 47–55, 2008.

[182] C. S. Yan, Z. C. Zhao, J. Hou, and K. Maiese, "The forkhead transcription factor FOXO3a controls microglial inflammatory activation and eventual apoptotic injury through caspase 3," *Current Neurovascular Research*, vol. 6, no. 1, pp. 20–31, 2009.

[183] M. Anitha, C. Gondha, R. Sutliff et al., "GDNF rescues hyperglycemia-induced diabetic enteric neuropathy through activation of the PI3K/Akt pathway," *The Journal of Clinical Investigation*, vol. 116, no. 2, pp. 344–356, 2006.

[184] W.-H. Zheng, S. Kar, and R. Quirion, "FKHRL1 and its homologs are new targets of nerve growth factor Trk receptor signaling," *Journal of Neurochemistry*, vol. 80, no. 6, pp. 1049–1061, 2002.

[185] W. Zhu, G. N. Bijur, N. A. Styles, and X. Li, "Regulation of FOXO3a by brain-derived neurotrophic factor in differentiated human SH-SY5Y neuroblastoma cells," *Molecular Brain Research*, vol. 126, no. 1, pp. 45–56, 2004.

[186] Z. Tothova, R. Kollipara, B. J. Huntly et al., "FoxOs are critical mediators of hematopoietic stem cell resistance to physiologic oxidative stress," *Cell*, vol. 128, no. 2, pp. 325–339, 2007.

[187] H. Liu, J. Yin, H. Wang et al., "FOXO3a modulates WNT/β-catenin signaling and suppresses epithelial-to-mesenchymal transition in prostate cancer cells," *Cellular Signalling*, vol. 27, no. 3, pp. 510–518, 2015.

[188] S. Bayod, I. Menella, S. Sanchez-Roige et al., "Wnt pathway regulation by long-term moderate exercise in rat hippocampus," *Brain Research*, vol. 1543, pp. 38–48, 2014.

[189] D. C. Berwick and K. Harvey, "The regulation and deregulation of Wnt signaling by PARK genes in health and disease," *Journal of Molecular Cell Biology*, vol. 6, no. 1, pp. 3–12, 2014.

[190] K. Maiese, F. Li, Z. Z. Chong, and Y. C. Shang, "The Wnt signaling pathway: aging gracefully as a protectionist?" *Pharmacology and Therapeutics*, vol. 118, no. 1, pp. 58–81, 2008.

[191] B. Marchetti and S. Pluchino, "Wnt your brain be inflamed? Yes, it Wnt!," *Trends in Molecular Medicine*, vol. 19, no. 3, pp. 144–156, 2013.

[192] T. J. Sun, R. Tao, Y. Q. Han, G. Xu, J. Liu, and Y. F. Han, "Therapeutic potential of umbilical cord mesenchymal stem cells with Wnt/beta-catenin signaling pathway pre-activated for the treatment of diabetic wounds," *European Review for Medical and Pharmacological Sciences*, vol. 18, no. 17, pp. 2460–2464, 2014.

[193] Z. Z. Chong, F. Li, and K. Maiese, "Cellular demise and inflammatory microglial activation during β-amyloid toxicity are governed by Wnt1 and canonical signaling pathways," *Cellular Signalling*, vol. 19, no. 6, pp. 1150–1162, 2007.

[194] F. L'Episcopo, C. Tirolo, N. Testa et al., "Reactive astrocytes and Wnt/beta-catenin signaling link nigrostriatal injury to repair in 1-methyl-4-phenyl-1,2,3,6-tetrahydropyridine model of Parkinson's disease," *Neurobiology of Disease*, vol. 41, no. 2, pp. 508–527, 2011.

[195] B. Marchetti, F. L'Episcopo, M. C. Morale et al., "Uncovering novel actors in astrocyte-neuron crosstalk in Parkinson's disease: the Wnt/β-catenin signaling cascade as the common final pathway for neuroprotection and self-repair," *European Journal of Neuroscience*, vol. 37, no. 10, pp. 1550–1563, 2013.

[196] C. González-Fernández, C. M. Fernández-Martos, S. D. Shields, E. Arenas, and F. J. Rodríguez, "Wnts are expressed in the spinal cord of adult mice and are differentially induced after injury," *Journal of Neurotrauma*, vol. 31, no. 6, pp. 565–581, 2014.

[197] Z. Z. Chong, Y. C. Shang, J. Hou, and K. Maiese, "Wnt1 neuroprotection translates into improved neurological function during oxidant stress and cerebral ischemia through AKT1 and mitochondrial apoptotic pathways," *Oxidative Medicine and Cellular Longevity*, vol. 3, no. 2, pp. 153–165, 2010.

[198] D. Xu, W. Zhao, G. Pan et al., "Expression of nemo-like kinase after spinal cord injury in rats," *Journal of Molecular Neuroscience*, vol. 52, no. 3, pp. 410–418, 2014.

[199] F. L'Episcopo, C. Tirolo, N. Testa et al., "Plasticity of subventricular zone neuroprogenitors in MPTP (1-Methyl-4-Phenyl-1,2,3,6-tetrahydropyridine) mouse model of Parkinson's disease involves cross talk between inflammatory and Wnt/β-catenin signaling pathways: functional consequences for neuroprotection and repair," *Journal of Neuroscience*, vol. 32, no. 6, pp. 2062–2085, 2012.

[200] B. He, N. Reguart, L. You et al., "Blockade of Wnt-1 signaling induces apoptosis in human colorectal cancer cells containing downstream mutations," *Oncogene*, vol. 24, no. 18, pp. 3054–3058, 2005.

[201] S. Pandey, "Targeting Wnt-Frizzled signaling in cardiovascular diseases," *Molecular Biology Reports*, vol. 40, no. 10, pp. 6011–6018, 2013.

[202] Y. Xing, X. Zhang, K. Zhao et al., "Beneficial effects of sulindac in focal cerebral ischemia: a positive role in Wnt/β-catenin pathway," *Brain Research*, vol. 1482, pp. 71–80, 2012.

[203] F. L'Episcopo, M. F. Serapide, C. Tirolo et al., "A Wnt1 regulated Frizzled-1/β-catenin signaling pathway as a candidate regulatory circuit controlling mesencephalic dopaminergic neuron-astrocyte crosstalk: therapeutical relevance for neuron survival and neuroprotection," *Molecular Neurodegeneration*, vol. 6, no. 1, article 49, 2011.

[204] L. P. Sowers, L. Loo, Y. Wu et al., "Disruption of the non-canonical Wnt gene PRICKLE2 leads to autism-like behaviors with evidence for hippocampal synaptic dysfunction," *Molecular Psychiatry*, vol. 18, no. 10, pp. 1077–1089, 2013.

[205] Y. Yang, Y. Su, D. Wang et al., "Tanshinol attenuates the deleterious effects of oxidative stress on osteoblastic differentiation via wnt/FoxO3a signaling," *Oxidative Medicine and Cellular Longevity*, vol. 2013, Article ID 351895, 18 pages, 2013.

[206] P. Esmaeili Tazangi, S. M. Moosavi, M. Shabani, and M. Haghani, "Erythropoietin improves synaptic plasticity and memory deficits by decrease of the neurotransmitter release probability in the rat model of Alzheimer's disease," *Pharmacology Biochemistry and Behavior*, vol. 130, pp. 15–21, 2015.

[207] T. Yu, L. Li, T. Chen, Z. Liu, H. Liu, and Z. Li, "Erythropoietin attenuates advanced glycation endproducts-induced toxicity of schwann cells in vitro," *Neurochemical Research*, vol. 40, no. 4, pp. 698–712, 2015.

[208] K. Maiese, J. Hou, Z. Z. Chong, and Y. C. Shang, "Erythropoietin, forkhead proteins, and oxidative injury: biomarkers and biology," *The Scientific World Journal*, vol. 9, pp. 1072–1104, 2009.

[209] D. J. Klinke II, "Induction of Wnt-inducible signaling protein-1 correlates with invasive breast cancer oncogenesis and reduced type 1 cell-mediated cytotoxic immunity: a retrospective study," *PLoS Computational Biology*, vol. 10, no. 1, Article ID e1003409, 2014.

[210] K. Knoblich, H. X. Wang, C. Sharma, A. L. Fletcher, S. J. Turley, and M. E. Hemler, "Tetraspanin TSPAN12 regulates tumor growth and metastasis and inhibits beta-catenin degradation," *Cellular and Molecular Life Sciences*, vol. 71, no. 7, pp. 1305–1314, 2014.

[211] A. Maeda, M. Ono, K. Holmbeck et al., "WNT1 induced secreted protein-1 (WISP1) : a novel regulator of bone turnover

and Wnt signaling," The Journal of Biological Chemistry, vol. 290, no. 22, pp. 14004–14018, 2015.

[212] K. Maiese, "WISP1: clinical insights for a proliferative and restorative member of the CCN family," *Current Neurovascular Research*, vol. 11, no. 4, pp. 378–389, 2014.

[213] V. Murahovschi, O. Pivovarova, I. Ilkavets et al., "WISP1 is a novel adipokine linked to inflammation in obesity," *Diabetes*, vol. 64, no. 3, pp. 856–866, 2015.

[214] K. R. Kelly, S. T. Nawrocki, C. M. Espitia et al., "Targeting Aurora A kinase activity with the investigational agent alisertib increases the efficacy of cytarabine through a FOXO-dependent mechanism," *International Journal of Cancer*, vol. 131, no. 11, pp. 2693–2703, 2012.

[215] D. Hoogeboom, M. A. G. Essers, P. E. Polderman, E. Voets, L. M. M. Smits, and B. M. T. Burgering, "Interaction of FOXO with beta-catenin inhibits beta-catenin/T cell factor activity," *The Journal of Biological Chemistry*, vol. 283, no. 14, pp. 9224–9230, 2008.

[216] T. Hosaka, W. H. Biggs III, D. Tieu et al., "Disruption of forkhead transcription factor (FOXO) family members in mice reveals their functional diversification," *Proceedings of the National Academy of Sciences of the United States of America*, vol. 101, no. 9, pp. 2975–2980, 2004.

[217] Y. Kamei, S. Miura, M. Suzuki et al., "Skeletal muscle FOXO1 (FKHR) transgenic mice have less skeletal muscle mass, down-regulated type I (slow twitch/red muscle) fiber genes, and impaired glycemic control," *The Journal of Biological Chemistry*, vol. 279, no. 39, pp. 41114–41123, 2004.

[218] D. H. Castrillon, L. Miao, R. Kollipara, J. W. Horner, and R. A. DePinho, "Suppression of ovarian follicle activation in mice by the transcription factor Foxo3a," *Science*, vol. 301, no. 5630, pp. 215–218, 2003.

[219] L. Liu, S. Rajareddy, P. Reddy et al., "Infertility caused by retardation of follicular development in mice with oocyte-specific expression of Foxo3a," *Development*, vol. 134, no. 1, pp. 199–209, 2007.

[220] N. H. Uhlenhaut and M. Treier, "Forkhead transcription factors in ovarian function," *Reproduction*, vol. 142, no. 4, pp. 489–495, 2011.

[221] W. J. Watkins, A. J. Umbers, K. J. Woad et al., "Mutational screening of FOXO3A and FOXO1A in women with premature ovarian failure," *Fertility and Sterility*, vol. 86, no. 5, pp. 1518–1521, 2006.

[222] K. Miyamoto, K. Y. Araki, K. Naka et al., "Foxo3a is essential for maintenance of the hematopoietic stem cell pool," *Cell Stem Cell*, vol. 1, no. 1, pp. 101–112, 2007.

[223] M. Dentice, A. Marsili, R. Ambrosio et al., "The FoxO3/type 2 deiodinase pathway is required for normal mouse myogenesis and muscle regeneration," *Journal of Clinical Investigation*, vol. 120, no. 11, pp. 4021–4030, 2010.

[224] J. Palazuelos, M. Klingener, and A. Aguirre, "TGFβ signaling regulates the timing of CNS myelination by modulating oligodendrocyte progenitor cell cycle exit through SMAD3/4/FoxO1/Sp1," *The Journal of Neuroscience*, vol. 34, no. 23, pp. 7917–7930, 2014.

[225] C. Kibbe, J. Chen, G. Xu, G. Jing, and A. Shalev, "FOXO1 competes with carbohydrate response element-binding protein (ChREBP) and inhibits thioredoxin-interacting protein (TXNIP) transcription in pancreatic beta cells," *Journal of Biological Chemistry*, vol. 288, no. 32, pp. 23194–23202, 2013.

[226] M. Almeida, L. Han, M. Martin-Millan, C. A. O'Brien, and S. C. Manolagas, "Oxidative stress antagonizes Wnt signaling in osteoblast precursors by diverting β-catenin from T cell factor- to forkhead box O-mediated transcription," *The Journal of Biological Chemistry*, vol. 282, no. 37, pp. 27298–27305, 2007.

[227] H.-D. Chae and H. E. Broxmeyer, "SIRT1 deficiency downregulates PTEN/JNK/FOXO1 pathway to block reactive oxygen species-induced apoptosis in mouse embryonic stem cells," *Stem Cells and Development*, vol. 20, no. 7, pp. 1277–1285, 2011.

[228] S. Iyer, L. Han, S. M. Bartell et al., "Sirtuin1 (Sirt1) promotes cortical bone formation by preventing beta-catenin sequestration by FoxO transcription factors in osteoblast progenitors," *The Journal of Biological Chemistry*, vol. 289, no. 35, pp. 24069–24078, 2014.

[229] E. C. Genin, N. Caron, R. Vandenbosch, L. Nguyen, and B. Malgrange, "Concise review: forkhead pathway in the control of adult neurogenesis," *Stem Cells*, vol. 32, no. 6, pp. 1398–1407, 2014.

[230] A. Domanskyi, H. Alter, M. A. Vogt, P. Gass, and I. A. Vinnikov, "Transcription factors Foxa1 and Foxa2 are required for adult dopamine neurons maintenance," *Frontiers in Cellular Neuroscience*, vol. 8, article 275, 2014.

[231] D. Lough, H. Dai, M. Yang et al., "Stimulation of the follicular bulge lgr5+ and lgr6+ stem cells with the gut-derived human alpha defensin 5 results in decreased bacterial presence, enhanced wound healing, and hair growth from tissues devoid of adnexal structures," *Plastic and Reconstructive Surgery*, vol. 132, no. 5, pp. 1159–1171, 2013.

[232] D.-W. Jung, W.-H. Kim, and D. R. Williams, "Reprogram or reboot: small molecule approaches for the production of induced pluripotent stem cells and direct cell reprogramming," *ACS Chemical Biology*, vol. 9, no. 1, pp. 80–95, 2014.

[233] C.-S. Yang, C. G. Lopez, and T. M. Rana, "Discovery of nonsteroidal anti-inflammatory drug and anticancer drug enhancing reprogramming and induced pluripotent stem cell generation," *Stem Cells*, vol. 29, no. 10, pp. 1528–1536, 2011.

[234] N. Case, Z. Xie, B. Sen et al., "Mechanical activation of β-catenin regulates phenotype in adult murine marrow-derived mesenchymal stem cells," *Journal of Orthopaedic Research*, vol. 28, no. 11, pp. 1531–1538, 2010.

[235] J. Heo, E.-K. Ahn, H.-G. Jeong et al., "Transcriptional characterization of Wnt pathway during sequential hepatic differentiation of human embryonic stem cells and adipose tissue-derived stem cells," *Biochemical and Biophysical Research Communications*, vol. 434, no. 2, pp. 235–240, 2013.

[236] R. Castaneda-Arellano, C. Beas-Zarate, A. I. Feria-Velasco, E. W. Bitar-Alatorre, and M. C. Rivera-Cervantes, "From neurogenesis to neuroprotection in the epilepsy: signalling by erythropoietin," *Frontiers in Bioscience*, vol. 19, pp. 1445–1455, 2014.

[237] K. Maiese, Z. Z. Chong, F. Li, and Y. C. Shang, "Erythropoietin: elucidating new cellular targets that broaden therapeutic strategies," *Progress in Neurobiology*, vol. 85, no. 2, pp. 194–213, 2008.

[238] K. Maiese, Z. Z. Chong, and Y. C. Shang, "Raves and risks for erythropoietin," *Cytokine and Growth Factor Reviews*, vol. 19, no. 2, pp. 145–155, 2008.

[239] A. M. Messier and R. K. Ohls, "Neuroprotective effects of erythropoiesis-stimulating agents in term and preterm neonates," *Current Opinion in Pediatrics*, vol. 26, no. 2, pp. 139–145, 2014.

[240] A. Palazzuoli, G. Ruocco, M. Pellegrini et al., "The role of erythropoietin stimulating agents in anemic patients with heart failure: solved and unresolved questions," *Therapeutics and Clinical Risk Management*, vol. 10, pp. 641–650, 2014.

[241] L. Wang, L. Di, and C. T. Noguchi, "Erythropoietin, a novel versatile player regulating energy metabolism beyond the erythroid system," *International Journal of Biological Sciences*, vol. 10, no. 8, pp. 921–939, 2014.

[242] W. J. Bakker, T. B. van Dijk, M. P.-V. Amelsvoort et al., "Differential regulation of Foxo3a target genes in erythropoiesis," *Molecular and Cellular Biology*, vol. 27, no. 10, pp. 3839–3854, 2007.

[243] N. Kaushal, S. Hegde, J. Lumadue, R. F. Paulson, and K. S. Prabhu, "The regulation of erythropoiesis by selenium in mice," *Antioxidants and Redox Signaling*, vol. 14, no. 8, pp. 1403–1412, 2011.

[244] S. Srinivasan, M. Anitha, S. Mwangi, and R. O. Heuckeroth, "Enteric neuroblasts require the phosphatidylinositol 3-kinase/Akt/Forkhead pathway for GDNF-stimulated survival," *Molecular and Cellular Neuroscience*, vol. 29, no. 1, pp. 107–119, 2005.

[245] K. Maiese, Z. Z. Chong, Y. C. Shang, and H. Jinling, "Rogue proliferation versus restorative protection: where do we draw the line for Wnt and Forkhead signaling?" *Expert Opinion on Therapeutic Targets*, vol. 12, no. 7, pp. 905–916, 2008.

[246] V. Exil, L. Ping, Y. Yu et al., "Activation of MAPK and FoxO by manganese (Mn) in rat neonatal primary astrocyte cultures," *PLoS ONE*, vol. 9, no. 5, Article ID e94753, 2014.

[247] P. K. Bahia, V. Pugh, K. Hoyland, V. Hensley, M. Rattray, and R. J. Williams, "Neuroprotective effects of phenolic antioxidant tBHQ associate with inhibition of FoxO3a nuclear translocation and activity," *Journal of Neurochemistry*, vol. 123, no. 1, pp. 182–191, 2012.

[248] K. Y. Yoo, S. H. Kwon, C. H. Lee et al., "FoxO3a changes in pyramidal neurons and expresses in non-pyramidal neurons and astrocytes in the gerbil hippocampal CA1 region after transient cerebral ischemia," *Neurochemical Research*, vol. 37, no. 3, pp. 588–595, 2012.

[249] G. Xu, J. Liu, K. Yoshimoto et al., "2,3,7,8-Tetrachlorodibenzo-p-dioxin (TCDD) induces expression of $p27^{kip1}$ and FoxO3a in female rat cerebral cortex and PC12 cells," *Toxicology Letters*, vol. 226, no. 3, pp. 294–302, 2014.

[250] A. Wilk, K. Urbanska, S. Yang et al., "Insulin-like growth factor-I-forkhead box O transcription factor 3a counteracts high glucose/tumor necrosis factor-α-mediated neuronal damage: implications for human immunodeficiency virus encephalitis," *Journal of Neuroscience Research*, vol. 89, no. 2, pp. 183–198, 2011.

[251] S. F. Eddy, S. E. Kane, and G. E. Sonenshein, "Trastuzumab-resistant HER2-driven breast cancer cells are sensitive to epigallocatechin-3 gallate," *Cancer Research*, vol. 67, no. 19, pp. 9018–9023, 2007.

[252] F. Gao and W. Wang, "MicroRNA-96 promotes the proliferation of colorectal cancer cells and targets tumor protein p53 inducible nuclear protein 1, forkhead box protein O1 (FOXO1) and FOXO3a," *Molecular Medicine Reports*, vol. 11, no. 2, pp. 1200–1206, 2015.

[253] J. Wang, X. Zheng, G. Zeng, Y. Zhou, and H. Yuan, "Purified vitexin compound 1 inhibits growth and angiogenesis through activation of FOXO3a by inactivation of Akt in hepatocellular carcinoma," *International Journal of Molecular Medicine*, vol. 33, no. 2, pp. 441–448, 2014.

[254] A. Kafka, S. Bašić-Kinda, and N. Pećina-Šlaus, "The cellular story of dishevelleds," *Croatian Medical Journal*, vol. 55, no. 5, pp. 459–46667, 2014.

[255] F. Li, Z. Z. Chong, and K. Maiese, "Winding through the WNT pathway during cellular development and demise," *Histology and Histopathology*, vol. 21, no. 1–3, pp. 103–124, 2006.

[256] H. Y. Park, K. Toume, M. A. Arai, S. K. Sadhu, F. Ahmed, and M. Ishibashi, "Calotropin: a cardenolide from calotropis gigantea that inhibits Wnt signaling by increasing casein kinase 1alpha in colon cancer cells," *ChemBioChem*, vol. 15, no. 6, pp. 872–878, 2014.

[257] Z.-H. Yang, R. Zheng, Y. Gao, Q. Zhang, and H. Zhang, "Abnormal gene expression and gene fusion in lung adenocarcinoma with high-throughput RNA sequencing," *Cancer Gene Therapy*, vol. 21, no. 2, pp. 74–82, 2014.

[258] C. Tan, S. Liu, S. Tan et al., "Polymorphisms in MicroRNA target sites of forkhead box O genes are associated with hepatocellular carcinoma," *PLOS ONE*, vol. 10, no. 3, Article ID e0119210, 2015.

[259] A. O. Estevez, K. L. Morgan, N. J. Szewczyk, D. Gems, and M. Estevez, "The neurodegenerative effects of selenium are inhibited by FOXO and PINK1/PTEN regulation of insulin/insulin-like growth factor signaling in *Caenorhabditis elegans*," *NeuroToxicology*, vol. 41, pp. 28–43, 2014.

[260] Y. K. Hong, S. Lee, S. H. Park et al., "Inhibition of JNK/dFOXO pathway and caspases rescues neurological impairments in *Drosophila* Alzheimer's disease model," *Biochemical and Biophysical Research Communications*, vol. 419, no. 1, pp. 49–53, 2012.

[261] E. Pino, R. Amamoto, L. Zheng et al., "FOXO3 determines the accumulation of α-synuclein and controls the fate of dopaminergic neurons in the substantia nigra," *Human Molecular Genetics*, vol. 23, no. 6, pp. 1435–1452, 2014.

[262] N. Ferrara, B. Rinaldi, G. Corbi et al., "Exercise training promotes SIRT1 activity in aged rats," *Rejuvenation Research*, vol. 11, no. 1, pp. 139–150, 2008.

[263] R. R. Alcendor, S. Gao, P. Zhai et al., "Sirt1 regulates aging and resistance to oxidative stress in the heart," *Circulation Research*, vol. 100, no. 10, pp. 1512–1521, 2007.

[264] M. Li, J.-F. Chiu, B. T. Mossman, and N. K. Fukagawa, "Down-regulation of manganese-superoxide dismutase through phosphorylation of FOXO3a by Akt in explanted vascular smooth muscle cells from old rats," *Journal of Biological Chemistry*, vol. 281, no. 52, pp. 40429–40439, 2006.

[265] H. Miyauchi, T. Minamino, K. Tateno, T. Kunieda, H. Toko, and I. Komuro, "Akt negatively regulates the in vitro lifespan of human endothelial cells via a p53/p21-dependent pathway," *EMBO Journal*, vol. 23, no. 1, pp. 212–220, 2004.

12

Role of Natural Radiosensitizers and Cancer Cell Radioresistance: An Update

Arif Malik,[1] Misbah Sultana,[1] Aamer Qazi,[2] Mahmood Husain Qazi,[2] Gulshan Parveen,[1] Sulayman Waquar,[1] Abdul Basit Ashraf,[3] and Mahmood Rasool[4]

[1] *Institute of Molecular Biology and Biotechnology (IMBB), The University of Lahore, Pakistan*
[2] *Center for Research in Molecular Medicine (CRiMM), The University of Lahore, Pakistan*
[3] *University College of Medicine and Dentistry, The University of Lahore, Pakistan*
[4] *Center of Excellence in Genomic Medicine Research (CEGMR), King Abdulaziz University, Jeddah, Saudi Arabia*

Correspondence should be addressed to Arif Malik; arifuaf@yahoo.com

Academic Editor: Francesco Marampon

Cancer originates from genetic mutations accumulation. Cancer stem cells have been depicted as tumorigenic cells that can differentiate and self-renew. Cancer stem cells are thought to be resistant to conventional therapy like chemotherapy and radiation therapy. Radiation therapy and chemotherapy damage carcinomic DNA cells. Because of the ability of cancer stem cells to self-renew and reproduce malignant tumors, they are the subject of intensive research. In this review, CSCs radioresistant mechanisms which include DNA damage response and natural radiosensitizers have been summed up. Reactive oxygen species play an important role in different physiological processes. ROS scavenging is responsible for regulation of reactive oxygen species generation. A researcher has proved that microRNAs regulate tumor radiation resistance. Ionizing radiation does not kill the cancer cells; rather, IR just slows down the signs and symptoms. Ionizing radiation damages DNA directly/indirectly. IR is given mostly in combination with other chemo/radiotherapies. We briefly described here the behavior of cancer stem cells and radioresistance therapies in cancer treatment. To overcome radioresistance in treatment of cancer, strategies like fractionation modification, treatment in combination, inflammation modification, and overcoming hypoxic tumor have been practiced. Natural radiosensitizers, for example, curcumin, genistein, and quercetin, are more beneficial than synthetic compounds.

1. Introduction

Cancer is now the most common cause of human death. Although many advances have been made in the treatment of cancer, still mortality rate of cancer malignancies remains the same, due to the tumor resistance to radiation therapy. The most common cause of failure is the development of secondary tumors and metastasis. Cancer is widely characterized by the abnormal growth of cells having genetic/epigenetic changes, which results in high rate of morbidity and mortality. With the declaration of cancer war, substantial steps are made in the battle of cancer biology for more understanding. Thus, antitumor therapy showed evident results against the genetic material of tumor destruction. Usually, the carcinomic DNA cells are damaged during radiation and chemotherapy. Commonly, cancer treatment includes both radiation and chemotherapy depending on the patient condition and wound type. Still, cancer is found to be one of the incurable diseases. The inadequate prognosis and late detection of malignancy made the survival rate lower.

Oncologists face another problem during treatment when renewal of tumor takes place. Metastasis happens by evading the DNA-damaged induced cells and makes the tumor cells able to regrow; thus, they are termed cancer stem cells. Although the mechanisms are still not clear, worldwide work is going on to illuminate CSC's resistance. Cancer stem cells due to their ability to self-renew and reproduce malignant tumors are the subject of intensive research. Stem cells by

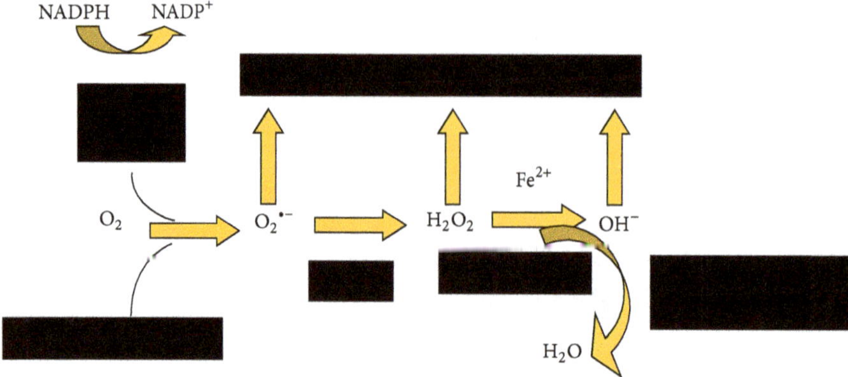

FIGURE 1: ROS have superoxide anion, hydrogen peroxide, and hydroxyl radical. Superoxide anion ($O_2^{\bullet -}$) generated from NADPH oxidation through NADPH oxidases. It reduces to hydrogen peroxide (H_2O_2) where superoxide dismutase (SOD) acts as catalyst. Hydrogen peroxide further reduces to H_2O via catalase/oxidized iron (Fe^{2+}) to highly reactive hydroxyl ion (OH^-). During oxidative stress, when generation of reactive oxygen species spaces out their scavenging system, levels of oxidized reactive oxygen species accumulate and this damages many cellular factors.

asymmetric cell division give rise to progenitor cell into differentiated cells. Cancer stem cells as compared with progenitor cells have very low rate of development [1]. Normally, origin of cancer occurs after genetic and epigenetic changes within the cell as a result abrogating genomic instability. It has been suggested that hierarchical original tissue structure is preserved by abnormal clones, at the start of malignancy. Through model of cancer stem cell, it is proposed that differentiated cells are produced by transit-amplifying cells [2].

2. Cancer Stem Cells and Radiation Therapy Response

Radiation therapy provides cure in many types of tumors. Radiotherapy in the initial stage of tumor procession can control tumor [3]. Radiation therapy is one of the effective treatments for glioblastoma, but still tumor renewal causes death of the patient. It was analyzed that cancer stem cells survive more during radiotherapy than noncancer stem cells. Although radiotherapy damages the same amount of DNA in both cancer stem cells and noncancer stem cells, cancer stem cells robustness ability to repair damage was dominant. After radiotherapy, noncancer stem cells showed more apoptosis. Genotoxic stress which is produced due to the damage to organism genome triggers ATM, CHK1, and CHK2 (serine/threonine-protein kinase) proteins which further triggers DNA repair pathway. Cancer stem cells exhibit basic level of checkpoint activation and are always ready against genotoxic stress. Using CHK1 and CHK2 inhibitors helps in radiation sensitivity of cancer stem cells [4]. During radioresistance, Wnt/β-catenin plays an important role. Radiation improves stem cells of murine mammary epithelial cell line that had antiapoptotic proteins, that is, activated β-catenin and survivin. These cells have the ability to self-renew elevation in mammosphere formation assay [5, 6]. Radiotherapy results in low reactive oxygen species (ROS) in breast cancer stem cells as compared to noncancer stem cells. This decrease in ROS level of breast could be the result of raised radical scavenger properties.

3. Reactive Oxygen Species (ROS)

Reactive oxygen species have a very important role in the physiological developmental processes, for example, emergence of embryonic stem cells/differentiation of embryonic cardiomyocytes [7–9]. It has been demonstrated that reactive oxygen species are concerned with many biological processes like expression of genes, translational proteins, and protein-protein interactions [10]. ROS function in cellular signaling, signals propagation, and balancing of cellular input. They function as variable resistor to organize several cellular processes and set the cellular activity [11]. With the growing advancement in genomics and proteomics, many pathways give information about the balancing of reactive oxygen species and how cellular processes are controlled. Particularly in stem cells, change in state of oxidation, also called redox regulation, may be responsible for communicating mitochondria and nucleus [12–14]. Redox-mediated communication between mitochondria and nucleus explains the cellular metabolism coordination with remodulation of chromatin, cell cycling, expression of gene, repairing of DNA, and cell differentiation. Reactive oxygen species are also concerned with the process of ageing but much is not known about the involvement of ROS in stem cells ageing [15, 16].

4. Genesis and Scavenging of Reactive Oxygen Species

Reactive oxygen species originate from molecular oxygen reducing one electron (Figure 1). Mainly intracellular ROS are of three kinds: hydrogen peroxide (H_2O_2), superoxide anion (O_2^-), and hydroxyl radical (OH^-). Superoxide anion comprises unpaired electron that rapidly reacts and reduces to hydrogen peroxide through superoxide dismutase (SOD), an antioxidant enzyme [17]. Hydrogen peroxide further reduces to water (H_2O) and oxide ion (O_2) through several cellular antioxidants (Figure 1). Reactive oxygen species can be observed intracellularly through many techniques, but still many tries have failed to discriminate within different ROS species. Hydrogen peroxide (H_2O_2) is considered as the major ROS species in signaling of intracellular molecules and in particular circumstances can directly play a role as second messenger and in integration of environmental cues and finally pass them to signal transduction cascade down. This is usually due to longer half-life of hydrogen peroxide (H_2O_2) and ability to discriminate via membranes comparatively with other kinds of reactive oxygen species [10].

During normal physiological conditions, ROS scavenging regulates the reactive oxygen species generation. ROS scavenging system includes such antioxidant enzymes that have the ability to directly neutralize reactive oxygen species and electron acceptance from reactive oxygen species. The abnormal production of ROS leads to OS (oxidative stress) which affects adversely multiple cellular components, that is, proteins, lipids, and DNA. Within the cell, specific antioxidants are specific for ROS species that prevents pathological levels of reactive oxygen species and repairs the cellular oxidative damage. Superoxide dismutase (SOD), catalase, peroxiredoxins (PRX), thioredoxin (TRX), glutathione peroxidase (GPX), and glutathione reductase (GRX) are included. Among all of these antioxidants, glutathione (a tripeptide) is mostly synthesized by the cell. Glutaredoxin and thioredoxin reduce the oxidized proteins and hydrogen peroxides while superoxides and catalases reduce O_2^- and H_2O_2. The other subcellular antioxidants present at increased generation of ROS, like mitochondria, raise the ROS scavenging efficiency.

5. Reactive Oxygen Species in Metabolism of Stem Cell

The process of catabolism and anabolism is termed cellular metabolism in which chemical carbon converts substrates for energy generation in the form of ATP. The reduction of cofactors is called catabolism and production of macromolecules precursors like lipids, nucleotides, and amino acids is known as anabolism. The cellular processes can shift the balance of catabolic and anabolic processes. The cellular processes may include growth and proliferation which mostly yield building blocks of deoxyribonucleic acids (DNA), proteins, and membranes through anabolism. Metabolic pathways can directly affect stem cells by remaining inactive, self-renew, or differentiate [18–20]. The changes in ROS levels can affect signaling pathways. The regulation of cell-cycle progression, apoptosis, and quiescence/differentiation can be altered through ROS by reacting with proteins like kinases and phosphatases/transcription factor [21–23]. The metabolic enzymes/proteins that direct the metabolic flux in nutrient-sensing pathways can be modified directly by ROS [24–26]. As a result, reactive oxygen species can be the signaling molecules that can play a role in both metabolism and stem cell. Significantly, cell membrane can be affected via different ROS-independent mechanisms. Mechanisms like epigenesis and functioning of metabolic enzymes can be changed [27–31]. Still, comparing the ROS effects, the discussions on metabolism and cell membrane methods are not considerably characterized in the stem cells.

6. Damaged DNA Response/DNA Signaling

Radiation-induced cell death may take place through direct/indirect transfer of energy to cellular structures that include plasma membrane, mitochondria, and chromatin. During replication stress or DSBs, proteins/enzymes like Ataxia Telangiectasia Mutated (ATM), Ataxia Telangiectasia/Rad3-related kinase (ATR), and CHK1 and CHK2 also get engaged. These mechanisms of cell-cycle arrest allow the enlistment of repair failure and irreversible damage of proapoptotic molecules [32]. The common observation for cancer stem cells resistance to radiation therapy is believed to occur due to their DNA damage repairing ability that is provoked by radiation/chemical drugs. This repairing of DNA damage can be by elevation of DNA repair mechanism directly or by cell-cycle progression indirectly. During DDR, in normal and malignant cells, one of the important DNA DSBs sensors is called MRN complex, that is, proteins like MRE11, RAD50, and NBS. MRN complex has a major role in binding and stabilization of broken DNA ends and also activates ATM. The functioning of MRN complex by BMI is interlinked with cancer stem cell molecules like Notch1, ALDH1A1, CD44, and Sonic Hedgehog, along with telomere biology, deregulation, tumor behavior, and prognosis of disease [33].

It has been observed that ATM kinase, the important signaling effector of DDR, plays a major role in DNA damage resistance of cancer stem cells. ATM contains an important sensor of DNA damage and kinase effector downstream that plays the major role in cell-cycle control regulation, DNA repair, senescence development, and apoptosis. It has been indicated that ATM also plays its role in maintenance and proliferation of normal stem cells. ATM plays two major roles: a role in the survival of stem cell and significantly in DDR part, in stem cell maintenance pathway [34, 35]. By considering the first role, ATM is concerned for the survival of neuronal stem cells (NSCs). According to the exact mechanism, although the expression of ATM in neuronal stem cells is abundant, during cell differentiation, it reduces gradually. This hypothesis indicates that for NSC functioning and survival ATM is very important [36]. For maintenance of normal self-renewal and proliferation of neuronal stem cells, ATM is involved by controlling redox status. NSCs become defective for proliferation with ATM loss through oxidative-stress-dependent p38 MAPK signaling, which suggests that p38 is the main key in the ATM/NSCs defective proliferation caused by oxidative stress [37, 38]. Furthermore, it has been depicted that ATM by its function in DDR plays the key role in human neural stem cell terminal differentiation [39]. Moreover, for maintenance of stem cell, ATM protein plays the major role in signaling pathways. Further, ITCH E3-ubiquitin ligases activity is regulated by ATM. ITCH belongs to the family of NEDD4, which is the protein family taking part in different signaling pathways like

TNFα, DNA damage response, Notch, and Sonic Hedgehog [40].

7. miRNAs CSC Resistance

MicroRNAs are a type of endogenous noncoding RNAs. Modifications during regulation of cancer stem cells against genotoxic insults include gene expression, which is regulated by microRNAs (miRNAs). Through the invention of miRNAs, many new ways have been opened in the world of science about gene expression regulation and functioning of various cells, like differentiation, apoptosis, therapy resistance, and proliferation [41]. For many years, it has been proved that cancer development is linked with these tiny genetic regulators. The miRNAs indicated huge information regarding history and tumors state differentiation and thus molecular link has been provided between cancer stem cells and normal stem cells. The expression of miRNAs might have adverse results for functioning of cancer cells for tumor radiation resistance. Yan and coworkers were the first to present the notion that DNA repair machinery could be targeted by miRNAs and thus tumor cells sensitized to radiation [42]. Now researchers proved that miRNAs can regulate tumor radiation resistance [43–46].

8. Radiotherapy

Radiation therapy is the most effective tool against treatment of cancer. High doses of radiation are used in radiation therapy to halt growth of tumor. Ionizing radiation (IR), like X-rays and gamma-rays, is commonly used for the treatment of cancer because it has the ability to pass through tissues and can break chemical bonds and help in the removal of electrons from atoms to get ionized. The ionized ions as a result damage cancer cells. Cancer cells are not killed immediately by ionizing radiation; in fact, substantial time is required for killing of cancer cells. Ionizing radiation can decrease the signs and symptoms induced by a growing tumor. To increase the effect of therapies, ionizing radiation is often given before, during, and even after the surgery. The exposure of ionizing radiation can be external and internal. External beam radiation like X-rays or γ-rays targets the particular part of the cancerous patient. Therapies of internal radiation have neutrons, electrons, protons, α or β particles, and carbon ions in which solid or liquid radiation is placed within the body. The use of ionizing radiation to kill cancer cells biologically depends on the kind of radiation being given, amount of dosage, rate of fractionation, and the organ to be targeted [47].

Although radiotherapy is one of the most effective treatments for cancer, still a large number of patients had radioresistance of their cancers. Ionizing radiation if given alone is found to be more effective against few cancers like non-small-cell lung cancer, cervical cancer, larynx cancer, skin cancer, head and neck cancer, prostate cancer, and lymphomas, but it is not found to be effective for the cancers like breast cancer, glioblastoma, advanced non-small-cell lung cancer, bladder cancer, and soft tissue carcinoma, maybe because of intrinsic radioresistance of cancer cells [48]. Ionizing radiation combined with other modes of treatment gives hope against radioresistant cancers. Ionizing radiation can cause DNA damage directly or indirectly. Basically, the radiation-induced bystander effect is the major part of ionizing radiation mediated damage which transfers the irradiated damage signals to unirradiated cells of cancer. Another hypothesis is that bystander effect also plays its role in imbalance of genome and carcinogenesis [49]. The most important constituents of IR-induced bystander effect are reactive oxygen species [50, 51]. This phenomenon also involves cytokines, activated macrophages, and nitric oxide (NO) [52].

Cellular senescence by permanently arresting the cells growth maintains a substantial tumor-suppressive effect and also damages the surrounding microenvironment. Among cellular senescence, the senescence-associated secretory phenotype (SASP) causes deleterious effects, promotes the proinflammatory responses, and results in progression of tumor [53]. Senescent cells activate the factors of senescence-associated secretory phenotype, that is, soluble signaling and proteases, to maintain potential effects. The major factors of SASP are interleukins, angiogenic factors, inflammatory cytokines, and growth and also have an impact on the neighboring cells. Senescent cells also release proteases like matrix metalloproteinases (MMPs) which contributes to remodeling of tissue [54]. Further, cells which undergo senescence enhance expression of fibronectin [55]. Different biological processes are maintained by fibronectin, that is, adhesion of cell, growth, migration, survival, and differentiation. Moreover, other than proteins, senescent cells can secrete molecules that can maintain tissue microenvironment. Collectively, all of the SASPs which are released by senescent cells have the ability to modify microenvironment by changing the receptors of cell-surface signal transduction. SASP can cause reinforcement of senescence in damaged cells. It has been suggested that IR-induced damage and premature senescence can be developed by the rise in secretory inflammatory signals [56]. Thus, IR-DNA damage activates secretory program. The activation of secretory program determines the radioresistance tumor response by affecting the microenvironment and interaction with other cells of tumor.

9. Overcoming Resistance Schemes to Ionizing Radiation

Radiation-induced programmed cell death is one of the major forms of death in tumors which are derived from lymphoid, hematopoietic, and germ cells. Still, epithelial solid tumors show wide resistance to apoptosis induced by ionizing radiation. Radioresistance is a serious concern, inducing failure of radiotherapy and consequent tumor relapse. Thus, new therapeutic radiosensitizers are desperately required to overcome tumor radioresistance and to improve radiotherapy outcome. Inhibitors which have the ability to target particular constituent of radioresistance pathways are developed for clinical purpose. Further, to compensate synthetic inhibitors limitations, natural radiosensitizers have been formulated. Various strategies have been proposed in the treatment of cancer to overcome resistance to ionizing radiation (Figure 2).

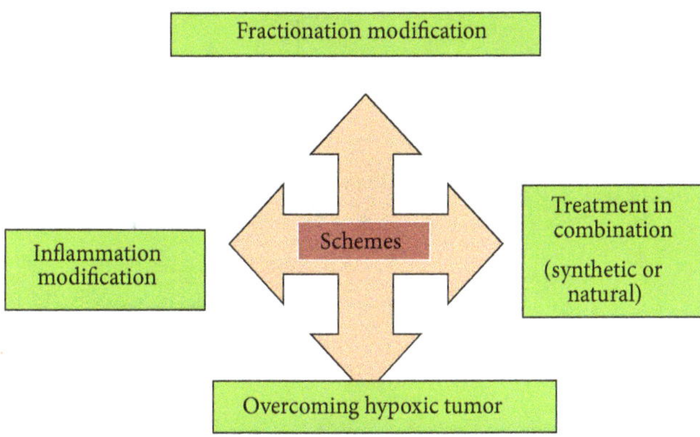

FIGURE 2: Schemes in treatment of cancer to overcome radioresistance. This includes fractionation modification, treatment in combination, inflammation modification, and overcoming hypoxic tumor.

10. Fractionation Modification

Radiation fractionated therapy for treatment of cancer has many advantages over single radiation administration as it raises the effect of anticancer therapy and decreases the chances of side effects occurrence in normal tissues. Formally, a total of 2.0 Gy per day, 10 Gy per week, with almost 60 Gy of radiation, is given for six weeks. Unluckily, this scheme cannot control locally elevated cancers sufficiently and because of efficacy limitation and side effects occurrence is not acceptable to patients. Hypofractionation, a novel strategy, has been advised to compensate fractionated radiation therapy limitations. At the beginning, clinical trials are to evaluate the administration per fraction of larger doses in fewer fractions of radiotherapy. Thus, next, hypofractionated radiation therapy will be largely in use compared with conventional strategy, as hypofractionation gives potent results; radiation beams are more focused to tumors. Hypofractionated radiation therapy has higher single dose of fraction but comparing with conventional radiation therapy total dose given is lower. The treatment of hypofractionation radiotherapy is expected to be beneficial in future use. Still researches are being made to investigate more ways of external beam radiation therapy which involves hyperfractionation and also hypofractionation. Hypofractionation treatment has shorter duration as compared with conventional treatment. Hypofractionated radiotherapy is very advantageous, especially for tumors growing rapidly.

11. Treatment in Combination

To defeat tumor radioresistance, researchers are much focused to develop tumor-specific radiosensitizers. For clinical practice, combined anticancer therapy is found to be more effective. For treating solid tumors, chemotherapy and radiotherapy in combination have more good results rather than treating with single therapy. The basic principle of this is that single agents of chemotherapy or radiotherapy have lower activity while combined agents show synergistic, anticancer effects.

12. Synthetic Targets

So, to target clinically developed DNA DSB repair pathways, many radiosensitizing agents have been formulated. Since the entire HR much correlate with radioresistance, searching ways to inhibit HR repair pathway might be beneficial in cancer cells. For inhibition of HR, many radiosensitizers have been discovered, for example, nucleoside and base analogs like gimeracil, gemcitabine, pentoxifylline, TAS-106, and caffeine [57]. Cox-2 inhibition, the most fundamental enzyme of inflammatory response, uses pharmacological inhibitors like celecoxib, SC-236, and coxibs, to act as radiosensitizers [58]. The HDAC inhibitor PCI-24781, the HSP90 inhibitor 17-allylamino-17-demethoxygeldanamycin, the tyrosine kinase inhibitors imatinib and erlotinib, and the proteasome inhibitor MG132 all target HR repair pathway to radiosensitize cancer cells [57]. Radiotherapy shows novel role as therapeutic partner of cancer immunotherapy. Ionizing radiation plays its role as immune adjuvant, leading to systemic antitumor immunity. IR activates various immunological proteins and transcription factors that regulate immune mediators expression that might elevate development of cancer. Therefore, targeting ionizing radiation-induced inflammatory signaling pathways improves radiotherapy by increasing radiosensitivity. During the treatment, radiotherapy and cisplatin in combination may redistribute calreticulin (a cisplatin-binding protein) by complementing the intrinsic inability of cisplatin drug and thus affect the cell death. The combined treatment of radiotherapy and poly(ADP-ribose), which is the polymerase inhibitor veliparib, through the elevation of tumor immunogenicity maintains its effect [59]. Many studies have proved that radiation therapy and immune stimulation in combination stimulate antitumor immunity, increasing cell death.

13. Natural Radiosensitizers

The synthetic inhibitors show limited improvement in treatment and also have more side effects. For these limitations, more and new radiosensitizers are needed to be developed. Radiosensitizers found naturally in foods are believed to be safer than synthetic compounds. Furthermore, natural products because of antioxidant and immune-enhancing effects have improved effects as biological and radiation protectors for normal cells. Few natural radiation sensitizers are curcumin, genistein, and quercetin. Their effect and action as radioprotector in cancer treatment are shown in Figures 3(a), 3(b), and 3(c).

14. Inflammation Modification

Recently, to enhance efficacy of radiation therapy, oncologists are paying attention to tumor stroma. Reducing tumor-associated macrophages increases IR antitumor effects; for example, VEGF-neutralizing antibodies in macrophages through IR-induced VEGF downregulation increase antitumor response to ionizing radiation [60]. Immune strategy along with local radiation maintains synergistic antitumor activity. As radiation therapy raises in situ vaccination, few

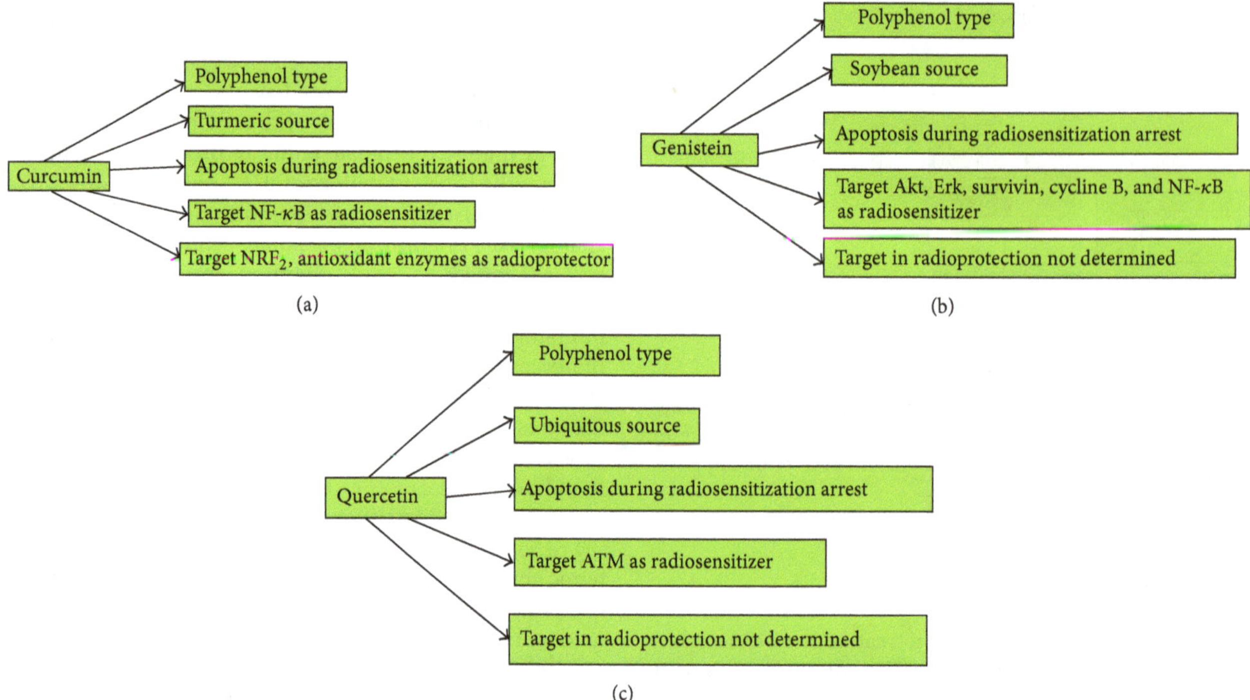

FIGURE 3: (a) Curcumin is a type of polyphenol. It has many anticancer activities. The source of curcumin is turmeric. It targets NF-κB as radiosensitizers. Curcumin has radioprotective effect and targets Nrf_2. (b) Genistein, a natural radiosensitizer, is a type of polyphenol. Genistein is a derivative of soybean. It has the ability to inhibit the growth of cancer cell through apoptosis. It can elevate the efficacy of radiation therapy by combining with ionizing radiation. Genistein suppresses Akt and Erk, reduces survivin and cyclin B expression in cervical cancer, and inhibits NF-κB. It acts as radioprotector but the target is not yet determined. (c) Quercetin is the main flavonoid component. It can behave as antioxidant, anti-inflammatory, and antiviral. Quercetin causes apoptosis and arrests the cell cycle. Quercetin by inhibiting ATM elevates radiosensitization. It has radioprotective effect against radiation therapy.

tries have tested radiation therapy and cancer vaccines in combination [61].

15. Overcoming Hypoxic Tumor

Tumor hypoxia is believed to be the major problem for radiotherapy as tumor cells of hypoxia are likely to survive ionizing radiation. Various strategies have been introduced against tumor hypoxia. Methods commonly used against tumor hypoxia-related resistance are radiation fractionation, high linear energy transfer (LET), and bioreductive drugs implementation.

16. Conclusions

Cancer is the leading cause of death in the world among different diseases. Radiation therapy is beneficial for those patients in whom surgery cannot be done by shrinking or damaging tumor. Tumor exposure to ionizing radiation activates changes, from biochemical changes to various forms of death. The number of doses and fractionation of ionizing radiation determine the level of cellular damage. Anticancer activity maintained by IR is through DNA lesions, like double strand breaks (DSBs), single strand breaks (SSBs), and DNA and base modifications. As radiation is effective for some tumors, other types of tumors are resistant to conventional radiotherapy like glioblastoma multiforme and pancreatic carcinoma, which creates difficulty in targeting. Radiosensitizers are urgently needed to elevate the radiotherapy effects and defeat tumor radioresistance. During treatment, chemotherapy and radiation therapy in combination were found to be successful for various types of tumors. Radiosensitization also targeted DNA damage response. Various trials made with drugs to destroy cancer cells have been found to be effective after radiation but radiosensitizers drugs have shown disappointing results. It has been concluded that novel ways and strategies are still needed to overcome radioresistance in cancer treatment.

Conflict of Interests

The authors declare that they have no conflict of interests.

Acknowledgments

The authors thank Professor Dr. M. H. Qazi, Director, Centre for Research in Molecular Medicine (CRiMM) and Institute of Molecular Biology and Biotechnology (IMBB), the University of Lahore, Pakistan, for the technical/financial support provided in writing and critical review of this paper.

The authors also wish to thank all the students of Lab-313-IMBB/CRiMM for their valuable questions, which made it possible to write this updated review.

References

[1] J. M. Reiman, K. L. Knutson, and D. C. Radisky, "Immune promotion of epithelial-mesenchymal transition and generation of breast cancer stem cells," *Cancer Research*, vol. 70, no. 8, pp. 3005–3008, 2010.

[2] P. Valent, D. Bonnet, R. De Maria et al., "Cancer stem cell definitions and terminology: the devil is in the details," *Nature Reviews Cancer*, vol. 12, no. 11, pp. 767–775, 2012.

[3] M. Krause, A. Yaromina, W. Eicheler, U. Koch, and M. Baumann, "Cancer stem cells: targets and potential biomarkers for radiotherapy," *Clinical Cancer Research*, vol. 17, no. 23, pp. 7224–7229, 2011.

[4] S. Bao, Q. Wu, R. E. McLendon et al., "Glioma stem cells promote radioresistance by preferential activation of the DNA damage response," *Nature*, vol. 444, no. 7120, pp. 756–760, 2006.

[5] M. S. Chen, W. A. Woodward, F. Behbod et al., "Wnt/β-catenin mediates radiation resistance of Sca1$^+$ progenitors in an immortalized mammary gland cell line," *Journal of Cell Science*, vol. 120, no. 3, pp. 468–477, 2007.

[6] W. A. Woodward, M. S. Chen, F. Behbod, M. P. Alfaro, T. A. Buchholz, and J. M. Rosen, "WNT/β-catenin mediates radiation resistance of mouse mammary progenitor cells," *Proceedings of the National Academy of Sciences of the United States of America*, vol. 104, no. 2, pp. 618–623, 2007.

[7] J. M. Harris, V. Esain, G. M. Frechette et al., "Glucose metabolism impacts the spatiotemporal onset and magnitude of HSC induction in vivo," *Blood*, vol. 121, no. 13, pp. 2483–2493, 2013.

[8] D. Hernández-García, C. D. Wood, S. Castro-Obregón, and L. Covarrubias, "Reactive oxygen species: a radical role in development?" *Free Radical Biology and Medicine*, vol. 49, no. 2, pp. 130–143, 2010.

[9] J. R. Hom, R. A. Quintanilla, D. L. Hoffman et al., "The permeability transition pore controls cardiac mitochondrial maturation and myocyte differentiation," *Developmental Cell*, vol. 21, no. 3, pp. 469–478, 2011.

[10] K. M. Holmström and T. Finkel, "Cellular mechanisms and physiological consequences of redox-dependent signalling," *Nature Reviews Molecular Cell Biology*, vol. 15, no. 6, pp. 411–421, 2014.

[11] R. Liang and S. Ghaffari, "Stem cells, redox signaling, and stem cell aging," *Antioxidants and Redox Signaling*, vol. 20, no. 12, pp. 1902–1916, 2014.

[12] A. P. Gomes, N. L. Price, A. J. Y. Ling et al., "Declining NAD$^+$ induces a pseudohypoxic state disrupting nuclear mitochondrial communication during aging," *Cell*, vol. 155, no. 7, pp. 1624–1638, 2013.

[13] L. Mouchiroud, R. H. Houtkooper, N. Moullan et al., "The NAD$^+$/sirtuin pathway modulates longevity through activation of mitochondrial UPR and FOXO signaling," *Cell*, vol. 154, no. 2, pp. 430–441, 2013.

[14] P. Rimmelé, C. L. Bigarella, R. Liang et al., "Aging-like phenotype and defective lineage specification in SIRT1-deleted hematopoietic stem and progenitor cells," *Stem Cell Reports*, vol. 3, no. 1, pp. 44–59, 2014.

[15] K. B. Beckman and B. N. Ames, "The free radical theory of aging matures," *Physiological Reviews*, vol. 78, no. 2, pp. 547–581, 1998.

[16] D. Harman, "Free radical theory of aging: dietary implications," *American Journal of Clinical Nutrition*, vol. 25, no. 8, pp. 839–843, 1972.

[17] W. Dröge, "Aging-related changes in the thiol/disulfide redox state: implications for the use of thiol antioxidants," *Experimental Gerontology*, vol. 37, no. 12, pp. 1333–1345, 2002.

[18] K. Takubo, G. Nagamatsu, C. I. Kobayashi et al., "Regulation of glycolysis by Pdk functions as a metabolic checkpoint for cell cycle quiescence in hematopoietic stem cells," *Cell Stem Cell*, vol. 12, no. 1, pp. 49–61, 2013.

[19] W.-M. Yu, X. Liu, J. Shen et al., "Metabolic regulation by the mitochondrial phosphatase PTPMT1 is required for hematopoietic stem cell differentiation," *Cell Stem Cell*, vol. 12, no. 1, pp. 62–74, 2013.

[20] J. Zhang, I. Khvorostov, J. S. Hong et al., "UCP2 regulates energy metabolism and differentiation potential of human pluripotent stem cells," *The EMBO Journal*, vol. 30, no. 24, pp. 4860–4873, 2011.

[21] T. B. Dansen, L. M. M. Smits, M. H. van Triest et al., "Redox-sensitive cysteines bridge p300/CBP-mediated acetylation and FoxO4 activity," *Nature Chemical Biology*, vol. 5, no. 9, pp. 664–672, 2009.

[22] Z. Guo, S. Kozlov, M. F. Lavin, M. D. Person, and T. T. Paull, "ATM activation by oxidative stress," *Science*, vol. 330, no. 6003, pp. 517–521, 2010.

[23] C. S. Velu, S. K. Niture, C. E. Doneanu, N. Pattabiraman, and K. S. Srivenugopal, "Human p53 is inhibited by glutathionylation of cysteines present in the proximal DNA-Binding domain during oxidative stress," *Biochemistry*, vol. 46, no. 26, pp. 7765–7780, 2007.

[24] D. Anastasiou, G. Poulogiannis, J. M. Asara et al., "Inhibition of pyruvate kinase M2 by reactive oxygen species contributes to cellular antioxidant responses," *Science*, vol. 334, no. 6060, pp. 1278–1283, 2011.

[25] J. K. Brunelle, E. L. Bell, N. M. Quesada et al., "Pxygen sensing requires mitochondrial ROS but not oxidative phosphorylation," *Cell Metabolism*, vol. 1, no. 6, pp. 409–414, 2005.

[26] D. D. Sarbassov and D. M. Sabatini, "Redox regulation of the nutrient-sensitive raptor-mTOR pathway and complex," *The Journal of Biological Chemistry*, vol. 280, no. 47, pp. 39505–39509, 2005.

[27] K. De Bock, M. Georgiadou, S. Schoors et al., "Role of PFKFB3-driven glycolysis in vessel sprouting," *Cell*, vol. 154, no. 3, pp. 651–663, 2013.

[28] P. Gut and E. Verdin, "The nexus of chromatin regulation and intermediary metabolism," *Nature*, vol. 502, no. 7472, pp. 489–498, 2013.

[29] C. R. Lew and D. R. Tolan, "Aldolase sequesters WASP and affects WASP/Arp2/3-stimulated actin dynamics," *Journal of Cellular Biochemistry*, vol. 114, no. 8, pp. 1928–1939, 2013.

[30] G. Sutendra, A. Kinnaird, P. Dromparis et al., "A nuclear pyruvate dehydrogenase complex is important for the generation of acetyl-CoA and histone acetylation," *Cell*, vol. 158, no. 1, pp. 84–97, 2014.

[31] W. Yang, Y. Xia, H. Ji et al., "Nuclear PKM2 regulates β-catenin transactivation upon EGFR activation," *Nature*, vol. 480, no. 7375, pp. 118–122, 2011.

[32] Y. Dai and S. Grant, "New insights into checkpoint kinase 1 in the DNA damage response signaling network," *Clinical Cancer Research*, vol. 16, no. 2, pp. 376–383, 2010.

[33] Anuranjani and M. Bala, "Concerted action of Nrf2-ARE pathway, MRN complex, HMGB1 and inflammatory cytokines—implication in modification of radiation damage," *Redox Biology*, vol. 2, no. 1, pp. 832–846, 2014.

[34] V. Stagni, V. Oropallo, G. Fianco, M. Antonelli, I. Cinà, and D. Barilà, "Tug of war between survival and death: exploring ATM function in cancer," *International Journal of Molecular Sciences*, vol. 15, no. 4, pp. 5388–5409, 2014.

[35] V. Stagni, S. Santini, and D. Barilà, "ITCH E3 ligase in ATM network," *Oncoscience*, vol. 1, pp. 394–395, 2014.

[36] D. M. Allen, H. van Praag, J. Ray et al., "Ataxia telangiectasia mutated is essential during adult neurogenesis," *Genes and Development*, vol. 15, no. 5, pp. 554–566, 2001.

[37] J. Kim and P. K. Y. Wong, "Loss of ATM impairs proliferation of neural stem cells through oxidative stress-mediated p38 MAPK signaling," *STEM CELLS*, vol. 27, no. 8, pp. 1987–1998, 2009.

[38] J. Kim, J. Hwangbo, and P. K. Y. Wong, "P38 mapk-mediated bmi-1 down-regulation and defective proliferation in atm-deficient neural stem cells can be restored by akt activation," *PLoS ONE*, vol. 6, no. 1, Article ID e16615, 2011.

[39] L. Carlessi, L. De Filippis, D. Lecis, A. Vescovi, and D. Delia, "DNA-damage response, survival and differentiation in vitro of a human neural stem cell line in relation to ATM expression," *Cell Death and Differentiation*, vol. 16, no. 6, pp. 795–806, 2009.

[40] F. Bernassola, M. Karin, A. Ciechanover, and G. Melino, "The HECT family of E3 ubiquitin ligases: multiple players in cancer development," *Cancer Cell*, vol. 14, no. 1, pp. 10–21, 2008.

[41] E. van Schooneveld, H. Wildiers, I. Vergote, P. B. Vermeulen, L. Y. Dirix, and S. J. Van Laere, "Dysregulation of micro RNAs in breasts cancer and their potential role as prognostic and predictive biomarkers in patient management," *Breast Cancer Research*, vol. 17, article 21, 2015.

[42] D. Yan, W. L. Ng, X. Zhang et al., "Targeting DNA-PKcs and ATM with miR-101 sensitizes tumors to radiation," *PLoS ONE*, vol. 5, no. 7, Article ID e11397, 2010.

[43] C. Qu, Z. Liang, J. Huang et al., "MiR-205 determines the radioresistance of human nasopharyngeal carcinoma by directly targeting PTEN," *Cell Cycle*, vol. 11, no. 4, pp. 785–796, 2012.

[44] S. Grosso, J. Doyen, S. K. Parks et al., "MiR-210 promotes a hypoxic phenotype and increases radioresistance in human lung cancer cell lines," *Cell Death & Disease*, vol. 4, no. 3, article e544, 2013.

[45] M. Svoboda, J. Sana, P. Fabian et al., "MicroRNA expression profile associated with response to neoadjuvant chemoradiotherapy in locally advanced rectal cancer patients," *Radiation Oncology*, vol. 7, article 195, 2012.

[46] M. Mognato and L. Celotti, "MicroRNAs used in combination with anti-cancer treatments can enhance therapy efficacy," *Mini-Reviews in Medicinal Chemistry*, vol. 15, no. 13, pp. 1052–1062, 2015.

[47] E. J. Hall, "Cancer caused by x-rays—a random event?" *The Lancet Oncology*, vol. 8, no. 5, pp. 369–370, 2007.

[48] A. C. Begg, F. A. Stewart, and C. Vens, "Strategies to improve radiotherapy with targeted drugs," *Nature Reviews Cancer*, vol. 11, no. 4, pp. 239–253, 2011.

[49] R. Baskar, "Emerging role of radiation induced bystander effects: cell communications and carcinogenesis," *Genome Integrity*, vol. 1, article 13, 2010.

[50] B. J. Blyth and P. J. Sykes, "Radiation-induced bystander effects: what are they, and how relevant are they to human radiation exposures?" *Radiation Research*, vol. 176, no. 2, pp. 139–157, 2011.

[51] R.-A. M. Panganiban, A. L. Snow, and R. M. Day, "Mechanisms of radiation toxicity in transformed and non-transformed cells," *International Journal of Molecular Sciences*, vol. 14, no. 8, pp. 15931–15958, 2013.

[52] M. Najafi, R. Fardid, G. Hadadi, and M. Fardid, "The mechanisms of radiation-induced bystander effect," *Journal of Biomedical Physics and Engineering*, vol. 4, no. 4, pp. 163–172, 2014.

[53] J.-P. Coppe, P.-Y. Desprez, A. Krtolica, and J. Campisi, "The senescence-associated secretory phenotype: the dark side of tumor suppression," *Annual Review of Pathology: Mechanisms of Disease*, vol. 5, pp. 99–118, 2010.

[54] A. R. Davalos, J.-P. Coppe, J. Campisi, and P.-Y. Desprez, "Senescent cells as a source of inflammatory factors for tumor progression," *Cancer and Metastasis Reviews*, vol. 29, no. 2, pp. 273–283, 2010.

[55] T. Kumazaki, R. S. Robetorye, S. C. Robetorye, and J. R. Smith, "Fibronectin expression increases during in vitro cellular senescence: correlation with increased cell area," *Experimental Cell Research*, vol. 195, no. 1, pp. 13–19, 1991.

[56] R. J. Sabin and R. M. Anderson, "Cellular Senescence-its role in cancer and the response to ionizing radiation," *Genome Integrity*, vol. 2, article 7, 2011.

[57] E. Mladenov, S. Magin, A. Soni, and G. Iliakis, "DNA double-strand break repair as determinant of cellular radiosensitivity to killing and target in radiation therapy," *Frontiers in Oncology*, vol. 3, article 113, 2013.

[58] F. M. Di Maggio, L. Minafra, G. I. Forte et al., "Portrait of inflammatory response to ionizing radiation treatment," *Journal of Inflammation*, vol. 12, article 14, 2015.

[59] Y. Meng, E. V. Efimova, K. W. Hamzeh et al., "Radiation-inducible immunotherapy for cancer: senescent tumor cells as a cancer vaccine," *Molecular Therapy*, vol. 20, no. 5, pp. 1046–1055, 2012.

[60] Y. R. Meng, M. A. Beckett, H. Liang et al., "Blockade of tumor necrosis factor α signaling in tumor-associated macrophages as a radiosensitizing strategy," *Cancer Research*, vol. 70, no. 4, pp. 1534–1543, 2010.

[61] S. C. Formenti and S. Demaria, "Combining radiotherapy and cancer immunotherapy: a paradigm shift," *Journal of the National Cancer Institute*, vol. 105, no. 4, pp. 256–265, 2013.

13

Hepatoma-Targeted Radionuclide Immune Albumin Nanospheres: ^{131}I-antiAFPMcAb-GCV-BSA-NPs

Mei Lin,[1,2] Junxing Huang,[1] Dongsheng Zhang,[2,3] Xingmao Jiang,[4] Jia Zhang,[2] Hong Yu,[1] Yanhong Xiao,[1] Yujuan Shi,[1] and Ting Guo[1]

[1]*Clinical Medical Institute, Taizhou People's Hospital Affiliated to Nantong University, Taizhou, Jiangsu 225300, China*
[2]*Medical School, Southeast University, Nanjing, Jiangsu 210009, China*
[3]*Jiangsu Key Laboratory for Biomaterials and Devices, Nanjing, Jiangsu 210009, China*
[4]*Key Laboratory of Advanced Catalytic Material and Technology, Changzhou University, Changzhou, Jiangsu 213000, China*

Correspondence should be addressed to Mei Lin; l_mei@163.com and Dongsheng Zhang; zdszds1222@163.com

Academic Editor: Francesco Marampon

An effective strategy has been developed for synthesis of radionuclide immune albumin nanospheres (^{131}I-antiAFPMcAb-GCV-BSA-NPs). *In vitro* as well as *in vivo* targeting of ^{131}I-antiAFPMcAb-GCV-BSA-NPs to AFP-positive hepatoma was examined. In cultured HepG2 cells, the uptake and retention rates of ^{131}I-antiAFPMcAb-GCV-BSA-NPs were remarkably higher than those of ^{131}I alone. As well, the uptake rate and retention ratios of ^{131}I-antiAFPMcAb-GCV-BSA-NPs in AFP-positive HepG2 cells were also significantly higher than those in AFP-negative HEK293 cells. Compared to ^{131}I alone, ^{131}I-antiAFPMcAb-GCV-BSA-NPs were much more easily taken in and retained by hepatoma tissue, with a much higher T/NT. Due to good drug-loading, high encapsulation ratio, and highly selective affinity for AFP-positive tumors, the ^{131}I-antiAFPMcAb-GCV-BSA-NPs are promising for further effective radiation-gene therapy of hepatoma.

1. Introduction

Undoubtedly, an ideal cancer treatment must meet two aspects: good therapeutic effect and no or little side effect [1, 2]. However, most current therapies, such as radiation and chemotherapy, destroy normal tissue and cause serious side effects while killing tumor cells. Traditional administration by intravenous injection ensures that drugs are uniformly distributed in the system. Generally, once administered, a drug undergoes many steps where loss can occur, including combination with plasma proteins, metabolism, and decomposition, before it gets to the tumor site. Only a small proportion of drugs finally reaches the tumor due to lack of specific affinity for tumor tissues or cells. This not only greatly decreases the therapeutic effect, but also increases the nonspecific side effect on normal tissue [3]. Traditional external radiation is currently well accepted as one of the most effective remedies for cancer, but it may inflict severe damage on normal tissue. Compared to external radiation, internal nuclide radiation provides prolonged low dose rate exposure and shows some advantages, but only a small minority of cancers can actively absorb nuclides unassisted. For example, thyroid carcinoma can take in ^{131}I by itself, but most tumors are nonselective to this treatment. In recent years, suicide gene therapy has been explored for cancer treatment. Among suicide genes, herpes simplex virus type thymidine kinase (HSV-TK) is most commonly used. It can express thymidine kinase to convert nontoxic prodrug ganciclovir (GCV) into toxic GCV-TP to kill tumor cells by blocking DNA synthesis. Studies have shown that better curative effects can be obtained when the anticancer effects of the HSV-TK/GCV system are combined with radiotherapy [4]. In our previous study, we succeeded in constructing recombinant plasmids of pEgr1-HSV-TK and transferring them into hepatoma cells. Upon irradiation, radiation promoter Egr1 could induce HSV-TK gene to express efficiently and the encoded products could convert GCV into a tumor killing drug [4, 5]. However, the ultimate goal to kill the cancer without damage to normal tissue cannot be achieved unless the radiation is localized to the tumor site and suicide genes only express effectively in tumor cells not in normal cells or the prodrugs are delivered selectively to the tumor. Therefore, it is important to develop drugs or nuclides into tumor-targeted agents to improve curative effect and minimize side effect.

Monoclonal antibody (McAb) is a very powerful cancer-targeted tool and has been widely used in targeting treatment [6–9]. Owing to its high specificity, strong affinity for the corresponding tumor, and little injury to normal cells, great progress in cancer-targeted therapy has been made. Studies have shown that monoclonal antibodies can specifically target tumor cells with the corresponding antigen and can carry therapeutic agents such as nuclides or drugs to tumor site to kill the tumor [10, 11]. McAb has become a preferred choice for a guiding drug vector because of its unique superiority, but the lethality of drugs carried by a single monoclonal antibody molecule is poor.

Nanoparticle drug delivery system using nanospheres as delivery vectors can accommodate much more antitumor drug molecule and increase the drug-loading significantly. In particular, bovine serum albumin (BSA) nanospheres, which use BSA as vectors to encapsulate drugs, show very good qualities for a delivery vector including good stability, high drug-loading, and slow release. BSA nanospheres bearing paclitaxel, adriamycin, or nuclides (^{125}I and ^{188}R) showed a much improved antitumor effect [12–15]. As a result of good targeting, drug-loaded nanospheres cross-linked with monoclonal antibodies have a greater ability to kill target cells specifically [16, 17]. Drug-loaded immune nanospheres have been used to label or separate cells and diagnose or treat disease because of the antibody adsorbed on the particles which results in nanospheres' immunocompetence [18]. For example, if combined with fluorescent protein, drug-loaded immune nanospheres can be used for detection and diagnosis.

At present, nanosized BSA targeting agents mediated by McAb and radioimmune therapy are active areas in tumor-targeted therapy. Advances in protein cross-linking technology have paved the way for construction of radioactive targeting immune nanospheres by applying drug-loaded BSA nanospheres to radiation immunotherapy. As a type of specific tumor antigen in the membrane and cytoplasm of cells, α-fetoprotein (AFP) is positive in over 70% of primary hepatic carcinomas, but negative in normal liver or other normal tissues [19, 20]. Consequently, it is a good potential antigen for hepatic cancer treatment. Owing to its high specificity and affinity for AFP antigen in hepatic cancer cells, anti-AFP monoclonal antibody (antiAFPMcAb) can carry various "warheads" such as chemotherapy agents, radionuclides, or toxins to selectively attack AFP-positive cancer cells [21–23].

Based on the above, it can be conceived that if drug-loaded nanospheres are combined with ^{131}I-labeled antiAFPMcAb, they could play a dual role of targeted radiotherapy and drug therapy on hepatoma. The drugs delivered in the nanospheres can be released slowly, which is crucial for improvement of the curative effect and reduction of side effect. If the drug is a prodrug such as GCV, in addition to the targeted radiation therapy, ^{131}I can activate the promoter Egrl to induce HSV-TK expression, converting GCV into a toxic drug for targeted radiation-gene therapy.

In the present study, ^{131}I-antiAFPMcAb-GCV-BSA nanospheres targeted to AFP-positive tumors were constructed and their characteristics and hepatoma-targeting *in vitro* and *in vivo* were investigated, with the aim of providing theoretical and experimental insights for further high-efficiency radiation-gene therapy of hepatoma.

2. Material and Methods

2.1. Main Material. DMEM, 0.25% trypsase/0.038% EDTA, and fetal bovine serum were purchased from Gibco; BSA, GCV, and SPDP (N-succinimidyl-3-(2-pyridyldithiol) propionate) were purchased from Sigma; ^{131}I was purchased from Nanjing Senke Company; chloramine-T and glutaraldehyde were purchased from Jiaxing Chenlong Chemical Co. Ltd.; antiAFPMcAb was purchased from Shanghai Yemin Biotechnology Company; HepG2 cells (AFP-positive) and HEK293 cells (AFP-negative) were purchased from the Institute of Biochemistry and Cell Biology, Shanghai Institute of Biological Sciences, Chinese Academy of Sciences, China.

2.2. Preparation and Characterization of GCV-BSA-NPs. GCV-BSA-NPs were prepared by the desolvation method [24] as follows: (1) GCV solution with a concentration of 10 mg/mL was prepared; (2) 200 mg BSA was dissolved in 23 mL twice-distilled H_2O; (3) 2 mL of (1) was added to (2) and the mixture was stirred magnetically. NaOH was used to adjust the pH of the solution to 9; (4) while being stirred magnetically, 100 mL EtOH was added slowly (1 mL/min) to (3), and the stirring was continued for additional 5 min; (5) 50 μL of 25% glutaraldehyde was added to (4), and then the mixture was stirred magnetically for 24 h; (6) the solution was centrifuged, and the precipitate was washed three times with distilled water.

The morphology of GCV-BSA-NPs was checked by a transmission electron microscope (TEM) (JEM-200CX, Japan).

2.3. GCV Standard Curve. 200 μg/mL of GCV stock solution was used to prepare standard solutions with GCV concentrations of 10, 20, 30, 40, 50, and 60 μg/mL. Using distilled water as a blank, the optical density (OD) values of each GCV standard solution were measured at a wavelength of 252 nm using a microplate reader (Multiskan MK3-353, USA). A standard curve was drawn, using the OD values as an ordinate and concentrations as abscissa, and a linear regression equation was established based on the data.

2.4. Drug-Loading (DL) and Encapsulation Ratio (ER) of GCV-BSA-NPs. 10 mg GCV-BSA-NPs were transferred to a 50 mL volumetric flask with 0.5% pepsin solution, and the mixture was digested and dissolved in water bath at 37°C for 2 h. After being cooled to room temperature, distilled water was added to 50 mL, and then the solution was filtered, and the OD was measured at 252 nm, GCV content was calculated according to the above standard curve, and DL and ER were calculated according to the following formulas:

Drug-loading efficiency = (GCV mass of the nanospheres/the total mass of the nanospheres) × 100%.

Encapsulation ratio = (GCV mass of the nanospheres/the total mass of GCV) × 100%.

2.5. Preparation and Purification ^{131}I-antiAFPMcAb. ^{131}I-antiAFPMcAb was prepared by chloramine-T method [25, 26] and purified on a gel chromatographic column. Trichloroacetic acid was used to precipitate the protein to test the labeling rate, radioactive concentration, and radioactive activity. The radiochemical purity was assessed by testing the chromatography paper.

2.6. Preparation, Purification, and Characterization of ^{131}I-antiAFPMcAb-GCV-BSA-NPs. ^{131}I-antiAFPMcAb-GCV-BSA-NPs were prepared by the following chemical cross-linking. (1) ^{131}I-antiAFP-McAb was modified by SPDP: 1 mL of purified ^{131}I-antiAFP-McAb was dialyzed for 12 h and then its volume was adjusted to 4 mL with PBS. While being mixed magnetically, 13.7 μL of SPDP solution in EtOH (20 mmol/L) was added to the mixture. After reaction for 30 min at room temperature, the reactant was transferred into a dialysis bag and dialyzed with acetate buffer (0.01 mmol/L, pH 4.5) to remove excess SPDP. Then it was enriched with PEG6000 to 4 mL and some DTT was added to make its concentration reach 50 mmol/L. Finally, the ^{131}I-antiAFPMcAb-SH was obtained after this reaction mixture was dialyzed using PBS as dialyzate to remove redundant DTT; (2) 1 mg of GCV-BSA-NPs was dispersed in 3.0 mL acetic acid salt solution (pH 4.5) and then added to 50 μL SPDP solution in EtOH (20 mmol/L). After being stirred for 30 min at room temperature, the reactant was centrifuged for three times for 1 min at 12,000 rpm and then washed with Hank's solution to remove redundant SPDP. Then the activatory albumin nanospheres (GCV-BSA-PDP-NPs) were obtained; (3) after (2) and (1) were mixed immediately and reacted for 15 h at 4°C with slow stirring, the crude ^{131}I-antiAFPMcAb-GCV-BSA-NPs were obtained.

After the ^{131}I-antiAFPMcAb-GCV-BSA-NPs were separated and purified, their labeling rate was measured by the same protocol with ^{131}I-antiAFPMcAb. Their radiochemical purity was tested by paper chromatography at 0, 1, 6, 12, and 24 h in air at room temperature and at 1, 6, 12, and 24 h in serum incubated at 37°C.

A transmission electron microscope (TEM, JEM-200CX, Japan) was used to observe the morphology of ^{131}I-antiAFPMcAb-GCV-BSA-NPs. The size distribution and average size of the particles were examined by a laser particle size analyzer (Malvern HPPS5001, England).

2.7. Cellular Uptake Experiment In Vitro. HepG2 cells and HEK293 cells in the logarithmic phase were digested with 0.25% trypsin and diluted into single cells (5 × 10^5 cells/mL) with the fresh complete culture medium and then seeded in 24-well plates (1 mL/well). The ^{131}I-antiAFPMcAb-GCV-BSA-NPs and ^{131}I absorbed by HepG2 cells were grouped as (1) and (2); groups (3) and (4) were labeled as ^{131}I-antiAFPMcAb-GCV-BSA-NPs and ^{131}I absorbed by HEK293 cells, respectively. Three replicates were done in every group. The above cells were incubated in air containing 5% CO_2 at 37°C. When the cells were attached well, the original culture medium in each well was replaced with 1 mL of fresh complete culture medium. 20 μCi of ^{131}I-antiAFPMcAb-GCV-BSA-NPs was added to each well of groups (1) and (3), and 20 μCi of ^{131}I was added to each well of groups (2) and (4). The plates continued to be incubated and the cell uptake rate of every group was tested at 0.5 h, 1 h, 2 h, 3 h, and 4 h. The culture medium in every well was taken out and the cells were washed three times with PBS. The culture medium and PBS used for washing were admixed and the radioactive counts of the mixture (C1) were measured by a γ counter. After the adherent cells in each well were lysed by lysis buffer (0.5 M NaOH + 1% SDS) and removed, each well was washed with PBS three times. Then the lysate and the corresponding PBS used for wash were mixed together and the radioactive counts of the mixture (C2) were measured by a γ counter. Cellular uptake rate was calculated using the following formula: cellular uptake rate = [C2/(C1 + C2)] × 100%. Radioactive uptake curves of ^{131}I-antiAFPMcAb-GCV-BSA-NPs and ^{131}I absorbed in HepG2 cells and in HEK293 cells at different time were drawn. This experiment was repeated three times.

2.8. Cell Retention Experiment In Vitro. Experiment grouping and the first half procedure were the same as those for cellular uptake experiment. Number of cells in each well in the cell retention experiment was 5 × 10^5 and three replicates were done in every group. ^{131}I-antiAFPMcAb-GCV-BSA-NPs and ^{131}I were added into the corresponding wells. After incubation for 2 h, the culture medium of every well was removed and each well was washed three times with PBS. Then the same volume of fresh culture medium was added into each well and the plates continued to be incubated. The culture medium and cells in each well were collected together at 0.5 h, 1 h, 2 h, 4 h, and 6 h, and the total radioactive counts of every group were determined. After centrifugation for 10 min at 1000 rpm, the supernatant was removed and radioactive counts in cells from each well were measured. Radioactive retention rate was calculated by the following formula: retention rate (%) = ((radioactive counts in cells)/(radioactive counts in cells + radioactive counts in culture medium)) × 100%. The radioactive retention curves for ^{131}I-antiAFPMcAb-GCV-BSA-NPs and ^{131}I retained in HepG2 cells and HEK293 cells at different times were drawn, using time as the abscissa and retention rate as the ordinate. This experiment was performed three times.

2.9. Nude Mice Model of Transplanted Hepatocarcinoma. Female 6-week-old BALB/c nude mice with body weight of 20–22 grams, purchased from the Institute of Biochemistry and Cell Biology, Shanghai Institute of Biological Sciences, Chinese Academy of Sciences, China, were used for the experiments. All experiments were approved by the Animal Care Committee of Jiangsu Province and were performed in accordance with the institutional guidelines. All the mice

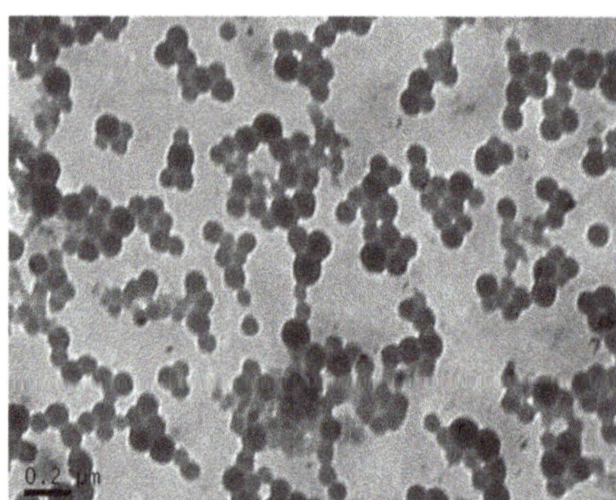

FIGURE 1: TEM image of GCV-BSA-NPs. GCV-BSA-NPs were nearly spherical, about 100–130 nm in diameter.

were maintained in the sterile barrier system of Medical School, Southeast University, China. Exponentially growing HepG2 cells (2×10^6 cells) were injected subcutaneously around the right posterior limb rump of the nude mice. All the mice were maintained in a sterile barrier system. After tumor diameters reached about 0.5 cm, the nude mice were used for the following experiments.

2.10. Radioactive Distribution Assay In Vivo. Twenty-four nude mice with tumors were randomly divided into two groups of twelve mice each: (1) ^{131}I-antiAFPMcAb-GCV-BSA-NPs group and (2) ^{131}I group. ^{131}I-antiAFPMcAb-GCV-BSA-NPs and ^{131}I (7.4 MBq/mouse) were injected into the tail vein of mice of group 1 and group 2. At 1 h, 8 h, 24 h, and 48 h after the injection, three mice were picked out randomly from group 1, and their blood was obtained by eyeball extraction. The same was done in group 2. All the mice were killed and their livers, spleens, kidneys, hearts, lungs, stomachs, intestines, muscles, bones, brains, and tumors were taken out to weigh and measure their radioactivity. Meanwhile, the radiocounts of the standard source were tested. The radioactive intake per gram of every organ (% ID/g) was calculated according to the following formula: ID/g = (tissue radiocounting (cpm)/tissue weight (g)/standard source radiocounting (cpm)) × 100%. T/NT (radioactivity ratio of tumor versus nontumor) was calculated with the following formula: T/NT = ID/g of tumor tissue/ID/g of nontumor tissue.

2.11. Statistical Analysis. Experimental values are reported as mean ± SD. The data were analyzed with the SPSS 16.0 program. A p value of <0.05 was considered significant.

3. Results

3.1. Characteristics of ^{131}I-antiAFPMcAb-GCV-BSA-NPs. As shown in Figure 1, GCV-BSA-NPs were nearly spherical, about 100–130 nm in diameter and uniform in size. The effective drug-loading rate of GCV-BSA-NPs was 22.70%, and the GCV embedding rate was 70.63%.

As a rule, when radionuclide is employed in clinical treatment or *in vivo* analysis, its radiochemical purity is required to be more than 90% [27, 28]. In this study, chloramine-T was used to prepare ^{131}I-antiAFPMcAb. The labeling yield was (72.97 ± 1.28)% and the radiochemical purity was (99.63 ± 0.11)%. ^{131}I-antiAFPMcAb-GCV-BSA-NPs were obtained by connecting ^{131}I-antiAFPMcAb to GCV-BSA-NPs by SPDP. The labeling yield of ^{131}I-antiAFPMcAb-GCV-BSA-NPs was (61.5 ± 1.92)%. The radiochemical purity in air at room temperature for 0 h, 1 h, 6 h, 12 h, and 24 h was (96.05 ± 1.92)%, (94.87 ± 1.41)%, (93.60 ± 1.06)%, (91.71 ± 0.85)%, and (90.44 ± 0.28)%, respectively. The radiochemical purity in serum at 37°C for 1 h, 6 h, 12 h, and 24 h was (92.61 ± 1.63)%, (91.04 ± 0.92)%, (90.71 ± 0.56)%, and (90.11 ± 0.10)%, respectively. All were >90%, which met the requirement for the further radionuclide research *in vivo*.

The shape, the size, and diameter distribution of ^{131}I-antiAFPMcAb-GCV-BSA-NPs were detected by TEM and laser particle size analyzer. As shown in Figure 2(a) (TEM

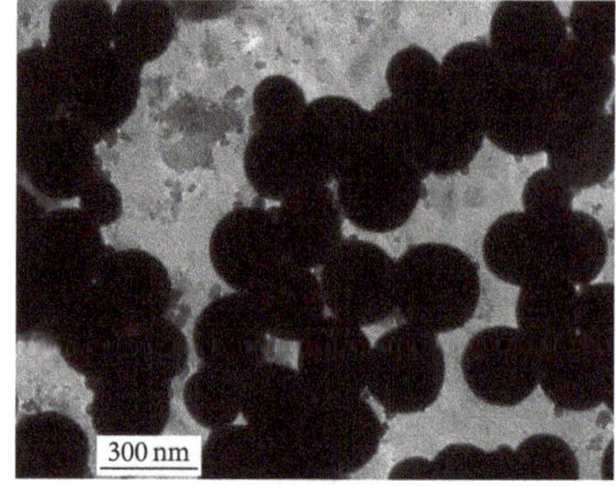

(a)

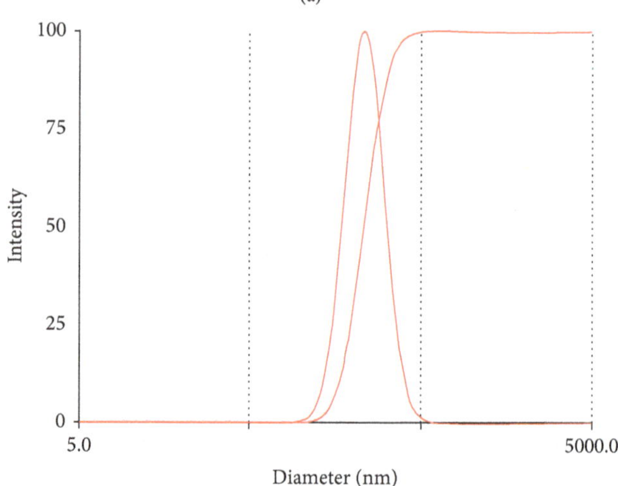

Effective diameter: 233.9 nm
Polydispersity: 0.059

(b)

FIGURE 2: Size and distribution of ^{131}I-antiAFPMcAb-GCV-BSA-NPs. (a) TEM image of ^{131}I-antiAFPMcAb-GCV-BSA-NPs. The particles were approximately spherical and their diameters were about 220–280 nm. (b) Diameter and particle distribution of ^{131}I-antiAFPMcAb-GCV-BSA-NPs examined by laser particle size analyzer. The average diameter was 233.9 nm. The polydispersity index (PDI) of the particles was 0.059.

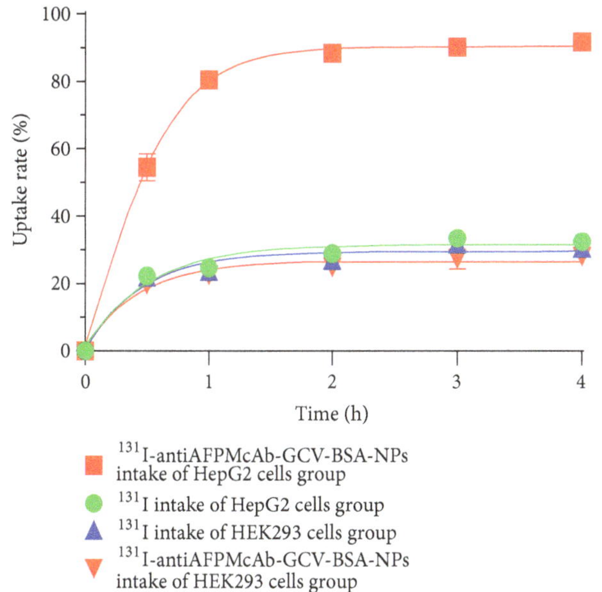

FIGURE 3: Uptake curves of ^{131}I and ^{131}I-antiAFP-GCV-BSA-NPs in HepG2 cells and HEK293 cells. The intake ratios of ^{131}I-antiAFPMcAb-GCV-BSA-NPs in HepG2 cells group are far higher than those of ^{131}I in HepG2 cells group, ^{131}I-antiAFPMcAb-GCV-BSA-NPs in HEK293 cells group, and ^{131}I in HEK293 cells group.

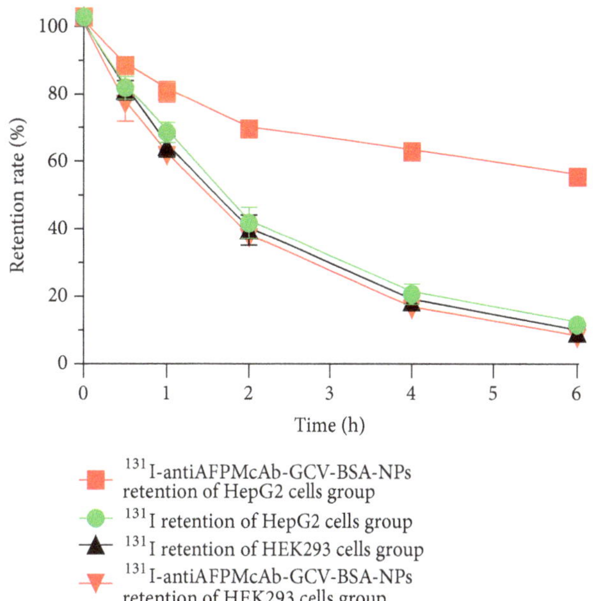

FIGURE 4: Retention curves of ^{131}I and ^{131}I-antiAFP-GCV-BSA-NPs in HepG2 cells and HEK293 cells. The radioactive retention rates of ^{131}I-antiAFPMcAb-GCV-BSA-NPs in HepG2 cells group are obviously higher than those of other three groups at the same time point.

image), ^{131}I-antiAFPMcAb-GCV-BSA-NPs were approximately spherical and their diameters were about 220–280 nm. The average size of ^{131}I-antiAFPMcAb-GCV-BSA-NPs examined by laser particle size analyzer was 233.9 nm, and the polydispersity index (PDI) of the particles was 0.059, indicating being largely uniform in size (Figure 2(b)).

3.2. Cellular Uptake and Retention In Vitro. To detect the targeting of ^{131}I-antiAFPMcAb-GCV-BSA-NPs to hepatoma, we compared the uptake and the retention of ^{131}I-anti-AFPMcAb-GCV-BSA-NPs in AFP-positive HepG2 cells with those in AFP-negative HEK293 cells *in vitro*. As controls, the uptake and the retention of ^{131}I in AFP-positive HepG2 cells and in AFP-negative HEK293 cells were also tested *in vitro*.

The cellular uptake test showed that the intake of ^{131}I-antiAFPMcAb-GCV-BSA-NPs in HepG2 cells gradually increased, reaching (91.7 ± 1.9)% at 4 h, while the intake of ^{131}I at 4 h was only (32.4 ± 2.1)%, far less than that of ^{131}I-antiAFPMcAb-GCV-BSA-NPs at the corresponding time point. The intakes of ^{131}I-antiAFPMcAb-GCV-BSA-NPs and ^{131}I in HEK293 cells were both much less than that of ^{131}I-antiAFPMcAb-GCV-BSA-NPs in HepG2 cells and there was little change with time. The statistics of ^{131}I-antiAFP-GCV-BSA-NPs in HepG2 cells group differed significantly from those of the other three groups ($p < 0.001$ or 0.000) (Figure 3).

As shown in Figure 4, the radioactive retention rates of four groups decreased as time progressed, but the retention rate of ^{131}I-antiAFPMcAb-GCV-BSA-NPs in HepG2 cells group was obviously higher than that of the other three groups (^{131}I in HepG2 cells group, ^{131}I-antiAFPMcAb-GCV-BSA-NPs in HEK293 cells group, and ^{131}I in HEK293 cells group) at the same time point ($p < 0.05$, 0.01, 0.001, or 0.000), indicating that ^{131}I-antiAFPMcAb-GCV-BSA-NPs are more easy to be taken in and retained in HepG2 cells with overexpressing AFP.

3.3. Radioactivity Distribution in Nude Mice with Transplanted Hepatoma. To validate the targeting of ^{131}I-anti-AFPMcAb-GCV-BSA-NPs to hepatoma *in vivo*, we investigated the nanospheres' dynamic radioactivity distribution in nude mice with transplanted hepatocellular carcinoma and calculated the radioactivity ratios of tumor versus nontumor (T/NT), using ^{131}I alone as control. The results showed that the majority of ^{131}I-antiAFPMcAb-GCV-BSA-NPs were distributed in blood, liver, and kidney at an early stage. As time progressed, the radioactivity in tumor tissue gradually increased while that in nontumor tissue decreased. ^{131}I alone mainly concentrated in blood, liver, and kidney at early stages and distributed slightly in the tumor as time advanced, but its distribution in tumor tissue was far below that of ^{131}I-antiAFPMcAb-GCV-BSA-NPs in tumor tissue at the same stage. Table 1 shows T/NT values at different stages after ^{131}I or ^{131}I-antiAFPMcAb-GCV-BSA-NPs were injected into nude mice with transplanted hepatoma. All T/NT values in the groups of ^{131}I-antiAFPMcAb-GCV-BSA-NPs gradually increased, indicating that ^{131}I-antiAFPMcAb-GCV-BSA-NPs gradually gathered in tumor tissue. Compared to the ^{131}I-antiAFPMcAb-GCV-BSA-NPs groups, all T/NT values in

Table 1: T/NT of ^{131}I-antiAFPMcAb-GCV-BSA-NPs and ^{131}I in nude mice with transplanted hepatoma (mean ± SD, $n = 3$).

Time	4 h		12 h		24 h		48 h	
Groups	^{131}I-antiAFP-GCV-BSA-NPs	^{131}I	^{131}I-antiAFP-GCV-BSA-NPs	^{131}I	^{131}I-antiAFP-GCV-BSA-NPs	^{131}I	^{131}I-antiAFP-GCV-BSA-NPs	^{131}I
Heart	1.26 ± 0.04[1]	1.12 ± 0.14	2.26 ± 0.17[2]	1.16 ± 0.07	4.16 ± 0.21[3]	1.30 ± 0.21	8.77 ± 0.19[4]	1.65 ± 0.26
Liver	0.46 ± 0.04[5]	0.35 ± 0.04	0.86 ± 0.06[6]	0.39 ± 0.09	1.36 ± 0.16[7]	0.41 ± 0.02	2.35 ± 0.40[8]	0.46 ± 0.06
Spleen	1.02 ± 0.06[9]	0.91 ± 0.05	1.78 ± 0.06[10]	0.97 ± 0.12	3.08 ± 0.16[11]	1.14 ± 0.12	9.02 ± 1.42[12]	1.57 ± 0.12
Lung	1.19 ± 0.04[13]	1.07 ± 0.14	2.26 ± 0.20[14]	1.18 ± 0.24	4.65 ± 0.52[15]	1.29 ± 0.10	9.38 ± 2.21[16]	1.90 ± 0.60
Kidney	0.64 ± 0.03	0.56 ± 0.10	1.29 ± 0.07[17]	0.66 ± 0.17	2.31 ± 0.08[18]	0.77 ± 0.10	5.91 ± 0.29[19]	0.99 ± 0.21
Stomach	1.22 ± 0.11[20]	0.98 ± 0.11	2.37 ± 0.03[21]	1.18 ± 0.06	5.11 ± 0.45[22]	1.53 ± 0.28	9.75 ± 1.80[23]	1.99 ± 0.24
Intestine	1.58 ± 0.08[24]	1.25 ± 0.17	3.04 ± 0.03[25]	1.40 ± 0.18	7.44 ± 1.01[26]	2.07 ± 0.16	12.29 ± 0.56[27]	2.45 ± 0.45
Brain	3.85 ± 0.19[28]	2.58 ± 0.41	8.76 ± 0.20[29]	3.28 ± 0.82	15.67 ± 2.10[30]	3.42 ± 0.36	30.68 ± 5.36[31]	3.32 ± 0.41
Bone	0.97 ± 0.05	0.89 ± 0.12	2.24 ± 0.15[32]	1.00 ± 0.29	4.22 ± 0.15[33]	1.24 ± 0.06	7.05 ± 0.42[34]	1.52 ± 0.42
Muscle	1.16 ± 0.04	1.08 ± 0.04	2.74 ± 0.21[35]	1.34 ± 0.20	5.65 ± 0.57[36]	1.74 ± 0.21	10.88 ± 0.53[37]	2.09 ± 0.36
Blood	0.18 ± 0.01	0.15 ± 0.01	0.40 ± 0.03[38]	0.19 ± 0.03	0.66 ± 0.03[39]	0.22 ± 0.04	1.70 ± 0.12[40]	0.33 ± 0.08

[1]$p < 0.05$ versus the heart group of 4 h ^{131}I; [2]$p < 0.01$ versus the heart group of 12 h ^{131}I; [3]$p < 0.001$ versus the heart group of 24 h ^{131}I; [4]$p < 0.000$ versus the heart group of 48 h ^{131}I; [5]$p < 0.05$ versus the liver group of 4 h ^{131}I; [6]$p < 0.01$ versus the liver group of 12 h ^{131}I; [7]$p < 0.001$ versus the liver group of 24 h ^{131}I; [8]$p < 0.000$ versus the liver group of 48 h ^{131}I; [9]$p < 0.05$ versus the spleen group of 4 h ^{131}I; [10]$p < 0.001$ versus the spleen group of 12 h ^{131}I; [11]$p < 0.000$ versus the spleen group of 24 h ^{131}I; [12]$p < 0.000$ versus the spleen group of 48 h ^{131}I; [13]$p < 0.05$ versus the lung group of 4 h ^{131}I; [14]$p < 0.001$ versus the lung group of 12 h ^{131}I; [15]$p < 0.000$ versus the lung group of 24 h ^{131}I; [16]$p < 0.000$ versus the lung group of 48 h ^{131}I; [17]$p < 0.001$ versus the kidney group of 12 h ^{131}I; [18]$p < 0.000$ versus the kidney group of 24 h ^{131}I; [19]$p < 0.000$ versus the kidney group of 48 h ^{131}I; [20]$p < 0.05$ versus the stomach group of 4 h ^{131}I; [21]$p < 0.001$ versus the stomach group of 12 h ^{131}I; [22]$p < 0.000$ versus the stomach group of 24 h ^{131}I; [23]$p < 0.000$ versus the stomach group of 48 h ^{131}I; [24]$p < 0.05$ versus the intestine group of 4 h ^{131}I; [25]$p < 0.000$ versus the intestine group of 12 h ^{131}I; [26]$p < 0.000$ versus the intestine group of 24 h ^{131}I; [27]$p < 0.000$ versus the intestine group of 48 h ^{131}I; [28]$p < 0.01$ versus the brain group of 4 h ^{131}I; [29]$p < 0.000$ versus the brain group of 12 h ^{131}I; [30]$p < 0.000$ versus the brain group of 24 h ^{131}I; [31]$p < 0.000$ versus the brain group of 48 h ^{131}I; [32]$p < 0.001$ versus the bone group of 12 h ^{131}I; [33]$p < 0.000$ versus the bone group of 24 h ^{131}I; [34]$p < 0.000$ versus the bone group of 48 h ^{131}I; [35]$p < 0.001$ versus the muscle group of 12 h ^{131}I; [36]$p < 0.000$ versus the muscle group of 24 h ^{131}I; [37]$p < 0.000$ versus the muscle group of 48 h ^{131}I; [38]$p < 0.001$ versus the blood group of 12 h ^{131}I; [39]$p < 0.000$ versus the blood group of 24 h ^{131}I; [40]$p < 0.000$ versus the blood group of 48 h ^{131}I.

the ^{131}I groups after 12 h were much lower at the same time point ($p < 0.01$, 0.001, or 0.000).

4. Discussion

There are many methods with which to prepare albumin drug-loading nanospheres, such as ultrasonic emulsifying, desolvation, polymer dispersion, and mechanical grinding. Among these, the desolvation method is the simplest and rapidest. In the present study, we prepared GCV-BSA-NPs by this method. TEM revealed that the nanospheres were 100–130 nm in diameter, smaller than 200 nm of BSA-NPs prepared by ultrasonic emulsification, a technique developed by Müller et al. [29]. The small size as well as hydrophilic surface is helpful to decrease opsonization, which in turn assists particles not easily engulfed by macrophages.

Drug-loading (DL) is one of important indicators with which to evaluate carrier performance for loading drugs. Generally, the higher the DL, the less the carriers that have to be used, and the better the effect [30]. The encapsulation ratio (ER) refers to the percentage of the total mass of drug embedded in the carriers accounting for the total mass of drugs, which is an assessment of drug utilization, reflecting the maturity of the preparation technology. As a rule, the higher the ER, the less the free drugs, and the higher the utilization. In this study, the effective drug-loading rate of GCV-BSA-NPs was 22.70%, and the GCV embedding rate reached 70.63%.

^{131}I has become one of the most commonly used radionuclides as a result of its superior properties, such as abundant sources, low price, and moderate half-life. In order to enhance targeting in radionuclide therapy, some special anti-McAb or ligand is often attached to the radionuclide. In the present study, chloramine-T technique was used to prepare ^{131}I-antiAFPMcAb. The labeling yield was (72.97 ± 1.28)%, and the radiochemical purity reached (99.63 ± 0.11)%.

Protein connecting technology can link the drug-loading protein nanosphere and radiation immune antibody. The antibody can guide radionuclide-bearing drug-loading nanosphere to kill lesions selectively, and the nanosphere can thus play a double "bio-missile" role of radionuclide and drug. This dual local treatment can greatly improve killing effect for tumor and minimize systemic side effect.

SPDP is a different bifunctional protein cross-linking agent, at whose termini a disulfide pyridine group and amber imide resin group are sensitive to sulfhydryl and amino groups and can easily cross-link two proteins containing thiol and amino groups. We used SPDP in the current study to connect GCV-BSA-NPs and ^{131}I-antiAFPMcAb, obtaining ^{131}I-antiAFPMcAb-GCV-BSA-NPs. Their diameters were 220–280 nm with average diameter 233.9 nm. After separation and purification, the labeling yield of ^{131}I-antiAFPMcAb-GCV-BSA-NPs was (61.5 ± 1.92)%. Their radiochemical purity both in air at room temperature and in serum at 37°C within 24 h was all in excess of 90%, indicating serum causes little damage to the radioactive stability. These ^{131}I-antiAFPMcAb-GCV-BSA-NPs therefore can be used for targeting analysis and treatment *in vivo*.

Cellular uptake ratio is an important parameter with which to evaluate drug targeting *in vitro*. Generally, the more the uptake, the stronger the targeting. The uptake rate of ^{131}I-antiAFPMcAb-GCV-BSA-NPs in HepG2 cells gradually increased with exposure, much greater than that of ^{131}I alone in HepG2 cells at the corresponding time point. The uptake rate of ^{131}I-antiAFPMcAb-GCV-BSA-NPs in HepG2 cells was far greater than that in HEK293 cells at the same time point. These indicate that ^{131}I-antiAFPMcAb-GCV-BSA-NPs have good selectivity to HepG2 cells. It may result from the fact that the antiAFPMcAb on the nanospheres specifically binds to AFP antigen on the HepG2 cell membrane, which facilitates the cells to endocytose ^{131}I-antiAFPMcAb-GCV-BSA-NPs, thus greatly improving the intake. The reason for the small change of ^{131}I intake may be that its radioactivity in cells represents nonspecific adsorption.

After it is taken up into cells, some ^{131}I-antiAFPMcAb-GCV-BSA-NPs may be retained in the cells; the rest is excreted. The retention time and the retention ratio are important factors influencing targeting. The cell retention test showed that the retention rate of ^{131}I-antiAFPMcAb-GCV-BSA-NPs in HepG2 cells was much higher than that in HEK293 cells and clearly higher than that of ^{131}I alone in HepG2 cells and HEK293 cells, suggesting better retention of ^{131}I-antiAFPMcAb-GCV-BSA-NPs in HepG2 cells. This may also be related to antiAFPMcAb. To be specific, the antiAFPMcAb on the nanospheres specifically binds to AFP antigen in the cytoplasm of HepG2 cells. This leads to more ^{131}I-antiAFPMcAb-GCV-BSA-NPs retained in HepG2 cells and longer retention time. By contrast, the entrance of ^{131}I alone into HepG2 or HEK293 cells and ^{131}I-antiAFPMcAb-GCV-BSA-NPs into HEK293 cells is passive, and they may quickly flush out of the cells.

The nuclides or drugs carried by nanospheres play a crucial role in killing tumor cells, and their concentration and residence time in tumor cells and T/NT are all crucial for the curative effect. T/NT is one of the main parameters which embody the ability of an antibody to concentrate specifically in tumor tissue. It reveals the relative ratio of affinities for antibody to tumor tissue and antibody to nontumor tissue. The nuclide distribution experiments *in vivo* showed that while most of ^{131}I-antiAFPMcAb-GCV-BSA-NPs and ^{131}I alone were distributed in blood, liver, and kidney at an early stage, the radioactivity in tumor tissue gradually increased and that in nontumor tissue decreased as time progressed in the ^{131}I-antiAFPMcAb-GCV-BSA-NPs group. In comparison, radioactive distribution had no clear difference between tumor tissue and nontumor tissue in ^{131}I alone group; both presented a gradually decreasing trend as time passed. Consistently, T/NT values of each ^{131}I-antiAFPMcAb-GCV-BSA-NPs group all showed an obviously increasing trend as time went on, significantly higher than that of the corresponding ^{131}I group at 12, 24, and 48 h. These data demonstrate that ^{131}I-antiAFPMcAb-GCV-BSA-NPs have a strong selectivity to AFP-positive hepatoma and the high affinity between antiAFPMcAb and AFP antigen can assist ^{131}I and GCV carried by the nanospheres to concentrate in hepatoma tissue.

In summary, ^{131}I-antiAFPMcAb-GCV-BSA-NPs have been prepared successfully for the first time in the present study. *In vitro* and *in vivo* experiments confirmed the highly selective targeting of ^{131}I-antiAFPMcAb-GCV-BSA-NPs to AFP-positive hepatocellular carcinoma tissue or cells. This is significant for the further radiation-gene therapy to selectively treat hepatoma and also provides a new strategy for other cancer-targeted treatment.

Conflict of Interests

The authors declare that there is no conflict of interests.

Acknowledgments

The work is financially supported by National Natural Science Foundation of China (81571797), Natural Science Foundation of Jiangsu, China (BK2010357), 333 Plan Foundation of Jiangsu, China (BRA2014183), Six Talents Peak Foundation of Jiangsu, China (2011-WS-023), Key Talent's Foundation in Science and Education of Jiangsu, China (RC2011212), and Social Development Plan of Taizhou (TS201345).

References

[1] T. M. Allen, "Long-circulating (sterically stabilized) liposomes for targeted drug delivery," *Trends in Pharmacological Sciences*, vol. 15, no. 7, pp. 215–220, 1994.

[2] E. M. Tazi, I. Essadi, H. M'rabti, A. Touyar, and P. H. Errihani, "Systemic treatment and targeted therapy in patients with advanced hepatocellular carcinoma," *North American Journal of Medical Sciences*, vol. 3, no. 4, pp. 167–175, 2011.

[3] I. Jemel, K. Jellali, J. Elloumi, and S. Aifa, "The offer of chemistry to targeted therapy in cancer," *Recent Patents on Biotechnology*, vol. 5, no. 3, pp. 174–182, 2011.

[4] M. Lin, J. X. Huang, J. Zhang et al., "The therapeutic effect of PEI-$Mn_{0.5}Zn_{0.5}Fe_2O_4$ nanoparticles/pEgr1-HSV-TK/GCV associated with radiation and magnet-induced heating on hepatoma," *Nanoscale*, vol. 5, no. 3, pp. 991–1000, 2013.

[5] M. Lin, D. Zhang, J. Huang et al., "An evaluation on transfection efficiency of pHRE-Egr1-EGFP in hepatocellular carcinoma cells Bel-7402 mediated by PEI-MZF-NPs," *Journal of Nanomaterials*, vol. 2011, Article ID 136052, 10 pages, 2011.

[6] T. Noguchi, G. Ritter, and H. Nishikawa, "Antibody-based therapy in colorectal cancer," *Immunotherapy*, vol. 5, no. 5, pp. 533–545, 2013.

[7] I. Tazi, H. Nafil, and L. Mahmal, "Monoclonal antibodies in hematological malignancies: past, present and future," *Journal of Cancer Research and Therapeutics*, vol. 7, no. 4, pp. 399–407, 2011.

[8] R. Perez, T. Crombet, J. de Leon, and E. Moreno, "A view on EGFR-targeted therapies from the oncogene-addiction perspective," *Frontiers in Pharmacology*, vol. 4, article 53, 2013.

[9] A. Chillemi, G. Zaccarello, V. Quarona et al., "Anti-CD38 antibody therapy: windows of opportunity yielded by the functional characteristics of the target molecule," *Molecular Medicine*, vol. 19, no. 1, pp. 99–108, 2013.

[10] J. Chen, H. Wu, D. Han, and C. Xie, "Using anti-VEGF McAb and magnetic nanoparticles as double-targeting vector for the radioimmunotherapy of liver cancer," *Cancer Letters*, vol. 231, no. 2, pp. 169–175, 2006.

[11] G.-P. Li, H. Zhang, C.-M. Zhu, J. Zhang, and X.-F. Jiang, "Avidin-biotin system pretargeting radioimmunoimaging and radioimmunotherapy and its application in mouse model of human colon carcinoma," *World Journal of Gastroenterology*, vol. 11, no. 40, pp. 6288–6294, 2005.

[12] Y. Zu, L. Meng, X. Zhao et al., "Preparation of 10-hydroxycamptothecin-loaded glycyrrhizic acid-conjugated bovine serum albumin nanoparticles for hepatocellular carcinoma-targeted drug delivery," *International Journal of Nanomedicine*, vol. 8, no. 1, pp. 1207–1222, 2013.

[13] L. Rastogi and J. Arunachalam, "Synthesis and characterization of bovine serum albumin-copper nanocomposites for antibacterial applications," *Colloids and Surfaces B: Biointerfaces*, vol. 108, pp. 134–141, 2013.

[14] H. Hao, Q. Ma, C. Huang, F. He, and P. Yao, "Preparation, characterization, and in vivo evaluation of doxorubicin loaded BSA nanoparticles with folic acid modified dextran surface," *International Journal of Pharmaceutics*, vol. 444, no. 1-2, pp. 77–84, 2013.

[15] C. Yu, F. Wo, Y. Shao, X. Dai, and M. Chu, "Bovine serum albumin nanospheres synchronously encapsulating "gold selenium/gold" nanoparticles and photosensitizer for high-efficiency cancer phototherapy," *Applied Biochemistry and Biotechnology*, vol. 169, no. 5, pp. 1566–1578, 2013.

[16] J.-M. Qin, P.-H. Yin, Q. Li et al., "Anti-tumor effects of brucine immuno-nanoparticles on hepatocellular carcinoma," *International Journal of Nanomedicine*, vol. 7, pp. 369–379, 2012.

[17] J. Gautier, E. Munnier, A. Paillard et al., "A pharmaceutical study of doxorubicin-loaded PEGylated nanoparticles for magnetic drug targeting," *International Journal of Pharmaceutics*, vol. 423, no. 1, pp. 16–25, 2012.

[18] L. Yu, Z. Dai, J. Zhou, and J. Fan, "Current advances in molecular targeted therapy of primary hepatocellular carcinoma," *Zhonghua Gan Zang Bing Za Zhi*, vol. 17, no. 6, pp. 475–477, 2009.

[19] G. J. Mizejewski, "Alpha-fetoprotein (AFP)-derived peptides as epitopes for hepatoma immunotherapy: a commentary," *Cancer Immunology, Immunotherapy*, vol. 58, no. 2, pp. 159–170, 2009.

[20] V. Wiwanitkit, "AFP and hepatoma staging," *European Journal of Surgical Oncology*, vol. 36, no. 10, p. 1015, 2010.

[21] Y. Liu, M. C. Wu, and G. X. Qian, "The experimental study of anti-human AFP variant McAb in radioimmuno-detection and radioimmuno-therapy of human hepatocellular carcinoma model in nude mice," *Zhonghua Wai Ke Za Zhi*, vol. 32, no. 11, pp. 650–653, 1994.

[22] Y. Liu, M. C. Wu, and B. Zhang, "Anti-human AFP variant McAb in radioimmunodetection for primary hepatocellular carcinoma," *Zhonghua Wai Ke Za Zhi*, vol. 34, no. 9, pp. 530–532, 1996.

[23] S. E. Severin, A. V. Rodina, M. B. Nitsvetov et al., "Regulation of anti-tumor activity using monoclonal antibodies to alpha-fetoprotein receptor and after immunization with this protein," *Russian Journal of Immunology*, vol. 6, no. 3, pp. 249–256, 2001.

[24] H. Y. Zhan, Q. S. Tang, Y. P. Tang, and D. Z. Chen, "Labeling bovine serum albumin-coated ganciclovir nanoparticles with 188Re," *Suzhou University Journal of Medical Science*, vol. 29, no. 1, pp. 105–115, 2009.

[25] D. S. C. Lee and B. W. Griffiths, "Comparative studies of iodo-bead and chloramine-T methods for the radioiodination of human alpha-fetoprotein," *Journal of Immunological Methods*, vol. 74, no. 1, pp. 181–189, 1984.

[26] Q. Zhao, P. Yan, L. Yin et al., "Validation study of ^{131}I-RRL: assessment of biodistribution, SPECT imaging and radiation dosimetry in mice," *Molecular Medicine Reports*, vol. 7, no. 4, pp. 1355–1360, 2013.

[27] Z. Y. Yang, *Radioimmunoimaging application and nuclide radiation therapy on pulmonary tumor [Ph.D. thesis]*, Peking Union Medical College Hospital, Beijing, China, 1994.

[28] http://wenku.baidu.com/view/f9a9a7f54028915f804dc2cf.html?from=search.

[29] B. G. Müller, H. Leuenberger, and T. Kissel, "Albumin nanospheres as carriers for passive drug targeting: an optimized manufacturing technique," *Pharmaceutical Research*, vol. 13, no. 1, pp. 32–37, 1996.

[30] F. Peng, Y. Su, X. Wei et al., "Silicon-nanowire-based nanocarriers with ultrahigh drug-loading capacity for in vitro and in vivo cancer therapy," *Angewandte Chemie—International Edition*, vol. 52, no. 5, pp. 1457–1461, 2013.

14

Fracture Forces of Dentin after Surface Treatment with High Speed Drill Compared to Er:YAG and Er,Cr:YSGG Laser Irradiation

Rene Franzen,[1,2] Nasrin Kianimanesh,[2] Rudolf Marx,[3] Asma Ahmed,[2] and Norbert Gutknecht[1]

[1] *Department of Conservative Dentistry, Periodontology and Preventive Dentistry, RWTH Aachen University Hospital, Pauwelsstrasse 30, 52074 Aachen, Germany*
[2] *AALZ Aachen Dental Laser Center, Center for Biomedical Technology, RWTH Aachen Campus, Pauwelsstrasse 17, 52074 Aachen, Germany*
[3] *Medical Material Science, RWTH Aachen University Hospital, Pauwelsstrasse 30, 52074 Aachen, Germany*

Correspondence should be addressed to Rene Franzen; rfranzen@ukaachen.de

Academic Editor: Kenji Yoshida

Dental tooth restorative procedures may weaken the structural integrity of the tooth, with the possibility of leading to fracture. In this study we present findings of coronal dentin strength after different techniques of surface modification. The fracture strength of dentin beams after superficial material removal with a fine diamond bur high speed drill hand piece, Er:YAG (2.94 μm, 8 J/cm^2), and Er,Cr:YSGG (2.78 μm, 7.8 J/cm^2) laser irradiation slightly above the ablation threshold was measured by a four-point bending apparatus. Untreated dentin beams served as a control. A total of 58 dentin beams were manufactured from sterilized human extracted molars using the coronal part of the available dentin. Mean values of fracture strength were calculated as 82.0 ± 27.3 MPa for the control group (n = 10), 104.5 ± 26.3 MPa for high speed drill treatment (n = 10), 96.1 ± 28.1 MPa for Er,Cr:YSGG laser irradiation (n = 20), and 89.1 ± 36.3 MPa for Er:YAG laser irradiation (n = 18). Independent Student's t-tests showed no significant difference between each two groups ($p > 0.05$). Within the parameter settings and the limits of the experimental setup used in this study, both lasers systems as well as the high speed drill do not significantly weaken coronal dentin after surface treatment.

1. Introduction

Factors related to tooth fracture have been investigated in different studies [1–3]. It is one of the most dramatic clinical situations which might be of concern to both dentists and patients, because it may consequently end up in loss of tooth structure. Therefore, the structural integrity of teeth under stress and how it may be jeopardized by different types of cracks is a very important issue [4]. The maximum stress by itself does not contribute to crack growth but the process of fatigue cycling results in producing cracks on the tooth surface [5]. The fatigue crack growth in human dentin is dependent on variables such as age, tubule orientation and density, and depth below the dentin-enamel junction [6–8].

Understanding the mechanical behavior of dentin under different conditions is crucial. Nevertheless, tooth fracture is multifactorial and restored teeth are more subject to experience cracks and damage during cutting and cavity preparation. Since cracking of teeth can have serious clinical consequences, the technique of cutting has a significant influence on the mechanical properties of the tooth by introducing and initiating cracks during cutting [1, 5, 9–11].

Though cracks of depths up to 71 μm were observed after diamond preparation in enamel, Banerjee et al. (2000) did not find cracks in dentin resulting from the use of burs but reported that sono-abrasion and Carisolv gels "caused flaws" [1, 3]. Yan et al. (2009) on the other hand did not observe flaws within dentin after bur treatment but nevertheless stated that material removal may be related to the cause of fracture [12]. Majd et al. (2012) evaluated the influence of 6-flute tungsten carbide bur and abrasive air-jet with 50 μm abrasive particles for cavity preparations on the mechanical behavior of coronal

TABLE 1: Exact dimensions, breaking force, and bending strength of the untreated control (group 1). The mean value of the bending strength is 82.02 MPa with a standard deviation of 27.25 MPa.

Number	Thickness/mm	Width/mm	Breaking force/N	Bending strength/MPa
1	1.20	1.90	37.90	112.20
2	1.96	1.60	84.00	110.70
3	1.36	1.90	32.00	73.76
4	1.44	1.88	6.58	13.67
5	1.77	1.66	55.30	86.13
6	1.58	1.86	45.20	78.85
7	1.37	1.85	37.20	86.78
8	1.40	1.86	38.00	84.43
9	1.30	1.75	34.40	94.21
10	1.88	1.77	61.40	79.50

dentin. The results were compared with the strength of intact control beams. Both methods significantly decreased the fatigue strength of dentin. In the same study, for the bur treatment an overall degradation in the endurance limit of nearly 40% was reported together with an accompanying decrease in fatigue life. It was considered a "critical issue" since this may hinder the dentin to provide a sound foundation for restorative materials [13]. When mechanical instrumentation is used, friction generates heat and hence elevated temperatures, which may cause irreversible damage to the tooth, while the tooth surface shows signs of thermal and mechanical damage in conjunction with a mechanically created smear layer that is formed as a consequence of this technique [14].

Current lasers for hard tissue preparation have been investigated for their abilities to ablate human enamel, dentin, and bone. Among the current commercially available laser systems, the radiation of the erbium lasers (Er:YAG 2.94 μm and Er,Cr:YSGG 2.78 μm) is strongly absorbed in water and mineral components and therefore offers the possibility for removal of hard tissues, caries removal, and cavity preparation with minimally invasive concept and more patient comfort. These lasers allow ablation of hard dental tissues without causing injury to the pulp or significant thermal side effects such as cracking, melting, or charring of the adjacent tissues at rates comparable with high speed dental drills and with less pain and vibration, as long as they are used with correct laser parameters and water sprays [15–20].

In a study by Maung et al. only 2 of the 15 samples ablated with the laser showed the formation of small cracks while 9 out of 15 samples exhibited crack formation with the dental hand piece [21]. Sehy and Drummond (2004) prepared class I or class II MOD cavities in molars using either a high speed hand piece with coarse diamond bur or an Er:YAG laser. The preparation was followed by placement of a resin composite, bulk curing to maximize interfacial stresses, and evaluation of the tooth-composite interface by scanning electron microscopy was performed. Neither method of preparation resulted in consistent or significant evidence of microcracking in dentin [22].

Staninec et al. compared a free-running pulsed Er:YAG laser (pulse duration 135 μs) with a q-switched Er,Cr:YSGG laser (pulse duration 0.5 μs). The 135 μs pulsed did not create any visible cracks on the irradiated surfaces while the q-switched systems with a 270 times shorter pulse duration, which was additionally operated without an air/water spray, created significant surface cracks from which fractures formed under bending of the specimens [23], pointing out the importance of pulse duration (nanosecond versus microsecond domain) and sufficient water sprays.

The present study addresses the question whether erbium laser surface treatment with fluencies close to the ablation threshold as found for a stopping ablation front in a free-running mode (microsecond domain) may cause weakening of dentin.

2. Materials and Methods

Caries-free extracted human molars were collected and completely cleaned of calculus and debris and then sterilized by γ-irradiation (Co^{60}) minimum absorbed dose of 29 KG. The teeth had been extracted for orthodontic reasons by cooperating dental offices and were donated to science.

The teeth were embedded in resin (Technovit 4000/4002: Heraeus-Kulzer, Wehrheim, Germany) and sectioned in buccolingual direction and then in mesiodistal direction to prepare dentin beams approximately 1.5 mm × 1.5 mm × 9 mm. The beams were roughly shaped with 400 grit and finished with 800 grit. The procedure of preparing dentin beams was adopted from the description of Staninec et al. [23]. The final dimensions after polishing are listed in Tables 1–4. The buccal surface was marked for later orientation of the specimen. The teeth and beam samples were stored in distilled water throughout the experiment with 0.9% NaCl.

The beams were assigned to two laser groups each containing 20 samples (groups 3 and 4) and two control groups each containing 10 samples (groups 1 and 2). In the control groups beams were kept either untreated (group 1), serving as a negative control, or treated with a fine diamond bur in a high speed hand piece under water cooling (group 2), serving as a positive control.

In the laser groups 3 and 4 beams were irradiated by either a free-running Er:YAG laser system 2.94 μm (Lightwalker system, Fotona d.d., Slovenia) or a free-running Er,Cr:YSGG

TABLE 2: Exact dimensions, breaking force, and bending strength of the Er,Cr:YSGG irradiated specimens (group 2). The mean value of the bending strength is 96.08 MPa with a standard deviation of 28.08 MPa.

Number	Thickness/mm	Width/mm	Breaking force/N	Bending strength/MPa
1	1.49	1.90	35.70	68.55
2	1.65	1.80	59.80	98.84
3	1.54	1.87	67.70	123.65
4	1.83	1.46	89.10	147.61
5	1.16	1.88	21.20	67.88
6	1.64	1.95	72.10	111.35
7	1.27	1.75	37.30	107.04
8	1.38	1.89	33.10	74.49
9	1.50	1.83	61.20	120.39
10	1.20	1.80	18.00	56.25
11	1.44	1.74	27.40	61.51
12	0.93	1.70	20.30	111.83
13	1.07	1.86	27.90	106.12
14	1.14	1.87	21.20	70.66
15	1.68	1.88	79.30	121.05
16	1.55	1.73	76.50	149.09
17	1.14	1.90	24.90	81.68
18	1.13	2.37	25.50	68.25
19	1.98	1.00	53.70	110.95
20	1.65	1.80	48.20	79.67

TABLE 3: Exact dimensions, breaking force, and bending strength of the Er:YAG irradiated specimens (group 2). The mean value of the bending strength is 89.12 MPa with a standard deviation of 36.32 MPa.

Number	Thickness/mm	Width/mm	Breaking force/N	Bending strength/MPa
1	1.27	1.76	33.00	94.16
2	1.02	1.86	36.00	150.69
3	1.24	1.88	25.90	72.57
4	2.00	1.22	70.50	117.02
5	1.86	1.22	30.70	58.92
6	1.57	1.70	60.00	115.98
7	1.45	1.92	60.10	120.59
8	1.64	1.85	38.60	62.84
9	1.26	1.90	27.70	74.38
10	1.75	1.84	43.00	61.81
11	1.59	1.50	62.40	133.29
12	1.14	1.60	18.40	71.68
13	1.75	1.57	31.50	53.07
14	1.97	1.80	90.60	105.05
15	1.94	1.04	29.00	60.01
16	1.98	1.65	118.00	147.76
17	1.81	1.80	63.10	86.67
18	2.00	1.42	38.90	55.47

2.79 μm (iPlus system, Biolase Inc., Irvine, CA, USA) both with a total radiation exposure of 10 seconds while their laser beams were scanned along the whole length of the dentin beams with one back and forth motion in mesiodistal direction and vice versa.

Parameters used in the groups were as follows:

(i) Group 1: untreated control (negative control).

(ii) Group 2: fine diamond bur in a high speed hand piece with water cooling (positive control).

(iii) Group 3: Er,Cr:YSGG used with a "*Gold*" type hand piece, MZ6 glass tip (diameter 600 μm), pulse duration 60 μs, 25 mJ, 10 Hz, water 80%, air 50% (adjustable spray), and fluence 8 J/cm^2 on the specimen's surface.

(iv) Group 4: Er:YAG laser used with an "*H14*" hand piece, glass tip (diameter 800 μm), pulse duration 100 μs, 40 mJ, 10 Hz, water 60%, air 40% (adjustable spray), and fluence 7.8 J/cm^2 on the specimen's surface.

TABLE 4: Exact dimensions, breaking force, and bending strength of the specimens treated by fine diamond bur in a high speed hand piece (group 1). The mean value of the bending strength is 104.47 MPa with a standard deviation of 26.31 MPa.

Number	Thickness/mm	Width/mm	Breaking force/N	Bending strength/MPa
1	1.15	2.12	39.90	115.27
2	1.75	1.05	34.20	86.15
3	1.12	1.89	24.40	83.36
4	1.55	1.81	44.10	82.15
5	1.56	1.67	49.10	97.86
6	1.35	1.79	48.20	119.68
7	1.40	1.79	33.60	77.57
8	1.65	1.87	55.90	88.94
9	2.00	1.09	78.70	146.21
10	1.57	1.86	83.50	147.52

Note that different pulse energies were chosen in groups 2 and 3 to compensate for different glass tip diameters of the laser systems in order to achieve a similar fluence. Around 4 J/cm^2 has been reported for the ablation threshold of dentin for Er:YAG laser irradiation [23, 24].

Laser parameters for groups 3 and 4 were chosen in such a way that the treated surface of the dentin beams was exposed to fluencies similar to those at the bottom of laser created cavities. While such cavities are obviously being created with significantly higher fluencies (in the order of 60 J/cm^2 for typical clinically used energies of 300 mJ and a beam cross section of 800 μm), the point where the ablation front stops moving into the dentin, hence the ablative process stopping, is where the newly created cavity floor is found. Therefore, the decision to use fluencies slightly above the ablation thresholds of 7-8 J/cm^2 was chosen to allow a slight ablative material removal with the ablation front stopping just inside the specimens. Only very little material is expected to be removed from the specimens themselves as due to their dimension for the fracture tests, they would be damaged or broken by the laser pulses if higher fluencies or removal rates are used. Instead, a dentin surface such as being found at a cavity floor is being simulated. Additionally, the dentin beam is irradiated on one surface side only, similar to that in a clinical dentin laser preparation, and the dentin is irradiated from one side.

In a similar fashion, the use of the diamond bur in the control group was moved manually along the length of the dentin beam, allowing it to remove material close to the surface and hence again simulating the floor of a bur-prepared excavation. Note that no EDTA or any similar agent was used to remove the created smear layer. Additionally, we point out that within the limits of our study design we cannot factor in additional sources of stress that could be found in a clinical situation such as forceful movement of the bur creating microfractures or high pulse energies for the laser systems creating similar incidences; however, to our knowledge the latter incidences have not been reported in the literature for free-running pulsed lasers.

Treated surfaces were oriented perpendicularly to the marked buccal surface; hence the direction of dentinal tubules was perpendicular to the treated surface and parallel to the direction of force of the bending test. That would be the same direction as the functional force naturally occurs. Each dentin beam was placed in a mechanical testing machine in a four-point bending apparatus (Zwick/Roell Z5.0, Zwick GmbH, Ulm, Germany) and tested with increasing load at a displacement rate of 1 mm/min until failure. The bending strength B can be calculated as shown in what follows:

$$B = \frac{3(l-c)F}{2bh^2} \tag{1}$$

using the following variables: l = lower distance of loading points = 7.2 mm, c = upper distance of loading points = 1.8 mm, b = width of the samples, h = thickness of the samples, and F = breaking force.

Each beam was positioned in a four-point bending apparatus with 1.8 mm distance to the upper loading points and 7.2 mm to the lower loading points until fracture occurred under the load. Load at fracture recorded as breaking force F and bending strength B of each beam was calculated accordingly.

3. Results

Final dimensions of the dentinal beams after preparation, breaking force, and bending strength are shown in Tables 1–4.

Mean values of bending strength were calculated as 82.0 ± 27.3 MPa for the unprepared control group, 96.1 ± 28.1 MPa for Er,Cr:YSGG laser irradiation, 89.1 ± 36.3 MPa for Er:YAG laser irradiation, and 104.5 ± 26.3 MPa for high speed drill conditioned surfaces. These values are presented in Figure 1. Independent t-tests showed that there were no significant differences between each two groups ($p > 0.05$).

4. Discussion

The effect of erbium family lasers on tooth structure during cavity preparation has been investigated in several studies. Various pulse durations and repetition rates and different energy and power parameters were investigated in these studies regarding the micromorphological aspect of enamel and dentin, ablation speed, depth, and/or volume [15, 25–31].

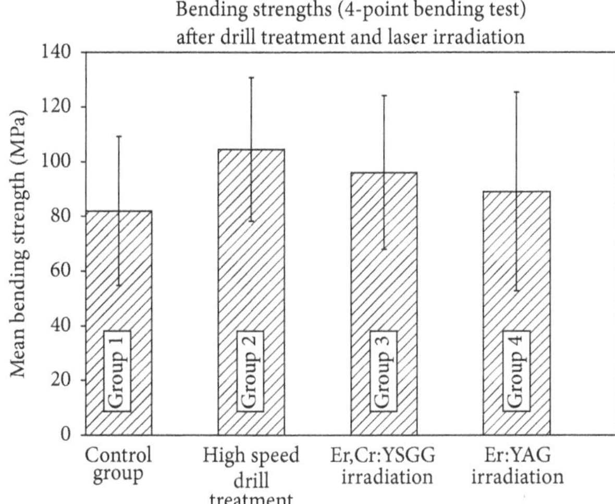

FIGURE 1: Illustration of the 4-point bending test results showing bending strengths for the control and the 3 test groups.

On the other hand, bur tooth preparation is associated with metallic noise and vibration that might cause discomfort and anxiety of the patient, as well as cracks and tooth weakening [1, 13, 21]. Less pain, noise, and vibration have been reported with laser cavity preparation [17, 32]. Bactericidal and anti-infective effects are the other aspects that could be expected [33].

Staninec et al. described a difference regarding fracture under bending between a free-running Er:YAG laser of 135 μs and a q-switched Er,Cr:YSGG laser of 0.5 μs pulse duration. While the Er:YAG treated surfaces did not show visible cracks, the Er,Cr:YSGG treated surfaces showed significant surface cracks. They reported that this resulted in significant weakening for the Er,Cr:YSGG treated specimens. This was explained by the q-switch laser generating mechanical and thermal shock waves, thermal expansion, and recoiling ablation debris [23]. It is to be noted that in addition to the drastically reduced pulse duration (135 versus 0.5 μs) the irradiation with the Er,Cr:YSGG laser was also performed without a water spray which represents an experimental setup which does not simulate a clinical situation.

Therefore, in the presented study, the pulse durations meet clinical requirements for dentin preparation with pulse durations of 50–100 μs typically found on free-running systems (flash-lamp operated). It is noteworthy that q-switched erbium lasers are so far not used clinically in dentistry and that it is well known that water sprays must be used during hard tissue preparations.

In our study, fracture strengths of dentinal beams irradiated with Er:YAG and Er,Cr:YSGG laser were compared with bur preparation and untreated intact beams in a 4-point bending test. There were no significant differences among groups. 4 J/cm^2 for Er:YAG laser irradiation has already been reported as the ablation threshold for dentin preparation [23, 24]. The fluencies above the ablation threshold for dentin preparation were selected in order to simulate a cavity floor on the surface of the dentin beams within the limits of our experimental setup. With the settings used in the present investigation laser irradiation did not weaken the dentinal beams in comparison with intact beams or bur treated beams.

The Er:YAG laser was compared by Sehy and Drummond with coarse diamond bur for preparation of class I and II MOD cavities that were restored by bulk curing composite restoration and no visible evidence of microcracking was found [22].

However in a study of fatigue crack growth rates by Nalla et al. in human dentin, it was concluded that, under simulated physiologic conditions, small flaws in teeth, in the order of 250 μm, will not radically affect their structural integrity as the predicted fatigue lifetime will exceed that of the patient [34]. For this reason we included group 2 (fine diamond bur in a high speed hand piece with water cooling) as positive control to include the possible effect of structural weakening under mechanical treatment of the surface. Another study by Bosa et al. utilizing a q-switched Er:YSGG laser reported on minimal thermal damage to the specimens while observing mechanical damage at higher fluencies [35].

Near infrared imaging of enamel samples irradiated by an industrial marking laser, operating at a wavelength of 9.3 μm with a repetition rate of 300 Hz, compared the peripheral thermal and mechanical damage produced by a standard dental hand piece with a high speed air turbine with the laser. Here 2 out of 15 (13.3%) irradiated samples were reported to have small cracks next to the ablation craters [21]. Without a water spray, mechanical as well as thermal damage occurred. Compared to this, 9 of 15 (60%) samples prepared with a high speed bur exhibited mechanical damage in the form of cracking and evidence of thermal damage [21].

In the present study, constant water spray was used during the whole laser irradiation process for both Er:YAG and Er,Cr:YSGG lasers, as it is also used in clinical treatments of enamel and dentin, either for cavity preparation or for other surface modifications. The importance of continuous spray application is also confirmed by Darling et al. who observed "very clean without large cracks" ablation craters and no accompanying thermal side effects [19]. The water spray acts as a mediator for efficient ablation and minimizes the risk of adverse thermal effects in the pulp tissue. The excessive increase of intrapulpal temperature and the possible thermal damage to the hard dental tissues have restricted Er:YAG laser ablation on dry teeth. Water sprays are, therefore, essential to reduce the side effects of temperature rise on biological tissues during clinical applications of Er:YAG lasers [36–39]. It has been shown that water cooling is essential to avoid destructive temperature increase whether an erbium laser or a high speed hand piece is used for cavity preparation [40]. The water spray is used to clean the irradiated surface, supply a cooling effect, and assist the ablation process [41, 42]. Additionally, the use of Er:YAG lasers without water spray has been reported to cause formation of non-apatite calcium phosphate phases which may be prone to acid dissolution and demineralization and may eventually lead to insufficient bonding of restorations [43].

In a study by Arola and Rouland the rate of fatigue crack growth was evaluated in terms of the dentin tubule orientation and tubule density. They concluded that fatigue crack growth in dentin is dependent on the tubule orientation [7]. For this reason the treated surface of dentin beams in our study was marked in such a way that tubules were perpendicular to the treated surface and in the same orientation for all samples. During the bending test the treated surfaces of the samples were positioned on the tensile side so the load is applied in the same direction in which it occurs naturally.

However, it is important to note that the presented study is to be interpreted with its limitations in mind. We investigated the influence of treatments and irradiations which are expected to influence the material close to the surface for the reason of simulating a standardized cavity floor. However, this situation does not include all effects that may be present in a clinical cavity preparation. For instance, effects such as shock or pressure waves created with higher fluencies and pulse powers are not present in our model. For flash-lamp pumped erbium lasers these shock waves are unlikely to have an effect, if present at all, as was described by Hibst and Keller [44]. Shock waves are more of a concern when pulse durations drop below 1 μs as is the case when using q-switched lasers [23]. Another effect not modeled in our in vitro situation is the act of mechanical drilling into the tooth during an actual cavity preparation; however, this may be partly compensated with the mechanical stress the teeth had experienced when being sawed apart to manufacture the dentin beam specimens from them. Additionally, the thermal influence of drilling into a tooth with clinical parameters has to be taken into account. While thermal weakening of the substance may in principle be possible, the appropriate use of the water sprays of free-running erbium lasers prevents a thermal increase, as was confirmed experimentally by Rizoiu et al. for the case of the Er,Cr:YSGG type system, where even a decrease in temperature of approx. 2°C was observed [45].

5. Conclusion

Within the conditions and limitations used in this study no statistically significant difference could be observed in the fracture strength of dentin beams when treating them either with Er:YAG and Er,Cr:YSGG laser irradiation or mechanically by a fine diamond bur in a high speed hand piece. Additionally, no statistically significant difference could be observed between treated and untreated specimens.

Conflict of Interests

The authors declare that there is no conflict of interests regarding the publication of this paper.

References

[1] H. H. K. Xu, J. R. Kelly, S. Jahanmir, V. P. Thompson, and E. D. Rekow, "Enamel subsurface damage due to tooth preparation with diamonds," *Journal of Dental Research*, vol. 76, no. 10, pp. 1698–1706, 1997.

[2] D. Arola, M. P. Huang, and M. B. Sultan, "The failure of amalgam dental restorations due to cyclic fatigue crack growth," *Journal of Materials Science: Materials in Medicine*, vol. 10, no. 6, pp. 319–327, 1999.

[3] A. Banerjee, E. A. M. Kidd, and T. F. Watson, "Scanning electron microscopic observations of human dentine after mechanical caries excavation," *Journal of Dentistry*, vol. 28, no. 3, pp. 179–186, 2000.

[4] J. J.-W. Lee, J.-Y. Kwon, H. Chai, P. W. Lucas, V. P. Thompson, and B. R. Lawn, "Fracture modes in human teeth," *Journal of Dental Research*, vol. 88, no. 3, pp. 224–228, 2009.

[5] J. J. Kruzic, R. K. Nalla, J. H. Kinney, and R. O. Ritchie, "Mechanistic aspects of in vitro fatigue-crack growth in dentin," *Biomaterials*, vol. 26, no. 10, pp. 1195–1204, 2005.

[6] D. Arola and R. K. Reprogel, "Effects of aging on the mechanical behavior of human dentin," *Biomaterials*, vol. 26, no. 18, pp. 4051–4061, 2005.

[7] D. D. Arola and J. A. Rouland, *The Effects of Tubule Orientation on Fatigue Crack Growth in Dentin*, John Wiley & Sons, New York, NY, USA, 2003.

[8] J. Ivancik, N. K. Neerchal, E. Romberg, and D. Arola, "The reduction in fatigue crack growth resistance of dentin with depth," *Journal of Dental Research*, vol. 90, no. 8, pp. 1031–1036, 2011.

[9] S. Ratcliff, I. M. Becker, and L. Quinn, "Type and incidence of cracks in posterior teeth," *Journal of Prosthetic Dentistry*, vol. 86, no. 2, pp. 168–172, 2001.

[10] H. Ryou, N. Amin, A. Ross et al., "Contributions of microstructure and chemical composition to the mechanical properties of dentin," *Journal of Materials Science: Materials in Medicine*, vol. 22, no. 5, pp. 1127–1135, 2011.

[11] T. F. Watson and R. J. Cook, "The influence of bur blade concentricity on high-speed tooth-cutting interactions: a video-rate confocal microscopic study," *Journal of Dental Research*, vol. 74, no. 11, pp. 1749–1755, 1995.

[12] J. Yan, B. Taskonak, and J. J. Mecholsky Jr., "Fractography and fracture toughness of human dentin," *Journal of the Mechanical Behavior of Biomedical Materials*, vol. 2, no. 5, pp. 478–484, 2009.

[13] H. Majd, J. Viray, J. A. Porter, E. Romberg, and D. Arola, "Degradation in the fatigue resistance of dentin by bur and abrasive air-jet preparations," *Journal of Dental Research*, vol. 91, no. 9, pp. 894–899, 2012.

[14] M. C. L. Luengo, M. Portillo, J. M. Sánchez et al., "Evaluation of micromorphological changes in tooth enamel after mechanical and ultrafast laser preparation of surface cavities," *Lasers in Medical Science*, vol. 28, no. 1, pp. 267–273, 2013.

[15] S. A. M. Corona, A. E. De Souza, M. A. Chinelatti, M. C. Borsatto, J. D. Pécora, and R. G. Palma-Dibb, "Effect of energy and pulse repetition rate of Er: YAG laser on dentin ablation ability and morphological analysis of the laser-irradiated substrate," *Photomedicine and Laser Surgery*, vol. 25, no. 1, pp. 26–33, 2007.

[16] C. Fornaini, S. Petruzzella, R. Podda, E. Merigo, S. Nammour, and P. Vescovi, "Er:YAG laser and fractured incisor restorations: an *in vitro* study," *International Journal of Dentistry*, vol. 2012, Article ID 617264, 6 pages, 2012.

[17] K. Takamori, H. Furukawa, Y. Morikawa, T. Katayama, and S. Watanabe, "Basic study on vibrations during tooth preparations caused by high-speed drilling and Er:YAG laser irradiation," *Lasers in Surgery and Medicine*, vol. 32, no. 1, pp. 25–31, 2003.

[18] R. J. G. De Moor and K. I. M. Delmé, "Laser-assisted cavity preparation and adhesion to erbium-lased tooth structure: part 1. Laser-assisted cavity preparation," *The Journal of Adhesive Dentistry*, vol. 11, no. 6, pp. 427–438, 2009.

[19] C. L. Darling, M. E. Maffei, W. A. Fried, and D. Fried, "Near-IR imaging of erbium laser ablation with a water spray," in *Proceedings of the 14th World Congress for Laser Dentistry*, vol. 6843 of *Proceedings of SPIE*, San Jose, Calif, USA, January 2003.

[20] V. Colucci, F. L. B. do Amaral, J. D. Pécora, R. G. Palma-Dibb, and S. A. Milori Corona, "Water flow on erbium:yttrium-aluminum-garnet laser irradiation: effects on dental tissues," *Lasers in Medical Science*, vol. 24, no. 5, pp. 811–818, 2009.

[21] L. H. Maung, C. Lee, and D. Fried, "Near-IR imaging of thermal changes in enamel during laser ablation," *Proceedings of the International Society for Optical Engineering*, vol. 7546, no. 1, p. 754902, 2010.

[22] C. Sehy and J. L. Drummond, "Micro-cracking of tooth structure," *American Journal of Dentistry*, vol. 17, no. 5, pp. 378–380, 2004.

[23] M. Staninec, N. Meshkin, S. K. Manesh, R. O. Ritchie, and D. Fried, "Weakening of dentin from cracks resulting from laser irradiation," *Dental Materials*, vol. 25, no. 4, pp. 520–525, 2009.

[24] B. Majaron, M. Lukac, D. Susteric, N. Funduk, and U. Skaleric, "Threshold and efficiency analysis in Er:YAG laser ablation of hard dental tissue," in *Laser Applications in Medicine and Dentistry*, vol. 2922 of *Proceedings of SPIE*, pp. 233–242, Vienna, Austria, September 1996.

[25] P. M. Freitas, R. S. Navarro, J. A. Barros, and C. D. P. Eduardo, "The use of Er:YAG laser for cavity preparation: an SEM evaluation," *Microscopy Research and Technique*, vol. 70, no. 9, pp. 803–808, 2007.

[26] K. I. M. Delmé and R. J. G. De Moor, "Scanning electron microscopic evaluation of enamel and dentin surfaces after Er:YAG laser preparation and laser conditioning," *Photomedicine and Laser Surgery*, vol. 25, no. 5, pp. 393–401, 2007.

[27] R. S. Navarro, S. Gouw-Soares, A. Cassoni, P. Haypek, D. M. Zezell, and C. De Paula Eduardo, "The influence of erbium:yttrium–aluminum–garnet laser ablation with variable pulse width on morphology and microleakage of composite restorations," *Lasers in Medical Science*, vol. 25, no. 6, pp. 881–889, 2010.

[28] W. Raucci-Neto, M. A. Chinelatti, and R. G. Palma-Dibb, "Ablation rate and morphology of superficial and deep dentin irradiated with different Er:YAG laser energy levels," *Photomedicine and Laser Surgery*, vol. 26, no. 6, pp. 523–529, 2008.

[29] W. Raucci-Neto, J. D. Pécora, and R. G. Palma-Dibb, "Thermal effects and morphological aspects of human dentin surface irradiated with different frequencies of Er:YAG laser," *Microscopy Research and Technique*, vol. 75, no. 10, pp. 1370–1375, 2012.

[30] A. Igarashi, J. Kato, Y. Takase, and Y. Hirai, "Influence of output energy and pulse repetition rate of the Er:YAG laser on dentin ablation," *Photomedicine and Laser Surgery*, vol. 26, no. 3, pp. 189–195, 2008.

[31] M. A. Chinelatti, W. Raucci-Neto, S. A. M. Corona, and R. G. Palma-Dibb, "Effect of erbium:yttrium–aluminum–garnet laser energies on superficial and deep dentin microhardness," *Lasers in Medical Science*, vol. 25, no. 3, pp. 317–324, 2010.

[32] J. Pelagalli, C. B. Gimbel, R. T. Hansen, A. Swett, D. W. Winn II, and M. Van Valen, "Investigational study of the use of Er:YAG laser versus dental drill for caries removal and cavity preparation—phase I," *Journal of Clinical Laser Medicine and Surgery*, vol. 15, no. 3, pp. 109–115, 1997.

[33] R. Lubart, G. Kesler, R. Lavie, and H. Friedmann, "Er:YAG laser promotes gingival wound repair by photo-dissociating water molecules," *Photomedicine and Laser Surgery*, vol. 23, no. 4, pp. 369–372, 2005.

[34] R. K. Nalla, V. Imbeni, J. H. Kinney, M. Staninec, S. J. Marshall, and R. O. Ritchie, "In vitro fatigue behavior of human dentin with implications for life prediction," *Journal of Biomedical Materials Research, Part A*, vol. 66, no. 1, pp. 10–20, 2003.

[35] A. D. Bosa, A. V. Sarma, C. Q. Le, R. S. Jones, and D. Fried, "Peripheral thermal and mechanical damage to dentin with microsecond and sub-microsecond 9.6 μm, 2.79 μm, and 0.355 μm laser pulses," *Lasers in Surgery and Medicine*, vol. 35, no. 3, pp. 214–228, 2004.

[36] E. J. Burkes Jr., J. Hoke, E. Gomes, and M. Wolbarsht, "Wet versus dry enamel ablation by Er:YAG laser," *The Journal of Prosthetic Dentistry*, vol. 67, no. 6, pp. 847–851, 1992.

[37] M. Hossain, Y. Nakamura, Y. Yamada, Y. Kimura, G. Nakamura, and K. Matsumoto, "Ablation depths and morphological changes in human enamel and dentin after Er:YAG laser irradiation with or without water mist," *Journal of Clinical Laser Medicine and Surgery*, vol. 17, no. 3, pp. 105–109, 1999.

[38] V. R. Geraldo-Martins, E. Y. Tanji, N. U. Wetter, R. D. Nogueira, and C. P. Eduardo, "Intrapulpal temperature during preparation with the Er:YAG laser: an in vitro study," *Photomedicine and Laser Surgery*, vol. 23, no. 2, pp. 182–186, 2005.

[39] J. Meister, R. Franzen, K. Forner et al., "Influence of the water content in dental enamel and dentin on ablation with erbium YAG and erbium YSGG lasers," *Journal of Biomedical Optics*, vol. 11, no. 3, Article ID 034030, 2006.

[40] B. N. Cavalcanti, J. L. Lage-Marques, and S. M. Rode, "Pulpal temperature increases with Er:YAG laser and high-speed handpieces," *Journal of Prosthetic Dentistry*, vol. 90, no. 5, pp. 447–451, 2003.

[41] K. Glockner, J. Rumpler, K. Ebeleseder, and P. Städtler, "Intrapulpal temperature during preparation with the Er:YAG laser compared to the conventional burr: an in vitro study," *Journal of Clinical Laser Medicine and Surgery*, vol. 16, no. 3, pp. 153–157, 1998.

[42] D. Oelgiesser, J. Blasbalg, and A. Ben-Amar, "Cavity preparation by Er:YAG laser on pulpal temperature rise," *American Journal of Dentistry*, vol. 16, no. 2, pp. 96–98, 2003.

[43] D. Fried, N. Ashouri, T. Breunig, and R. Shori, "Mechanism of water augmentation during IR laser ablation of dental enamel," *Lasers in Surgery and Medicine*, vol. 31, no. 3, pp. 186–193, 2002.

[44] R. Hibst and U. Keller, "Mechanism of Er:YAG laser-induced ablation of dental hard substances," in *Proceedings of the Lasers in Orthopedic, Dental, and Veterinary Medicine II*, vol. 1880 of *Proceedings of SPIE*, Los Angeles, Calif, USA, July 1993.

[45] I. Rizoiu, F. Kohanghadosh, A. I. Kimmel, and L. R. Eversole, "Pulpal thermal responses to an erbium,chromium:YSGG pulsed laser hydrokinetic system," *Oral Surgery, Oral Medicine, Oral Pathology, Oral Radiology, and Endodontics*, vol. 86, no. 2, pp. 220–223, 1998.

15

Insulin-Like Growth Factor and Epidermal Growth Factor Signaling in Breast Cancer Cell Growth: Focus on Endocrine Resistant Disease

Kallirroi Voudouri,[1] Aikaterini Berdiaki,[1] Maria Tzardi,[2] George N. Tzanakakis,[1] and Dragana Nikitovic[1]

[1]*Laboratory of Anatomy-Histology-Embryology, School of Medicine, University of Crete, 71003 Heraklion, Greece*
[2]*Laboratory of Pathology, School of Medicine, University of Crete, 71003 Heraklion, Greece*

Correspondence should be addressed to Dragana Nikitovic; dnikitovic@med.uoc.gr

Academic Editor: Matthias Stope

Breast cancer is the most common type of cancer for women worldwide with a lifetime risk amounting to a staggering total of 10%. It is well established that the endogenous synthesis of insulin-like growth factor (IGF) and epidermal growth factor (EGF) polypeptide growth factors are closely correlated to malignant transformation and all the steps of the breast cancer metastatic cascade. Numerous studies have demonstrated that both estrogens and growth factors stimulate the proliferation of steroid-dependent tumor cells, and that the interaction between these signaling pathways occurs at several levels. Importantly, the majority of breast cancer cases are estrogen receptor- (ER-) positive which have a more favorable prognosis and pattern of recurrence with endocrine therapy being the backbone of treatment. Unfortunately, the majority of patients progress to endocrine therapy resistant disease (acquired resistance) whereas a proportion of patients may fail to respond to initial therapy (de novo resistance). The IGF-I and EGF downstream signaling pathways are closely involved in the process of progression to therapy resistant disease. Modifications in the bioavailability of these growth factors contribute critically to disease progression. In the present review therefore, we will discuss in depth how IGF and EGF signaling participate in breast cancer pathogenesis and progression to endocrine resistant disease.

1. Introduction

Breast cancer is the most common type of cancer for women worldwide. Its lifetime risk amounts to a staggering total of 10% where approximately 15–20% of all breast cancers are associated with genetic predisposition [1]. It is well established that breast cancer growth is regulated by the endogenous synthesis of polypeptide growth factors [2] and by growth factors produced at distant sites [3]. Both growth factors and steroids can stimulate proliferation of steroid-dependent tumor cells, and interaction between these signaling pathways occurs at several levels. Indeed, breast cancer is categorized into histopathologic subtypes based on estrogen (ER) and progesterone (PR) hormone receptor status and HER2/ErbB2 epidermal growth factor (EGF) receptors' expression levels. Namely, about 75% of all breast cancers are estrogen receptor- (ER-) positive [4]. This type of breast cancer generally has a more favorable prognosis and pattern of recurrence with endocrine therapy being the backbone of treatment. Antiestrogens and aromatase inhibitors can effectively induce tumor responses in a large proportion of these patients. However, the majority of patients progress during endocrine therapy to resistant disease (acquired resistance) and a proportion of patients may fail to respond to initial therapy (de novo resistance) [4]. Importantly, several steroid responses have now been functionally linked to other intracellular signaling pathways, including c-Src or tyrosine kinase receptors [5]. Moreover, endocrine resistant breast cancer has been correlated to the activation of other signaling pathways, including insulin-like growth factor (IGF) and epidermal growth factor (EGF) pathway [4]. Indeed, endocrine resistance is associated with overexpression of IGF and EGF signaling pathway components, including EGFR, HER2, IGF-IR, and c-Src [6]. Dissecting signaling pathways involved in endocrine and targeted therapy resistant disease is critical for developing novel, more efficient strategies.

2. Epidermal Growth Factors Family

The significant role of EGF family members and their respective ErbB receptors in breast cancer cell pathogenesis is well established [7]. The EGF family consists of EGF, transforming growth factor-alpha (TGF-α), heparin-binding epidermal growth factor (HB-EGF), amphiregulin (AR), epiregulin (EPR), betacellulin (BTC) and neuregulins (NRGs) [8, 9]. All family members are synthesized as membrane-anchored precursors and their ectodomains cleaved to release the soluble form of growth factor, subsequent to a proteolytic process [7, 10].

The ErbB family of receptors structurally related to EGFR, is composed of ErbB1 (also known as EGFR or HER1), ErbB2 (HER2/Neu), ErbB3 (HER3), and ErbB4 (HER4) [8, 11]. Structurally, the ErbB receptors are composed of an extracellular domain rich in cysteine, a single membrane region and a large cytoplasmic domain [7]. All specific ErbB ligands have an EGF-like domain that endows them with high binding specificity [11, 12]. The extracellular domain is the ligand-binding site of ErbB receptors whereas the cytoplasmic domain has tyrosine protein kinase activity. Mechanistically, the binding of ligands to ErbB receptors leads to their dimerization and subsequent tyrosine phosphorylation of specific tyrosine residues within the cytoplasmic tail [11]. These structural modifications enhance docking of effector proteins whose recruitment induces the activation of downstream signal transduction pathways, including Mitogen-Activated Protein Kinase (MAPK) and Phospatidylinositol-3 Kinase (PI-3K) pathways [7, 13, 14].

2.1. EGF Signaling in Breast Cancer Cell Proliferation. ErbB receptors are positively correlated with breast cancer cell proliferation [15, 16]. They are activated by the EGF ligands, EGF, a potent mitogen, being the basic ligand of these receptors, particularly in cells overexpressing EGFR [17, 18]. In addition the ErbB receptors can autophosphorylate or be phosphorylated by other kinases [11]. The activated ErbB receptors bind to Grb2 and Sos downstream mediators, resulting in the activation of intracellular signaling pathways such as Ras/Raf, MAPK, and the PI-3K/Akt pathways which are involved in cell growth, apoptosis, invasion, and migration of breast cancer cells [13, 14, 19, 20]. Specifically, the formation of EGFR-Grb7-Ras complex enhances breast cancer cell proliferation [21].

The key role of EGFR in tumor growth is evident from the antiproliferative effects of monoclonal antibodies specific for this receptor [22]. Furthermore, there is evidence that EGFR activator proteins contribute to EGFR-dependent breast cancer cell proliferation. For example, ERp57 protein, a member of the disulfide isomerase family, participates in the activation of EGFR signaling and in the modulation of its internalization leading to enhanced breast cancer cell proliferation [23]. Moreover, the stimulation of proliferation through activation of EGFR promotes degradation of Fhit protein (the product of tumor suppressor gene *FHIT*) [24].

A concentration-dependent effect of EGF on breast cancer cell proliferation has also been proposed [25–27]. Thus, EGF at concentrations that stimulate most other cell lines reduced the growth of MDA-468 breast cancer cells [25]. Additionally Zhang et al. [28] indicated a biphasic effect of EGF on breast cancer cell proliferation and demonstrated that Src functions as a switch of EGF signaling, depending on EGF concentration. Moreover, EGF seems to induce an inhibition of proliferation through the stimulation of an interleukin 6 type cytokine, oncostatin M, in both estrogen receptor positive and negative breast cancer cells [26]. A novel role for EGF has been proposed by Adams et al. [27]. Specifically, it was found that EGF treatments enhanced miR-206 (microRNA-206) levels in MCF-7 cells, which resulted in reduced cell proliferation, enhanced apoptosis, and reduced expression of multiple estrogen-responsive genes [27].

On the other hand, ezrin-radixin-moesin-binding phosphoprotein-50 (EBP50) suppresses breast cancer cell proliferation [29]. Indeed, EBP50 can suppress EGF-induced proliferation of breast cancer cells by inhibiting EGFR phosphorylation and blocking EGFR downstream signaling [30].

3. Insulin-Like Growth Factor Family Members

The biological activities of IGF family not only affect the normal development of the organism but have been strongly implicated in tumorigenesis [31, 32]. This important signaling family consists of the IGF ligands (IGF-I and IGF-II), *their cell membrane* receptors (IGF-IR, IGF-IIR, and IR), and a group of IGF-binding proteins (IGFBPs) [33].

Structurally, whereas insulin is composed of two domains denominated A and B, the IGFs are single-chain molecules that maintain the equivalent of the connecting C-peptide of proinsulin between A and B domains [34]. IGFs are reported to play significant role in cancer progression and according to LeRoith et al. [33] high levels of circulating IGF-I *have been indicated* to constitute a risk factor for the development of breast, prostate, colon, and lung cancer. However, further clinical studies are needed to clarify these first indications.

Importantly, the expression of IGF-I is predictive of breast cancer progression, prognosis, and outcome [32]. The antiapoptotic and mitogenic actions of IGF-I are mediated by its receptor IGF-IR [33, 35]. The IGF-IR activation and overexpression have been implicated in many cellular processes, including cell migration, proliferation, and attenuation of cell survival and are related to the malignant phenotype [31, 36, 37]. IGF-IR is a heterotetrameric transmembrane glycoprotein. Structurally, it forms a $\alpha_2\beta_2$ structure, the β subunits endowed with intrinsic tyrosine kinase activity, whereas the α subunits are the ligand-binding sites [38, 39]. Binding of ligands to the receptor results in its conformational change and a subsequent autophosphorylation of tyrosine residues 1131, 1135, and 1136 in the kinase domain, juxtamembrane tyrosines, and C-terminal serines [40].

IGF-binding proteins and their respective concentrations regulate the bioavailability of the IGFs and IGF-induced proliferation through IGF/IGFBP complex formation [41–43]. Six high-affinity IGFBPs have been identified to date. Specifically, IGFBP-1 to IGFBP-4 have similar affinities for IGF-I and IGF-II, whereas IGFBP-5 and IGFBP-6 bind IGF-II with higher affinity [44, 45]. All IGFBPs (six proteins) are expressed in mammary tumors [46, 47]. Specifically, IGFBP-4 and IGFBP-5 are expressed in primary breast cancer [46, 47]. Thus, IGFBP-3 provides most of the IGF-binding capacity of serum and greatly prolongs the circulating half-life of the IGFs [48]. Generally, IGFBPs modulate the interactions between IGF ligands and cell-surface receptors [48].

3.1. IGF Signaling in Breast Cancer Cell Proliferation. IGF family members (including IGF-I, IGF-II, and their receptors) are overexpressed in breast cancer tumor cells and were shown to promote these cells' survival and growth through various signaling pathways [32]. The principal transduction routes of the IGF signaling are MAPK and PI-3K pathways [49–51]. It is noteworthy that the MAPK and PI-3K/Akt are key mediators of cell proliferation [52–54]. Also, recent data have shown that ERK (MAPK44/42) plays an important role in the resistance of MCF-7 cells to cell apoptosis, which shows the importance of ERK signaling in the extended survival of breast cancer cells [54]. On the other hand, there is evidence that c-Jun N-terminal kinase (JNK) signaling negatively regulates IGF-I induced breast cancer cell proliferation [55].

The majority of IGF-I cellular actions are mediated by the key signaling component of the IGF-I system, the IGF-IR [33]. The activation of IGF-IR by IGF-I results in its autophosphorylation at tyrosine residues [33, 56]. Consecutively, the activated IGF-IR directly phosphorylates other substrates such as IRS-1, IRS-2, and IRS-4 [57]. Upon activation IRS-1 becomes a "docking" protein for other molecules, exhibiting binding sites for SH2 domain-containing proteins [58]. As a consequence, after IRS-1 phosphorylation, many downstream signaling pathways associated with mitogenesis, such as PI-3K [59] and MAPK cascade [60, 61], are activated. Other substrates which are phosphorylated by IGF-IR are src-homology 2/collagen-α proteins (Shc) [62], growth factor receptor-binding protein 10 [63], focal adhesion kinase (FAK) [64], and carboxyl-terminal src kinase (CSK) [65].

The importance of IGF signaling in breast cancer is highlighted by reports showing that the IGF-I induced proliferation of MCF-7 breast cancer cells is attenuated with the PI-3K inhibitor LY294002 and the antiestrogen ICI 182780 [66]. In addition, Ahmad et al. [49] suggested that Akt is a downstream mediator of estrogen- and IGF-I-dependent proliferation in hormone-responsive MCF-7 breast carcinoma cells. IGF-I also upregulates Cyr61, a family member of CCN family proteins with many roles in cancer progression, which is characterized by various homologous domains, including the IGF-binding protein domain, through activation of the PI-3K/Akt pathway [67]. This increase in Cyr61 leads to stimulation of breast cancer cell growth and invasion [67]. Furthermore, the inhibition of MAPK or Akt pathways prior to IGF-I stimulation prevents the expression of specific tumor suppressor miRNAs. In a novel report, [51] suggest that IGF-I signaling regulates the expression of specific miRNAs in the estrogen receptor positive MCF-7 breast cancer cell line and indicate kinase signaling as a modulator of expression for a small subset of microRNAs.

Burtrum et al. [68] show that the inhibition of IGF-I signaling, via IGF-IR blockade (generation of specific monoclonal antibody), inhibits the activation of downstream MAPK and Akt signaling pathways. As a result, the proliferative potential effect of IGF-I and IGF-II was reduced. Moreover, IGF-IR deficient mice show a reduced rate of tumor growth and cell migration [69], indicating the central role of IGF-IR in breast cancer cell proliferation. Additionally, the IGF-IR suppression increases apoptosis through p38MAPK phosphorylation in MCF-7 cells [70]. Preclinical findings however have not been translated to date in effective treatment strategies [71]. The function of tumor suppressor genes influences the IGF-IR signals and their downstream proliferative effects on breast cancer cells [48]. Transcription of IGF-IR gene is negatively regulated by tumor suppressors, including the Breast Cancer Gene-1 (BRCA1), p53, and Wilms' tumor protein-1 (WT1) [72, 73]. The role of BRCA1 and BRCA2 in breast cancer progression and prognosis is well documented [74]. BRCA1 inhibits IGF-I action, so *BRCA1* deficiency also leads to increased expression of several IGF-I signaling pathway components in multiple experimental systems, including mice, mammary tumors, and cultured human cells [75, 76]. As a result, mutation or deficiency of *BRCA1* leads to stimulated IGF-I activity and, consequently, increased cell proliferation. Apart from this, the loss of p53 tumor suppressor gene has also been demonstrated to increase IGF-IR expression [77, 78]. This mechanism however does not involve direct DNA binding to IGF-IR promoter sequences [73]. Another example is loss of function of tumor suppressor gene *PTEN* which encodes a phosphatase that attenuates signals originating at tyrosine kinase receptors such as IGF-IR [32, 48].

3.2. Insulin-Like Growth Factor and Epidermal Growth Factor Signaling in Endocrine and Targeted Therapy Resistant Breast Cancer Proliferation. It is well established that both steroids and growth factors stimulate proliferation of steroid-dependent tumor cells and that the interaction between these signaling pathways occurs at several levels [6, 49]. The steroid ligands are transferred to the nucleus where they bind steroid receptors, which are classified as ligand-activated transcription factors, to activate target gene transcription and cell growth. Several steroid responses have now been functionally linked to other intracellular signaling pathways, including tyrosine kinase receptors or c-Src. Steroids such as 17 beta-estradiol (E2) via binding to cytoplasmic or membrane-associated receptors were also shown to rapidly activate intracellular signaling cascades including ERK, PI-3K, and STATs [79]. These E2-stimulated phosphorylation-mediated cascades can then contribute to altered tumor cell function [80]. ER-α targeted therapy is routinely used to treat breast cancer. However, patient responses are limited by resistance to endocrine therapy [81, 82]. The development of resistance to endocrine therapy often results in uncontrollable growth and dissemination of breast cancer

[82]. Therefore, identifying mechanisms that drive endocrine resistance is a high clinical priority.

A large body of experimental evidence indicates that oncogenic signaling pathways underlie endocrine resistance, including EGFR, HER2, IGF-IR, c-Src, and ER itself [6]. The crosstalk between estrogen, IGF-I, and EGF signaling pathways and its involvement in endocrine resistance is well documented in breast cancer [83, 84]. Indeed, breast cancer cells resistant to the pure steroidal ER antagonist fulvestrant demonstrate increased activation of EGFR family members and downstream ERK signaling. Moreover, EGFR has been identified as one of main genes conferring estrogen independence to human breast cancer cells [85]. E2 signaling interacts with IGF-I and EGF pathways, at different levels, for example, through the rapid activation of IGF-IR and EGFR receptors and with the consequent induction of MAPK activation in breast cancer cells [86–88]. Thus, E2 and EGF cues are obligatory in the proliferation of ductal epithelial breast cancer cells and they have synergistic effects [5, 80]. Furthermore, the knockout of EGFR (or IGF-IR) abolished the E2-proliferative response in mice, and the inhibition of EGFR activity suppressed the proliferative effect of E2 in breast cancer cells *in vitro* [79, 89]. In addition, the selective inhibitors or knockdown of both receptors diminished E2-induced MAPK activation but also blocked E2-proliferative action [90]. It is proposed that E2 stimulates the expression of IGF and EGF ligands and receptors in rodent tissues and human cell lines [91]. The ER suppression in breast cancer cells prevents both EGF (and E2) stimulation of DNA synthesis [92]. However, the mitogenic effects of EGF are not mediated by ER, but it is suggested that the crosstalk between the estrogen and EGF signaling pathways may occur by other mechanisms [93]. Notably, both EGFR and c-Src stimulated pathways can induce activation of a transcription factor STAT5, which is needed for E2-induced breast cancer cell proliferation, in some cell lines [79]. Growth factor mediated ER activation is a major route through which breast cancer cells exhibit endocrine resistance to antiestrogen therapies [94]. During the genomic action of E2, binding of E2 to ERα results in its activation through separation from heat-shock protein 90 (Hsp90). Active ER-E2 dimer binds directly or indirectly to ERE genes (genes containing estrogen response elements) [95]. On the other hand, the nongenomic actions of E2 lead to the rapid activation of independent signaling pathways, such as IGF-IR and EGFR, depending on cell type [96]. In MCF-7 cells, estrogen potentiates the effect of IGF-I on IGF-IR signaling in the promotion of cell proliferation and protection against apoptosis [97]. Specifically, ERα binds to the IGF-IR and activates downstream signaling pathways [98]. Moreover, Yu et al. [99] recently reported the IGF-I induced association of IGF-IR and ERα. Furthermore, ERα regulates the IGF-I signaling pathways through phosphorylation of ERK1/2 and Akt where the interaction of ER-IGF-IR potentiates breast cancer cell growth [99]. Selective inhibitors or knockdown of IGF-IR (and EGFR) decreased E2-induced MAPK activation and blocked E2 mitogenic effect, confirming crosstalk signaling between IGF-IR, E2, and EGFR [90]. Moreover, E2 was found to utilize a signaling pathway which involves the interactions between ERα, IGF-IR, matrix metalloproteinases, and EGF-R to activate MAPK phosphorylation [88]. A consecutive study indicated that the transcriptional activity of ligand free ER is sufficient to complement the mitogenic action of IGF-IR-induced PI-3K/Akt activation [100]. On the other hand, Amin et al. [101] suggested that proliferation of MCF-7 breast cancer cells is suppressed by IGF-I-activated JNK MAPK pathway, through the induction of the SHP1 phosphatase expression.

Approximately, 15% of breast tumors are classified as triple-negative breast cancers (TNBC), a term that denotes their lack of estrogen receptor and progesterone receptor and nonamplification of the HER2 [102]. Therefore, TNBC patients cannot be treated with endocrine therapy or targeted therapies due to lack of related receptors which results in the poor prognosis. Characteristically, these patients overexpress the EGFR and IGFBP-3 proteins [103] but are resistant to tyrosine kinase inhibitors (TKIs) and anti-EGFR therapies. Up to date different mechanisms have been suggested for resistance to TKIs including EGFR independence, mutations and alterations in EGFR, and its downstream signaling pathways [104]. Efforts have focused on overcoming targeted therapy resistance. Thus, in TNBC cells a Src Family Kinases (SFKs) influenced EGFR translocation to nucleus has been reported, which in turn enhances breast cancer cell growth [105]. Within the nucleus, EGFR can function as a cotranscription factor to regulate genes involved in tumor progression [106], which has been linked to anti-EGFR therapies resistance [107]. Importantly, EGFR contributes to chemo- and radioresistance by enhancing DNA damage repair [107]. Inhibition of EGFR translocation led to a subsequent accumulation of EGFR on the plasma membrane, which greatly enhanced sensitivity of TNBC cells to anti-EGFR therapy [105]. Therefore, targeting both the nuclear EGFR signaling pathway, through the inhibition of its nuclear transport, and the classical EGFR signaling pathway may prove a viable therapeutic approach. Moreover, recently it has been demonstrated that the scaffolding protein NHERF1 sensitizes EGFR-dependent tumor growth, motility, and invadopodia function to anti-EGFR (gefitinib) treatment in TNBC cells [104]. Inhibition of IGFB-3 signaling through sphingosine kinase-1 sensitizes TNBC cells to EGF receptor blockade [108]. Furthermore, the blocking of annexin A2 (a calcium-dependent phospholipid binding protein, present at the surface of triple-negative breast cancer cells) by a specific antibody suppressed the EGF-induced EGFR tyrosine phosphorylation and internalization. Treatment with this antibody also inhibited the EGFR-dependent PI3K-Akt and Raf-MEK-ERK downstream pathways, resulting in reduced cell proliferation [109]. The main IGF/EGF-related signaling mechanisms in breast cancer disease are schematically depicted in Figure 1.

4. Bioavailability of Growth Factors

The cellular microenvironment and modifications of extracellular matrix components (ECM) are closely correlated to malignant transformation and all the steps of the metastatic cascade [110, 111]. Namely, the tumor cells do not exist

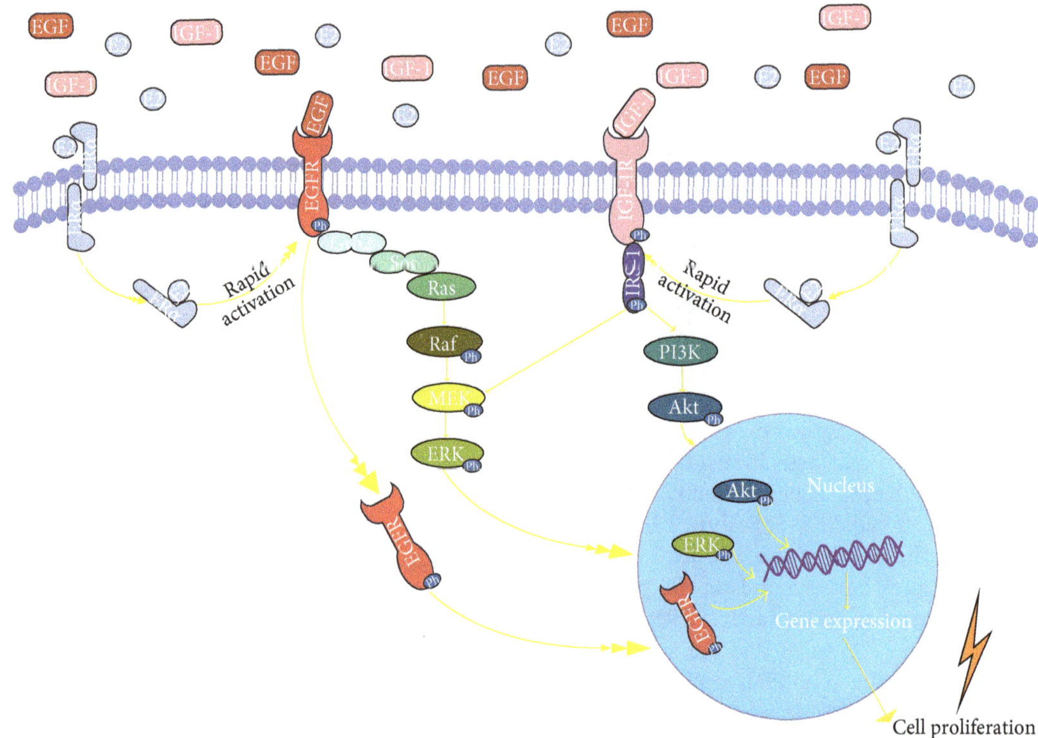

Figure 1: Schematic representation of IGF/EGF signaling, crosstalk with ERs. IGF-I binding to IGF-IR results in its activation and the consequent activation of PI-3K and ERK mediators. EGF-induced activation of EGFR activates the ERK and may lead to gene expression of proliferative genes via internalization of activated EGFR to nucleus. E2-ERα binding leads to rapid activation of EGFR and/or IGF-IR. The activation of IGF/EGF signaling pathways stimulates cell proliferation.

in isolation but rather subsist in a rich microenvironment provided by resident fibroblasts, endothelial cells, pericytes, leukocytes, and ECM components. Indeed, interactions with the tumor microenvironment or stroma are recognized as one of important "hallmarks of cancer."

In addition the ECM is characterized as a big "tank" containing various mediators including growth factors and cytokine which are either soluble or bound into structural ECM components [112]. We discuss here the fact that bioavailability of EGF and IGF-I, provided by the tumor microenvironment, modulates phenotypic plasticity, gene expression, and the recurrence rate of certain TNBC tumors. Combinatorial therapy with EGFR and IGF-IR inhibitors prevents disease progression by interrupting paracrine interactions between TNBC tumor cells and their microenvironment.

The ECM turnover and remodeling are extremely active in the tumor microenvironment [111]. The ECM components are modified through the actions of various proteases and glycosidases which results in altered ECM structure and bioavailability of key mediators [113]. Indeed, the proteolytic action of various enzymes modulates the bioavailability of soluble growth factors which via the activation of specific intracellular signaling pathways regulate critical tumor cell functions, such as migration and proliferation. The matrix metalloproteinase's family (MMP) which consists of 24 (known) zinc-dependent endopeptidases has a key role in the ECM reorganization that occurs during cancer progression [114]. Specifically, the MMPs' action in the tumor microenvironment creates space for cancer cell migration and regulates their cell proliferation by proteolytical release and activation of the ECM-stored growth factors [114].

5. Therapeutic Approach

Targeting of EGF/IGF signaling pathway components has been characterized as a promising approach for breast cancer treatment. Many research groups have focused on the utilization of natural and synthetic inhibitors as well as specific antibodies for EGF family proteins as a strategy to attenuate breast cancer cell proliferation [115–117]. Gefitinib, a tyrosine kinase inhibitor, has been shown to reduce cell proliferation and tumor growth in breast cancer cell lines or *in vivo* conditions in xenografted animals with different levels of EGFR or HER2 expression [118]. Different combinatorial regimes have been approached; thus, the combination of gefitinib with calcitriol or their synthetic analogs resulted in a greater antiproliferative effect than with either of the agents alone in EGFR and HER2 positive breast cancer cells. These effects were due to downregulation of MAPK signaling pathway, decrease of cells in G2/M phase, and induction of apoptosis mediated by upregulation of BIM and activation of caspase 3 [119]. The utilization of monoclonal antibodies is a well-documented approach. Thus, trastuzumab, pertuzumab, and ado-trastuzumabemtansine, which are given intravenously, are monoclonal antibodies that target the ErbB extracellular domains and are used for the treatment of ErbB2-positive breast cancer [120]. The effects of natural products on EGF signaling have also been investigated. Indeed, HMQ1611, a taspine derivative, with anticancer properties, has been shown to reduce the phosphorylation of EGFR and the activation of its downstream signaling mediators ERK1/2 and Akt [117]. Additionally, extracts of *Livistona chinensis* R seeds, with both anticancer and protein kinase inhibitor activity, can attenuate EGF signaling events mainly through EGFR modification [121]. Another agent, (+)-aeroplysinin-1 (a natural metabolite from a type of marine sponge), abolished the proliferative effect of EGF on breast cancer cells and inhibited the ligand-induced endocytosis of the EGFR *in vitro* [122]. However, even though anti-EGFR or combinatorial treatments have been endorsed they are unfortunately meeting with resistance. Current research is focused on increasing our understanding on the mechanisms of response and the discovery of predictive markers. Due to overlapping and redundancy targeting several pathways simultaneously seem essential [123].

Many research groups have endeavored to inhibit the IGF-I signaling, via IGF-IR blockade [68, 124, 125]. This strategy resulted in antiproliferative effects and conclusion that IGF-IR blockade may provide a number of clinical benefits [68]. Furthermore, the effects of natural products on IGF-induced cell proliferation have also been widely studied [124–126]. Thus, it has been reported that samsum ant venom (SAV) inhibits the IGF-I mediated phosphorylation of ERK and AKT, but not p38MAPK [126]. Moreover, deguelin, a natural product isolated from several plant species, has antitumor activity, targeting IGF-IR signaling pathway via upregulation of IGFBP-3 expression [124]. Nimbolide is a terpenoid lactone derived from *Azadirachta indica* (Neem tree) displaying a variety of biological activities. Nimbolide decreases the proliferation of breast cancer cells by modulating the IGF signaling molecules [125]. Calycosin, a natural phytoestrogen with similar structure to estrogen, successfully induced apoptosis of MCF-7 breast cancer cells. Calycosin tends to inhibit growth by ERβ-induced inhibition of IGF-IR, along with the selective regulation of MAPK and phosphatidylinositol 3-kinase (PI-3K)/Akt pathways [127]. However, even though IGF-IR appeared to be one of promising new targets and early results from clinical trials that targeted the IGF-IR and showed some evidence of response, larger randomized phase III trials have not shown clear clinical benefit of targeting this pathway in combination with conventional strategies [71, 128]. These findings may partly be explained by the complexity of the IGF/insulin system. Thus, surface composition of the receptors, preferential expressions of IRS adaptor proteins, and expression of respective ligands may affect therapeutic outcomes and disease prognosis [129–131]. Therefore, assessment of above factors may be necessary for identification of patients who would benefit from anti-IGFR therapy.

6. Conclusions

The bridging between preclinical studies and useful clinical strategies seems to demand a deeper understanding of these complex pathways. Development of predictive molecular biomarkers and optimal inhibitory approaches of the IGF/EGF systems should yield better clinical strategies. In conclusion, unraveling the interaction between the critical signaling pathways in breast cancer biology including ERα, EGFR, and IGF components should provide additional new concepts in designing combination therapies.

Conflict of Interests

The authors declare that there is no conflict of interests regarding the publication of this paper.

Acknowledgments

Part of this research has been cofinanced by the European Union (European Social Fund (ESF)) and Greek national funds through the Operational Program "Education and Lifelong Learning" of the National Strategic Reference Framework (NSRF), Research Funding Program THALES, investing in knowledge society through the European Social Fund MIS 380222.

References

[1] M. W. Beckmann, M. R. Bani, P. A. Fasching, R. Strick, and M. P. Lux, "Risk and risk assessment for breast cancer: molecular and clinical aspects," *Maturitas*, vol. 57, no. 1, pp. 56–60, 2007.

[2] R. B. Dickson and M. E. Lippman, "Estrogenic regulation of growth and polypeptide growth factor secretion in human breast carcinoma," *Endocrine Reviews*, vol. 8, no. 1, pp. 29–43, 1987.

[3] C. L. Arteaga, L. J. Kitten, E. B. Coronado et al., "Blockade of the type I somatomedin receptor inhibits growth of human breast cancer cells in athymic mice," *The Journal of Clinical Investigation*, vol. 84, no. 5, pp. 1418–1423, 1989.

[4] A. Milani, E. Geuna, G. Mittica et al., "Overcoming endocrine resistance in metastatic breast cancer: current evidence and future directions," *World Journal of Clinical Oncology*, vol. 5, no. 5, pp. 990–1001, 2014.

[5] M. A. Shupnik, "Crosstalk between steroid receptors and the c-Src-receptor tyrosine kinase pathways: implications for cell proliferation," *Oncogene*, vol. 23, no. 48, pp. 7979–7989, 2004.

[6] J. M. Gee, J. F. Robertson, E. Gutteridge et al., "Epidermal growth factor receptor/HER2/insulin-like growth factor receptor signalling and oestrogen receptor activity in clinical breast cancer," *Endocrine-Related Cancer*, vol. 12, supplement 1, pp. S99–S111, 2005.

[7] D. J. Riese II and D. F. Stern, "Specificity within the EGF family/ErbB receptor family signaling network," *BioEssays*, vol. 20, no. 1, pp. 41–48, 1998.

[8] N. E. Hynes and D. F. Stern, "The biology of erbB-2/neu/HER-2 and its role in cancer," *Biochimica et Biophysica Acta*, vol. 1198, no. 2-3, pp. 165–184, 1994.

[9] D. Meyer and C. Birchmeier, "Multiple essential functions of neuregulin in development," *Nature*, vol. 378, no. 6555, pp. 386–390, 1995.

[10] J. Massagué and A. Pandiella, "Membrane-anchored growth factors," *Annual Review of Biochemistry*, vol. 62, pp. 515–541, 1993.

[11] T. Holbro, G. Civenni, and N. E. Hynes, "The ErbB receptors and their role in cancer progression," *Experimental Cell Research*, vol. 284, no. 1, pp. 99–110, 2003.

[12] R. Pinkas-Kramarski, L. Soussan, H. Waterman et al., "Diversification of Neu differentiation factor and epidermal growth factor signaling by combinatorial receptor interactions," *The EMBO Journal*, vol. 15, no. 10, pp. 2452–2467, 1996.

[13] M. A. Olayioye, R. M. Neve, H. A. Lane, and N. E. Hynes, "The ErbB signaling network: receptor heterodimerization in development and cancer," *The EMBO Journal*, vol. 19, no. 13, pp. 3159–3167, 2000.

[14] Y. Yarden and M. X. Sliwkowski, "Untangling the ErbB signalling network," *Nature Reviews Molecular Cell Biology*, vol. 2, no. 2, pp. 127–137, 2001.

[15] B. Bucci, I. D'Agnano, C. Botti et al., "EGF-R expression in ductal breast cancer: proliferation and prognostic implications," *Anticancer Research*, vol. 17, no. 1, pp. 769–774, 1997.

[16] S. S. Skandalis, N. Afratis, G. Smirlaki et al., "Cross-talk between estradiol receptor and EGFR/IGF-IR signaling pathways in estrogen-responsive breast cancers: focus on the role and impact of proteoglycans," *Matrix Biology*, vol. 35, pp. 182–193, 2014.

[17] D. F. Stern, P. A. Heffernan, and R. A. Weinberg, "P185, a product of the neu proto-oncogene, is a receptorlike protein associated with tyrosine kinase activity," *Molecular and Cellular Biology*, vol. 6, no. 5, pp. 1729–1740, 1986.

[18] X.-F. Dong, Y. Berthois, and P. M. Martin, "Effect of epidermal growth factor on the proliferation of human epithelial cancer cell lines: correlation with the level of occupied EGF receptor," *Anticancer Research*, vol. 11, no. 2, pp. 737–743, 1991.

[19] E. R. Levin, "Bidirectional signaling between the estrogen receptor and the epidermal growth factor receptor," *Molecular Endocrinology*, vol. 17, no. 3, pp. 309–317, 2003.

[20] X. Fu, C. K. Osborne, and R. Schiff, "Biology and therapeutic potential of PI3K signaling in ER+/HER2-negative breast cancer," *The Breast*, vol. 22, pp. S12–S18, 2013.

[21] P.-Y. Chu, T.-K. Li, S.-T. Ding, I.-R. Lai, and T.-L. Shen, "EGF-induced Grb7 recruits and promotes ras activity essential for the tumorigenicity of Sk-Br3 breast cancer cells," *The Journal of Biological Chemistry*, vol. 285, no. 38, pp. 29279–29285, 2010.

[22] J. Mendelsohn and J. Baselga, "The EGF receptor family as targets for cancer therapy," *Oncogene*, vol. 19, no. 56, pp. 6550–6565, 2000.

[23] E. Gaucci, F. Altieri, C. Turano, and S. Chichiarelli, "The protein ERp57 contributes to EGF receptor signaling and internalization in MDA-MB-468 breast cancer cells," *Journal of Cellular Biochemistry*, vol. 114, no. 11, pp. 2461–2470, 2013.

[24] F. Bianchi, A. Magnifico, C. Olgiati et al., "FHIT-proteasome degradation caused by mitogenic stimulation of the EGF receptor family in cancer cells," *Proceedings of the National Academy of Sciences of the United States of America*, vol. 103, no. 50, pp. 18981–18986, 2006.

[25] J. Filmus, M. N. Pollak, R. Cailleau, and R. N. Buick, "MDA-468, a human breast cancer cell line with a high number of epidermal growth factor (EGF) receptors, has an amplified EGF receptor gene and is growth inhibited by EGF," *Biochemical and Biophysical Research Communications*, vol. 128, no. 2, pp. 898–905, 1985.

[26] S. L. Grant, A. Hammacher, A. M. Douglas et al., "An unexpected biochemical and functional interaction between gp130 and the EGF receptor family in breast cancer cells," *Oncogene*, vol. 21, no. 3, pp. 460–474, 2002.

[27] B. D. Adams, D. M. Cowee, and B. A. White, "The role of miR-206 in the epidermal growth factor (EGF) induced repression of estrogen receptor-alpha (EERalpha) signaling and a luminal phenotype in MCF-7 breast cancer cells," *Molecular Endocrinology*, vol. 23, no. 8, pp. 1215–1230, 2009.

[28] X. Zhang, J. Meng, and Z.-Y. Wang, "A switch role of Src in the biphasic EGF signaling of ER-negative breast cancer cells," *PLoS ONE*, vol. 7, no. 8, Article ID e41613, 2012.

[29] J.-F. Zheng, L.-C. Sun, H. Liu, Y. Huang, Y. Li, and J. He, "EBP50 exerts tumor suppressor activity by promoting cell apoptosis and retarding extracellular signal-regulated kinase activity," *Amino Acids*, vol. 38, no. 4, pp. 1261–1268, 2010.

[30] W. Yao, D. Feng, W. Bian et al., "EBP50 inhibits EGF-induced breast cancer cell proliferation by blocking EGFR phosphorylation," *Amino Acids*, vol. 43, no. 5, pp. 2027–2035, 2012.

[31] R. Baserga, A. Hongo, M. Rubini, M. Prisco, and B. Valentinis, "The IGF-I receptor in cell growth, transformation and apoptosis," *Biochimica et Biophysica Acta*, vol. 1332, no. 3, pp. F105–F126, 1997.

[32] D. LeRoith and C. T. Roberts Jr., "The insulin-like growth factor system and cancer," *Cancer Letters*, vol. 195, no. 2, pp. 127–137, 2003.

[33] D. LeRoith, H. Werner, D. Beitner-Johnson, and C. T. Roberts Jr., "Molecular and cellular aspects of the insulin-like growth factor I receptor," *Endocrine Reviews*, vol. 16, no. 2, pp. 143–163, 1995.

[34] W. H. Daughaday and P. Rotwein, "Insulin-like growth factors I and II. Peptide, messenger ribonucleic acid and gene structures, serum, and tissue concentrations," *Endocrine Reviews*, vol. 10, no. 1, pp. 68–91, 1989.

[35] L. Sepp-Lorenzino, "Structure and function of the insulin-like growth factor I receptor," *Breast Cancer Research and Treatment*, vol. 47, no. 3, pp. 235–253, 1998.

[36] E. Surmacz, "Function of the IGF-I receptor in breast cancer," *Journal of Mammary Gland Biology and Neoplasia*, vol. 5, no. 1, pp. 95–105, 2000.

[37] E. A. Bohula, M. P. Playford, and V. M. Macaulay, "Targeting the type 1 insulin-like growth factor receptor as anti-cancer treatment," *Anti-Cancer Drugs*, vol. 14, no. 9, pp. 669–682, 2003.

[38] A. Ullrich, A. Gray, A. W. Tam et al., "Insulin-like growth factor I receptor primary structure: comparison with insulin receptor suggests structural determinants that define functional specificity," *The EMBO Journal*, vol. 5, no. 10, pp. 2503–2512, 1986.

[39] R. Baserga, F. Peruzzi, and K. Reiss, "The IGF-1 receptor in cancer biology," *International Journal of Cancer*, vol. 107, no. 6, pp. 873–877, 2003.

[40] H. Kato, T. N. Faria, B. Stannard, C. T. Roberts Jr., and D. LeRoith, "Essential role of tyrosine residues 1131, 1135, and 1136 of the insulin-like growth factor-I (IGF-I) receptor in IGF-I action," *Molecular Endocrinology*, vol. 8, no. 1, pp. 40–50, 1994.

[41] A. Grimberg and P. Cohen, "Role of insulin-like growth factors and their binding proteins in growth control and carcinogenesis," *Journal of Cellular Physiology*, vol. 183, no. 1, pp. 1–9, 2000.

[42] S. M. Firth and R. C. Baxter, "Cellular actions of the insulin-like growth factor binding proteins," *Endocrine Reviews*, vol. 23, no. 6, pp. 824–854, 2002.

[43] L. S. Laursen, K. Kjaer-Sorensen, M. H. Andersen, and C. Oxvig, "Regulation of insulin-like growth factor (IGF) bioactivity by sequential proteolytic cleavage of IGF binding protein-4 and -5," *Molecular Endocrinology*, vol. 21, no. 5, pp. 1246–1257, 2007.

[44] J. I. Jones and D. R. Clemmons, "Insulin-like growth factors and their binding proteins: biological actions," *Endocrine Reviews*, vol. 16, no. 1, pp. 3–34, 1995.

[45] C. M. Perks and J. M. P. Holly, "Insulin-like growth factor binding proteins (IGFBPs) in breast cancer," *Journal of Mammary Gland Biology and Neoplasia*, vol. 5, no. 1, pp. 75–84, 2000.

[46] F. Pekonen, T. Nyman, V. Ilvesmaki, and S. Partanen, "Insulin-like growth factor binding proteins in human breast cancer tissue," *Cancer Research*, vol. 52, no. 19, pp. 5204–5207, 1992.

[47] S. E. McGuire, S. G. Hilsenbeck, J. A. Figueroa, J. G. Jackson, and D. Yee, "Detection of insulin-like growth factor binding proteins (IGFBPs) by ligand blotting in breast cancer tissues," *Cancer Letters*, vol. 77, no. 1, pp. 25–32, 1994.

[48] M. N. Pollak, E. S. Schernhammer, and S. E. Hankinson, "Insulin-like growth factors and neoplasia," *Nature Reviews Cancer*, vol. 4, no. 7, pp. 505–518, 2004.

[49] S. Ahmad, N. Singh, and R. I. Glazer, "Role of AKT1 in 17beta-estradiol- and insulin-like growth factor I (IGF-I)-dependent proliferation and prevention of apoptosis in MCF-7 breast carcinoma cells," *Biochemical Pharmacology*, vol. 58, no. 3, pp. 425–430, 1999.

[50] T. E. Adams, V. C. Epa, T. P. J. Garrett, and C. W. Ward, "Structure and function of the type 1 insulin-like growth factor receptor," *Cellular and Molecular Life Sciences*, vol. 57, no. 7, pp. 1050–1093, 2000.

[51] E. C. Martin, M. R. Bratton, Y. Zhu et al., "Insulin-like growth factor-1 signaling regulates miRNA expression in MCF-7 breast cancer cell line," *PLoS ONE*, vol. 7, no. 11, Article ID e49067, 2012.

[52] J. A. McCubrey, L. S. Steelman, S. L. Abrams et al., "Roles of the RAF/MEK/ERK and PI3K/PTEN/AKT pathways in malignant transformation and drug resistance," *Advances in Enzyme Regulation*, vol. 46, no. 1, pp. 249–279, 2006.

[53] J. Whyte, O. Bergin, A. Bianchi, S. McNally, and F. Martin, "Key signalling nodes in mammary gland development and cancer. Mitogen-activated protein kinase signalling in experimental models of breast cancer progression and in mammary gland development," *Breast Cancer Research*, vol. 11, no. 5, article 209, 2009.

[54] E. K. Jeong, S. Y. Lee, H. M. Jeon, M. K. Ju, C. H. Kim, and H. S. Kang, "Role of extracellular signal-regulated kinase (ERK)1/2 in multicellular resistance to docetaxel in MCF-7 cells," *International Journal of Oncology*, vol. 37, no. 3, pp. 655–661, 2010.

[55] C. L. Mamay, A. M. Mingo-Sion, D. M. Wolf, M. D. Molina, and C. L. Van Den Berg, "An inhibitory function for JNK in the regulation of IGF-I signaling in breast cancer," *Oncogene*, vol. 22, no. 4, pp. 602–614, 2003.

[56] H. Kato, T. N. Faria, B. Stannard, C. T. Roberts Jr., and D. LeRoith, "Role of tyrosine kinase activity in signal transduction by the insulin-like growth factor-I (IGF-I) receptor: characterization of kinase-deficient IGF-I receptors and the action of an IGF-I-mimetic antibody (αIR-3)," *Journal of Biological Chemistry*, vol. 268, no. 4, pp. 2655–2661, 1993.

[57] M. G. Myers Jr., X. J. Sun, and M. F. White, "The IRS-1 signaling system," *Trends in Biochemical Sciences*, vol. 19, no. 7, pp. 289–293, 1994.

[58] M. G. Myers Jr., X. J. Sun, B. Cheatham et al., "IRS-1 is a common element in insulin and insulin-like growth factor-I signaling to the phosphatidylinositol 3′-kinase," *Endocrinology*, vol. 132, no. 4, pp. 1421–1430, 1993.

[59] M. G. Myers Jr., L.-M. Wang, X. J. Sun et al., "Role of IRS-1-GRB-2 complexes in insulin signaling," *Molecular and Cellular Biology*, vol. 14, no. 6, pp. 3577–3587, 1994.

[60] E. Y. Skolnik, C. H. Lee, A. Batzer et al., "The SH2/SH3 domain-containing protein GRB2 interacts with tyrosine-phosphorylated IRS1 and Shc: implications for insulin control of ras signalling," *The EMBO Journal*, vol. 12, no. 5, pp. 1929–1936, 1993.

[61] R. Baserga, C. Sell, P. Porcu, and M. Rubini, "The role of the IGF-I receptor in the growth and transformation of mammalian cells," *Cell Proliferation*, vol. 27, no. 2, pp. 63–71, 1994.

[62] S. Giorgetti, P. G. Pelicci, G. Pelicci, and E. Von Obberghen, "Involvement of Src-homology/collagen (SHC) proteins in signaling through the insulin receptor and the insulin-like-growth-factor-I-receptor," *European Journal of Biochemistry*, vol. 223, no. 1, pp. 195–202, 1994.

[63] A. Morrione, B. Valentinis, S. Li, J. Y. T. Ooi, B. Margolis, and R. Baserga, "Grb10: a new substrate of the insulin-like growth factor I receptor," *Cancer Research*, vol. 56, no. 14, pp. 3165–3167, 1996.

[64] V. Baron, V. Calléja, P. Ferrari, F. Alengrin, and E. Van Obberghen, "p125(Fak) focal adhesion kinase is a substrate for the insulin and insulin-like growth factor-I tyrosine kinase receptors," *The Journal of Biological Chemistry*, vol. 273, no. 12, pp. 7162–7168, 1998.

[65] C. Arbet-Engels, S. Tartare-Deckert, and W. Eckhart, "C-terminal Src kinase associates with ligand-stimulated insulin-like growth factor-I receptor," *The Journal of Biological Chemistry*, vol. 274, no. 9, pp. 5422–5428, 1999.

[66] S. Zhang, X. Li, R. Burghardt, R. Smith III, and S. H. Safe, "Role of estrogen receptor (ER) alpha in insulin-like growth factor (IGF)-I-induced responses in MCF-7 breast cancer cells," *Journal of Molecular Endocrinology*, vol. 35, no. 3, pp. 433–447, 2005.

[67] S. Sarkissyan, M. Sarkissyan, Y. Wu, J. Cardenas, H. P. Koeffler, and J. V. Vadgama, "IGF-1 regulates Cyr61 induced breast cancer cell proliferation and invasion," *PLoS ONE*, vol. 9, no. 7, Article ID e103534, 2014.

[68] D. Burtrum, Z. Zhu, D. Lu et al., "A fully human monoclonal antibody to the insulin-like growth factor I receptor blocks ligand-dependent signaling and inhibits human tumor growth in vivo," *Cancer Research*, vol. 63, no. 24, pp. 8912–8921, 2003.

[69] S. Yakar, D. LeRoith, and P. Brodt, "The role of the growth hormone/insulin-like growth factor axis in tumor growth and progression: lessons from animal models," *Cytokine and Growth Factor Reviews*, vol. 16, no. 4-5, pp. 407–420, 2005.

[70] R. A. Mendoza, E. E. Moody, M. I. Enriquez, S. M. Mejia, and G. Thordarson, "Tumorigenicity of MCF-7 human breast cancer cells lacking the p38alpha mitogen-activated protein kinase," *Journal of Endocrinology*, vol. 208, no. 1, pp. 11–19, 2011.

[71] D. Yee, "Insulin-like growth factor receptor inhibitors: baby or the bathwater?" *Journal of the National Cancer Institute*, vol. 104, no. 13, pp. 975–981, 2012.

[72] S. Abramovitch and H. Werner, "Functional and physical interactions between BRCA1 and p53 in transcriptional regulation of the IGF-IR gene," *Hormone and Metabolic Research*, vol. 35, no. 11-12, pp. 758–762, 2003.

[73] R. Sarfstein, S. Maor, N. Reizner, S. Abramovitch, and H. Werner, "Transcriptional regulation of the insulin-like growth factor-I receptor gene in breast cancer," *Molecular and Cellular Endocrinology*, vol. 252, no. 1-2, pp. 241–246, 2006.

[74] Q. Wang, H. Zhang, R. Fishel, and M. I. Greene, "BRCA1 and cell signaling," *Oncogene*, vol. 19, no. 53, pp. 6152–6158, 2000.

[75] V. Shukla, X. Coumoul, L. Cao et al., "Absence of the full-length breast cancer-associated gene-1 leads to increased expression of insulin-like growth factor signaling axis members," *Cancer Research*, vol. 66, no. 14, pp. 7151–7157, 2006.

[76] G. Hudelist, T. Wagner, M. Rosner et al., "Intratumoral IGF-I protein expression is selectively upregulated in breast cancer patients with BRCA1/2 mutations," *Endocrine-Related Cancer*, vol. 14, no. 4, pp. 1053–1062, 2007.

[77] N. J. G. Webster, J. L. Resnik, D. B. Reichart, B. Strauss, M. Haas, and B. L. Seely, "Repression of the insulin receptor promoter by the tumor suppressor gene product p53: a possible mechanism for receptor overexpression in breast cancer," *Cancer Research*, vol. 56, no. 12, pp. 2781–2788, 1996.

[78] H. Werner and S. Maor, "The insulin-like growth factor-I receptor gene: a downstream target for oncogene and tumor suppressor action," *Trends in Endocrinology and Metabolism*, vol. 17, no. 6, pp. 236–242, 2006.

[79] E. M. Fox, T. M. Bernaciak, J. Wen, A. M. Weaver, M. A. Shupnik, and C. M. Silva, "Signal transducer and activator of transcription 5b, c-Src, and epidermal growth factor receptor signaling play integral roles in estrogen-stimulated proliferation of estrogen receptor-positive breast cancer cells," *Molecular Endocrinology*, vol. 22, no. 8, pp. 1781–1796, 2008.

[80] E. M. Fox, J. Andrade, and M. A. Shupnik, "Novel actions of estrogen to promote proliferation: integration of cytoplasmic and nuclear pathways," *Steroids*, vol. 74, no. 7, pp. 622–627, 2009.

[81] S. Ali, L. Buluwela, and R. C. Coombes, "Antiestrogens and their therapeutic applications in breast cancer and other diseases," *Annual Review of Medicine*, vol. 62, pp. 217–232, 2011.

[82] C. Barrios, J. F. Forbes, W. Jonat et al., "The sequential use of endocrine treatment for advanced breast cancer: where are we?" *Annals of Oncology*, vol. 23, no. 6, pp. 1378–1386, 2012.

[83] V.-I. Alexaki, I. Charalampopoulos, M. Kampa et al., "Estrogen exerts neuroprotective effects via membrane estrogen receptors and rapid Akt/NOS activation," *The FASEB Journal*, vol. 18, no. 13, pp. 1594–1596, 2004.

[84] B. Dufourny, J. Alblas, H. A. A. M. van Teeffelen et al., "Mitogenic signaling of insulin-like growth factor I in MCF-7 human breast cancer cells requires phosphatidylinositol 3-kinase and is independent of mitogen-activated protein kinase," *The Journal of Biological Chemistry*, vol. 272, no. 49, pp. 31163–31171, 1997.

[85] T. van Agthoven, J. Veldscholte, M. Smid et al., "Functional identification of genes causing estrogen independence of human breast cancer cells," *Breast Cancer Research and Treatment*, vol. 114, no. 1, pp. 23–30, 2009.

[86] S. Kahlert, S. Nuedling, M. van Eickels, H. Vetter, R. Meyer, and C. Grohé, "Estrogen receptor alpha rapidly activates the IGF-1 receptor pathway," *Journal of Biological Chemistry*, vol. 275, no. 24, pp. 18447–18453, 2000.

[87] R. J. Pietras, "Interactions between estrogen and growth factor receptors in human breast cancers and the tumor-associated vasculature," *Breast Journal*, vol. 9, no. 5, pp. 361–373, 2003.

[88] R. X.-D. Song, Y. Chen, Z. Zhang et al., "Estrogen utilization of IGF-1-R and EGF-R to signal in breast cancer cells," *The Journal of Steroid Biochemistry and Molecular Biology*, vol. 118, no. 4-5, pp. 219–230, 2010.

[89] J. M. Hall, J. F. Couse, and K. S. Korach, "The multifaceted mechanisms of estradiol and estrogen receptor signaling," *The Journal of Biological Chemistry*, vol. 276, no. 40, pp. 36869–36872, 2001.

[90] R. X.-D. Song, Z. Zhang, Y. Chen, Y. Bao, and R. J. Santen, "Estrogen signaling via a linear pathway involving insulin-like growth factor I receptor, matrix metalloproteinases, and epidermal growth factor receptor to activate mitogen-activated protein kinase in MCF-7 breast cancer cells," *Endocrinology*, vol. 148, no. 8, pp. 4091–4101, 2007.

[91] M. H. Faulds, H. Olsen, L. A. Helguero, J.-Å. Gustafsson, and L.-A. Haldosén, "Estrogen receptor functional activity changes during differentiation of mammary epithelial cells," *Molecular Endocrinology*, vol. 18, no. 2, pp. 412–421, 2004.

[92] A. Migliaccio, M. Di Domenico, G. Castoria et al., "Steroid receptor regulation of epidermal growth factor signaling through Src in breast and prostate cancer cells: steroid antagonist action," *Cancer Research*, vol. 65, no. 22, pp. 10585–10593, 2005.

[93] B. D. Gehm, J. M. McAndrews, V. C. Jordan, and J. L. Jameson, "EGF activates highly selective estrogen-responsive reporter plasmids by an ER-independent pathway," *Molecular and Cellular Endocrinology*, vol. 159, no. 1-2, pp. 53–62, 2000.

[94] Y. Hawsawi, R. El-Gendy, C. Twelves, V. Speirs, and J. Beattie, "Insulin-like growth factor—oestradiol crosstalk and mammary gland tumourigenesis," *Biochimica et Biophysica Acta—Reviews on Cancer*, vol. 1836, no. 2, pp. 345–353, 2013.

[95] S. Nilsson, S. Mäkelä, E. Treuter et al., "Mechanisms of estrogen action," *Physiological Reviews*, vol. 81, no. 4, pp. 1535–1565, 2001.

[96] D. Yee and A. V. Lee, "Crosstalk between the insulin-like growth factors and estrogens in breast cancer," *Journal of Mammary Gland Biology and Neoplasia*, vol. 5, no. 1, pp. 107–115, 2000.

[97] J. Dupont and D. Le Roith, "Insulin-like growth factor 1 and oestradiol promote cell proliferation of MCF-7 breast cancer cells: new insights into their synergistic effects," *Journal of Clinical Pathology: Molecular Pathology*, vol. 54, no. 3, pp. 149–154, 2001.

[98] R. X. Song, C. J. Barnes, Z. Zhang, Y. Bao, R. Kumar, and R. J. Santen, "The role of Shc and insulin-like growth factor 1 receptor in mediating the translocation of estrogen receptor α to the plasma membrane," *Proceedings of the National Academy of Sciences of the United States of America*, vol. 101, no. 7, pp. 2076–2081, 2004.

[99] Z. Yu, W. Gao, E. Jiang et al., "Interaction between IGF-IR and ER Induced by E2 and IGF-I," *PLoS ONE*, vol. 8, no. 5, Article ID e62642, 2013.

[100] A.-M. Gaben, M. Sabbah, G. Redeuilh, M. Bedin, and J. Mester, "Ligand-free estrogen receptor activity complements IGF1R to induce the proliferation of the MCF-7 breast cancer cells," *BMC Cancer*, vol. 12, article 291, 2012.

[101] S. Amin, A. Kumar, L. Nilchi, K. Wright, and M. Kozlowski, "Breast cancer cells proliferation is regulated by tyrosine phosphatase SHP1 through c-jun N-terminal kinase and cooperative induction of RFX-1 and AP-4 transcription factors," *Molecular Cancer Research*, vol. 9, no. 8, pp. 1112–1125, 2011.

[102] K. N. Stevens, C. M. Vachon, and F. J. Couch, "Genetic susceptibility to triple-negative breast cancer," *Cancer Research*, vol. 73, no. 7, pp. 2025–2030, 2013.

[103] N. M. Probst-Hensch, J. H. B. Steiner, P. Schraml et al., "IGFBP2 and IGFBP3 protein expressions in human breast cancer: association with hormonal factors and obesity," *Clinical Cancer Research*, vol. 16, no. 3, pp. 1025–1032, 2010.

[104] A. Bellizzi, M. R. Greco, R. Rubino et al., "The scaffolding protein NHERF1 sensitizes EGFR-dependent tumor growth,

motility and invadopodia function to gefitinib treatment in breast cancer cells," *International Journal of Oncology*, vol. 46, no. 3, pp. 1214–1224, 2015.

[105] T. M. Brand, M. Iida, E. F. Dunn et al., "Nuclear epidermal growth factor receptor is a functional molecular target in triple-negative breast cancer," *Molecular Cancer Therapeutics*, vol. 13, no. 5, pp. 1356–1368, 2014.

[106] T. M. Brand, M. Iida, C. Li, and D. L. Wheeler, "The nuclear epidermal growth factor receptor signaling network and its role in cancer," *Discovery Medicine*, vol. 12, no. 66, pp. 419–432, 2011.

[107] W.-C. Huang, Y.-J. Chen, L.-Y. Li et al., "Nuclear translocation of epidermal growth factor receptor by Akt-dependent phosphorylation enhances breast cancer-resistant protein expression in gefitinib-resistant cells," *The Journal of Biological Chemistry*, vol. 286, no. 23, pp. 20558–20568, 2011.

[108] J. L. Martin, H. C. De Silva, M. Z. Lin, C. D. Scott, and R. C. Baxter, "Inhibition of insulin-like growth factor-binding protein-3 signaling through sphingosine kinase-1 sensitizes triple-negative breast cancer cells to egf receptor Blockade," *Molecular Cancer Therapeutics*, vol. 13, no. 2, pp. 316–328, 2014.

[109] P. Chaudhary, S. I. Thamake, P. Shetty, and J. K. Vishwanatha, "Inhibition of triple-negative and Herceptin-resistant breast cancer cell proliferation and migration by Annexin A2 antibodies," *British Journal of Cancer*, vol. 111, no. 12, pp. 2328-2341, 2014.

[110] N. Afratis, C. Gialeli, D. Nikitovic et al., "Glycosaminoglycans: key players in cancer cell biology and treatment," *The FEBS Journal*, vol. 279, no. 7, pp. 1177–1197, 2012.

[111] D. Nikitovic, K. Kouvidi, K. Voudouri et al., "The motile breast cancer phenotype roles of proteoglycans/glycosaminoglycans," *BioMed Research International*, vol. 2014, Article ID 124321, 13 pages, 2014.

[112] C. A. Kirkpatrick and S. B. Selleck, "Heparan sulfate proteoglycans at a glance," *Journal of Cell Science*, vol. 120, no. 11, pp. 1829–1832, 2007.

[113] C. Gialeli, A. D. Theocharis, and N. K. Karamanos, "Roles of matrix metalloproteinases in cancer progression and their pharmacological targeting," *The FEBS Journal*, vol. 278, no. 1, pp. 16–27, 2011.

[114] K. Kessenbrock, V. Plaks, and Z. Werb, "Matrix metalloproteinases: regulators of the tumor microenvironment," *Cell*, vol. 141, no. 1, pp. 52–67, 2010.

[115] S. Ghosh, R. K. Narla, Y. Zheng et al., "Structure-based design of potent inhibitors of EGF-receptor tyrosine kinase as anti-cancer agents," *Anti-Cancer Drug Design*, vol. 14, no. 5, pp. 403–410, 1999.

[116] O. M. Fattah, S. M. Cloutier, C. Kündig et al., "Peptabody-EGF: a novel apoptosis inducer targeting ErbB1 receptor overexpressing cancer cells," *International Journal of Cancer*, vol. 119, no. 10, pp. 2455–2463, 2006.

[117] Y. Zhan, Y. Zhang, C. Liu et al., "A novel taspine derivative, HMQ1611, inhibits breast cancer cell growth via estrogen receptor α and EGF receptor signaling pathways," *Cancer Prevention Research*, vol. 5, no. 6, pp. 864–873, 2012.

[118] J. Anido, P. Matar, J. Albanell et al., "ZD1839, a specific epidermal growth factor receptor (EGFR) tyrosine kinase inhibitor, induces the formation of inactive EGFR/HER2 and EGFR/HER3 heterodimers and prevents heregulin signaling in HER2-overexpressing breast cancer cells," *Clinical Cancer Research*, vol. 9, no. 4, pp. 1274–1283, 2003.

[119] M. Segovia-Mendoza, L. Díaz, M. E. González-González et al., "Calcitriol and its analogues enhance the antiproliferative activity of gefitinib in breast cancer cells," *The Journal of Steroid Biochemistry and Molecular Biology*, vol. 148, pp. 122–131, 2015.

[120] R. Roskoski, "The ErbB/HER family of protein-tyrosine kinases and cancer," *Pharmacological Research*, vol. 79, pp. 34–74, 2014.

[121] W.-C. Huang, R.-M. Hsu, L.-M. Chi, Y.-L. Leu, Y.-S. Chang, and J.-S. Yu, "Selective downregulation of EGF receptor and downstream MAPK pathway in human cancer cell lines by active components partially purified from the seeds of *Livistona chinensis* R. Brown," *Cancer Letters*, vol. 248, no. 1, pp. 137–146, 2007.

[122] M.-H. Kreuter, R. E. Leake, F. Rinaldi et al., "Inhibition of intrinsic protein tyrosine kinase activity of EGF-receptor kinase complex from human breast cancer cells by the marine sponge metabolite (+)-aeroplysinin-1," *Comparative Biochemistry and Physiology—Part B: Biochemistry and*, vol. 97, no. 1, pp. 151–158, 1990.

[123] A. Lluch, P. Eroles, and J.-A. Perez-Fidalgo, "Emerging EGFR antagonists for breast cancer," *Expert Opinion on Emerging Drugs*, vol. 19, no. 2, pp. 165–181, 2014.

[124] Y.-A. Suh, J.-H. Kim, M. A. Sung et al., "A novel antitumor activity of deguelin targeting the insulin-like growth factor (IGF) receptor pathway via up-regulation of IGF-binding protein-3 expression in breast cancer," *Cancer Letters*, vol. 332, no. 1, pp. 102–109, 2013.

[125] P. Elumalai, R. Arunkumar, C. S. Benson, G. Sharmila, and J. Arunakaran, "Nimbolide inhibits IGF-I-mediated PI3K/Akt and MAPK signalling in human breast cancer cell lines (MCF-7 and MDA-MB-231)," *Cell Biochemistry & Function*, vol. 32, no. 5, pp. 476–484, 2014.

[126] G. Badr, O. Garraud, M. Daghestani, M. S. Al-Khalifa, and Y. Richard, "Human breast carcinoma cells are induced to apoptosis by samsum ant venom through an IGF-1-dependant pathway, PI3K/AKT and ERK signaling," *Cellular Immunology*, vol. 273, no. 1, pp. 10–16, 2012.

[127] J. Chen, R. Hou, X. Zhang, Y. Ye, Y. Wang, and J. Tian, "Calycosin suppresses breast cancer cell growth via ERβ-dependent regulation of IGF-1R, p38 MAPK and PI3K/Akt pathways," *PLoS ONE*, vol. 9, no. 3, Article ID e91245, 2014.

[128] Y. Yang and D. Yee, "Targeting insulin and insulin-like growth factor signaling in breast cancer," *Journal of Mammary Gland Biology and Neoplasia*, vol. 17, no. 3-4, pp. 251–261, 2012.

[129] S. A. Byron, K. B. Horwitz, J. K. Richer, C. A. Lange, X. Zhang, and D. Yee, "Insulin receptor substrates mediate distinct biological responses to insulin-like growth factor receptor activation in breast cancer cells," *British Journal of Cancer*, vol. 95, no. 9, pp. 1220–1228, 2006.

[130] A. Gualberto, M. L. Hixon, D. D. Karp et al., "Pre-treatment levels of circulating free IGF-1 identify NSCLC patients who derive clinical benefit from figitumumab," *British Journal of Cancer*, vol. 104, no. 1, pp. 68–74, 2011.

[131] M. A. Becker, X. Hou, S. C. Harrington et al., "IGFBP ratio confers resistance to IGF targeting and correlates with increased invasion and poor outcome in breast tumors," *Clinical Cancer Research*, vol. 18, no. 6, pp. 1808–1817, 2012.

16

Fractal Analysis and the Diagnostic Usefulness of Silver Staining Nucleolar Organizer Regions in Prostate Adenocarcinoma

Alex Stepan,[1] Cristiana Simionescu,[1] Daniel Pirici,[1,2] Raluca Ciurea,[1] and Claudiu Margaritescu[1]

[1]*Department of Pathology, University of Medicine and Pharmacy of Craiova, Petru Rares Street 2, Dolj, 200349 Craiova, Romania*
[2]*Department of Research Methodology, University of Medicine and Pharmacy of Craiova, Petru Rares Street 2, Dolj, 200349 Craiova, Romania*

Correspondence should be addressed to Daniel Pirici; danielpirici@yahoo.com

Academic Editor: Anant Madabhushi

Pathological diagnosis of prostate adenocarcinoma often requires complementary methods. On prostate biopsy tissue from 39 patients including benign nodular hyperplasia (BNH), atypical adenomatous hyperplasia (AAH), and adenocarcinomas, we have performed combined histochemical-immunohistochemical stainings for argyrophilic nucleolar organizer regions (AgNORs) and glandular basal cells. After ascertaining the pathology, we have analyzed the number, roundness, area, and fractal dimension of individual AgNORs or of their skeleton-filtered maps. We have optimized here for the first time a combination of AgNOR morphological denominators that would reflect best the differences between these pathologies. The analysis of AgNORs' roundness, averaged from large composite images, revealed clear-cut lower values in adenocarcinomas compared to benign and atypical lesions but with no differences between different Gleason scores. Fractal dimension (FD) of AgNOR silhouettes not only revealed significant lower values for global cancer images compared to AAH and BNH images, but was also able to differentiate between Gleason pattern 2 and Gleason patterns 3–5 adenocarcinomas. Plotting the frequency distribution of the FDs for different pathologies showed clear differences between all Gleason patterns and BNH. Together with existing morphological classifiers, AgNOR analysis might contribute to a faster and more reliable machine-assisted screening of prostatic adenocarcinoma, as an essential aid for pathologists.

1. Introduction

Prostate cancer is considered the second cause of death by malignant neoplasia in the male population around the world, over 95% of all diagnosed cases being represented by acinar adenocarcinoma [1–3]. The incidence of prostate cancer in Romania in 2012 was officially estimated at 20 cases per 100,000 males, these low incidence rates being largely due to underregistration of prostate cancer, as well as the lack of sensitive diagnostic tests for an early detection [4, 5].

Pathological diagnosis of prostate neoplasia is sometimes cumbersome and the differential diagnosis needs to be made with atypical benign lesions. In these cases, techniques such as immunohistochemistry for acinar basal cells [6, 7], the histochemical silver staining for the nucleolar organiser regions (AgNORs) [8], and genetic testings have brought an invaluable support in establishing the correct diagnosis [9, 10]. AgNOR silver impregnation protocols have been utilized and standardized [8, 11, 12] for counting and morphometry and may contribute to the differential diagnosis between benign and malignant prostate lesions, either alone [13–16] or in combination with immunohistochemistry and serologic markers [17–19], and have even been assessed as a prognostic factor for this pathology [20, 21]. Nucleolar organizing regions (NORs) represent fragments of ribosomal DNA involved in transcription of ribosomal RNA, which due to their association with nonhistonic argyrophilic proteins may be observed and quantified after precipitation of silver nitrate [8, 22].

AgNOR analysis is justified by the well-known morphological changes of nucleoli in prostate adenocarcinoma [6]. Beyond subjective observations, automated image analysis for diagnostic applications is currently a dynamically evolving domain, supporting an increasing standardization and an accuracy of the diagnostic process [23, 24]. While classical objective morphological denominators like areas and diameters have proved insufficient to describe highly variable and complex pathological processes, scale-invariant parameters like fractal dimension (FD) have been very useful in characterizing complex and nonregular objects [25]. Classical morphological features are based on Euclidean geometric system that has three dimensions as integers, while the FD of an object is a real (adimensional) number that expresses the morphological complexity and the inner self-similarity of the object or, in simple terms, it characterizes the space-filling properties of that object [25]. The closer this dimension is to the topological dimension of the space in which it resides, the greater its space-filling capacity is, and thus its FD value, with a bidimensional structure (like planar images) having FD values between 1 and 2.

This complexity-related concept is now widely used in pathology to describe tumor angiogenesis, chromatin distribution in malignant cells, or even prostate glands' morphology [26–28].

In this context, the advent of more powerful image analysis segmentation algorithms based on color, intensity, texture, and background contrast, coupled with fractal analysis of AgNOR regions might offer supplemental valuable classifiers for future machine-based diagnostic algorithms that will help the pathologist with classifying benign, atypical, and malignant prostate lesions.

2. Methods

2.1. Patients. Formalin-fixed paraffin-embedded archived prostate transurethral resection of the prostate (TURP) biopsies were selected from previously confirmed patients with benign nodular hyperplasia (number (N) = 8), atypical adenomatous hyperplasia (AAH) (N = 5), and Gleason grading of 2 (N = 5), 3 (N = 5), 4 (N = 7), and 5 (N = 9) conventional acinar adenocarcinoma. All selected cases belong to the archive of the Pathology Department from the Emergency County Hospital 1, Craiova, Romania, and were diagnosed without equivoque as belonging to the respective groups (Alex Stepan, Claudiu Margaritescu, and Daniel Pirici), following the latest WHO grading system [2]. All patients that have been included were at their first presentation, thus without any treatments. A written informed consent was obtained for each patient from their relatives, accepting tissue sampling for research purposes, and the study was approved by the responsible ethical committee.

2.2. Immunohistochemistry and AgNOR Staining. In order to stain for the nucleolar organizers and still identify the histopathology of the tissue with the best contrast, we have optimized a mixed protocol combining the silver staining protocol as proposed by the International Committee on AgNOR Quantitation with immunohistochemistry for basal cells and a Nuclear Red counter staining [12].

The slides were first dewaxed in xylene and rehydrated through graded alcohols to distilled water, and then antigen retrieval was performed by microwaving the sections in sodium-citrate buffer (0.01 M sodium-citrate monohydrate, pH 6.0) for 20 minutes at 650 W. After cooling, the sections were incubated for 30 minutes in a 1% hydrogen peroxide solution and then blocked for 1 hour in 3% skim milk (Bio-Rad, Medicalkit, Craiova, Romania). A mix of 34βE12 (1 : 100) and p63 (1 : 200) mouse anti-human primary antibodies (Dako, Redox, Bucharest, Romania) was added onto the slides for 18 hours at 4°C; the next day the signal was amplified utilizing a peroxidase polymer-based system (Nichirei-Histofine, Medicalkit, Craiova, Romania), and then the signal was detected with Permanent HRP Green substrate (Zytomed, Medicalkit, Craiova, Romania). After washing the slides in distillated water, a modified silver staining protocol was performed [12]. The slides were counterstained in 0.1% Nuclear Red prepared in a 5% aqueous aluminum sulphate solution. The slides were dehydrated fast, cleared in xylene, and mounted in DPX (Fluka, Medicalkit, Craiova, Romania).

2.3. Image Grabbing and Analysis. Light microscopy images were grabbed utilizing a Nikon Eclipse 55i microscope equipped with a 5-megapixel Nikon DS-Fi1 CCD cooled color camera, together with the Nikon NIS-Elements Basic Research image analysis software (Nikon, Apidrag, Bucharest, Romania). Three investigators (AS, CM, and DP) followed the sections individually and, based on the nuclear glandular-like histological staining and the immunohistochemistry for basal cells, respectively, collected suggestive images for Gleason gradings 2, 3, 4, and 5 as well as AAH and benign nodular hyperplasia (BNH), according to the latest WHO grading system. Images have been collected with a 40x objective, either as single frames (57.6583,69 μm^2) or as composites of 24 400x objective areas automatically merged as unique captures in the Nikon NIS-Elements software (Figures 1 and 2). More than 500 images have been captured, saved, and archived as uncompressed tiff files. After confirming once again the grading of the captured images and removing all images on which the investigators did not agree (AS, DP, and CM), AgNOR dots were first manually counted and averaged for epithelial nuclei, using the manual tag option in our image analysis software.

Next, nucleolar organizers have been selected as regions of interests (ROIs) and subtracted as binary images from the original RGB images, based on their color profile, intensity, texture, background, and morphological filters found under the "smart segmentation" command in the Image-Pro-Premier image analysis software package (trial version, Media Cybernetics, Bethesda, MD, USA) (Figures 1 and 2).

Moreover, in order to better address also the morphology and the relationships between nucleolar organizers rather than the individual ROIs, the binary images have also been processed through a pruning morphological filter reducing the images to their skeletons (Figure 3). All final images were analyzed regarding their fractal dimension, utilizing the same approach in Image-Pro-Premier.

2.4. Statistical Analysis. All the data were represented graphically and further analyzed utilizing Microsoft Excel 2010 and SPSS 10.0 (SPSS Inc., Chicago, IL, USA). All areas and roundness values equal to 0 and FDs equal to 1 have not been considered in this analysis in order to filter out smaller,

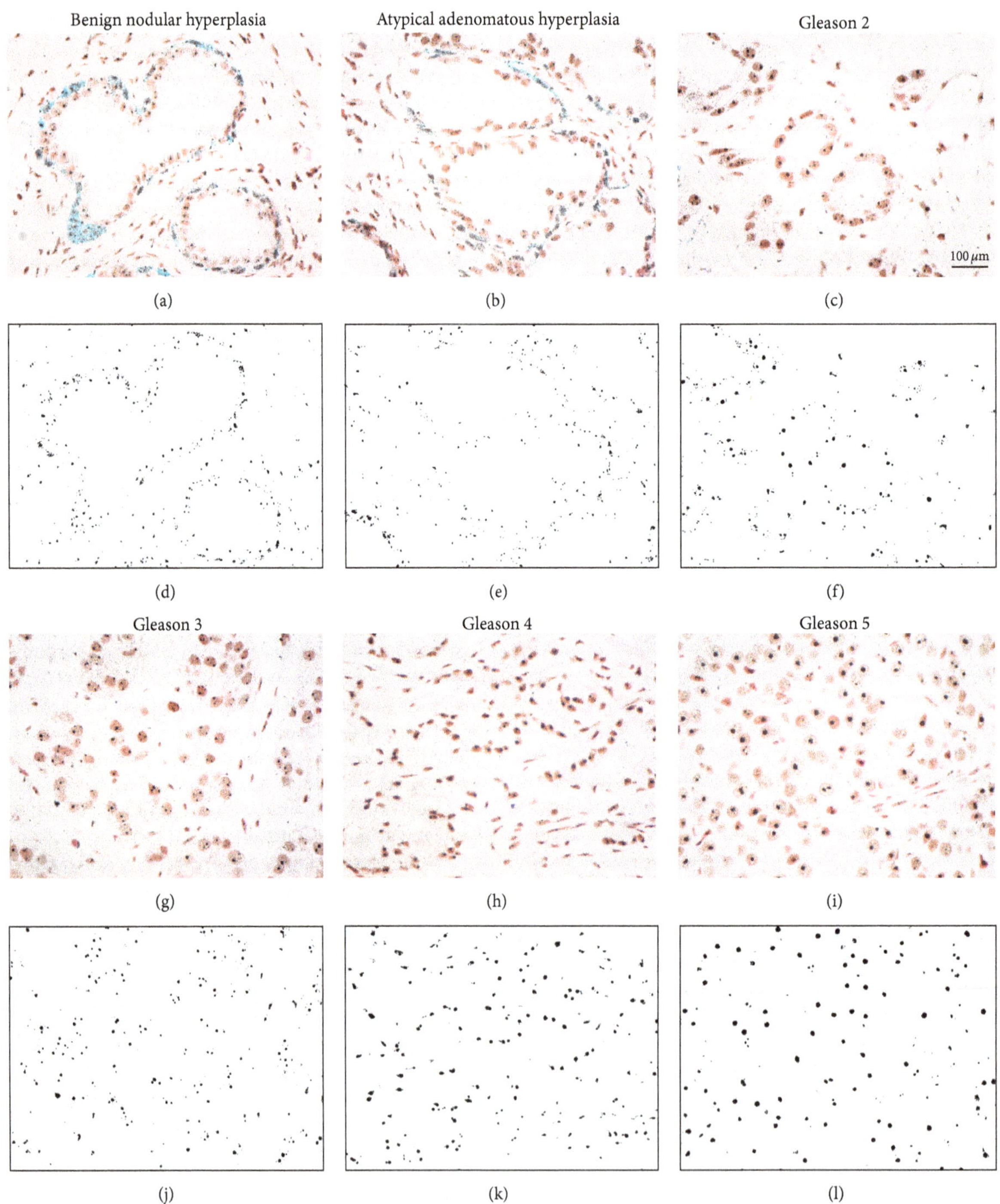

FIGURE 1: Segmentation and binarisation of argyrophilic nucleolar organizer regions (AgNORs). Histochemical-immunohistochemical stainings have been performed for AgNORs (dark dots) and glandular basal cells (a cocktail of p63 and 34βE12, visualized in green), with a Nuclear Red counterstaining in order to ensure a good pathological classification of nodular benign nodular hyperplasia (a), atypical adenomatous hyperplasia (b), and acinar adenocarcinoma Gleason grades 2 (c), 3 (g), 4 (h), and 5 (i). Following segmentation, binary images of AgNORs substractions have been generated ((d)–(f) and (j)–(l)). Scale bar represents 100 μm.

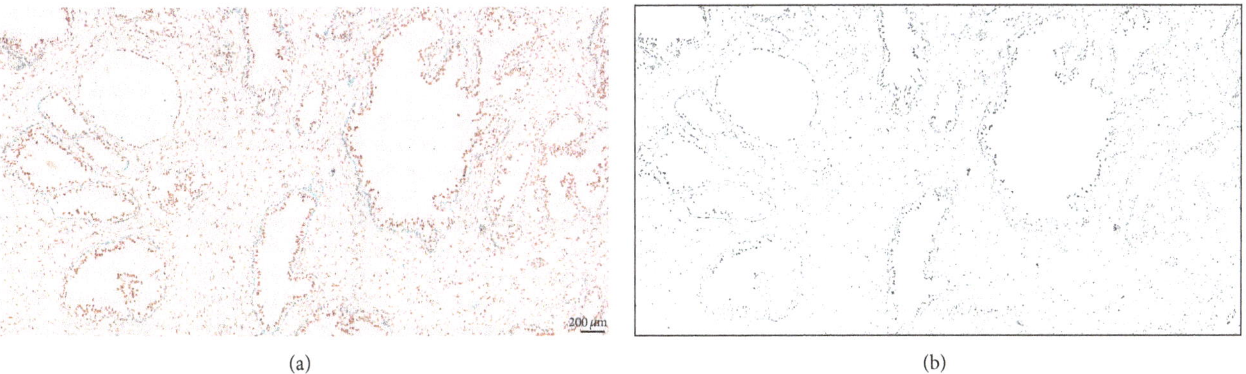

(a) (b)

FIGURE 2: Larger scan areas (24x 400x) utilized for segmentation and binarisation of argyrophilic nucleolar organizer regions (AgNORs). An area of benign nodular hyperplasia is shown ((a)-(b)). Scale bar represents 200 μm.

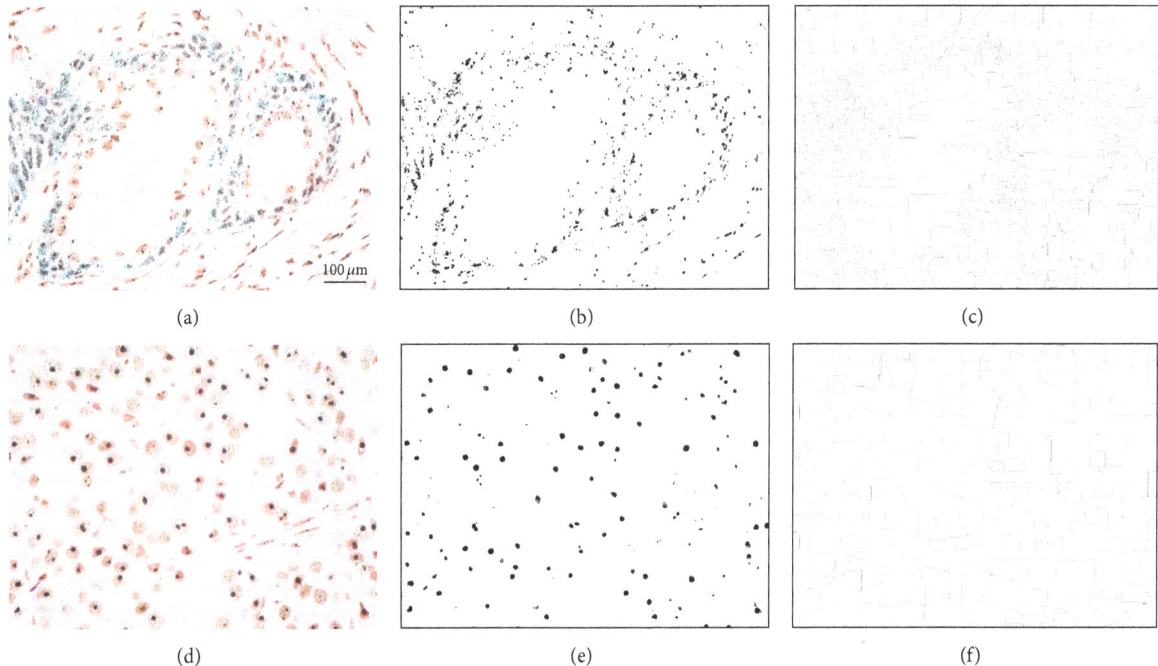

(a) (b) (c)

(d) (e) (f)

FIGURE 3: Example of binarisation and pruning filtering. After segmentation of original images ((a), (d)), argyrophilic nucleolar organizer regions (AgNORs) are binarised ((b), (e)) and then skeletons of the AgNOR dots are extracted ((c), (f)) in order to offer a quantifiable view of the glandular distribution of the dots. Scale bar represents 100 μm.

unequivocally stained particles. All measured values were averaged for each image, patient, and gradings and have been compared utilizing a one-way ANOVA with the Tukey correction as post hoc analysis. Pearson testing was utilized to explore correlations, and, in all cases, $P < 0.05$ was used to indicate statistical significance.

3. Results

After segmenting the nucleolar organizer regions, we have looked at multiple individual and integrative morphological parameters in order to evaluate the possibilities of stratification of the different pathological entities.

First of all, we have counted the individual nucleolar organizer regions as stained and segmented by our image analysis algorithm. The number of silver stained dots was first evaluated as an average per glandular epithelial cell nucleus, and although these averages tended to show higher values for Gleason patterns 4 and 5, they did not exhibit any statistical separation power ($P > 0.05$) (Figure 4(a)). Next, we looked at the total densities of AgNOR entities on both 40x individual images (Figure 4(b)) and composed collages, thus without separating epithelial cells from the stromal component (data not shown). AAH tended to show a somehow lower density of stained ROIs, but this difference was again not significant for both individual Gleason scores overall cancers pooled together versus benign conditions ($P > 0.05$) (Figure 3(b)).

Roundness analysis on high resolution images seemed to offer lower global values (1.554 ± 0.158) for carcinoma

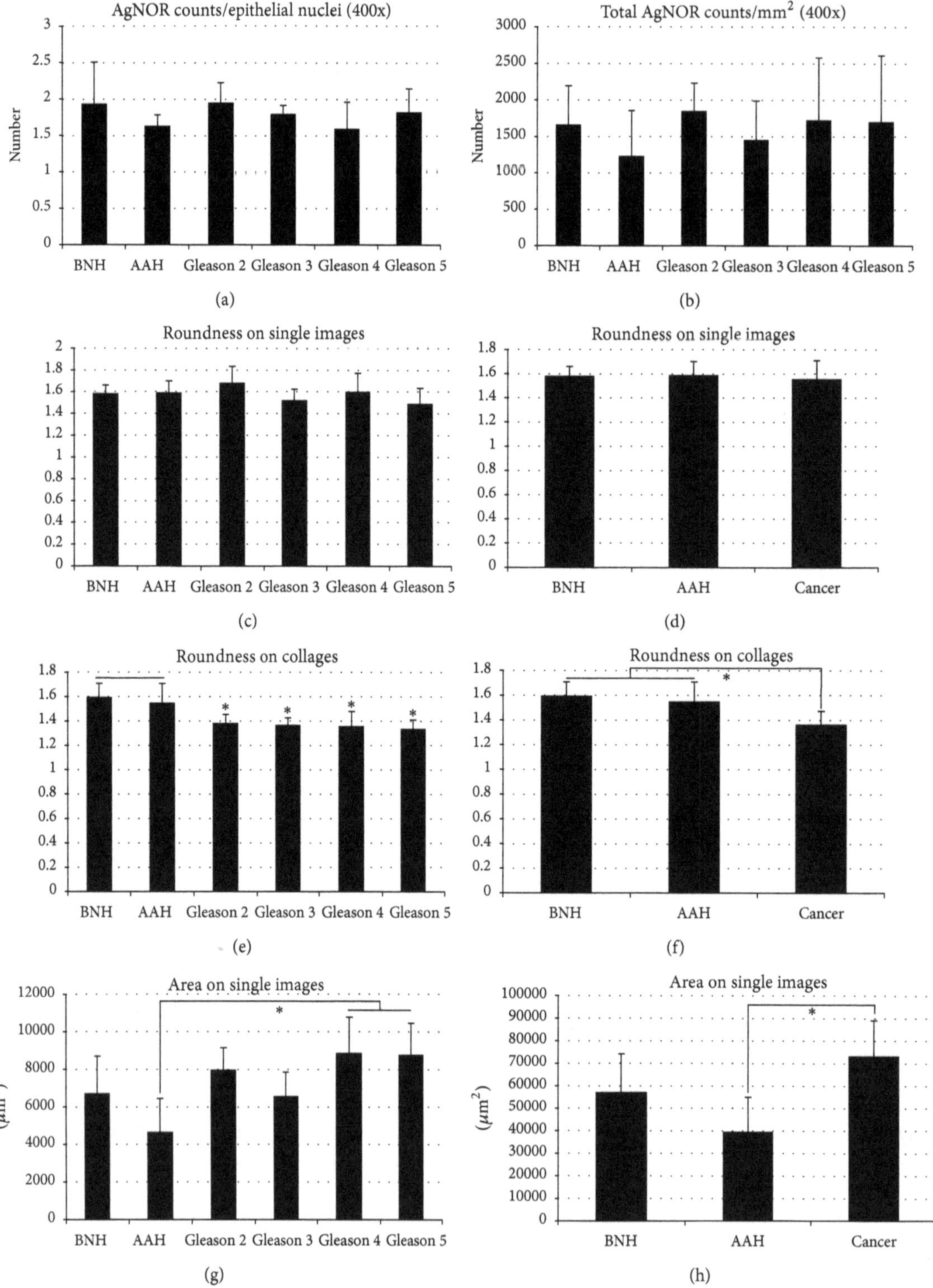

FIGURE 4: Morphometric assessment of argyrophilic nucleolar organizer regions (AgNORs). AgNORs, counted as average per epithelial cells' nuclei (a) or without discrimination for all the cells in the 40x area (b), show no difference between different pathologies. Roundness factor of the AgNOR dots on individual 40x images cannot account also for difference between pathologies ((c), (d)). Roundness factor of the AgNOR dots on collages, however, could differentiate each Gleason pattern from benign nodular hyperplasia (BNH) and atypical adenomatous hyperplasia (AAH) ((e), (f)). Averaged areas of AgNORs have a very limited value, being able to differentiate only AAH from Gleason patterns 4 and 5 ((g), (h)). Bars represent standard deviation. * represents significance on corrected ANOVA testing.

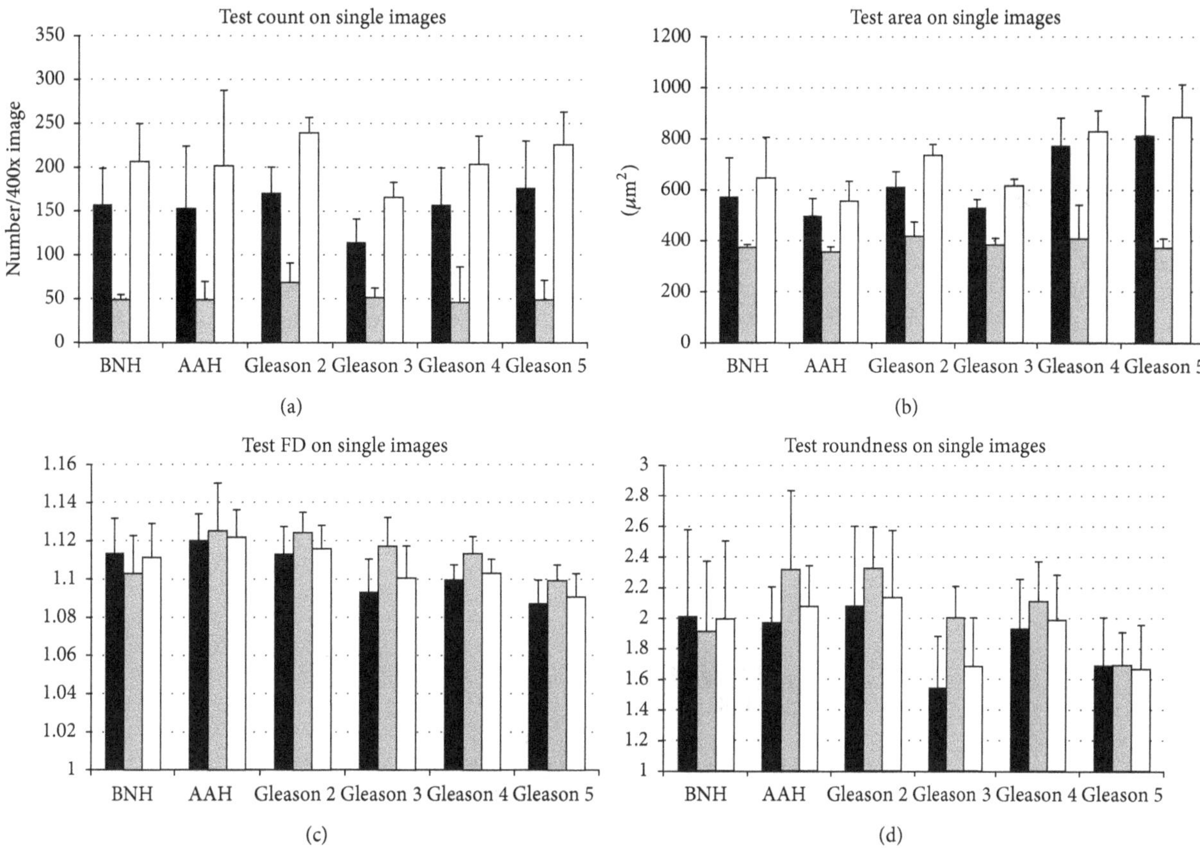

FIGURE 5: Testing different measurements for argyrophilic nucleolar organizer regions (AgNORs) for select epithelial, stromal, and complete 400x areas showed strong direct correlations between data coming from epithelia and complete tissue areas ($r > 0.89$ on Pearson testing).

compared to AAH (1.589 ± 0.110) and nodular benign hyperplasia (1.583 ± 0.077), although the high intracase variability leads to no statistical differences (Figures 4(c) and 4(d)). On composed images, however, acinar adenocarcinoma showed clearly lower values compared to AAH and BNH ($F(5, 54) = 5.887$, $P < 0.001$; with post hoc comparisons using the Tukey HSD test ($P < 0.01$)) (Figure 4(e)). Also, carcinoma cases pooled together (1.365 ± 0.107) showed clear-cut lower roundness values compared to atypical adenomatous hyperplasia (1.549 ± 0.248) and nodular benign hyperplasia (1.596 ± 0.109) ($F(2, 54) = 13.173$, $P < 0.001$; with post hoc comparisons using the Tukey HSD test ($P < 0.01$)) (Figure 4(f)). No significant differences could be found between any individual Gleason grading, AAH, and BNH on either single 40x images or composites.

A one-way ANOVA found a global difference between the total normalized areas of AgNOR positive pixels for different gradings ($F(5, 40) = 5.396$, $P < 0.001$), and post hoc comparisons indicated a difference only between AAH (545.91 ± 210.94) compared to Gleason grading 4 (1041.43 ± 221.94, $P < 0.01$) and, respectively, AAH compared to Gleason grading 5 (1030.89 ± 196.93, $P < 0.01$) (Figure 4(g)). Altogether, carcinoma cases (8592.98 ± 1723.62) showed higher total pixel areas compared to atypical adenomatous hyperplasia (4653.73 ± 1798.22) and nodular benign hyperplasia (6715.97 ± 1983.22) ($F(2, 40) = 11.820$, $P < 0.001$; with post hoc comparisons ($P < 0.05$)) (Figure 4(h)). The same trend was also identified for collage images (data not shown).

Besides the fact that analysis of complete images will add more objectivity rather than separating the glands only, we also assessed whether there was a correlation between the values for direct AgNOR counting, areas, roundness, and FD on a select set of images analyzed for epithelia, stroma, and complete areas (Figure 5). The result was that, for all approaches, epithelia variations could predict very closely overall tissue variations ($r > 0.89$) compared to stroma-complete tissue variations ($r < 0.64$).

We next looked at the averages of fractal dimensions of the silhouettes of nucleolar organizer regions (Figure 6(a)). On individual Gleason scoring, this approach revealed clear-cut differences between Gleason 2 (1.119 ± 0.0007) and Gleason 3–5 group (1.096±0.010; 1.097±0.014; 1.099±0.007), as well as between Gleason 3–5 group and AAH (1.132 ± 0.031) and, respectively, BNH (1.123 ± 0.011) ($F(5, 54) = 8.492$, $P < 0.001$; with post hoc comparisons ($P < 0.05$)). Upon grouping together the cases of acinar adenocarcinoma (1.101 ± 0.013), these were deemed lower than both AAH and BNH ($F(2, 54) = 14.999$, $P < 0.001$; with post hoc comparisons ($P < 0.01$)) (data not shown).

In order to evaluate as much as possible the morphological architecture of the glandular distribution of the silver dots,

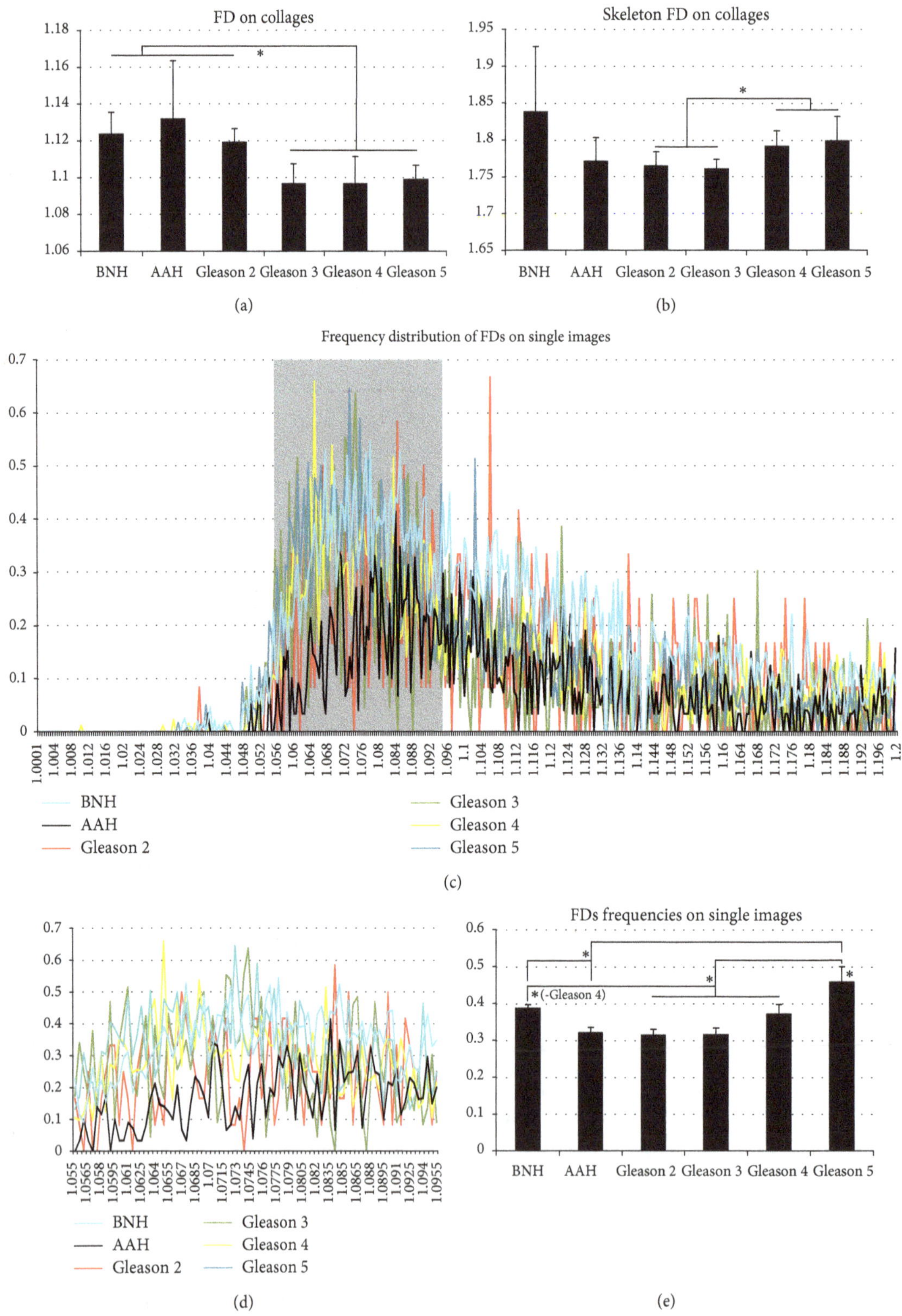

FIGURE 6: Fractal analysis assessment of argyrophilic nucleolar organizer regions (AgNORs). Benign nodular hyperplasia (BNH), atypical adenomatous hyperplasia (AAH), and Gleason pattern 2 have significantly higher fractal dimensions (FDs) compared to Gleason patterns 3–5 (a). Skeleton reductions of the AgNORs could show significant differences only between Gleason patterns 2-3 group and Gleason patterns 4-5 group (b). Frequency distribution of FDs reveals global maxim values for the interval of 1.05–1.09 (c), and after plotting the average values for this narrowed interval, the filtered data revealed significant differences between BNH, AAH, Gleason patterns 2–4 group, and Gleason pattern 5 group ((d)-(e)). Bars represent standard deviation ((a), (b)) or standard errors of the means (e). ∗ represents significance on corrected ANOVA testing.

we have next performed a fractal analysis of the skeleton-filter images extracted from the repartition of the nucleolar organizers. Gleason 2 and 3 patterns (1.765 ± 0.018; 1.1761 ± 0.012) were lower than Gleason 4-5 patterns (1.792 ± 0.020; 1.1799 ± 0.032) ($F(5, 54) = 4.552$, $P < 0.01$; with post hoc comparisons ($P < 0.05$)) (Figure 6(b)). Overall, carcinoma cases could not be differentiated from AAH and BNH utilizing this classifier only.

In a last attempt to evaluate the ruggedness of the silhouettes of nucleolar organizers, we have plotted the frequency distribution of the averaged fractal dimensions of the AgNORs from the individual high magnification images and collages (Figure 6(c)). The total data revealed no global significant differences between the seven pathological entities considered on ANOVA testing for individual images ($F(5, 1456) = 2.214$, $P = 0.051$) and, respectively, for composites ($F(5, 1435) = 1.388$, $P = 0.227$). Observing that the relative peaks of the distributions were concentrated in the 1.05–1.09 FD interval values, we have next analyzed only the data coming from this narrowed interval (Figures 6(d) and 6(e)). Narrowed data from composed images did not exhibit a great deal of differences ($F(5, 3395) = 4.443$, $P = 0.001$), with post hoc comparisons revealing a significant difference only between Gleason 4 and AAH ($P < 0.001$) (data not shown). Narrowed data from individual images, however, revealed not only a global difference between the trends ($F(5, 3184) = 19.832$, $P < 0.001$), but also significant differences between all Gleason stages and BNH, although AAH could be clearly differentiated only from Gleason 5 cases (post hoc comparisons, $P \leq 0.05$) (Figures 6(d) and 6(e)).

4. Discussion

Morphological features of AgNOR, as depicted by silver impregnation techniques, have been utilized to compare cancers with normal structures and nonmalignant neoplasia [29, 30]. For prostate cancer, besides algorithms that attempted to recognize glandular morphology in order to identify malignant prostate tissue areas, AgNOR silver impregnation has been utilized in various studies based on manual, semi-automatic, or fully automatic scoring methods, taking into account the number, aggregation, and size of argyrophilic dots in relation to clinicopathological prognostic parameters for prostatic carcinoma [13–16].

Our study was performed on a group of 39 cases that included BNH, AAH, and adenocarcinomas of the prostate, for which we have analyzed the number, roundness factor, area, and fractal dimension of individual AgNOR signals or of their skeleton reductions. In different other studies, the number of AgNOR signals provided significant [14, 15, 21, 29] or insignificant [30, 31] differences for malignant lesions of the prostate, with significantly higher values for high Gleason scores [14, 15, 21]. Compared to the direct counting of AgNOR signals, morphometric analysis allows a more objective and reproducible quantification on histological sections [17, 32].

In our study, AgNOR direct counting and averaging per nucleus of epithelial cells revealed no significant difference between the pathologies. This difference from studies finding to some extent differences between pathologies could be due to different issues, namely, the different histological techniques and assessment protocols. First, we have implemented here a standardized AgNOR staining, as recommended by the "International Committee on AgNOR Quantitation" [12]. On the other hand, in the present study, we have also performed a selective count only in the nuclei of luminal glandular cells, based on combined silver staining and basal cells immunohistochemistry. Moreover, morphometric analysis is recommended and is based on a common fixed threshold applied to all images to be segmented, resulting in more objective and constant results [33, 34].

Further Euclidian classifiers have been utilized for the differentiation and characterization of malignant lesions of the prostate based on AgNORs analyses, such as their average diameter, total area, or percentage area from the total area of the nucleus [17, 29]. In our study, the analysis of roundness (diameters ratio) and the areas of the AgNORs averaged for large composite images revealed significantly lower values in carcinomas compared to benign and atypical lesions. Both roundness and areas showed no differences for different Gleason scores, issues that are also supported by other published data [29]. In other studies, the analysis of the AgNOR diameters and areas, respectively, indicated significant differences both between benign, atypical, and malignant prostatic lesions and for different Gleason scores, clinical stage, and ploidy of the tumors [17]. All the morphological analysis was done here on all the cells present in the captured images, thus without the need of discriminating glands from parenchyma, greatly increasing the simplicity of the approach and eliminating any user interference that might be necessary to reliably select epithelial tissue from stroma. Also, by utilizing high resolution large composite images, this gave a much more homogenous and reliable approximation of the pathology compared to single high resolution images that might focus on areas with a lower morphological variation.

A relative recent published paper based on utilizing complex in-house software for automatic grading of prostate carcinomas reported correct classification rates of over 90% after employing fractal analysis of the intensity variations and texture complexity of the ROIs [35]. In our study we have both characterized the averaged individual FDs of AgNOR silhouettes and extracted the FDs of skeletonized AgNOR regions which reflected the general glandular disposition of the dots. To our knowledge, this is the first study to perform fractal analysis of silver impregnated nucleoli in prostate pathology [28, 36–38]. Fractal analysis of AgNOR silhouettes regularity not only revealed significant lower values for global cancer images compared to AAH and BNH images, but was also able to differentiate between Gleason 2 group and Gleason 3–5 group of carcinomas. Coupled with the fact that roundness alone could separate cancer samples from AAH and BNH, this leads to an increased selectivity for the combined use of the two denominators. Although this precise methodology has never been employed in the study of nucleolar organizers for prostate cancer, the increasing size and regularity of the nucleoli are a long-standing subjective observation in these tumors [4, 5, 39]. Moreover, a great variability exists regarding the association of large, multiple, and relatively round nucleoli in advanced Gleason stages of prostatic acinar adenocarcinoma [5, 36]. Our data sheds more light on the global morphological changes of nucleoli during prostate cancer progression, revealing that in fact the global tendency of nucleoli is to increase in size and to become less round and with a decreasing complexity of their boundaries, thus coining that the better description of their appearance would be of smoother ellipsoids or ovals rather than circles. Regarding the glandular repartition of the AgNORs, FD of skeleton images revealed significant lower values for carcinomas with Gleason score of 2-3 compared with those with a score of 4-5, but without being able to differentiate global malignant and hyperplastic lesions. However, if we looked again at averaged ROIs areas, FDs and skeleton FDs taken together, the added value is that we can separate almost all pathological states except BNH from AAH and Gleason 4 from 5.

Lastly, after plotting the frequency distribution of the FDs for different pathologies and observing that most of the values are in fact gathered in the interval of 1.05–1.09, we have compared the frequency distribution of FDs only for this narrow interval for all pathologies. Surprisingly, this could differentiate between Gleason 2, 3, and 4 group and Gleason 5, AAH, and BNH group. Most probably this limitation of separating Gleason 5 from AAH and BNH lies somehow in the influence of stromal cells which we have not separated in our algorithm; altogether averaged ROIs areas, FDs, and frequencies of FDs should allow an almost complete separation of each Gleason score from AAH and BNH.

There have been attempts to develop both texture-based [40–42] and fractal-based [35, 43] image analysis algorithms to automate the diagnosis of prostatic carcinoma. Most of these studies were based on color and texture morphological features of glandular and nuclear structures to characterize tissues. The introduction of neural networks and digital mapping led to increased rates of consensus for grading of prostatic carcinoma and achieving good quantification results [44–47]. In the direction of automated image analysis, AgNOR staining may be of interest and may contribute as an implementable parameter among other classifiers in existing image diagnostic software packages.

5. Conclusions

Based on a relatively simple staining technique, the present study presents the combined analysis of AgNORs roundness, averaged FDs, and FDs' frequency analysis as a suite of denominators able to differentiate between malignant and nonmalignant lesions of the prostate, as well as between different Gleason scores. Together with existing classifiers already in use such as nuclear, glandular, stromal, and other architectural features, these present data might contribute to faster and more reliable objective additive diagnosis tools of prostatic carcinoma and decreased reports of uncertain histological lesions, as an essential aid for pathologists.

Conflict of Interests

The authors declare that there is no conflict of interests regarding the publication of this paper.

References

[1] A. Jemal, F. Bray, M. M. Center, J. Ferlay, E. Ward, and D. Forman, "Global cancer statistics," *CA: A Cancer Journal for Clinicians*, vol. 61, no. 2, pp. 69–90, 2011.

[2] J. N. Eble, G. Sauter, J. I. Epstein, and I. A. Sesterhenn, *Pathology and Genetics of Tumours of the Urinary System and Male Genital Organs*, IARC Press, Lyon, France, 2008.

[3] J. T. Kwak, S. M. Hewitt, S. Sinha, and R. Bhargava, "Multimodal microscopy for automated histologic analysis of prostate cancer," *BMC Cancer*, vol. 11, article 62, 2011.

[4] J. Ferlay, E. Steliarova-Foucher, J. Lortet-Tieulent et al., "Cancer incidence and mortality patterns in Europe: estimates for 40 countries in 2012," *European Journal of Cancer*, vol. 49, no. 6, pp. 1374–1403, 2013.

[5] J. Ferlay, H.-R. Shin, F. Bray, D. Forman, C. Mathers, and D. M. Parkin, "Estimates of worldwide burden of cancer in 2008: GLOBOCAN 2008," *International Journal of Cancer*, vol. 127, no. 12, pp. 2893–2917, 2010.

[6] R. B. Shah and M. Zhou, *Prostate Biopsy Interpretation: An Illustrated Guide*, Springer, New York, NY, USA, 2012.

[7] K. A. Trujillo, A. C. Jones, J. K. Griffith, and M. Bisoffi, "Markers of field cancerization: proposed clinical applications in prostate biopsies," *Prostate Cancer*, vol. 2012, Article ID 302894, 12 pages, 2012.

[8] D. Ploton, M. Menager, P. Jeannesson, G. Himber, F. Pigeon, and J. J. Adnet, "Improvement in the staining and in the visualization of the argyrophilic proteins of the nucleolar organizer region at the optical level," *The Histochemical Journal*, vol. 18, no. 1, pp. 5–14, 1986.

[9] M. V. P. Fordham, A. H. Burdge, J. Matthews, G. Williams, and T. Cooke, "Prostatic carcinoma cell DNA content measured by flow cytometry and its relation to clinical outcome," *British Journal of Surgery*, vol. 73, no. 5, pp. 400–403, 1986.

[10] A. Pollack, D. J. Grignon, K. H. Heydon et al., "Prostate cancer DNA ploidy and response to salvage hormone therapy after radiotherapy with or without short-term total androgen blockade: an analysis of RTOG 8610," *Journal of Clinical Oncology*, vol. 21, no. 7, pp. 1238–1248, 2003.

[11] S. E. Bloom and C. Goodpasture, "An improved technique for selective silver staining of nucleolar organizer regions in human chromosomes," *Human Genetics*, vol. 34, no. 2, pp. 199–206, 1976.

[12] M. Aubele, S. Biesterfeld, M. Derenzini et al., "Guidelines of AgNOR quantitation. Committee on AgNOR Quantitation within the European Society of Pathology," *Zentralblatt für Pathologie*, vol. 140, no. 1, pp. 107–108, 1994.

[13] A. B. Hansen and B. Ostergard, "Nucleolar organiser regions in hyperplastic and neoplastic prostatic tissue," *Virchows Archiv. A Pathological Anatomy and Histopathology*, vol. 417, no. 1, pp. 9–13, 1990.

[14] S. Mamaeva, R. Lundgren, P. Elfving et al., "AgNOR staining in benign hyperplasia and carcinoma of the prostate," *Prostate*, vol. 18, no. 2, pp. 155–162, 1991.

[15] W. A. Sakr, F. H. Sarkar, P. Sreepathi, S. Drozdowicz, and J. D. Crissman, "Measurement of cellular proliferation in human prostate by AgNOR, PCNA, and SPF," *Prostate*, vol. 22, no. 2, pp. 147–154, 1993.

[16] A. R. Schned, "Nucleolar organizer regions as discriminators for the diagnosis of well-differentiated adenocarcinoma of the

prostate," *Archives of Pathology & Laboratory Medicine*, vol. 117, no. 10, pp. 1000–1004, 1993.

[17] D. Trere, A. Zilbering, D. Dittus, P. Kim, P. C. Ginsberg, and I. Daskal, "AgNOR quantity in needle biopsy specimens of prostatic adenocarcinomas: correlation with proliferation state, Gleason score, clinical stage, and DNA content," *Clinical Molecular Pathology*, vol. 49, no. 4, pp. M209–M213, 1996.

[18] M. Munda, T. Hajdinjak, R. Kavalar, and D. Štiblar Martinčič, "p53, Bcl-2 and AgNOR tissue markers: model approach in predicting prostate cancer characteristics," *Journal of International Medical Research*, vol. 37, no. 6, pp. 1868–1876, 2009.

[19] T. Goel and S. Garg, "Role of AgNOR count and its correlation with serum PSA levels in prostatic lesions," *Urologia Internationalis*, vol. 82, no. 3, pp. 286–290, 2009.

[20] H. Contractor, J. Ruschoff, T. Hanisch et al., "Silver-stained structures in prostatic carcinoma: evaluation of diagnostic and prognostic relevance by automated image analysis," *Urologia Internationalis*, vol. 46, no. 1, pp. 9–14, 1991.

[21] M. Eskelinen, P. Lipponen, and K. Syrjanen, "Nucleolar organiser regions (AgNORs) related to histopathological characteristics and survival in prostatic adenocarcinoma," *Anticancer Research*, vol. 12, no. 5, pp. 1635–1640, 1992.

[22] M. O. J. Olson, Z. M. Rivers, B. A. Thompson, W.-Y. Kao, and S. T. Case, "Interaction of nucleolar phosphoprotein C23 with cloned segments of rat ribosomal deoxyribonucleic acid," *Biochemistry*, vol. 22, no. 14, pp. 3345–3351, 1983.

[23] L. Mulrane, E. Rexhepaj, S. Penney, J. J. Callanan, and W. M. Gallagher, "Automated image analysis in histopathology: a valuable tool in medical diagnostics," *Expert Review of Molecular Diagnostics*, vol. 8, no. 6, pp. 707–725, 2008.

[24] D. J. Brennan, J. Brändstedt, E. Rexhepaj et al., "Tumour-specific HMG-CoAR is an independent predictor of recurrence free survival in epithelial ovarian cancer," *BMC Cancer*, vol. 10, article 125, 2010.

[25] B. B. Mandelbrot, "Stochastic models for the Earth's relief, the shape and the fractal dimension of the coastlines, and the number-area rule for islands," *Proceedings of the National Academy of Sciences of the United States of America*, vol. 72, no. 10, pp. 3825–3828, 1975.

[26] C. Margaritescu, M. Raica, D. Pirici et al., "Podoplanin expression in tumor-free resection margins of oral squamous cell carcinomas: an immunohistochemical and fractal analysis study," *Histology and Histopathology*, vol. 25, no. 6, pp. 701–711, 2010.

[27] J. W. Baish and R. K. Jain, "Fractals and cancer," *Cancer Research*, vol. 60, no. 14, pp. 3683–3688, 2000.

[28] P. F. F. de Arruda, M. Gatti, F. N. Facio Jr. et al., "Quantification of fractal dimension and Shannon's entropy in histological diagnosis of prostate cancer," *BMC Clinical Pathology*, vol. 13, article 6, 2013.

[29] J. Deschenes and N. Weidner, "Nucleolar organizer regions (NOR) in hyperplastic and neoplastic prostate disease," *The American Journal of Surgical Pathology*, vol. 14, no. 12, pp. 1148–1155, 1990.

[30] J. C. Cheville, G. H. Clamon, and R. A. Robinson, "Silver-stained nucleolar organizer regions in the differentiation of prostatic hyperplasia, intraepithelial neoplasia, and adenocarcinoma," *Modern Pathology*, vol. 3, no. 5, pp. 596–598, 1990.

[31] B. Helpap and C. Riede, "Nucleolar and AgNOR-analysis of prostatic intraepithelial neoplasia (PIN), atypical adenomatous hyperplasia (AAH) and prostatic carcinoma," *Pathology Research and Practice*, vol. 191, no. 5, pp. 381–390, 1995.

[32] D. Trere, "Quantitative analysis of silver stained nucleolar organiser regions: a reliable marker of cell proliferation and a promising prognostic parameter in tumour pathology," *Clinical Molecular Pathology*, vol. 48, no. 4, pp. M219–M220, 1995.

[33] J. Ruschoff, K. H. Plate, H. Contractor, S. Kern, R. Zimmermann, and C. Thomas, "Evaluation of nucleolus organizer regions (NORs) by automatic image analysis: a contribution to standardization," *The Journal of Pathology*, vol. 161, no. 2, pp. 113–118, 1990.

[34] M. Derenzini and D. Trere, "Standardization of interphase AgNOR measurement by means of an automated image analysis system using lymphocytes as an internal control," *The Journal of Pathology*, vol. 165, no. 4, pp. 337–342, 1991.

[35] P.-W. Huang and C.-H. Lee, "Automatic classification for pathological prostate images based on fractal analysis," *IEEE Transactions on Medical Imaging*, vol. 28, no. 7, pp. 1037–1050, 2009.

[36] P. Waliszewski, F. Wagenlehner, S. Kribus, W. Schafhauser, W. Weidner, and S. Gattenlöhner, "Objective grading of prostate carcinoma based on fractal dimensions: Gleason 3 + 4 = 7a ≠ Gleason 4 + 3 = 7b," *Der Urologe A*, vol. 53, no. 10, pp. 1504–1511, 2014.

[37] Y. Pu, W. Wang, M. Al-Rubaiee, S. K. Gayen, and M. Xu, "Determination of optical coefficients and fractal dimensional parameters of cancerous and normal prostate tissues," *Applied Spectroscopy*, vol. 66, no. 7, pp. 828–834, 2012.

[38] M. Tambasco, B. M. Costello, A. Kouznetsov, A. Yau, and A. M. Magliocco, "Quantifying the architectural complexity of microscopic images of histology specimens," *Micron*, vol. 40, no. 4, pp. 486–494, 2009.

[39] R. M. Hoffman, "Screening for prostate cancer," *The New England Journal of Medicine*, vol. 365, no. 21, pp. 2013–2019, 2011.

[40] R. Farjam, H. Soltanian-Zadeh, K. Jafari-Khouzani, and R. A. Zoroofi, "An image analysis approach for automatic malignancy determination of prostate pathological images," *Cytometry Part B: Clinical Cytometry*, vol. 72, no. 4, pp. 227–240, 2007.

[41] P. W. Hamilton, P. H. Bartels, R. Montironi et al., "Automated histometry in quantitative prostate pathology," *Analytical and Quantitative Cytology and Histology*, vol. 20, no. 5, pp. 443–460, 1998.

[42] J. Diamond, N. H. Anderson, P. H. Bartels, R. Montironi, and P. W. Hamilton, "The use of morphological characteristics and texture analysis in the identification of tissue composition in prostatic neoplasia," *Human Pathology*, vol. 35, no. 9, pp. 1121–1131, 2004.

[43] K. Jafari-Khouzani and H. Soltanian-Zadeh, "Multiwavelet grading of pathological images of prostate," *IEEE Transactions on Biomedical Engineering*, vol. 50, no. 6, pp. 697–704, 2003.

[44] R. Stotzka, R. Manner, P. H. Bartels, and D. Thompson, "A hybrid neural and statistical classifier system for histopathologic grading of prostatic lesions," *Analytical and Quantitative Cytology and Histology*, vol. 17, no. 3, pp. 204–218, 1995.

[45] M. Arif and N. Rajpoot, "Classification of potential nuclei in prostate histology images using shape manifold learning," in *Proceedings of the International Conference on Machine Vision (ICMV '07)*, pp. 113–118, IEEE, Islamabad, Pakistan, December 2007.

[46] K. Nguyen, A. K. Jain, and B. Sabata, "Prostate cancer detection: fusion of cytological and textural features," *Journal of Pathology Informatics*, vol. 2, supplement S1, article 3, 2011.

[47] S. Doyle, C. Rodriguez, A. Madabhushi, J. Tomaszeweski, and M. Feldman, "Detecting prostatic adenocarcinoma from digitized histology using a multi-scale hierarchical classification approach," in *Proceedings of the Annual International Conference of the IEEE Engineering in Medicine and Biology Society*, vol. 1, pp. 4759–4762, 2006.

17

Isolation and Time Lapse Microscopy of Highly Pure Hepatic Stellate Cells

Matthias Bartneck,[1] Klaudia Theresa Warzecha,[1] Carmen Gabriele Tag,[1,2] Sibille Sauer-Lehnen,[1,2] Felix Heymann,[1] Christian Trautwein,[1] Ralf Weiskirchen,[2] and Frank Tacke[1]

[1]*Department of Medicine III, RWTH University Hospital Aachen, Pauwelsstrasse 30, 52074 Aachen, Germany*
[2]*Institute of Molecular Pathobiochemistry, Experimental Gene Therapy and Clinical Chemistry, RWTH University Hospital Aachen, Pauwelsstrasse 30, 52074 Aachen, Germany*

Correspondence should be addressed to Frank Tacke; frank.tacke@gmx.net

Academic Editor: Nady Braidy

Hepatic stellate cells (HSC) are the main effector cells for liver fibrosis. We aimed at optimizing HSC isolation by an additional step of fluorescence-activated cell sorting (FACS) via a UV laser. HSC were isolated from livers of healthy mice and animals subjected to experimental fibrosis. HSC isolation by iohexol- (Nycodenz) based density centrifugation was compared to a method with subsequent FACS-based sorting. We assessed cellular purity, viability, morphology, and functional properties like proliferation, migration, activation marker, and collagen expression. FACS-augmented isolation resulted in a significantly increased purity of stellate cells (>99%) compared to iohexol-based density centrifugation (60–95%), primarily by excluding doublets of HSC and Kupffer cells (KC). Importantly, this method is also applicable to young animals and mice with liver fibrosis. Viability, migratory properties, and HSC transdifferentiation *in vitro* were preserved upon FACS-based isolation, as assessed using time lapse microscopy. During maturation of HSC in culture, we did not observe HSC cell division using time lapse microscopy. Strikingly, FACS-isolated, differentiated HSC showed very limited molecular and functional responses to LPS stimulation. In conclusion, isolating HSC from mouse liver by additional FACS significantly increases cell purity by removing contaminations from other cell populations especially KC, without affecting HSC viability, migration, or differentiation.

1. Introduction

Hepatic stellate cells (HSC) are the main effector cells in liver fibrosis [1]. In homeostatic conditions, they reside in the perisinusoidal space of Dissé, store vitamin A, and are involved in maintaining tissue integrity [2]. In case of liver injury, HSC can be activated by different stimuli such as macrophages [3] or danger-associated signals [4]. Activated HSC were found to release proinflammatory mediators and transdifferentiate into myofibroblasts, which are highly proliferative and produce large amounts of extracellular matrix proteins such as collagen types I and III. This process leads to the excess production of hepatic connective tissue, ultimately leading to hepatic fibrosis, and reduced in liver functionality [5].

Activated HSC are considered one of the major target cells for antifibrotic therapies, because they are the main contributors of hepatic extracellular matrix [6]. In order to study HSC biology and to evaluate therapeutic strategies affecting HSC activation or functionality, primary HSC isolation from human, mouse, or rat liver is an evitable tool in experimental fibrosis research. Early attempts to isolate HSC from mouse or rat livers were based on centrifugal fractionation and/or centrifugal elutriation [7, 8]. Subsequent methods incorporated the simultaneous isolation of different hepatic cell populations based on density gradient centrifugation with Stractan [9]. With the rise of flow cytometry and flow cytometric cell sorting, early attempts for flow cytometric cell sorting were based on the strong sideward scattering of HSC due to the specific intracellular (retinol) droplets [10]. Later strategies incorporated multiplex staining of surface markers and cell sorting to exclude cell types other than HSC from cell purifications. However, the purity of all these strategies for HSC isolation remained disputed, since antibody staining may affect cell populations [11]. Moreover, there is no reliable surface marker known that is generally expressed on HSC and myofibroblasts, which hampers positive selection strategies based on antibody staining [5]. Some surface markers that had been suggested for HSC isolation include platelet-derived growth factor β (PDGFR-β) or low-affinity nerve growth factor receptor (p75), while other investigators tested intracellular glial fibrillary acidic protein (GFAP) staining to identify Vitamin A^+ HSC [1, 5, 12]. FACS sorting of HSC has been lately employed by several groups, including ours, by using a UV laser that specifically excites the stored retinol droplets in resting HSC [12–18]. However, it remained unclear whether this technique would alter functional properties of HSC, such as migratory properties relevant to wound healing responses.

The current "gold standard" for HSC isolation is still based on density centrifugation using iohexol (also known under their brand names Nycodenz, Exypaque, or Omnipaque), which separates the HSC due to its physical properties from other hepatic cells and usually results in a high number of viable HSC applicable to cell culture experiments. We hypothesized that, via the "conventional" density gradient method, cell aggregates between HSC and other cell types, especially Kupffer cells (KC), may occur, which in turn result in cellular impurities that could lead to contradictory results on distinct HSC functions. For example, it is heavily debated in the field whether HSC can act as antigen-presenting cells, as studies have led to conflicting results on this topic [11, 19]. Also the notion that HSC strongly respond to bacterial products like lipopolysaccharides (LPS) [20, 21] requires that there is no relevant contamination with macrophages, which are equipped with manifold danger-recognition receptors [22].

In this study, we optimized the "conventional" methodology for the isolation of HSC, based on iohexol density centrifugation, and compared it to an additional step of fluorescence-activated cell sorting (FACS), based on antibodies and UV-autofluorescence, with respect to cellular purity, viability, yield, and cellular characteristics. We further analyzed the behavior of highly pure HSC *in vitro* by studying their cellular morphology and maturation over five days of culture using time lapse microscopy as well as migratory properties in an assay for cell migration and after stimulation with LPS. By implementing an additional step of cell sorting to the current "gold standard" HSC isolation method, our protocol results in significantly improved cellular purity, which helps to clarify HSC functions.

2. Materials and Methods

2.1. Ethics Statement. All *in vivo* experiments were performed following approval by the State Animal Protection Board at the Bezirksregierung Cologne, Germany. The investigation conforms to the Guide for the Care and Use of Laboratory Animals published by the US National Institutes of Health (NIH Publication Number 85-23, revised 1996).

2.2. Mice. C57BL/6J wild-type mice at 40–50 weeks of age, if not stated otherwise, were housed in a specific pathogen-free environment. To induce liver fibrosis, carbon tetrachloride (CCl_4, 0.6 mL/kg, Sigma-Aldrich, Taufkirchen, Germany) was injected intraperitoneally two times per week for six weeks; control animals received the vehicle (corn oil) [13]. All animal experiments have been approved by the Institutional Review Board and by the German legal authorities (LANUV, Recklinghausen, Germany).

2.3. Liver Perfusion, Enzymatic Digestion, and Density Gradient Centrifugation. Mice were anaesthetized using 7 mg/kg body weight xylazine and 105 mg/kg body weight of ketamine. The liver was perfused via the *Vena portae* using a 26 G needle (BD, Franklin Lakes, USA) that was fixed using a Bulldog clamp (Aesculap, Tuttlingen, Germany). Buffers were prewarmed to 37°C and pumped into the liver via the abdominal *Vena portae* and drained via the *Vena cava inferior* using a peristaltic pump at a flow rate of 6.5 mL/minute.

Initially, perfusion buffer 1 (8 g/L NaCl, 400 mg/L KCl, 78 mg/L $NaH_2PO_4 \times H_2O$, 151 mg/L $NaHPO_4 \times 2\ H_2O$, 2380 mg/L HEPES, 350 mg/L $NaHCO_3$, 190 mg/L EGTA, 900 mg/L glucose, and 6 mg/L phenol red, adjusted to pH 7.3–7.4 using 10 N NaOH, sterile filtered, and kept at 4°C until use) was injected into the liver for 4.5 minutes. Second, perfusion buffer 2 (8 g/L NaCl, 400 mg/L KCl, 78 mg/L $NaH_2PO_4 \times H_2O$, 151 mg/L $NaHPO_4 \times 2\ H_2O$, 2380 mg/L HEPES, 350 mg/L $NaHCO_3$, 560 mg/L $CaCl_2 \times 2\ H_2O$, and 6 mg/L phenol red, adjusted to pH 7.3–7.4 using 10 N NaOH, sterile filtered, and kept at 4°C until use) was applied for 4.5 minutes and supplemented with 0.5 mg/mL pronase E (Merck, Darmstadt, Germany). Third, perfusion buffer 2 which was supplemented with 0.75 U/mL collagenase P (Roche, Basel, Switzerland) was administered for 4.5 minutes. The perfused liver was removed, and the gall bladder and connective tissue sticking to the liver were detached. HSC were removed by tearing the liver into bits using two tweezers.

The liver cell suspension was further digested for 20 minutes in a 37°C water bath in perfusion buffer 2 supplemented with 0.4 mg/mL pronase E, 1.5 U/mL collagenase P, and 0.02 mg/mL DNase I (Roche, Basel, Switzerland), adjusted to a pH of 7.2–7.4 using NaOH. Cells were filtered using a 70 μm nylon gaze and rinsed using perfusion buffer 2 tempered at 4°C and centrifuged for ten minutes at 4°C at 600 g. The pellet was then washed using 4°C Gey's buffered salt solution (GBSS) (exact composition: 370 mg/L KCl, 210 mg/L $MgCl_2 \times 6\ H_2O$, 70 mg/L $MgSO_4 \times 7\ H_2O$, 75 mg/L $Na_2HPO_4 \times 2\ H_2O$, 30 mg/L KH_2PO_4, 991 mg/L glucose, 227 mg/L $NaHCO_3$, 225 mg/L $CaCl_2 \times H_2O$, 8000 mg/L NaCl, and 6 mg/L phenol red, adjusted to pH 7.3–7.4, sterile filtered, and kept at 4°C until use) supplemented with 0.01 mg/mL DNase I. Cells were then centrifuged for ten minutes at 4°C at 600 g and suspended in the same buffer (without NaCl, otherwise identical) that was supplemented with iohexol (Nycodenz, Axis-Shield, Dundee, Scotland) to a final concentration of 8%.

The mixture was then pipetted to the ground of a falcon containing GBSS and centrifuged at 4°C and 1500 g for 22 minutes without brake. The interphase containing enriched

HSC between the GBSS and iohexol layer was removed and washed using 4°C tempered GBSS (for cell culture) or 4°C Hank's complete (Hank's buffered salt solution without calcium or magnesium containing 10 mM 4-(2-hydroxyethyl)-1-piperazineethanesulfonic acid (HEPES), 0.06% bovine serum albumin (BSA), and 0.3 mM EDTA, adjusted to pH 7.3–7.4 (for FACS). The cells were then washed for ten minutes at 600 g and the supernatant was removed.

In case of optional F4/80 staining (here only done to identify HSC-KC doublets) that is not required routinely, the cell pellet was resuspended in 4°C FACS staining buffer (one part of phosphate-buffered saline without calcium or magnesium and one part of Hank's complete, supplemented with each 1% of mouse, human, and rabbit serum, and 1% BSA). Staining with anti-F4/80 antibody (diluted 1:400) conjugated with PE-Cy7 rat anti-mouse antibody was done for 30 minutes; antibody and staining buffer were removed by one time of washing in Hank's complete for ten minutes at 4°C and 500 g without brake and suspending in the same solution.

2.4. Fluorescence-Activated Cell Sorting. Cell sorting was done using a BD FACS Aria II SORP Cell Sorter (BD Biosciences, Franklin Lakes, NJ, USA). The pellet was resolved in 4°C Hank's complete and filtered using 40 μm nylon gaze. The sorting of the HSC required excitation via UV laser and measuring the emission in the Indo-1 channel based on a 505 nm long pass and a 530 ± 30 nm band-pass filter. The sample loading port was set to 4°C and 300 rpm. We used a 100 μm nozzle and a pressure of 20 psi. HBSS with calcium or magnesium was used as sheath fluid. The flow rate was set to 5000 events per second and the threshold was adjusted to 5000. The precision mode purity was set up using a yield mask of 32, a purity mask of 32, and a phase mask of 0. The collection device was set to 4°C. The collection tube was a 5 mL glass tube that contained 1 mL of Hank's BSS without calcium or magnesium, 10 mM HEPES, and 20% of fetal bovine serum (FBS). After sorting, cells were centrifuged for 10 minutes at 4°C and at 750 g without brake.

2.5. Cell Culture, Viability, and Purity. Cells were counted using a hemocytometer (Neubauer chamber) and 0.4% trypan blue (Sigma-Aldrich, St. Louis, MO, USA). The purity after sorting was determined by a BD FACS Aria II SORP Cell Sorter (BD Biosciences, Franklin Lakes, NJ, USA) and a hemocytometer. The cell pellet was suspended in DMEM cell culture medium supplemented with 25 mM HEPES, 4.5 g/L glucose, 4 mM glutamine, 1% penicillin/streptomycin, and 10% FBS (all Lonza, Basel, Switzerland). Cell culture was done in 24-well plates (Greiner, Kremsmünster, Austria) using 40,000 cells per well in a volume of 1 mL medium.

2.6. Fluorescence Microscopy. To stain cells for actin, phallotoxin staining was done. Therefore, cells were grown on glass slides that were precoated with poly-L-lysine as described earlier [23]. Cells were washed before and after each step using 4°C *Hank's buffered salt solution (HBSS)*. Cells were fixed using 4% paraformaldehyde for 20 minutes at 4°C. Permeabilization was done using 0.2% triton X-100 for 4 minutes at 4°C. A solution of 3% of BSA dissolved in PBS was used to inhibit unspecific binding. Actin staining was done for 20 minutes at room temperature (21°C) using rhodamine phalloidin (Invitrogen, Carlsbad, CA, USA) which was diluted 1:40 in PBS. Desmin staining was done by the same methods for fixation, permeabilization, and blocking. The primary antibody was antidesmin (Novus Biologicals, Littleton, Colorado, USA). Cells were then blocked again and the secondary antibody was Cy3 donkey anti-rabbit (Jackson Immuno Research, Bethesda, MD, USA) diluted 1:100 in 3% BSA in PBS for 90 minutes at room temperature. Nuclear staining was done using 0.1 μg/mL 4′,6-diamidino-2-phenylindole (DAPI) in HBSS for 5 minutes at room temperature. Finally, slides were mounted using Vectashield Mounting medium (Vector laboratories, Burlingame, CA, USA). Micrographs were made using a DMLB (Leica, Microsystems, Vienna, Austria).

2.7. Staining of Liver Sections. Paraffin-embedded liver sections were cleared from paraffin using xylene and ethanol in ascending line and distilled water for all staining procedures. Hematoxylin and eosin (H&E) staining was done by 15 minutes of incubation in hematoxylin, rinsing for 10 minutes using warm tap water, and 5 minutes of staining with eosin. Sirius red staining was performed using 100 mg Sirius Red (Polysciences Inc., Warrington, USA) in 100 mL saturated picric acid for staining, with the pH adjusted to 2 using 2 N NaOH. To differentiate, sections were incubated for two minutes in 0.01 N HCl and rinsed with tap water. Morphometric quantification of collagen fibres was done using Image J. Staining for α smooth muscle actin (αSMA) was done using the antibody M0851 and the Animal Research Kit, according to the instructions of the manufacturer (all Dako, Hamburg, Germany). All sections were dehydrated using a descending order of ethanol and xylene.

2.8. Quantitative Gene Expression Analysis. To isolate RNA from cells, peqGOLD (peqLab, Erlangen, Germany) was added to cell pellets, and RNA was purified as described before [24]. Complementary DNA was generated from 100 ng of RNA using the Transcriptor first strand cDNA synthesis kit (Roche, Basel, Switzerland). The quantitative real-time polymerase chain reaction (PCR) was performed using SYBR Green Reagent (Invitrogen, Carlsbad, CA, USA) using a 7500 PCR system (Applied Biosystems, Carlsbad, CA, USA). Exon-spanning primers were used, and β-actin regulation of transcripts was employed to normalize gene expression. Primer sequences are available upon request.

2.9. Time Lapse Microscopy and Migration Assays. Micrographs were taken using an Axio Observer Z1 equipped with an Axio Cam MR and an XLmulti S1 DARK LS incubator, providing identical conditions like in a normal incubator. To process data, we used the ZEN pro. 2012 software (Carl Zeiss MicroImaging GmbH, Göttingen, Germany). Pictures were made every 15 minutes. To evaluate the effects of cell culture on HSC proliferation, we normalized the cell number data to the starting point.

To study HSC migration into a defined area, we used culture inserts for self-insertion (IBIDI, Martinsried, Germany) that were inserted before adding the cells to 24-well plates (Greiner, Kremsmünster, Austria). Cells grow among these inserts and, to initiate the migration experiment, the inserts were removed and cells began to move to the empty space (similar to a "scratch assay," but with a well-defined area for the cells to migrate and as a big advantage, no cells are harmed in this assay).

2.10. Statistical Analysis. Statistical analysis was performed using Graph Pad Prism 5.0. Unpaired *t*-tests were performed to test significance of data.

3. Results

3.1. Effect of Additional Sorting on Stellate Cell Purity, Viability, and Differentiation. We first compared the standard method for HSC isolation to an optimized protocol based on additional sorting of HSC. This standard method includes digesting the liver in anaesthetized mice using pronase and collagenase containing buffers. Pronase reduces the abundance of other liver cells, especially of liver sinusoidal endothelial cells and hepatocytes (Figure 1(a)). Liver cells are then harvested into a cell culture dish (Figure 1(b)), and a postdigestion step is done (Figure 1(c)). The cellular mixture is then subjected to iohexol-based density centrifugation (Figure 1(d)). Cells can be cultured directly (Figure 1(e)), as shown by others [25], or be subjected to an additional step of FACS (Figure 1(f)). The FACS-based isolation of primary HSC from mouse livers has been reported from several groups [12–18] with considerable variations in the exact gating strategy.

Our FACS gating strategy is based on selecting cells that exhibit a high extent of sideward scattering due to their vitamin A droplets (Figure 2(a)). The next step consists of excluding cell doublets (Figures 2(b) and 2(c)). The most decisive step in our method is the selection of HSC based on their emission of retinol-based autofluorescence via UV excitation (Figure 2(d)). In the protocol, it is further important to exclude the larger retinol$^+$ cells (larger cells exhibit a higher forward scattering, FSC) from the HSC gate as these are HSC-KC doublets indicated by their expression of F4/80 (Figure 2(d), right side), whereas the smaller retinol$^+$ cells are F4/80$^-$ HSC (Figure 2(d), left hand side).

Using the iohexol density gradient centrifugation as standard method of HSC purification, we normally observe HSC purities of 60–95% HSC, strongly depending on the batch number of the enzymes (pronase, collagenase) used to digest the liver (which therefore has to be pretested extensively), the age of mice, genetic background, and the gender. By direct comparison, FACS of HSC resulted in final purities of up to 99.5% compared to 66.8% after iohexol-based density centrifugation only (Figure 3(a)). Earlier studies that were claiming to reach 95% or higher levels of purity in conventional HSC isolation may have reported on retinol$^+$ cells, which however might contain a considerable quantity of HSC-KC doublets [25]. As shown in Figure 2(d), these retinol$^+$ HSC-KC doublets cannot be removed completely by density gradient but only by stringent gating in flow cytometric cell sorting (Figure 2(d)).

This became more evident by statistical evaluations of four independent experiments, which showed that the number of retinol$^+$ cells was much higher than the number of pure HSC singlets (Figure 3(b)). Furthermore, the HSC derived from sorting were highly viable indicated by 89.3% living cells, similar to that after the iohexol gradient as retrieved from trypan blue staining (90%) (detailed data not shown). To our experience, it is not reliably possible to discriminate between singular HSC and HSC-KC doublets by microscopic analysis but it requires FACS to remove doublets (Figure 2(d)).

The dramatic improvement in HSC purity was corroborated by quantitative real-time PCR analyses. After flow cytometry-based sorting, mRNA expression of the HSC-specific decorin was further increased (Figure 3(c)) compared to standard density centrifugation isolation. On the other hand, the expression of mRNA characteristic of other hepatic cell types, such as the C-type lectin domain family 4f (Clec4f), which is expressed by macrophages, the platelet endothelial cell adhesion molecule 1 (Pecam-1, CD31) exhibited by liver sinusoidal endothelial cells, and albumin, reflective of hepatocytes, were strongly and significantly reduced by additional FACS (Figure 3(c)).

To further investigate the functionality of HSC after additional cell sorting *in vitro*, we isolated HSC via iohexol gradient and used half of these cells for an additional step of purification with FACS. Both cell isolates were subsequently cultured for up to four days. If only the iohexol gradient was performed, KC were found in the culture dishes after one day of culture (Figure 4(a)), and, more visibly, after four days, HSC could hardly be identified due to excessive growth of diverse cell types other than HSC, with KC being noticeable (Figure 4(b)). Performing an additional step of FACS-based cell isolation resulted in a significantly higher purity of cell populations, and HSC could clearly be identified due to their retinol droplets (Figure 4(c)). After four days of culture, HSC could still be identified and exhibited a rather stretched morphology, whereas KC or other contaminating cell types could not be observed (Figure 4(d)). Immunofluorescent staining for desmin (Figure 4(e)) and actin (Figure 4(f)) showed that the FACS-isolated cells expressed these characteristic markers of activated HSC at day 4, indicating that the sorting procedure did not negatively impact HSC differentiation *in vitro*.

3.2. Suitability of the Methodology for Stellate Cell Isolation from Experimental Liver Injury Models. To outline the activation of HSC *in vivo*, chronic toxic liver injury was induced in 8-week-old C57BL/6 mice using CCl_4 for six weeks and twice weekly, a standard method for fibrosis induction [13]. Liver damage was associated with necrotic areas and characteristic fibrotic bridging (Figure 5(a)), whereas Sirius red staining which marks collagen reflective of fibrosis confirmed fibrosis progression in the animals treated with CCl_4 (Figure 5(b)), similar to αSMA which stains for activated HSC (Figure 5(c)). Morphometric quantifications of Sirius

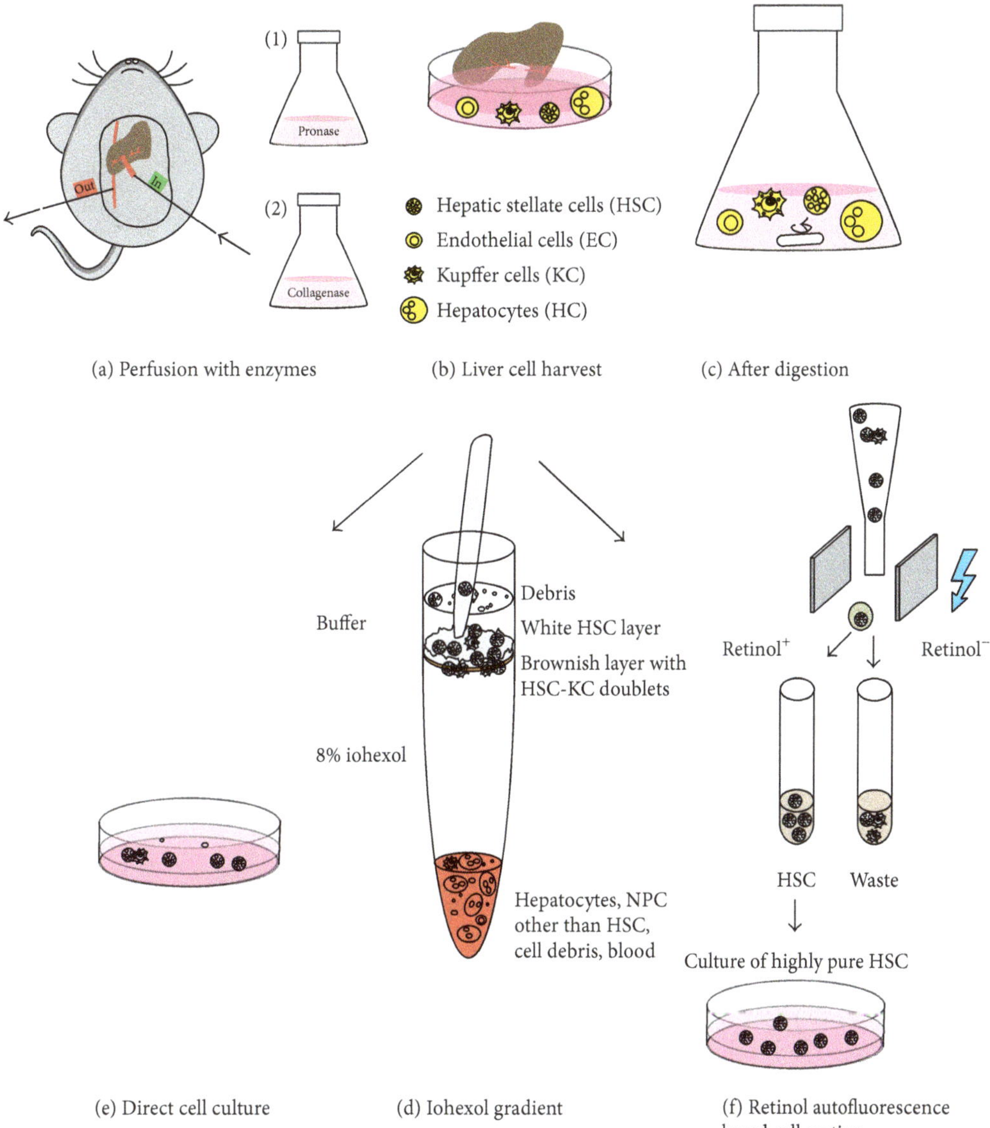

Figure 1: Optimization of the isolation of primary hepatic stellate cells (HSC) based on iohexol density gradient centrifugation and fluorescence-activated cell sorting (FACS) (schematic depiction). In both strategies for cell purification, the mouse is anaesthetized before surgery, and the liver is then perfused via the *Vena portae* and drained through the *Vena cava inferior* using a two-step perfusion of the enzymes pronase and collagenase (a). Liver cells are harvested by gently tearing the liver into bits (b), followed by a postdigestion using a combination of both enzymes (c). The liver cells are subjected to iohexol density gradient centrifugation, after which HSC and Kupffer cells are located in the interphase between iohexol and buffer (d). The enriched HSC layer containing HSC, HSC-Kupffer cell doublets, and cellular debris can be used directly for cell culture of HSC (e) or can be cleared from HSC-Kupffer cell doublets and cellular debris using FACS based on the autofluorescence of retinol, using the UV laser of the cell sorter, resulting in highly pure HSC (f).

red revealed a significant increase in the fibrotic areas in the liver of fibrotic mice (Figure 5(d)). Real-time PCR confirmed fibrosis development on the level of collagen 1 and αSMA mRNA expression (Figure 5(e)). To investigate whether our method is suitable to isolate HSC from the livers of younger control and diseased mice, HSC were then isolated from these via iohexol density gradient centrifugation and additional FACS. We observed that the gating strategy could also be applied to younger diseased (Figure 5(f)) and control mice (Figure 5(g)), which are known to have fewer numbers of HSC and in which HSC might contain fewer retinol droplets. In case of the diseased mice, the sorting step appeared to be even more important than in case of healthy mice, because after CCl_4 treatment the amount of debris or other cells compared to HSC (28.6%) was much higher than that for control littermates that were treated with the vehicle corn oil (65.6%) (Figure 5(h)). FACS helped to get rid of cellular debris relating to the toxic effects of CCl_4 and made it possible to increase the purity up to 99.1% (Figure 5(h)), thereby allowing comparable purity to that of healthy mice.

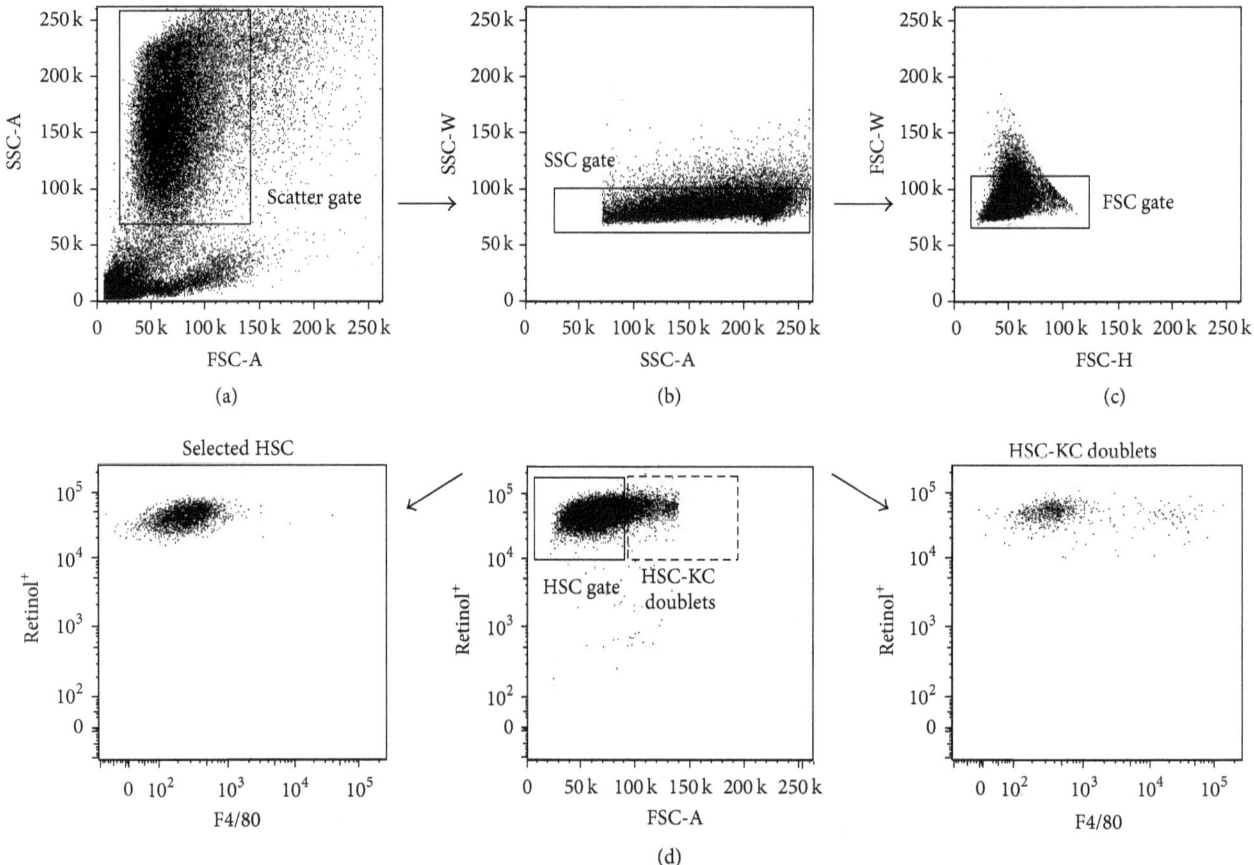

FIGURE 2: Gating strategy for the purification of hepatic stellate cells using fluorescence-activated cell sorting. Cells are first gated based on their forward and sideward scattering (a), doublets are excluded from sideward (b) and forward scattering (c), and hepatic stellate cells (HSC) are selected based on the UV light excitation of retinol (vitamin A) (d). A detailed cell-type specific staining of the Kupffer cell marker F4/80 demonstrated that the large (here: FSC-A > 100 in the plot, dotted gate) retinol$^+$ cells are Kupffer cell- (KC-) HSC doublets that stain positive for F4/80 (right hand side), whereas the smaller retinol$^+$ cells are F4/80$^-$ HSC (left hand side). By placing a sorting gate as depicted in (d) (middle plot, black line), selected HSC (left plot) are pure and do not contain contaminating KC.

3.3. Functional Studies of FACS-Isolated Stellate Cells In Vitro. To further characterize the HSC *in vitro*, we performed time lapse microscopy under different experimental conditions. During the first five days of HSC culture, retinol droplets moved within the HSC, but we did not observe proliferation of HSC (Video 1 in Supplementary Material available online at http://dx.doi.org/10.1155/2015/417023 and Figures 6(a) and 6(b)). During days five to seven, motility of intracellular retinol droplets was increased, but no HSC proliferation was noted (Video 2 and Figures 6(a) and 6(b)).

It is well established that HSC respond to bacterial products like lipopolysaccharide (LPS) via toll-like receptor 4 signaling [4]. When LPS was added to the cultures at the fourth day of culture for 24 hours, no changes in HSC morphology or in the spontaneous migration of HSC in the culture dishes were observed (Video 3, Figure 6(b)). A longer LPS incubation period from days five to seven did not result in any morphological differences compared to control conditions either (Figure 6(b) and Video 4). To further study HSC functionality, we performed a horizontal migration assay with the HSC (similar to a "scratch assay," but using culture inserts which results in well-defined regions) at day five until day seven of culture without (Video 5 and Figure 6(c)) and with LPS stimulation (Video 6 and Figure 6(d)). FACS-isolated HSC showed horizontal migration, and the migratory capacity of the HSC was slightly enhanced by LPS (Figure 6(d)).

To further study the differentiation and effector functions of HSC *in vitro*, we isolated mRNA from cells directly after cell sorting, after one day of culture, after five days, and after an additional stimulation with LPS at day four until day five of culture. We found that the HSC-characteristic activation markers collagen 1 (Col1A1) and αSMA were upregulated starting at the first day of culture and further increase at day 5, but with comparatively low increase after treatment with lipopolysaccharides (LPS). The transforming growth factor β (TGFβ), however, was only weakly affected during culture (Figure 6(e)).

4. Discussion

Mechanistic studies in liver fibrosis research using highly pure HSC rely on a robust method that guarantees cellular

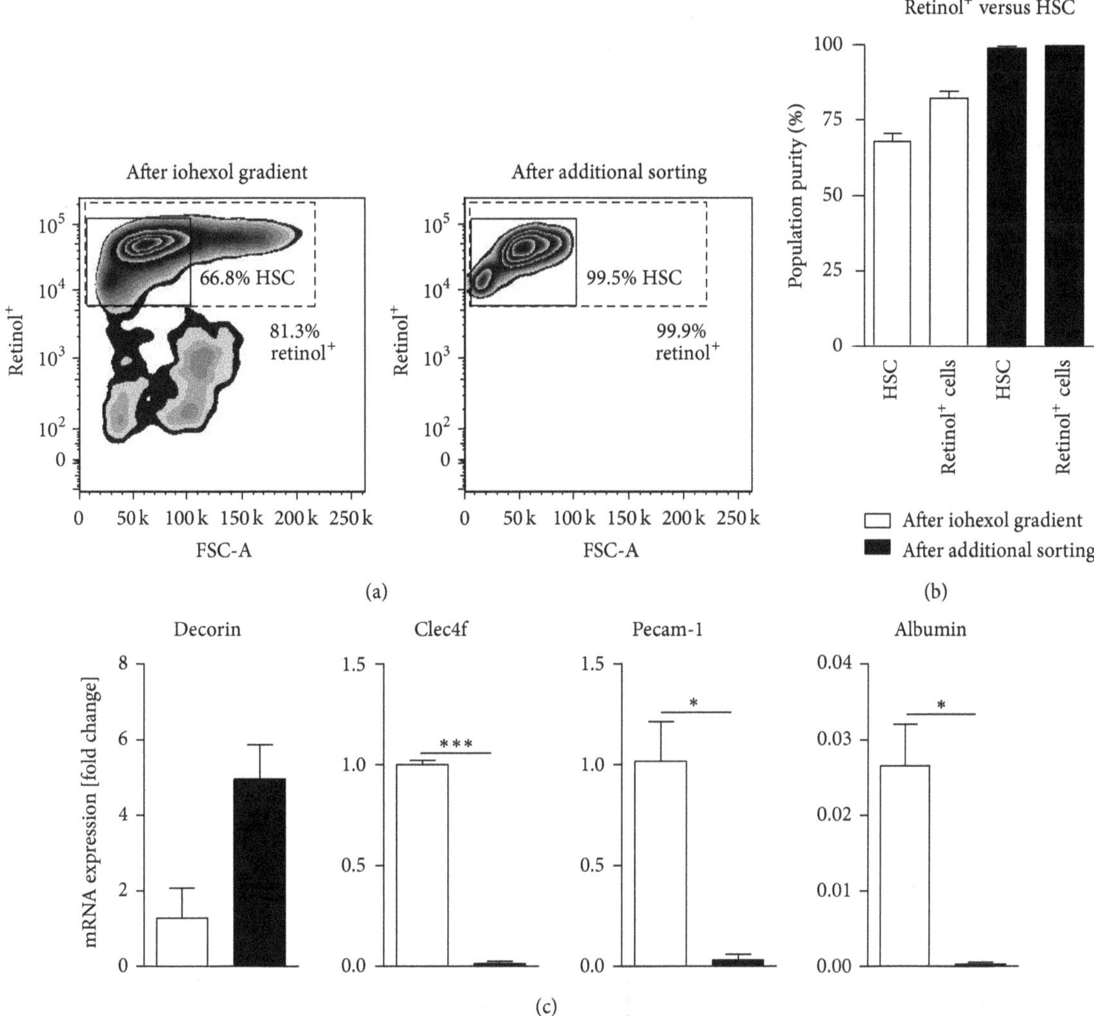

FIGURE 3: Comparison of the purity of hepatic stellate cells isolated via iohexol gradient without or with subsequent cell sorting. Purity of hepatic stellate cells (HSC) before (left top) and after fluorescence-activated cell sorting (FACS, right top) (a) based on their retinol autofluorescence only (dashed line) or additional exclusion of HSC-Kupffer cell doublets (highly pure real HSC, straight line). The statistical summary of retinol$^+$ cells compared to HSC (with HSC-KC doublets excluded) is depicted (b). Analysis of purity using cell type-specific markers for major cell populations. Decorin is considered as a marker for hepatic stellate cells, C-type lectin domain family 4f (Clec4f) is a gene expressed by Kupffer cells, the platelet/endothelial cell adhesion molecule 1 (Pecam-1, CD31) is mainly expressed by endothelial cells, and albumin is a marker for hepatocytes (c). Data are given relative to the expression of β-actin of the cells derived from perfusion and digestion. Mean data ± SD of $n = 4$ independent experiments.

purity and functionality. However, especially "conventional" HSC isolation suffers from high levels of variation caused by the batch-dependent quality of the enzymes used for liver digestion, age, gender, genetic background, and the treatment of the mice [5]. The FACS-based sorting of HSC has been reported from several groups, including ours, with considerable variations in the protocols and without comprehensive analyses on the functional properties of FACS-isolated HSC [12–18]. Many researchers in the field believe that FACS-based cell sorting is insufficient to retrieve high enough HSC numbers for functional *in vitro* experiments and, furthermore, may affect the viability of HSC.

In this study, we demonstrate that FACS is actually required to retrieve highly pure and functional HSC and that this methodology allows functional *in vitro* experimentations with sufficient cell numbers and unaffected viability over at least one week of culture. Moreover, this technique is also applicable to the isolation from young animals (e.g., 12 weeks of age) as well as to mice subjected to standard liver injury models like repetitive CCl_4 administration over 6 weeks. Especially the isolation of HSC from fibrotic livers using the density gradient centrifugation method without FACS has yielded conflicting results, because gene array analyses from these HSC did not match with culture-activated HSC [26]. At this time, the authors found that the addition of KC or LPS to cultured HSC shifted the gene expression pattern towards the *in vivo* activation, suggesting that macrophages and inflammatory cytokines drive HSC activation *in vivo* [26]. However,

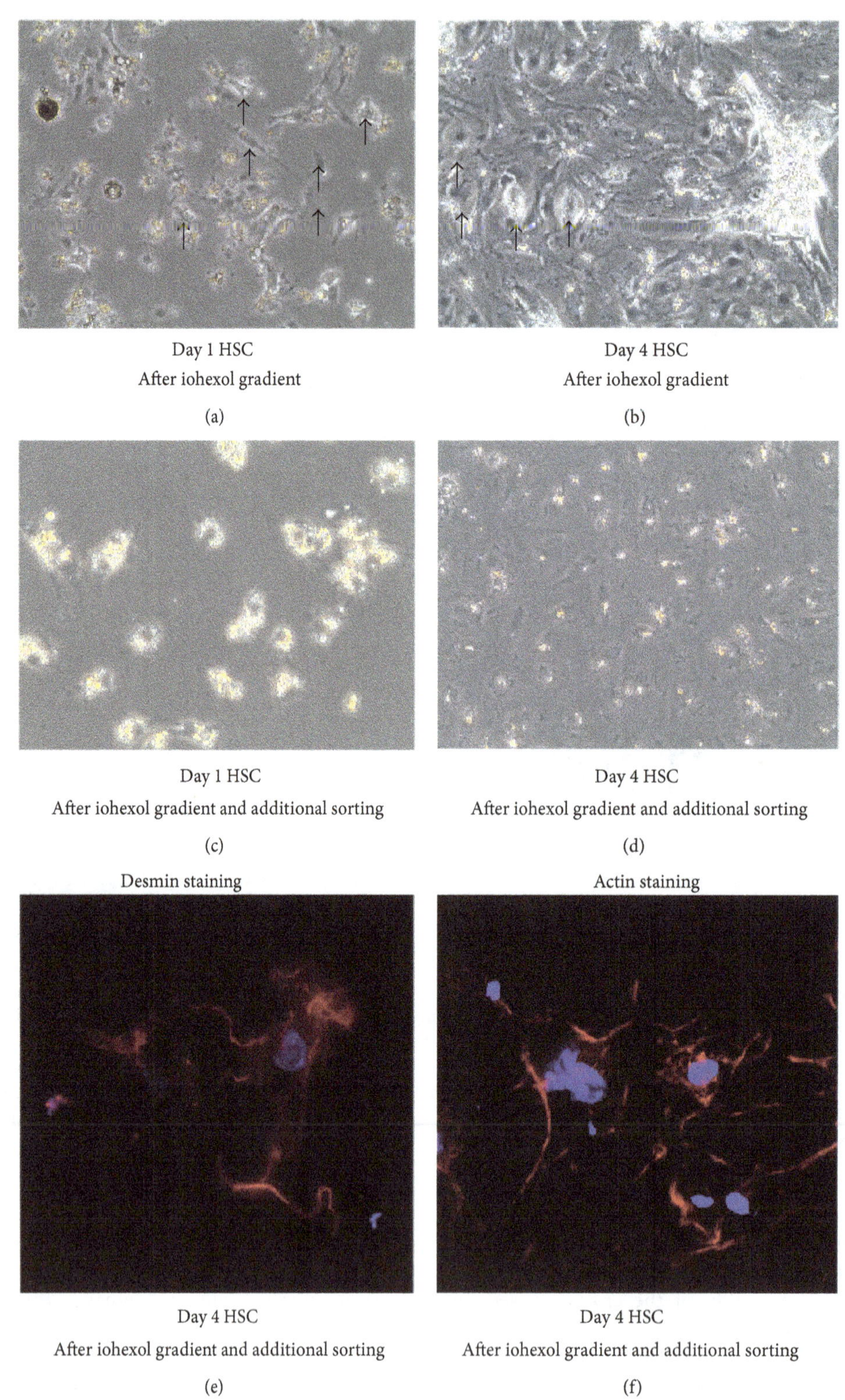

Figure 4: Cultures of hepatic stellate cells isolated via iohexol density gradient centrifugation without or with subsequent cell sorting. Hepatic stellate cells (HSC) were isolated from 40-week-old C57BL/6J mice using enzymatic digestion of the liver based on pronase and collagenase, followed by density gradient centrifugation in 8% iohexol. Cells were cultured directly after the gradient for one day (a) and four days (b), where Kupffer cells (indicated by arrows) can be found in the HSC culture. Highly pure HSC after additional fluorescence-activated cell sorting (FACS) after one (c) and four days of culture are shown (d). Expression analysis of desmin (e) and phalloidin (f) of HSC after four days of culture, indicating proper maturation of HSC.

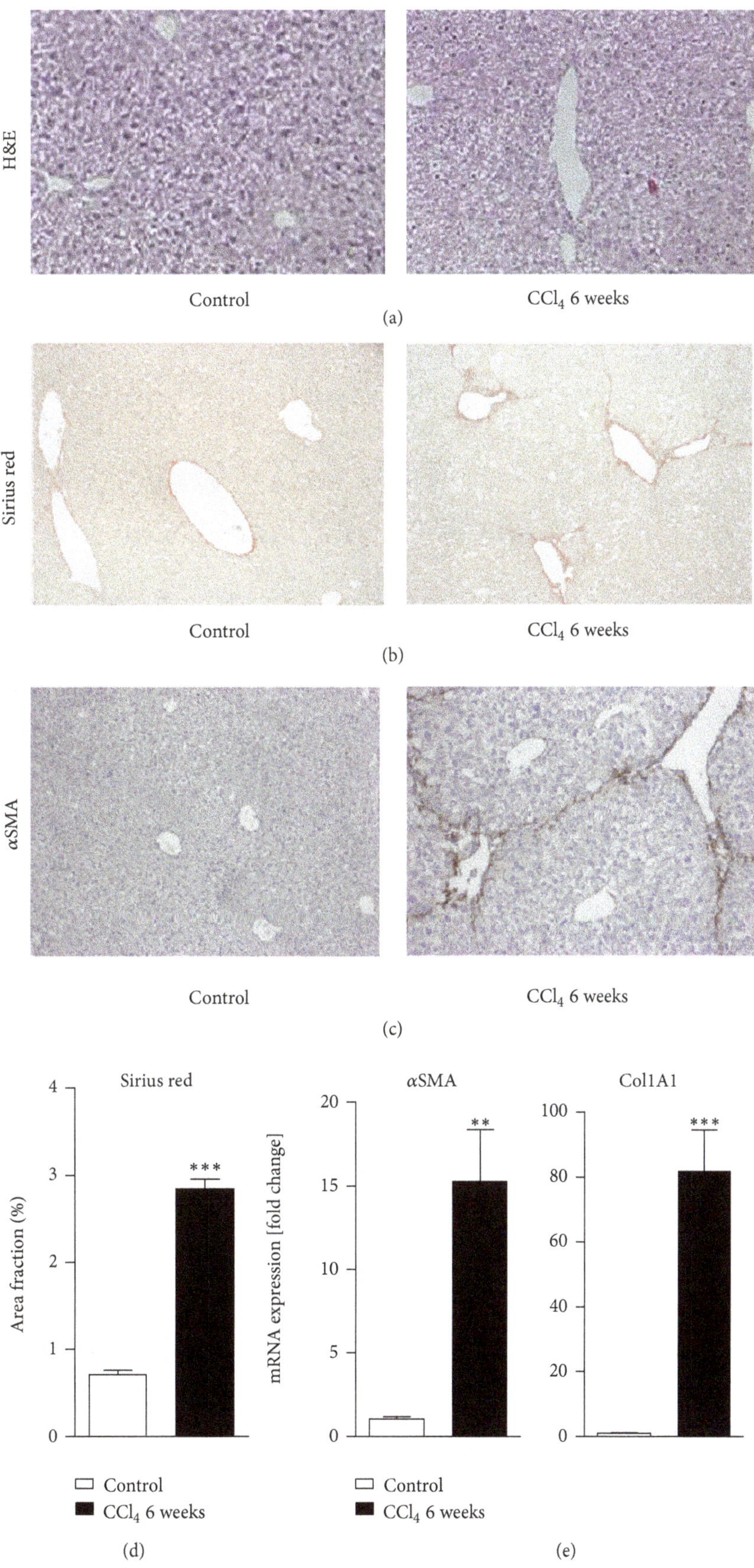

FIGURE 5: Continued.

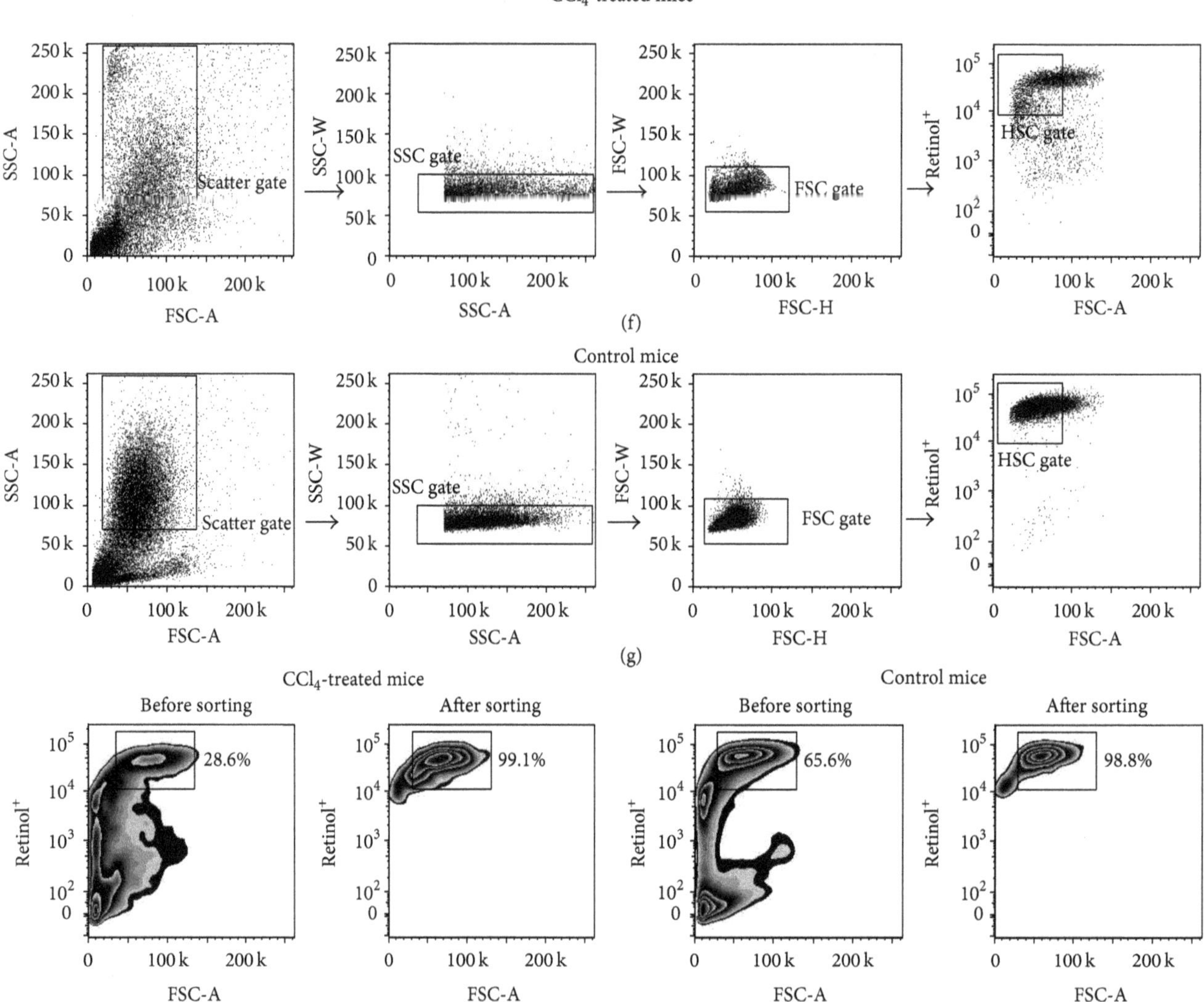

Figure 5: Hepatic stellate cell activation *in vivo* and isolation of hepatic stellate cells from livers of injured mice. Chronic toxic liver injury was induced in 8-week-old C57BL/6 mice by 6 weeks of carbon tetrachloride (CCl_4) treatment, and control treatment was done using corn oil. Mice were sacrificed 48 hours after the last injection of (CCl_4) and liver sections were stained for hematoxylin eosin (a), Sirius red (stains collagen fibres, a hallmark of fibrosis) (b), and α smooth muscle action (αSMA) which targets activated hepatic stellate cells, mediators of fibrosis. Morphometric quantification of Sirius red confirms fibrosis progression (d). Quantitative real-time PCR indicates upregulation of collagen 1 (Col1A1) and αSMA mRNA in liver sections (e). Application of the gating strategy of fluorescence-activated cell sorting (FACS) to isolate hepatic stellate cells from livers of mice that underwent six weeks of repetitive CCl_4-based liver injury (f) compared to vehicle corn oil-treated control mice (g). Flow cytometric analysis of HSC purity before and after sorting demonstrated that the purification was successful (h). Mean ± SD of three independent experiments, $n = 12$ for control and 16 for fibrotic mice; $^{***}P < 0.001$, $^{**}P < 0.005$, and $^{*}P < 0.05$ (unpaired Student's t-test).

our data show that, in addition to other nontarget cells, especially doublets of HSC with KC can considerably "contaminate" primary HSC isolates from mouse liver, if no additional FACS-based sorting is performed. Therefore, it is important to exclude that such doublets confounded prior conclusions on HSC gene expression profiles from fibrotic livers.

Along the same line, a solid body of literature exists demonstrating that HSC isolated from mouse or rat livers can produce large amounts of proinflammatory mediators synthesized by HSC [27] and respond vividly to bacterial products like LPS via toll-like receptor recognition [4]. Similarly, LPS was also found to activate human HSC *in vitro* [28]. It will be important to determine whether some of the LPS responsiveness reported for HSC might be partly related to contaminations with KC, which are known to be both efficient producers and responders to inflammatory mediators [22]. Using highly pure HSC cultures after FACS-based isolation, LPS had very limited effects on HSC behavior such as spontaneous migration as well as transdifferentiation or proliferation.

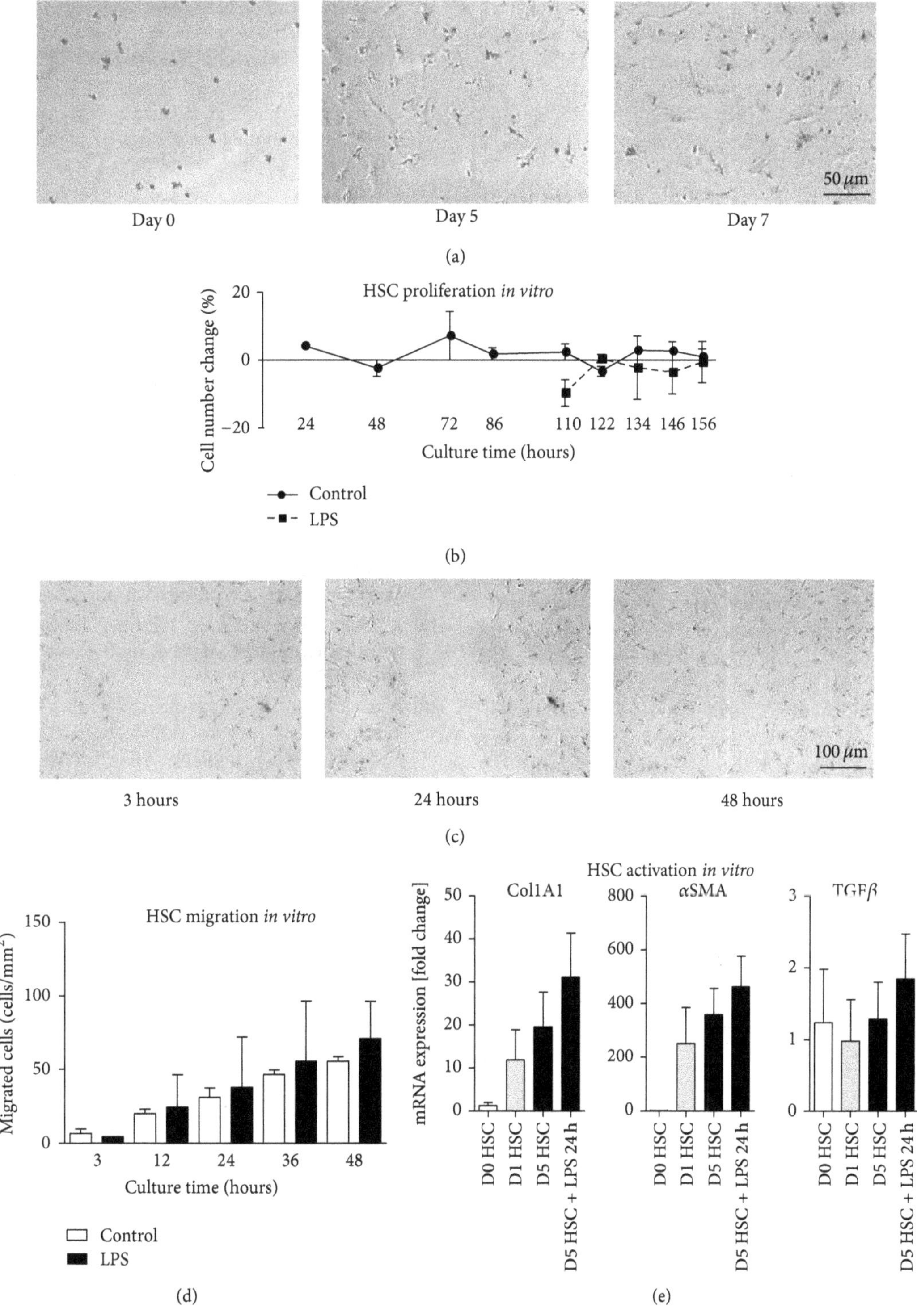

FIGURE 6: Hepatic stellate cell functionality *in vitro*. Hepatic stellate cells (HSC) were isolated from 40-week-old C57BL/6J mice using enzymatic digestion of the liver based on pronase and collagenase, followed by density gradient centrifugation in 8% iohexol and fluorescence-activated cell sorting (FACS). The HSC were cultured in DMEM with 10% fetal calf serum, and some plates were stimulated with lipopolysaccharides (LPS) at 100 ng/mL (after five days of culture) for another 48 hours. Changes in the cell number during culture were determined from time lapse microscopy (a) and statistical summary (b). HSC were cultured for five days on tissue culture-treated polystyrene in DMEM with 10% fetal calf serum including culture inserts for self-insertion ("scratch assay"). To start horizontal migration, the plastic inserts were removed and HSC migrated (c) and were quantified using software (d). HSC were cultured for designated periods and quantitative real-time PCR was performed to study the expression of α smooth muscle actin (αSMA), collagen 1 (ColIA1), or the transforming growth factor β (TGFβ) as markers of HSC activation. Gene expression was normalized to β-actin expression of cells that were lysed directly after isolation at day zero (e). Mean ± SD of three independent experiments.

Nevertheless, one should keep in mind that, upon contact with the tissue culture material, HSC begin to mature and do not reflect quiescent HSC but "culture-activated" HSC [29]. This is well reflected by the fact that HSC, isolated either by conventional methodology or with additional FACS, significantly upregulate activation and myofibroblast differentiation markers upon culture.

Another controversial aspect of HSC biology relates to the question whether HSC derived from noninjured liver microenvironment proliferate *in vitro*. It is known that LPS-stimulated peripheral blood mononuclear cells such as monocytes can stimulate HSC proliferation [30]. Moreover, different profibrogenic stimuli, such as TGF-β, can stimulate HSC proliferation *in vitro* [31]. However, it was not clear whether highly pure FACS-isolated HSC alone would proliferate. In our hands, highly pure HSC do not proliferate spontaneously, suggesting that they rely on external stimuli such as cytokines from inflamed liver or cell-cell contacts with macrophages [3]. Furthermore, one has to consider that also HSC exhibit heterogeneity and it was reported that retinol^{-} HSC proliferate whereas retinol^{+} cells do not [32].

In conclusion, we developed and validated an optimized isolation procedure for primary HSC from mouse livers, which results in a highly pure, viable, and functionally active population of HSC. Upcoming studies should validate controversial basic studies to unravel to which extent contaminations especially with KC may have confounded earlier conflicting data on HSC biology, as earlier studies suggest that KC release molecules which induce HSC proliferation [33].

Disclaimer

The funding agencies had no role in study design, collection, analysis, or interpretation of data.

Conflict of Interests

The authors declare that there is no conflict of interests regarding the publication of this paper.

Authors' Contribution

Matthias Bartneck and Klaudia Theresa Warzecha contributed equally to this work.

Acknowledgments

The authors thank Aline Roggenkamp for excellent technical assistance. This work was supported by the German Research Foundation (DFG/TRR57, cell isolation platform Q3) and a START grant of the medical faculty (to Matthias Bartneck).

References

[1] I. Mederacke, C. C. Hsu, J. S. Troeger et al., "Fate tracing reveals hepatic stellate cells as dominant contributors to liver fibrosis independent of its aetiology," *Nature Communications*, vol. 4, article 2823, 2013.

[2] A. Geerts, "History, heterogeneity, developmental biology, and functions of quiescent hepatic stellate cells," *Seminars in Liver Disease*, vol. 21, no. 3, pp. 311–335, 2001.

[3] J.-P. Pradere, J. Kluwe, S. De Minicis et al., "Hepatic macrophages but not dendritic cells contribute to liver fibrosis by promoting the survival of activated hepatic stellate cells in mice," *Hepatology*, vol. 58, no. 4, pp. 1461–1473, 2013.

[4] E. Seki, S. De Minicis, C. H. Österreicher et al., "TLR4 enhances TGF-β signaling and hepatic fibrosis," *Nature Medicine*, vol. 13, no. 11, pp. 1324–1332, 2007.

[5] F. Tacke and R. Weiskirchen, "Update on hepatic stellate cells: pathogenic role in liver fibrosis and novel isolation techniques," *Expert Review of Gastroenterology & Hepatology*, vol. 6, no. 1, pp. 67–80, 2012.

[6] D. Schuppan and Y. O. Kim, "Evolving therapies for liver fibrosis," *Journal of Clinical Investigation*, vol. 123, no. 5, pp. 1887–1901, 2013.

[7] D. L. Knook, A. M. Seffelaar, and A. M. de Leeuw, "Fat-storing cells of the rat liver: their isolation and purification," *Experimental Cell Research*, vol. 139, no. 2, pp. 468–471, 1982.

[8] A. Margreet de Leeuw, S. P. McCarthy, A. Geerts, and D. L. Knook, "Purified rat liver fat-storing cells in culture divide and contain collagen," *Hepatology*, vol. 4, no. 3, pp. 392–403, 1984.

[9] R. Weiskirchen and A. M. Gressner, "Isolation and culture of hepatic stellate cells," *Methods in Molecular Medicine*, vol. 117, pp. 99–113, 2005.

[10] A. Geerts, T. Niki, K. Hellemans et al., "Purification of rat hepatic stellate cells by side scatter-activated cell sorting," *Hepatology*, vol. 27, no. 2, pp. 590–598, 1998.

[11] S. Ichikawa, D. Mucida, A. J. Tyznik, M. Kronenberg, and H. Cheroutre, "Hepatic stellate cells function as regulatory bystanders," *Journal of Immunology*, vol. 186, no. 10, pp. 5549–5555, 2011.

[12] K. Iwaisako, C. Jiang, M. Zhang et al., "Origin of myofibroblasts in the fibrotic liver in mice," *Proceedings of the National Academy of Sciences of the United States of America*, vol. 111, no. 32, pp. E3297–E3305, 2014.

[13] C. Baeck, A. Wehr, K. R. Karlmark et al., "Pharmacological inhibition of the chemokine CCL2 (MCP-1) diminishes liver macrophage infiltration and steatohepatitis in chronic hepatic injury," *Gut*, vol. 61, no. 3, pp. 416–426, 2012.

[14] L. Hammerich, J. M. Bangen, O. Govaere et al., "Chemokine receptor CCR6-dependent accumulation of $\gamma\delta$ T cells in injured liver restricts hepatic inflammation and fibrosis," *Hepatology*, vol. 59, no. 2, pp. 630–642, 2014.

[15] T. Kisseleva, M. Cong, Y. Paik et al., "Myofibroblasts revert to an inactive phenotype during regression of liver fibrosis," *Proceedings of the National Academy of Sciences of the United States of America*, vol. 109, no. 24, pp. 9448–9453, 2012.

[16] I. Mederacke, D. H. Dapito, S. Affò, H. Uchinami, and R. F. Schwabe, "High-yield and high-purity isolation of hepatic stellate cells from normal and fibrotic mouse livers," *Nature Protocols*, vol. 10, no. 2, pp. 305–315, 2015.

[17] C. Roderburg, M. Luedde, D. Vargas Cardenas et al., "MiR-133a mediates TGF-β-dependent derepression of collagen synthesis in hepatic stellate cells during liver fibrosis," *Journal of Hepatology*, vol. 58, no. 4, pp. 736–742, 2013.

[18] J. S. Troeger, I. Mederacke, G.-Y. Gwak et al., "Deactivation of hepatic stellate cells during liver fibrosis resolution in mice," *Gastroenterology*, vol. 143, no. 4, pp. 1073.e22–1083.e22, 2012.

[19] F. Winau, G. Hegasy, R. Weiskirchen et al., "Ito cells are liver-resident antigen-presenting cells for activating T cell responses," *Immunity*, vol. 26, no. 1, pp. 117–129, 2007.

[20] B. Wang, M. Trippler, R. Pei et al., "Toll-like receptor activated human and murine hepatic stellate cells are potent regulators of hepatitis C virus replication," *Journal of Hepatology*, vol. 51, no. 6, pp. 1037–1045, 2009.

[21] Q. Zhu, L. Zou, K. Jagavelu et al., "Intestinal decontamination inhibits TLR4 dependent fibronectin-mediated cross-talk between stellate cells and endothelial cells in liver fibrosis in mice," *Journal of Hepatology*, vol. 56, no. 4, pp. 893–899, 2012.

[22] F. Tacke and H. W. Zimmermann, "Macrophage heterogeneity in liver injury and fibrosis," *Journal of Hepatology*, vol. 60, no. 5, pp. 1090–1096, 2014.

[23] M. Bartneck, H. A. Keul, G. Zwadlo-Klarwasser, and J. Groll, "Phagocytosis independent extracellular nanoparticle clearance by human immune cells," *Nano Letters*, vol. 10, no. 1, pp. 59–63, 2010.

[24] M. Bartneck, T. Ritz, H. A. Keul et al., "Peptide-functionalized gold nanorods increase liver injury in hepatitis," *ACS Nano*, vol. 6, no. 10, pp. 8767–8777, 2012.

[25] P. Maschmeyer, M. Flach, and F. Winau, "Seven steps to stellate cells," *Journal of Visualized Experiments*, no. 51, article e2710, 2011.

[26] S. de Minicis, E. Seki, H. Uchinami et al., "Gene expression profiles during hepatic stellate cell activation in culture and *in vivo*," *Gastroenterology*, vol. 132, no. 5, pp. 1937–1946, 2007.

[27] A. Dangi, T. L. Sumpter, S. Kimura et al., "Selective expansion of allogeneic regulatory T cells by hepatic stellate cells: role of endotoxin and implications for allograft tolerance," *Journal of Immunology*, vol. 188, no. 8, pp. 3667–3677, 2012.

[28] M. Mühlbauer, T. S. Weiss, W. E. Thasler et al., "LPS-mediated NFκB activation varies between activated human hepatic stellate cells from different donors," *Biochemical and Biophysical Research Communications*, vol. 325, no. 1, pp. 191–197, 2004.

[29] S. W. Woo, J.-X. Nan, S. H. Lee, E.-J. Park, Y. Z. Zhao, and D. H. Sohn, "Aloe emodin suppresses myofibroblastic differentiation of rat hepatic stellate cells in primary culture," *Pharmacology and Toxicology*, vol. 90, no. 4, pp. 193–198, 2002.

[30] K. Toda, N. Kumagai, K. Tsuchimoto et al., "Induction of hepatic stellate cell proliferation by LPS-stimulated peripheral blood mononuclear cells from patients with liver cirrhosis," *Journal of Gastroenterology*, vol. 35, no. 3, pp. 214–220, 2000.

[31] Y. He, C. Huang, X. Sun, X.-R. Long, X.-W. Lv, and J. Li, "MicroRNA-146a modulates TGF-beta1-induced hepatic stellate cell proliferation by targeting SMAD4," *Cellular Signalling*, vol. 24, no. 10, pp. 1923–1930, 2012.

[32] T. Ogawa, C. Tateno, K. Asahina et al., "Identification of vitamin A-free cells in a stellate cell-enriched fraction of normal rat liver as myofibroblasts," *Histochemistry and Cell Biology*, vol. 127, no. 2, pp. 161–174, 2007.

[33] X. Zhang, W.-P. Yu, L. Gao, K.-B. Wei, J.-L. Ju, and J.-Z. Xu, "Effects of lipopolysaccharides stimulated Kupffer cells on activation of rat hepatic stellate cells," *World Journal of Gastroenterology*, vol. 10, no. 4, pp. 610–613, 2004.

18

Comparison of the Manual, Semiautomatic, and Automatic Selection and Leveling of Hot Spots in Whole Slide Images for Ki-67 Quantification in Meningiomas

Zaneta Swiderska,[1] Anna Korzynska,[2] Tomasz Markiewicz,[1,3] Malgorzata Lorent,[3] Jakub Zak,[1,2] Anna Wesolowska,[2] Lukasz Roszkowiak,[2] Janina Slodkowska,[3] and Bartlomiej Grala[3]

[1] *Warsaw University of Technology, Pl. Politechniki 1, 00-661 Warsaw, Poland*
[2] *Nalecz Institute of Biocybernetics and Biomedical Engineering PAS, Trojdena 4, 02-109 Warsaw, Poland*
[3] *Military Institute of Medicine, Szaserow 128, 04-141 Warsaw, Poland*

Correspondence should be addressed to Zaneta Swiderska; swidersz@ee.pw.edu.pl

Academic Editor: Sebastian Wachsmann-Hogiu

Background. This paper presents the study concerning hot-spot selection in the assessment of whole slide images of tissue sections collected from meningioma patients. The samples were immunohistochemically stained to determine the Ki-67/MIB-1 proliferation index used for prognosis and treatment planning. *Objective.* The observer performance was examined by comparing results of the proposed method of automatic hot-spot selection in whole slide images, results of traditional scoring under a microscope, and results of a pathologist's manual hot-spot selection. *Methods.* The results of scoring the Ki-67 index using optical scoring under a microscope, software for Ki-67 index quantification based on hot spots selected by two pathologists (resp., once and three times), and the same software but on hot spots selected by proposed automatic methods were compared using Kendall's tau-b statistics. *Results.* Results show intra- and interobserver agreement. The agreement between Ki-67 scoring with manual and automatic hot-spot selection is high, while agreement between Ki-67 index scoring results in whole slide images and traditional microscopic examination is lower. *Conclusions.* The agreement observed for the three scoring methods shows that automation of area selection is an effective tool in supporting physicians and in increasing the reliability of Ki-67 scoring in meningioma.

1. Introduction

Immunohistochemistry (IHC) has become an important technique to both diagnostic pathology and clinical research, as it can help in the process of diagnosis, prognosis, and grading [1]. Furthermore, during a personalized cancer treatment various molecular markers coupled with specific antibodies allow the pattern of the growth of certain tumors and their response to the particular treatment to be predicted. For example, the proliferation marker Ki-67 is used in meningiomas to differentiate cancer into meningothelial (WHO I), atypical (WHO II), and anaplastic (WHO III) and correlates with tumor recurrences [1–5]. This is because the immunopositive signal expression is a surrogate measure of Ki-67 expression inside cells' nuclei. According to the World Health Organization (WHO) rules, the quantitative evaluation of the proliferation index is performed on a set of high power areas of hot spots selected in various places inside a whole specimen observed under a microscope. For each chosen area of selection, the number of immunopositive and immunonegative cell nuclei is counted to establish the Ki-67 index as the ratio of immunopositive cell nuclei to the whole number of cell nuclei. This routine practice lacks reproducibility from observer to observer because this definition is highly flexible. By definition, selected areas should represent fields of high Ki-67 index in different tumor localizations.

The significant variability of possible selection leads to inter- and intraobserver variability in quantitative results which should be investigated in observer based assessment [6–16].

There have been many attempts to help histopathologists in Ki-67 index quantification involving computers and digital versions of the glass slide, called the whole slide image (WSI). A review of papers concerning this subject published both in the days when only small images could be handled by computers [17–24] and nowadays when WSIs are available and computers or clusters of computers have the necessary computing power to manipulate them [25–34] shows that investigators propose the use of computers on at least 3 levels of the process of proliferation index quantification: (1) in region selection, (2) in immunopositive and immunonegative cell nuclei selection, and (3) in proliferation and other index counting. While the third level is obvious and the second is widely explored, the first level is still poorly represented in the literature. There are methods of region selection concerning Hematoxylin and Eosin staining [35–37], while for Ki-67 stained with DAB and counterstained by Hematoxylin there are the studies published by Potts [34] and coworkers, Lu and coworkers [35], and Gavrielides and coworkers [7, 8]. The third group of investigators performed a pooling study and concluded that "... for validation study should be focused on specific pathology tasks to eliminate sources of variability that might dilute findings." So, a validation study of a specific use of Digital Pathology, that is, in the quantification of the proliferation index based on Ki-67 used in meningiomas, is presented in this paper.

2. Materials and Methods

2.1. Glass Slide Preparation. The glass slides used in this study came from meningioma patients diagnosed or graded at the Department of Pathomorphology, the Military Institute of Medicine in Warsaw, Poland. They were divided into two sets of data according to two methods of preparation. In set A there were twenty-three glass slides (57%, 13 patients, in grade I; 30%, 7 patients, in grade II; and 13%, 3 patients, in grade III according to WHO scores) prepared from paraffin blocks which had been randomly chosen with respect to quality from the hospital archives. The Ki-67/MIB-1 immunohistochemical stained procedure was performed using a Dako Autostainer Link and the following chemical: FLEX Monoclonal Mouse Anti-Human Ki-67 Antigen Clone MIB-1 Ready-to-Use (Link) reference number IR626 from Dako. The staining was visualized using EnVision FLEX Target Retrieval Solution from Dako according to the procedure described in the user manual. All manual and mechanical activities were performed very carefully, because the samples were supposed to be model quality in comparison to the slides from set B.

In set B twenty-seven glass slides (70%, 19 patients, in grade I and 30%, 8 patients, in grade II) from routine hospital prognoses and grading using Ki-67/MIB were chosen to be involved in the study. All these slides had been prepared between 2011 and 2014 with or without Autostainer Link in a manual procedure using various chemicals purchased from Dako. Set B contained inhomogeneous WSI in terms of both the manner of preparation and the chemicals used. The overall quality of glass slides from set B was worse than that of glass slides from set A.

2.2. Microscope and Monitor Review of the Digitalized Glass Slides. The sets of glass slides were both scored by an experienced pathologist, henceforth known as expert, using an Olympus BX40 optical microscope with PlanApo objective. Then, the slides were digitalized using an Aperio ScanScope scanner for set A and a 3DHISTECH Panoramic II for set B. These were then reviewed on a calibrated EIZO FlexScan 22-inch monitor. The WSIs were acquired under 400x magnification with a resolution of 0.279 μm and 0.38895 μm per pixel for sets A and B, respectively. Digital images were reviewed using dedicated software prepared according to project requirements which allowed panning around with a mouse/trackball to view the WSI in various magnifications and to mark fields of quantification. This software was prepared in MATLAB using library Open Slide [38] to read WSI files.

To ensure comparability of an area examined by an expert under a microscope as one field of view and area of quantification chosen from digital WSI, the size of the rectangle which covered the same area as the microscopic circular field of view was determined. It was assumed that the microscopic field of view at 400x magnification represents around 0.12 mm^2 of a tissue; the size of the digitized field of view was 1424×1064 pixels in set A and 1024×766 pixels in set B.

2.3. Observer Training and Environmental Adjustments. Two pathologists with 7 and 3 years of practice in meningioma sections quantification were asked to support this study. To minimize sources of variability, both observers were trained on the software they were to use and their environments were controlled: they used the same computer, monitor, and light in the room in order to eliminate environmental influences on the pathologists work.

The pathologists had an introductory session to become familiar with all the controls and interfaces which were necessary in the selection of hot spots and proper size areas for quantification by automatic software. Pathologists had been instructed the following:

(i) The interpretation of Ki-67 does not include the classification of the intensity of staining but the percentage of tumor cells with positive staining.

(ii) They should find 20 areas of the size mentioned above with high populations of brown objects in comparison to the nearest neighborhoods, but these areas should be distributed among all hot spots which could be found in WSI.

(iii) Each area should be at least 80% covered by tumor lesion and without any artifacts.

Cases where even one of pathologists was unable to score (because of a lack or inadequacy of the region of a hot spot) were removed from the analysis. During the area selection the leader of the project assisted the pathologists by offering hardware and software support but did not make any suggestions as to how to gather information about hot spots or how to choose areas for quantification.

2.4. Textural Features Applied in the Proposed Method. To find hot-spot localizations, a texture analysis was performed on WSI. The normalized probabilities $\widehat{P}_s(i)$ and $\widehat{P}_d(i)$ of the ith intensity on the basis of histograms of the sum and difference images [37] were used. These images were formed from the original image by applying the relative translation (d_1, d_2). Let $f_{k,l}$ mean the intensity of a pixel at (k,l)th position in the gray scale (each of RGB channels) and the image was translated by a fixed displacement (d_1, d_2)

$$s_{k,l} = f_{k,l} + f_{k+d_1,l+d_2}, \quad d_{k,l} = f_{k,l} - f_{k+d_1,l+d_2}, \tag{1}$$

where s and d represent the sum and difference images. The normalized sum and difference probabilities were estimated by

$$\widehat{P}_s(i) = \frac{h_s(i)}{N}, \quad \widehat{P}_d(i) = \frac{h_d(i)}{N}, \tag{2}$$

where N is the total number of pixels in the image. We used the modified formulas of Unser features [37] which are presented in Table 1. They were applied over a given region Ω associated with each pixel of the image. In our notation, N_Ω represents the total number of pixels in Ω region, and $s(\mathbf{x})$ and $d(\mathbf{x})$ represent the pixel values of the sum and difference images.

The determination of the image resolution and Ω radius, which allow the best characterization of the local structures in images, was achieved.

The texture analysis was performed in the following steps. The sum and difference images on the basis of the original image and the original image translated by 3 pixels were calculated for each of the RGB channels. Then, the disk masks with a radius of 10 pixels selected the set of the neighborhood region masks for each pixel location. For a neighborhood of size of 5, 8, 10, 12, 15, and 20 pixels the radius size of 10 pixels appears to be the best and this was used in further experiments.

For the texture features defined in Table 1, the computation complexity problems were obvious. These were associated with the traveling location of the central pixel and its neighboring region Ω. This was solved by applying the array operations. The process of adding the pixel values in sum and difference images was realized quickly by applying the average filtering of the image (embedded *imfilter* function in MATLAB). Thereby, the mean mask for the whole image could be calculated in only one analysis. The (k,l)th coordinate of this mask represented the region center located in this point. To efficiently implement this method of feature calculation, the array form of operations was applied. For example, the variance feature (the second row in Table 1)

TABLE 1: Modified definitions of Unser features.

Name	Modified computational formula
Mean	$f_1 = \frac{\sum_{\mathbf{x}\in\Omega} s(\mathbf{x})}{2N_\Omega} = \mu_\Omega$
Variance	$f_2 = \frac{1}{2}\left(\frac{\sum_{\mathbf{x}\in\Omega}(s(\mathbf{x}) - 2\mu_\Omega)^2 + \sum_{\mathbf{x}\in\Omega} d(\mathbf{x})^2}{N_\Omega}\right)$
Energy	$f_3 = \frac{\sum_{\mathbf{x}\in\Omega} s(\mathbf{x})^2 \cdot \sum_{\mathbf{x}\in\Omega} d(\mathbf{x})^2}{N_\Omega^2}$
Correlation	$f_4 = \frac{1}{2}\left(\frac{\sum_{\mathbf{x}\in\Omega}(s(\mathbf{x}) - 2\cdot\mu_\Omega)^2 - \sum_{\mathbf{x}\in\Omega} d(\mathbf{x})^2}{N_\Omega}\right)$
Contrast	$f_5 = \frac{\sum_{\mathbf{x}\in\Omega} d(\mathbf{x})^2}{N_\Omega}$
Homogeneity	$f_6 = \frac{\sum_{\mathbf{x}\in\Omega}(1/1 + d(\mathbf{x})^2)}{N_\Omega}$
Cluster shade	$f_7 = \frac{\sum_{\mathbf{x}\in\Omega}(s(\mathbf{x}) - 2\mu_\Omega)^3}{N_\Omega}$
Cluster prominence	$f_8 = \frac{\sum_{\mathbf{x}\in\Omega}(s(\mathbf{x}) - 2\mu_\Omega)^4}{N_\Omega}$

could be computed according to the following (modified) expression:

$$f_2 = \frac{\sum_{\mathbf{x}\in\Omega} s(\mathbf{x})^2 - 4\mu_\Omega \sum_{\mathbf{x}\in\Omega} s(\mathbf{x}) + 4{\mu_\Omega}^2 N_\Omega + \sum_{\mathbf{x}\in\Omega} d(\mathbf{x})^2}{2N_\Omega}. \tag{3}$$

The first term of this relation was calculated by applying the filtering of the array-squared sum image (the Hadamard product) and the second by array-fashion multiplication of the mean of the image and the filtered sum image. In the same way, the other terms were calculated. Thereby, the texture feature computation time has been significantly decreased.

2.5. Automatic Hot Spot and Area of Quantification Selection. The proposed method for the hot-spot localization and area of quantification selection based on mathematical morphology, texture classification, and controlled dispersion was described in this section.

An analysis of the information contained in WSI after a resolution decrease on various scales showed that the texture in the original image is redundant and the resolution can be decreased. To localize hot spots, information about the ratio of brown (red) to blue pixels as a basic feature and some other features described below were needed. All features were also visible in images with the resolution decreased by up to 8x, while at a 16x decrease they were not visible. This is presented in Figure 1.

It appears that an eightfold reduction of the resolution does not disturb the required further textural features (size of object-cell nuclei is decreased from 128 ± 51 for brown and 102 ± 73 for blue in original image to 18 ± 9 and 10 ± 6 for the selected 8x decreased resolution, resp.) and enables the evaluation to be performed by a computer and by a pathologist with a direct visual examination.

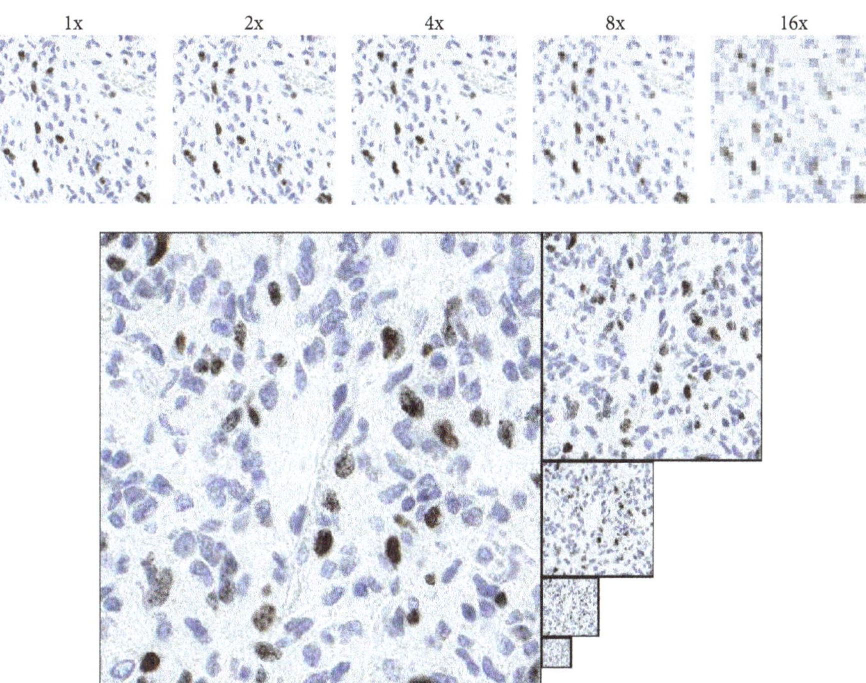

FIGURE 1: Fragments of WSI in original and decreased resolution: 2x, 4x, 8x, and 16x.

The proposed method of analysis of WSI in decreased resolutions uses the following steps: (1) the specimen map is established, (2) the texture quantification and classification are done to eliminate hemorrhage areas from the specimen map, (3) the hot spots are detected, and finally, (4) based on the proposed penalty function, selection of the area of quantification inside selected hot spots is performed. The general schema of the algorithm for steps 1–3 is presented in Figure 2.

In the first step, a map of the specimen was created using the thresholding procedure and morphological filtering [39–42]. To do this, a whole slide image was used to produce a supported image by the morphological operation of opening and brightness equalization. This was performed using a structuring element shaped like a disk with a large radius (100 pixels). The operation of the division of each RGB color component of the image by its version after morphological opening was performed independently for each channel. Afterwards, components from channels B and R were processed with the Otsu thresholding method [43]. Additionally, morphological operations, such as erosion, dilatation, and hole filling, were performed to filter the specimen map.

The next step, which eliminates hemorrhage areas from the specimen map, was performed by differentiating the tumor area from hemorrhage areas using texture analysis and classification. The local textural descriptors came from the Unser features [33, 40] and were applied independently for RGB and CMYK color channels and also for the combined u (from CIE Luv) and C (form CMYK) representation. A set of 64 textures was created as 8 features defined in Table 1 by 8 color channels or sums of channels as presented in Table 2. Next, based on Fisher's linear discriminant, the most significant 25 were selected on a teaching phase and then used in the classification phases (see Table 2).

Finally, the Support Vector Machine (SVM) with Gaussian kernel function [41–46] was applied as a classifier to recognize the hemorrhage areas and to eliminate them from the specimen map.

The third step of the algorithm was an estimate of the local density of immunopositive cells using the reduced resolution WSI. The local maxima of the immunopositive cell densities are hot spots. To select these, the mathematical morphology and proportion of the color components were used. It was found that u of the CIE Luv representation of colors is strictly associated with the red color and can be used to differentiate the immunopositive cells from the remainder of the image. The extended regional minima transformation is applied to evaluate the spatial relation of the stained brown objects to their neighboring environment. The density map was created, based on the isolated marks representing the immunoreactive tumor cells.

The fourth and final step of the proposed method focused on the fields of quantification selection based on an artificial model of field spatial dispersion. To prevent all fields of quantification being chosen, the penalty function was defined from one large dominant hot spot with a high Ki-67 index by the following formula:

$$\text{penalty} = 1 - \rho \sum_{i} \frac{1}{\left(\sqrt{(x - x_i)^2 + (y - y_i)^2}\right)^{0.5}} \quad (4)$$

TABLE 2: Significant texture features (features in 8 color channels or sum of channels (a), color channels or sum of channels in features (b)).

(a)

Color component	R (1–8)	G (9–16)	B (17–24)	u (luv) + C (CMYK) (25–32)	C (33–40)	M (41–48)	Y (49–56)	K (57–64)
Number of features	3, 5	11, 13	—	25, 26, 27, 29, 30, 32	33, 34, 35, 37, 38, 40	41, 42, 43, 45, 46, 48	49, 54	63
Feature name	(i) Energy (ii) Contrast	(i) Energy (ii) Contrast		(i) PSM (ii) Variance (iii) Energy (iv) Contrast (v) Homogeneity (vi) Cluster prominence	(i) PSM (ii) Variance (iii) Energy (iv) Contrast (v) Homogeneity (vi) Cluster prominence	(i) PSM (ii) Variance (iii) Energy (iv) Contrast (v) Homogeneity (vi) Cluster prominence	(i) PSM (ii) Homogeneity	Cluster shade

(b)

1	2	3	4	5	6	7	8
PSM (u + C), C, M, Y	Variance (u + C), C, M	Energy R, G, (u + C), C, M	Correlation —	Contrast R, G, (u + C), C, M	Homogeneity (u + C), C, M, Y	Cluster shade K	Cluster prominence (u + C), C, M

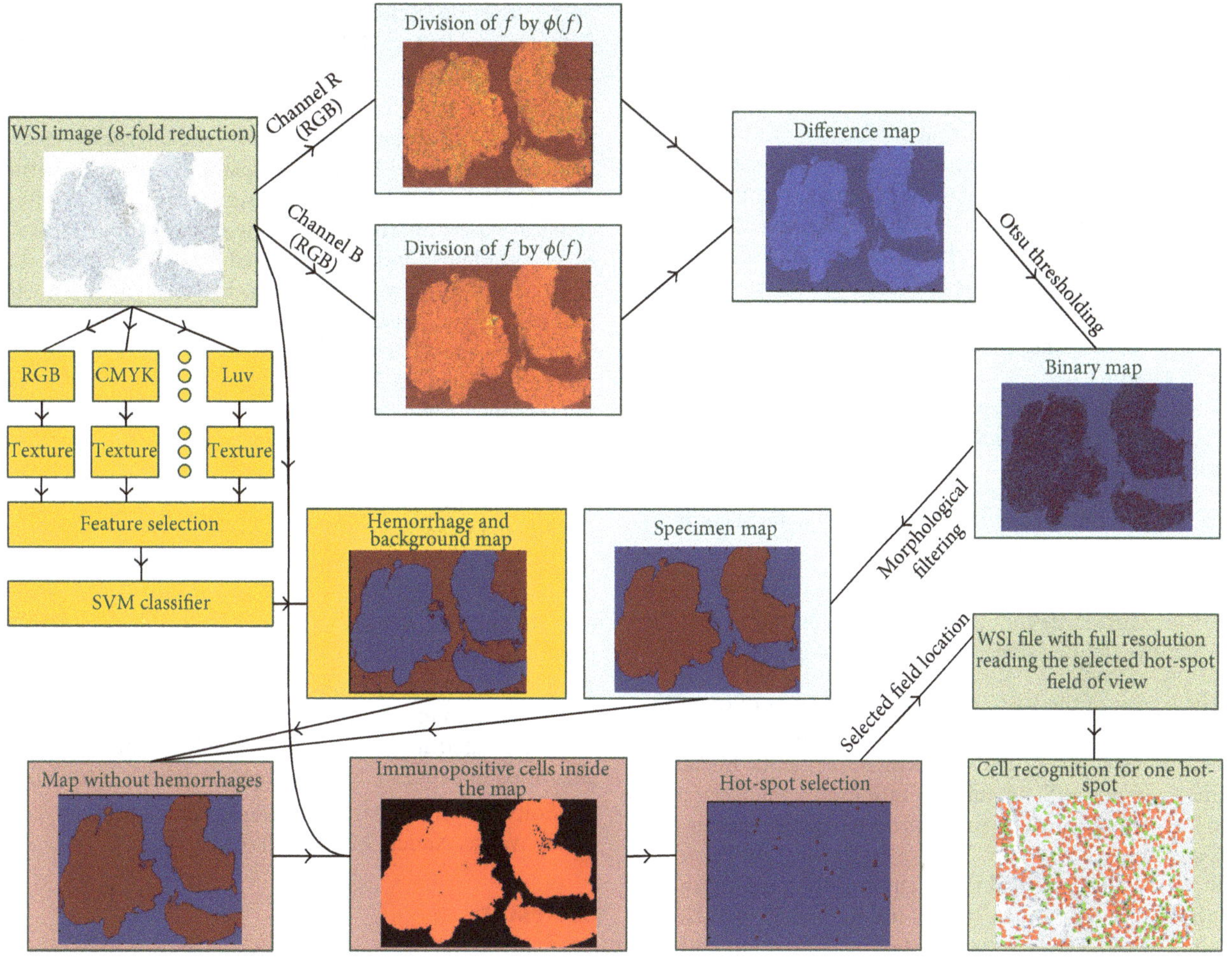

FIGURE 2: The schema of the algorithm for hot-spot localization.

which was based on information about the distance between the designated areas and the position of another candidate for hot spot.

An increase in the ρ value shows an increase in the scattering of the areas of quantification selection. The ρ value had been chosen experimentally (see Section 3). The proposed function combined selection of fields of quantification from different localization in the specimen according to a gradual reduction of the concentration of immunopositive cells. However, when hot-spot areas other than the dominant one show a significantly lower density of immunopositive nuclei, the candidates from dominant region will still be selected first. The final analysis of the Ki-67 index in all chosen areas of quantification was performed on full resolution images with the method published earlier and described in [45].

2.6. Evaluation of the Concordance of Selected Hot-Spot Fields. To evaluate the concordance of hot-spot field localization between the experts' and automatic results the localization concordance measure (LCM) was proposed. This measure assumed that (1) those fields at a shorter distance should have a reduced impact on the LCM and (2) the significance of fields should relate to their Ki-67 index. The localization concordance measure was calculated according to the following formula:

$$\text{LCM} = \sum_i \left(w_i * \text{sigm}\left(\min_j \left| \frac{\text{dist}\left[(x_j, y_j), (x_i, y_i) \right]}{(4\text{FOV}_{\text{size}})} \right| \right) \right), \quad (5)$$

$$\text{where: } w_i = \frac{L_{E_i}}{\overline{L}_E}$$

in which L_E is the level of the Ki-67 index for the expert and FOV_{size} is a one field of view size. A low value of the LCM shows a similarity in the areas of quantification selection by algorithm and expert. This means that the expert's selected fields of quantification are represented or near the fields selected by the proposed method; for example, they represent the same tumor area. If expert and algorithm select fields of view from different virtual slide areas, the localization measure LCM is high. The proposed measure allows both the evaluation of the similarity of choice of hot-spot fields and the identification of the best penalty factor. The proposed measure can be used in cases of both inter- and intraobservation variability.

2.7. *Study Design.* Both the proposed automated method of area of quantification selection and the two pathologists were used to review all the samples (A and B sets) using digital representation of glass slides with an 8x reduced WSI resolution while expert quantification was done in full resolution and for 10 areas of unknown location. The outcomes were then averaged to give the final result.

Each of the pathologists chose 20 fields of quantification for each WSI. One pathologist had two additional sessions for the WSI from set A to estimate interobserver variability. Each additional session was performed with at least a one-month delay between sessions. The order of samples was randomized for each session.

Then, automated hot-spot selection software was used to select 20 fields of quantification as an area which fulfill two criteria:

(i) Biggest number of immunopositive nuclei in comparison to the others.

(ii) That distances between new and previously found areas are large enough to meet the requirements of the above defined penalty function, that is, (4).

The scores of the Ki-67 index from the areas of quantification chosen by the pathologists and the automatic method were produced using software which segments nuclei in subimages from WSI in full resolution and then classifies them into immunopositive and immunonegative classes and estimates the Ki-67 index. This software was published in 2009 [45] by the principal investigator of the project who is coauthor of this paper. The ratio of immunopositive nuclei to the number of all cells in each area of quantification and the mean of these ratios for each WSI were sent for computer-enabled statistical analysis.

2.8. *Statistical Analysis.* The scores from the expert microscopic examination and all automatic scores from areas chosen by both pathologists and scores from the proposed automatic method of area of quantification selection were analyzed using agreement analysis, since IHC interpretation is a subjective process of evaluation. For this process, a true score is not available. Besides, agreement between digital and optical scores was not the primary objective of the study, but rather this is considered the reference value, while agreement between the automatic and pathologists' hot spots and area of quantification selection in IHC assessment was the main aim of the study.

The primary objective of the investigation was to find patterns of agreement between manual human and automated selection of the area of quantification in WSI. The commonly used concordance measure, Kendall's tau-b, was used as in Gavrielides and coworkers [7, 8]. The test was calculated separately for sets A and B in pooled and categorized/grouped versions in both pairwise and cumulated versions.

Kendall's tau-b is a rank-based correlation metric which calculates the difference between the rate of concordance and discordance [46–48]. The range of Kendall's tau-b is −1 to 1, where 1 indicates perfect agreement, −1 indicates data are inverted (perfect agreement inversion), and 0 indicates no relationship. Kendall's tau-b was computed according to Balboacă and Jäntschi [48] using dedicated software prepared in MATLAB.

Kendall's tau-b values were utilized to quantify *interobserver* and *intraobserver agreements.* The *interobserver agreement* was estimated between all pairs: (1) between pathologists themselves, ((2) and (3)) between each pathologist and classical expert microscopic reviewing, ((4) and (5)) between each pathologist and the proposed automated method and additionally in a grouped version between (6) the mean of pathologist and classical expert microscopic reviewing and (7) the mean of the pathologist and proposed automated method applied to WSI and (8) between classical expert microscopic reviewing and proposed automated method applied to WSI. The *intraobserver agreement* (agreement between the scores of the same observer in various sessions of area selection) was estimated between all pairs of three independent scorings from one pathologist: (1) the first and the second scores, (2) the second and the third scores, and (3) the first and the third scores, both in pooled data and in categorized data. Because of the small number of WSIs from patients in grade III, the results relate to only two categories: grade I and grade II in diagnosed meningioma patients. Confidence intervals for the overall agreement measures were calculated applying bootstrap analysis using a procedure described in detail in the study by Gavrielides et al. [7].

Software for bootstrap was implemented using MATLAB (MathWorks, Natick, MA, USA) functions.

3. Results

First, the influence of the ρ value on the penalty factor was examined. A subset of twelve WSIs from set A was chosen for this analysis. The hot-spot localization and areas of quantification selections performed by pathologists and the automated proposed method were compared using the LCM measure. The results of Ki-67 index estimations and LCM measures for ρ from 0.1 to 0.5 with an increment of 0.05 are presented in Figure 3. The best concordance between the automatically selected areas of quantification and those selected by pathologists is for a ρ value equal to 0.2. For this ρ value, LCM is minimal for a relatively high value of the Ki-67 index.

The dispersion of areas of quantification chosen by the proposed automatic method and pathologists can be observed in Figures 4 and 5.

Figure 4 presents the distribution of the areas of quantification selected in hot spots found for two WSIs by two pathologists (red and yellow rectangles) and by the proposed automatic method (black rectangles). In the top line (Figures 4(a) and 4(b)) it can be observed that there is no agreement between both pathologists and that the distribution of regions is different and inhomogeneous, so the measure of concordance, LCM, is 9. The distance between the proposed automatic method and the mean measure for both pathologists is 8.6. The bottom line (Figures 4(c) and 4(d)) shows good agreement in areas of quantification distribution. Their measure of concordance, LCM, is 2.9

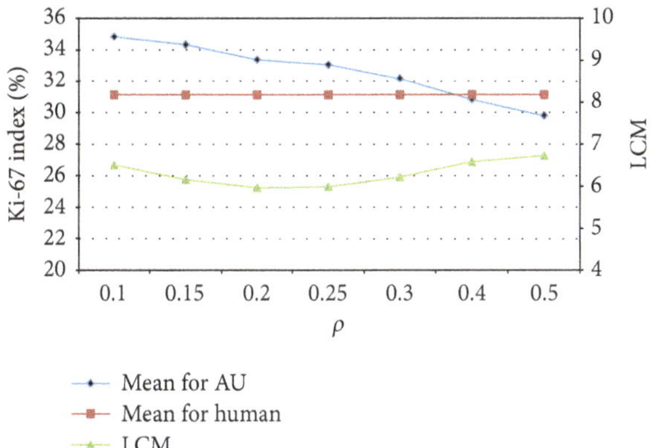

FIGURE 3: Examination of Ki-67 index and LCM in respect to the ρ factor of the penalty function.

between pathologists while between the proposed automatic method and the mean measure for both pathologists it is 3.4.

Figure 5 presents results of three repetitions of the selections of the areas of quantification from one pathologist (Figures 5(a), 5(b), and 5(c), blind trial) and from automated method (Figure 5(d)) using one of the WSIs from set A. It is visible that this one person chose a region of quantification in various parts of specimen. The third trial is significantly different from the previous two rather similar trials, but the Ki-67 indexes for each of them are similar (10.7%, 10.6%, and 11.9% for pathologist and 13.2% for automated method).

As the selected fields of quantification were previously quantified by the software, the Ki-67 index for each area and for each specimen becomes the data for statistical analysis.

In Figure 6, where all results for Ki-67 quantification using all early interdicted methods of its estimation (manually experts, by means of two pathologists' semiautomatic approach and fully automatic approach) are shown, the general tendency for a relationship between them can be observed. Quantification with the manual microscopic method produces the lowest Ki-67 proliferation index values, while the automatic methods produce the highest values of this index. This pattern is biased by one specimen from set A and for 3 specimens from set B. In the first case, the lower result for the pathologists is caused by an undervalued score from one pathologist. In the other cases from set B, the pattern is reversed and the highest values for this index appear for the manual microscopic method. Exposé control of WSI shows that there are very small hot spots in each of these three specimens. It seems that when hot spots do not cover the whole area of quantification (although they fulfill the criterion that about 80% of the area of quantification should be covered by a hot spot) it causes various results from the pathologists and automatic method. In such cases, an expert performing microscopic scoring used to deal with part of field of quantification restricted to hot spots, while the automatic method diluted the score by counting the number of cells from the whole area of the rectangle.

The results of inter- and intraobserver variability measurements are presented in Tables 3, 4, and 5.

Table 3 presents the results of pairwise agreement using Kendall's tau-b analysis for interobserver variability as a coefficient of concordance along with confidence intervals (95% confidence level) constructed using bootstrap analysis of the samples (100 order changes). It can be observed that all concordance between all pairs calculated for set A is bigger than the analogous values for set B. This can be explained by the fact that WSIs in set A were prepared using autostainer and the same set of new chemicals while WSIs in set B were regular glass slides prepared earlier, some with and some without autostainer, and using the chemicals available at the time. Visual examination shows that glasses in set A are of really good quality and homogenous in performance, while the glasses from set B are not. This inhomogeneity among glasses from set B led to differing interpretations by the two pathologists which is seen as a decrease in agreement between them (from 0.92 to 0.86) and between each of them and the automated method (from 0.82 and 0.81 to 0.78 and 0.76, resp.).

Both parts of Table 3, A and B, show an overall tendency for the highest correlation to be between both pathologists and the lowest agreement to be between a classical microscopic expert scoring and the proposed automated method employed on WSI. The concordance between both pathologists and the other two methods of scoring are between these two extremes, but the concordance is greater between the pathologist and the proposed automated method than between the pathologists and the classical microscopic score.

Table 4 presents the results of pooled expert agreement in two categories, grade I and grade II (WHO categorization of meningioma), using Kendall's tau-b analysis for interobserver variability. The coefficient of concordance is presented with confidence intervals (95% confidence level) calculated using bootstrap analysis of the samples (100 order changes). It can be observed that concordance is higher in category grade II than in grade I in both subsets: A and B. This fact can be explained as the reason that grade I patients' scores are usually lower (up to 8%; see Figure 4) than grade II patients' scores (up to 20%; see Figure 4). This means that the hot spots are more intensive and visible in comparison to the surrounding space in those specimens from patients diagnosed as grade II. This visibility is more important for the pathologists than for the automated method. So, coincidence between pathologists' digital scoring and the proposed automated method is very high (0.86 for set A and 0.8 for set B) if grade II patients' sections are analyzed, while for grade I patients' sections the coincidence is lower (0.79 and 0.78), but it still shows coincidence. For the coincidence between experts' digital scoring and the manual microscopic expert scoring the results show similar patterns, but the numbers are lower (0.87, 0.43 and 0.6, and 0.3, resp.).

The coincidence between the results of the proposed automatic method and manual microscopic expert scoring is ambiguous. This coincidence is rather low, except for grade II of set A.

Table 5 presents the results of pairwise agreement analysis for uncategorized and categorized data using Kendall's tau-b for intraobserver variability. One of the pathologists repeated the scoring procedure 3 times, with a delay long enough

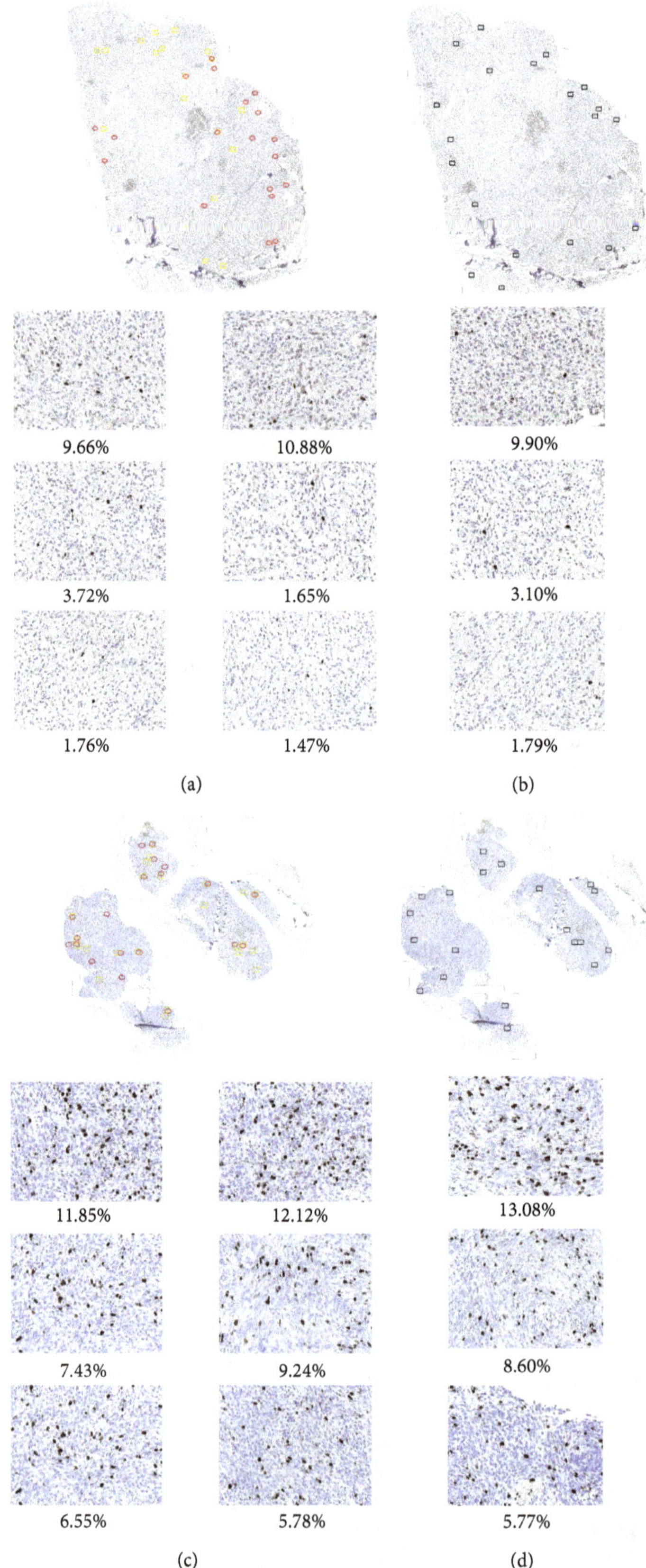

FIGURE 4: Two WSIs with an area of quantification inside a hot spot marked by two experts ((a) and (c): red and yellow rectangles) and chosen by the proposed automatic method ((b) and (d): black rectangles) with examples of 3 areas of quantification for each method and for both WSIs with large and small variation in Ki-67 index value calculated as percentage of immunopositive nuclei to the whole number of nuclei in presented area.

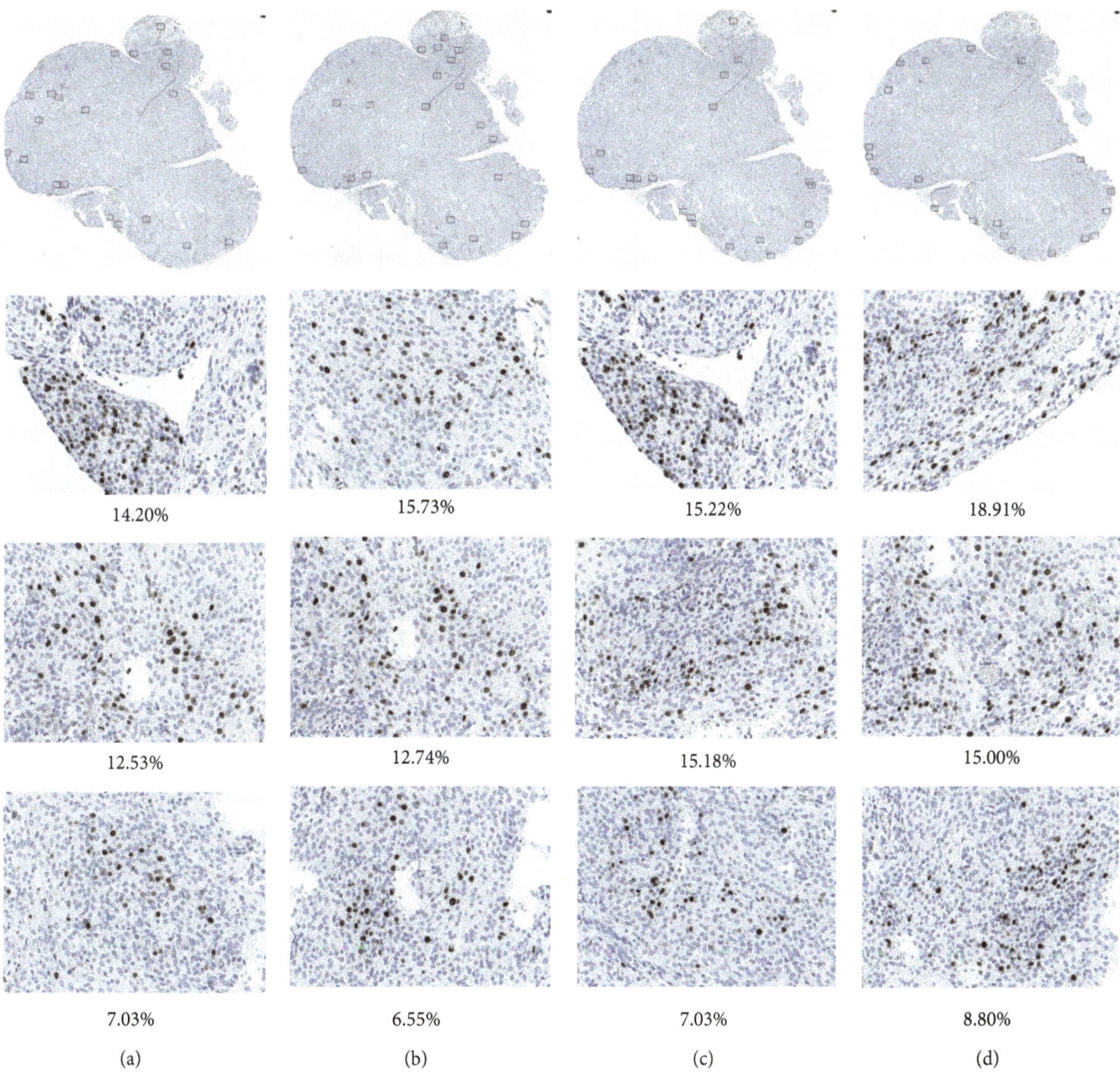

FIGURE 5: The results of hot spot and area of quantification selections by one pathologist ((a), (b), and (c)) and by proposed automated method (d) with examples of 3 areas of quantification chosen approximately in the same region (hot spot) for each selection. The Ki-67 index value calculated as percentage of immunopositive nuclei to the whole number of nuclei in presented area differs slightly.

TABLE 3: The results of the pairwise agreement analysis of data, without taking into account categorical information produced using Kendall's tau-b analysis for interobserver variability on the WSI from sets A and B separately: TM means classical expert microscopic review, P1 and P2 mean pathologists, and AU means proposed automatic method.

	TM	P1	P2	AU
		A		
TM		0.85281 (0.78355 : 0.87879)	0.79221 (0.71429 : 0.82684)	0.68831 (0.60173 : 0.68831)
P1	0.85281 (0.78355 : 0.87619)		0.92208 (0.88745 : 0.93074)	0.81818 (0.76623 : 0.81818)
P2	0.79221 (0.71429 : 0.82684)	0.92208 (0.88745 : 0.93074)		0.80952 (0.75758 : 0.80952)
AU	0.68831 (0.60173 : 0.68831)	0.81818 (0.76623 : 0.81818)	0.80952 (0.75758 : 0.80952)	
		B		
TM		0.67687 (0.65 : 0.70017)	0.58503 (0.55629 : 0.60697)	0.54762 (0.51888 : 0.56871)
P1	0.67687 (0.64966 : 0.70034)		0.86735 (0.85782 : 0.87398)	0.78231 (0.77262 : 0.78912)
P2	0.58503 (0.55629 : 0.60714)	0.86735 (0.85748 : 0.87381)		0.7551 (0.75 : 0.76531)
AU	0.54762 (0.51871 : 0.56871)	0.78231 (0.77228 : 0.78912)	0.7551 (0.75 : 0.76531)	

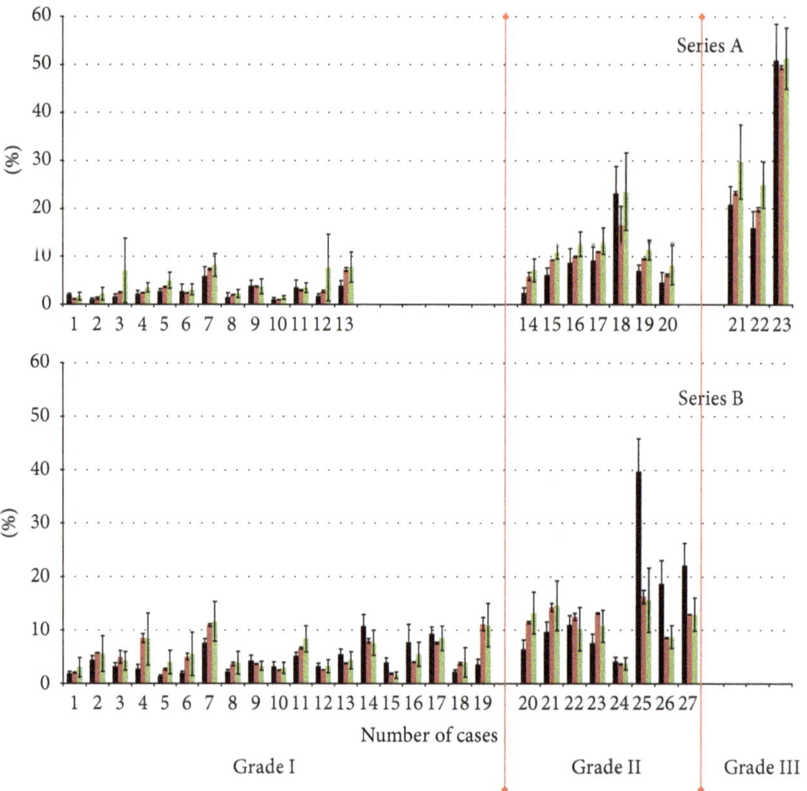

FIGURE 6: The mean and standard deviation of the scoring Ki-67 index for all 50 examined glass slides and their WSI derived from meningioma patients. Data are grouped according to the types of measurements, grade of malignance (grade I, grade II, and grade III), and type of sample preparation method (sets A and B). In each of the three bars the first, blue bar shows the result for the manual microscopic expert score and the second, red bar shows the result for the mean of the pathologists' quantifications using WSI, while the third, green bar presents results for the proposed automated method.

TABLE 4: The results of pooled (for all experts) agreement analysis of categorized data using Kendall's tau-b analysis for interobserver variability on the WSI from sets A and B separately. The data are grouped in categories, grade I and grade II, while grade III was excluded from the analysis because of the small number of WSIs (3) in this category. TM means classical expert microscopic review, Human means the mean of the pathologists, and AU means the proposed automatic method.

	Human	TM	AU
		A—grade I	
Human		0.60606 (0.54545 : 0.69697)	0.78788 (0.66667 : 0.78788)
TM	0.60606 (0.54545 : 0.69697)		0.39394 (0.27273 : 0.42424)
AU	0.78788 (0.66667 : 0.78788)	0.39394 (0.27273 : 0.42424)	
		A—grade II	
Human		0.86667 (0.46667 : 0.86667)	0.86667 (0.46667 : 0.86667)
TM	0.86667 (0.46667 : 0.86667)		1 (0.46667 : 1)
AU	0.86667 (0.46667 : 0.86667)	1 (0.46667 : 1)	
		B—grade I	
Human		0.33333 (0.28105 : 0.39608)	0.77778 (0.75163 : 0.80392)
TM	0.33333 (0.28105 : 0.39869)		0.32026 (0.26797 : 0.35948)
AU	0.77778 (0.75163 : 0.80392)	0.32026 (0.26928 : 0.35948)	
		B—grade II	
Human		0.42857 (0.2381 : 0.52381)	0.80952 (0.71429 : 0.90476)
TM	0.42857 (0.2381 : 0.52381)		0.2381 (0.047619 : 0.33333)
AU	0.80952 (0.71429 : 0.90476)	0.2381 (0.047619 : 0.33333)	

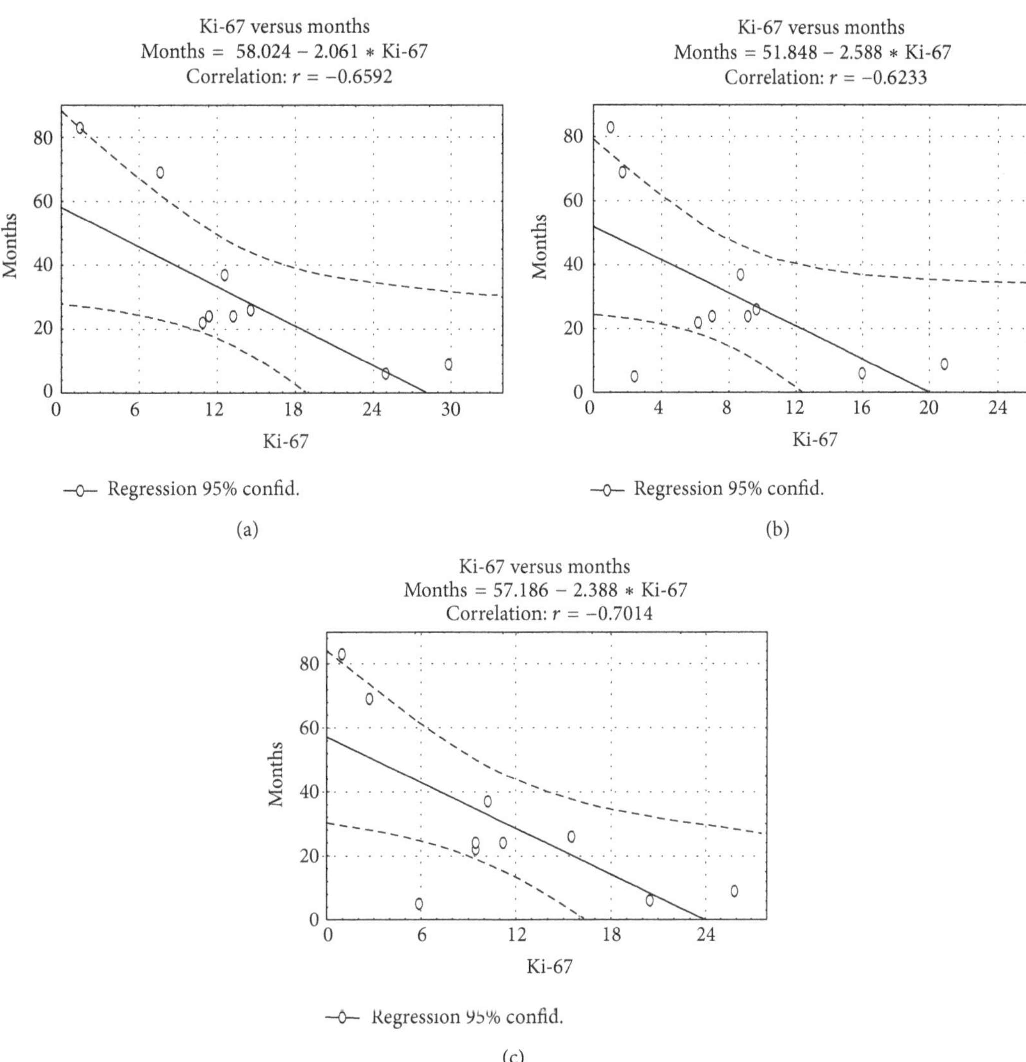

FIGURE 7: The regression function estimated for the number of months between recurrences of meningioma related to the value of Ki-67 index calculated based on (i) fully automatic method (a), (ii) traditional microscopic assessment (b), and (iii) semiautomatic human-computer hybrid approach (c).

to forget the samples. The results presented coefficients of concordance supported with confidence intervals (95% confidence level) calculated using bootstrap analysis of the samples (100 order changes). This shows very good agreement for all combinations of three scores performed by one observer (all coefficients are between 0.85 and 0.9 for data without categorization and between 0.7 and 0.85 for those categorized in grade I and between 0.73 and 1 for those categorized in grade II). Intraobserver variability is significantly smaller than analogous interobserver analysis results presented in Table 4.

4. Discussion and Conclusions

The Ki-67 index, obtained for each patient WSI, determines the downstream clinical decision which concerns patients' treatment and, in consequence, patients' recovery, recurrences of the disease, or patient death. To compare the Ki-67 index obtained using three methods, that is, traditional microscopic, human-computer hybrid method, and the fully automatic method proposed in this paper in the context of the final results of the therapy for the patients, there is a need to know full patients' case histories which are not available in the Polish Healthcare System. What appears to be available after exposé documentation review is data on the recurrence of meningioma in those patients who have been rehospitalized in the same hospital. Among 50 patients whose samples or glasses were used in these investigations, only 10 patients have currently returned to the same hospital with a recurrence of meningioma. So, the prediction of the probability of the meningioma recurrence based on the Ki-67 index for all three methods of estimation has been estimated. The regression functions calculated for the number of months between the cancer surgical treatment and its recurrence in relation to the value of the Ki-67 index calculated based on 10 patients' information are presented in Figure 7.

Table 5: The results of intraobserver agreement examinations using Kendall's tau-b analysis calculated based on pairwise analysis performed in uncategorized (top part) and categorized schemas. The results show coincidence between Ki-67 indexes based on 3 selections of fields of quantification by the same pathologist.

	P1 (1)	P1 (2)	P1 (3)
		All	
P1 (1)		0.85004 (0.8355 : 0.88658)	0.9032 (0.88398 : 0.91775)
P1 (2)	0.85948 (0.8329 : 0.88745)		0.88216 (0.85541 : 0.90649)
P1 (3)	0.86165 (0.83203 : 0.8961)	0.89835 (0.87965 : 0.92554)	
		Grade I	
P1 (1)		0.69697 (0.66667 : 0.72727)	0.84848 (0.72727 : 0.87879)
P1 (2)	0.69697 (0.66667 : 0.72727)		0.78788 (0.75758 : 0.84848)
P1 (3)	0.84848 (0.72727 : 0.87879)	0.78788 (0.75758 : 0.84848)	
		Grade II	
P1 (1)		0.73333 (0.73333 : 0.73333)	0.73333 (0.73333 : 0.73333)
P1 (2)	0.73333 (0.73333 : 0.73333)		1 (0.86667 : 1)
P1 (3)	0.73333 (0.73333 : 0.73333)	1 (0.86667 : 1)	

Comparing all three regression function parameters ($ax+b$) and the value of the correlation, there is no significant difference between them.

In summary, the results of both the above analysis and the analysis described in the previous section show that there is no evidence that either hybrid human-computer aided or fully automatic selection of the area of quantification is superior for quantifying the Ki-67 index in meningioma patient samples. The results of the study show close agreement in terms of their correlations with tumor recurrences and a relatively high overall agreement for quantification using both methods presented in the paper, while the results for each of the methods and traditional macroscopic estimation by an expert are not so high.

In this study, the time constraints were not examined but without any doubt the automatic area selection followed by automatic analyses would lead to time saving for pathologists.

The agreement observed for the three scoring methods, that is, traditional optical microscope and the method based on digital modalities used by pathologists to select the region of quantification, together with a fully automatic computer aided version of this selection, shows that automation of area selection in WSI is an effective tool in helping physicians and in increasing the reliability of diagnosis based on immunohistochemically stained tissue sections. Furthermore, discussion of the standardization of meningioma Ki-67 quantification is welcomed.

Conflict of Interests

The authors declare that there is no conflict of interests regarding the publication of this paper.

Acknowledgment

This study was supported by the National Centre for Research and Development, Poland (Grant PBS2/A9/21/2013).

References

[1] S. H. Swerdlow, International Agency for Research on Cancer, and World Health Organization, *WHO Classification of Tumours of Haematopoietic and Lymphoid Tissue*, World Health Organization Classification of Tumors, International Agency for Research on Cancer, 2008.

[2] D. L. Commins, R. D. Atkinson, and M. E. Burnett, "Review of meningioma histopathology," *Neurosurgical Focus*, vol. 23, no. 4, p. E3, 2007.

[3] H. Colman, C. Giannini, L. Huang et al., "Assessment and prognostic significance of mitotic index using the mitosis marker phospho-histone H3 in low and intermediate-grade infiltrating astrocytomas," *American Journal of Surgical Pathology*, vol. 30, no. 5, pp. 657–664, 2006.

[4] A. Terzi, E. A. Saglam, A. Barak, and F. Soylemezoglu, "The significance of immunohistochemical expression of Ki-67, p53, p21, and p16 in meningiomas tissue arrays," *Pathology Research and Practice*, vol. 204, no. 5, pp. 305–314, 2008.

[5] A. Cruz-Roa, F. González, J. Galaro et al., "A visual latent semantic approach for automatic analysis and interpretation of anaplastic medulloblastoma virtual slides," *Medical Image Computing and Computer-Assisted Intervention*, vol. 15, part 1, pp. 157–164, 2012.

[6] M. A. Gavrielides, B. D. Gallas, P. Lenz, A. Badano, and S. M. Hewitt, "Observer variability in the interpretation of HER2/neu immunohistochemical expression with unaided and computer-aided digital microscopy," *Archives of Pathology & Laboratory Medicine*, vol. 135, no. 2, pp. 233–242, 2011.

[7] M. A. Gavrielides, C. Conway, N. O'Flaherty, B. D. Gallas, and S. M. Hewitt, "Observer performance in the use of dgital and optical microscopy for the interpretation of tissue-based biomarkers," *Analytical Cellular Pathology*, vol. 2014, Article ID 157308, 10 pages, 2014.

[8] M. A. Gavrielides, B. D. Gallas, P. Lenz, A. Badano, and S. M. Hewitt, "Observer variability in the interpretation of HER2/neu immunohistochemical expression with unaided and computer-aided digital microscopy," *Archives of Pathology and Laboratory Medicine*, vol. 135, no. 2, pp. 233–242, 2011.

[9] T. Seidal, A. J. Balaton, and H. Battifora, "Interpretation and quantification of immunostains," *The American Journal of Surgical Pathology*, vol. 25, no. 9, pp. 1204–1207, 2001.

[10] G. Puppa, C. Senore, K. Sheahan et al., "Diagnostic reproducibility of tumour budding in colorectal cancer: a multicentre, multinational study using virtual microscopy," *Histopathology*, vol. 61, no. 4, pp. 562–575, 2012.

[11] D. S. A. Sanders, H. Grabsch, R. Harrison et al., "Comparing virtual with conventional microscopy for the consensus diagnosis of Barrett's neoplasia in the AspECT Barrett's chemoprevention trial pathology audit," *Histopathology*, vol. 61, no. 5, pp. 795–800, 2012.

[12] M. G. Rojo, G. Bueno, and J. Slodkowska, "Review of imaging solutions for integrated quantitative immunohistochemistry in the Pathology daily practice," *Folia Histochemica et Cytobiologica*, vol. 47, no. 3, pp. 349–354, 2009.

[13] K. E. Brick, J. C. Sluzevich, M. A. Cappel, D. J. Dicaudo, N. I. Comfere, and C. N. Wieland, "Comparison of virtual microscopy and glass slide microscopy among dermatology residents during a simulated in-training examination," *Journal of Cutaneous Pathology*, vol. 40, no. 9, pp. 807–811, 2013.

[14] L. Pantanowitz, J. H. Sinard, W. H. Henricks et al., "Validating whole slide imaging for diagnostic purposes in pathology: guideline fromthe College of American Pathologists Pathology and Laboratory Quality Center," *Archives of Pathology & Laboratory Medicine*, vol. 137, no. 12, pp. 1710–1722, 2013.

[15] M. G. Rojo, G. Bueno, and J. Slodkowska, "Review of imaging solutions for integrated quantitative immunohistochemistry in the Pathology daily practice," *Folia Histochemica et Cytobiologica*, vol. 47, no. 3, pp. 349–354, 2010.

[16] T. Markiewicz, S. Osowski, J. Patera, and W. Kozlowski, "Image processing for accurate cell recognition and count on histologic slides," *Analytical and Quantitative Cytology and Histology*, vol. 28, no. 5, pp. 281–291, 2006.

[17] M. Krótkiewicz and K. Wojtkiewicz, "An introduction to ontology based structured knowledge base system: knowledge acquisition module," in *Intelligent Information and Database Systems: 5th Asian Conference, ACIIDS 2013, Kuala Lumpur, Malaysia, March 18–20, 2013, Proceedings, Part I*, vol. 7802 of *Lecture Notes in Computer Science*, pp. 497–506, Springer, Berlin, Germany, 2013.

[18] M. Bator and L. J. Chmielewski, "Finding regions of interest for cancerous masses enhanced by elimination of linear structures and considerations on detection correctness measures in mammography," *Pattern Analysis and Applications*, vol. 12, no. 4, pp. 377–390, 2009.

[19] C. López, M. Lejeune, R. Bosch et al., "Digital image analysis in breast cancer: an example of an automated methodology and the effects of image compression.," *Studies in Health Technology and Informatics*, vol. 179, pp. 155–171, 2012.

[20] C. López, M. Lejeune, M. T. Salvadó et al., "Automated quantification of nuclear immunohistochemical markers with different complexity," *Histochemistry and Cell Biology*, vol. 129, no. 3, pp. 379–387, 2008.

[21] U. Neuman, A. Korzynska, C. Lopez, and M. Lejeune, "Segmentation of stained lymphoma tissue section images," in *Information Technologies in Biomedicine*, E. Piętka and J. Kawa, Eds., vol. 69 of *Advances in Intelligent and Soft Computing*, pp. 101–113, Springer, Berlin, Germany, 2010.

[22] A. Korzynska, L. Roszkowiak, C. Lopez, R. Bosch, L. Witkowski, and M. Lejeune, "Validation of various adaptive threshold methods of segmentation applied to follicular lymphoma digital images stained with 3,3′-diaminobenzidine&haematoxylin," *Diagnostic Pathology*, vol. 8, no. 1, article 48, 2013.

[23] U. Neuman, A. Korzynska, C. Lopez, M. Lejeune, Ł. Roszkowiak, and R. Bosch, "Equalisation of archival microscopic images from immunohistochemically stained tissue sections," *Biocybernetics and Biomedical Engineering*, vol. 33, no. 1, pp. 63–76, 2013.

[24] T. Markiewicz, P. Wisniewski, S. Osowski, J. Patera, W. Kozlowski, and R. Koktysz, "Comparative analysis of methods for accurate recognition of cells through nuclei staining of Ki-67 in neuroblastoma and estrogen/progesterone status staining in breast cancer," *Analytical and Quantitative Cytology and Histology*, vol. 31, no. 1, pp. 49–62, 2009.

[25] S. di Cataldo, E. Ficarra, and E. Macii, "Automated segmentation of tissue images for computerized IHC analysis," *Computer Methods and Programs in Biomedicine*, vol. 100, no. 1, pp. 1–15, 2010.

[26] S. Di Cataldo, E. Ficarra, A. Acquaviva, and E. Macii, "Achieving the way for automated segmentation of nuclei in cancer tissue images through morphology-based approach: a quantitative evaluation," *Computerized Medical Imaging and Graphics*, vol. 34, no. 6, pp. 453–461, 2010.

[27] M. M. Fernández-Carrobles, I. Tadeo, G. Bueno et al., "TMA vessel segmentation based on color and morphological features: application to angiogenesis research," *The Scientific World Journal*, vol. 2013, Article ID 263190, 11 pages, 2013.

[28] G. Bueno, R. González, O. Déniz et al., "A parallel solution for high resolution histological image analysis," *Computer Methods and Programs in Biomedicine*, vol. 108, no. 1, pp. 388–401, 2012.

[29] V. Roullier, O. Lézoray, V.-T. Ta, and A. Elmoataz, "Multiresolution graph-based analysis of histopathological whole slide images: application to mitotic cell extraction and visualization," *Computerized Medical Imaging and Graphics*, vol. 35, no. 7-8, pp. 603–615, 2011.

[30] S. Kothari, J. H. Phan, T. H. Stokes, and M. D. Wang, "Pathology imaging informatics for quantitative analysis of whole-slide images," *Journal of the American Medical Informatics Association*, vol. 20, no. 6, pp. 1099–1108, 2013.

[31] K. Kayser, D. Radziszowski, P. Bzdyl, R. Sommer, and G. Kayser, "Towards an automated virtual slide screening: theoretical considerations and practical experiences of automated tissue-based virtual diagnosis to be implemented in the internet," *Diagnostic Pathology*, vol. 1, article 10, 2006.

[32] J. R. Gilbertson, J. Ho, L. Anthony, D. M. Jukic, Y. Yagi, and A. V. Parwani, "Primary histologic diagnosis using automated whole slide imaging: a validation study," *BMC Clinical Pathology*, vol. 6, article 4, 2006.

[33] B. Molnar, L. Berczi, C. Diczhazy et al., "Digital slide and virtual microscopy based routine and telepathology evaluation of routine gastrointestinal biopsy specimens," *Journal of Clinical Pathology*, vol. 56, no. 6, pp. 433–438, 2003.

[34] S. J. Potts, D. A. Eberhard, and M. E. Salama, "Practical approaches to microvessel analysis: hotspots, microvessel density, and vessel proximity," in *Molecular Histopathology and Tissue Biomarkers in Drug and Diagnostic Development*, Methods in Pharmacology and Toxicology, pp. 87–100, Springer, 2014.

[35] H. Lu, T. G. Papathomas, D. van Zessen et al., "Automated Selection of Hotspots (ASH): enhanced automated segmentation and adaptive step finding for Ki67 hotspot detection in adrenal cortical cancer," *Diagnostic Pathology*, vol. 9, no. 1, article 216, 2014.

[36] S. Nakasu, D. H. Li, H. Okabe, M. Nakajima, and M. Matsuda, "Significance of MIB-1 staining indices in meningiomas: comparison of two counting methods," *The American Journal of Surgical Pathology*, vol. 25, no. 4, pp. 472–478, 2001.

[37] M. Unser, "Sum and difference histograms for texture classification," *IEEE Transactions on Pattern Analysis and Machine Intelligence*, vol. 8, no. 1, pp. 118–125, 1986.

[38] http://www.openslice.com.

[39] R. Koprowski and Z. Wrobel, "The cell structures segmentation," in *Computer Recognition Systems*, M. Kurzynski, E. Puchala, M. Wozniak, and A. Zolnierek, Eds., vol. 30 of *Advances in Soft Computing*, pp. 569–576, Springer, Berlin, Germany, 2005.

[40] A. Korzyńska, U. Neuman, C. Lopez, M. Lejeun, and R. Bosch, "The method of immunohistochemical images standardization," in *Image Processing and Communications Challenges 2*, vol. 84 of *Advances in Intelligent and Soft Computing*, pp. 213–221, Springer, Berlin, Germany, 2010.

[41] T. Álvaro-Naranjo, M. Lejeune, M.-T. Salvadó et al., "Immunohistochemical patterns of reactive microenvironment are associated with clinicobiologic behavior in follicular lymphoma patients," *Journal of Clinical Oncology*, vol. 24, no. 34, pp. 5350–5357, 2006.

[42] P. Soille, *Morphological Image Analysis—Principles and Applications*, Springer, Berlin, Germany, 2004.

[43] N. Otsu, "A threshold selection method from gray-level histograms," *IEEE Systems, Man, and Cybernetics Society*, vol. 9, no. 1, pp. 62–66, 1979.

[44] R. O. Duda, P. E. Hart, and P. Stork, *Pattern Classification and Scene Analysis*, Wiley, New York, NY, USA, 2003.

[45] B. Grala, T. Markiewicz, W. Kozłowski, S. Osowski, J. Słodkowska, and W. Papierz, "New automated image analysis method for the assessment of Ki-67 labeling index in meningiomas," *Folia Histochemica et Cytobiologica*, vol. 47, no. 4, pp. 587–592, 2009.

[46] M. Kendall, *Rank Correlation Methods*, Charles Griffin and Co. Limited, London, UK, 1948.

[47] R. F. Woolson and W. R. Clarke, *Statistical Methods for the Analysis of Biomedical Data*, John Wiley & Sons, New York, NY, USA, 1987.

[48] S. D. Balboacă and L. Jäntschi, "Pearson versus Spearman, Kendall's tau correlation analysis on structure-activity relationships of biologic active compounds," *Leonardo Journal of Sciences*, no. 9, pp. 179–200, 2006.

19

Ex Vivo Nicotine Stimulation Augments the Efficacy of Human Peripheral Blood Mononuclear Cell-Derived Dendritic Cell Vaccination via Activating Akt-S6 Pathway

Yan Yan Wang,[1] Yi Wen Yang,[1] Xiang You,[1] Xiao Qian Deng,[1] Chun Fang Hu,[1] Cong Zhu,[1] Jun Yao Wang,[1] Jiao Jiao Gu,[1] Yi Nan Wang,[1] Qing Li,[1] and Feng Guang Gao[1,2]

[1] *Department of Immunology, Basic Medicine Science, Medical College, Xiamen University, Xiamen 361102, China*
[2] *The State Key Laboratory for Oncogenes and Related Genes, Shanghai Jiao Tong University, Shanghai 200032, China*

Correspondence should be addressed to Qing Li; sunnymaylq@hotmail.com and Feng Guang Gao; gfengguang@xmu.edu.cn

Academic Editor: Consuelo Amantini

Our previous studies showed that $\alpha7$ nicotinic acetylcholine receptor (nAchR) agonist nicotine has stimulatory effects on murine bone marrow-derived semimature DCs, but the effect of nicotine on peripheral blood mononuclear cell- (PBMC-) derived human semimature dendritic cells (hu-imDCs) is still to be clarified. In the present study, hu-imDCs (cultured 4 days) were conferred with *ex vivo* lower dose nicotine stimulation and the effect of nicotine on surface molecules expression, the ability of cross-presentation, DCs-mediated PBMC priming, and activated signaling pathways were determined. We could demonstrate that the treatment with nicotine resulted in increased surface molecules expression, enhanced hu-imDCs-mediated PBMC proliferation, upregulated release of IL-12 in the supernatant of cocultured DCs-PBMC, and augmented phosphorylation of Akt and ribosomal protein S6. Nicotine associated with traces of LPS efficiently enhanced endosomal translocation of internalized ovalbumin (OVA) and increased TAP-OVA colocalization. Importantly, the upregulation of nicotine-increased surface molecules upregulation was significantly abrogated by the inhibition of Akt kinase. These findings demonstrate that *ex vivo* nicotine stimulation augments hu-imDCs surface molecules expression via Akt-S6 pathway, combined with increased Ag-presentation result in augmented efficacy of DCs-mediated PBMC proliferation and Th1 polarization.

1. Introduction

Dendritic cells (DCs) are professional antigen-presenting cells (APCs) that recognize extracellular antigens in the peripheral tissue. On recognition of microbial substances, DCs migrate toward the draining lymph node, where they can induce antigen-specific T-cell priming and reveal therapeutic and protective antitumor immunity [1, 2]. In previous studies, we have demonstrated that *ex vivo* nicotine stimulation has stimulatory effects on murine bone marrow-derived semimature DCs (imDCs), which reveal efficient upregulation of surface molecules through $\alpha7$ nicotinic acetylcholine receptor (nAchR) [3–6]. Further studies showed that the treatment with nicotine increases surface molecules expression via PI3K-Akt pathway and nicotine-treated murine imDCs has antitumor effects in both Lewis lung cancer and hepatocellular carcinoma [4, 5]. Although several groups have documented that nicotine has positive effects in the treatment of neurodegenerative diseases, ulcerative colitis, and Tourette syndrome [7–9], it is the first time of our studies demonstrating that nicotine-treated imDCs have preventive and therapeutic effects on murine tumor formation. However, the effect of *ex vivo* nicotine stimulation on human peripheral blood mononuclear cells- (PBMC-) derived imDCs (hu-imDCs) is still uncertain.

For T-cell activation, internalized antigens are degraded, and the resulting peptides are loaded to MHC molecules and transported to plasma membrane, where these complexes are recognized by antigen-specific T cells. While peptides which resulted from soluble antigen can be loaded to MHC class II molecules, it can also be loaded to MHC class I molecules, a process termed cross-presentation [10, 11]. Efficient cross-presentation requires antigen uptake-mediated entrance of antigen into early endosome [12], which was mediated by mannose receptor [13]. Meanwhile, the critical role of proteasome in generating epitopes and transporting internalized antigen across the endosomal membrane into cytoplasm was also documented [14]. Although previous studies revealed that *ex vivo* nicotine stimulation increases antigen internalization and promotes imDCs' cross-presentation [3–6], the exact effect of endosomal translocation of internalized antigen in nicotine-increased cross-presentation is still uncertain, nevertheless the effect of nicotine on the transporting internalized antigen to cytoplasm.

In the present study, hu-imDCs (cultured 4 days) were conferred with *ex vivo* lower dose nicotine stimulation and the effect of nicotine on surface molecules expression, the ability of cross-presentation, DCs-mediated PBMC priming, and activated signaling pathways were determined. We demonstrate that *ex vivo* nicotine stimulation results in increased surface molecules expression, enhanced hu-imDCs-mediated PBMC proliferation, upregulated the release of IL-12, increased the percentage of CD8/IFN-gamma double positive cell in cocultured DCs-PBMC, and augmented phosphorylation of Akt and ribosomal protein S6. Nicotine associated with traces of LPS efficiently enhanced endosomal translocation of internalized ovalbumin (OVA) and increased TAP-OVA colocalization. Importantly, nicotine-increased upregulation of surface molecules was significantly abrogated by the inhibition of Akt kinase. These findings demonstrate that *ex vivo* nicotine stimulation augments hu-imDCs surface molecules expression via Akt-S6 pathway, combined with increased Ag-presentation result in augmented efficacy of DCs-mediated PBMC proliferation and Th1 polarization.

2. Materials and Methods

2.1. Reagents. Reagents were purchased from the following companies: (−)-nicotine (N3876), lipopolysaccharide (LPS), α-bungarotoxin-tetramethylrhodamine from Bungarus multicinctus (Formosan Banded Krait) (T0195), and tubocurarine chloride were obtained from Sigma-Aldrich (St. Louis, MO, USA). Recombinant human GM-CSF and IL-4 were obtained from PeproTech (Rocky Hill, NJ, USA). Endotoxin-free EndoGrade-ovalbumin (OVA) was purchased from Hyglos GmbH (Regensburg, Germany). PI3K inhibitor LY294002 and Akt inhibitor Wortmannin were from Cayman Chemical (Ann Arbor, MI, USA). Purified anti-chicken ovalbumin (OVA) (Clone TOSGAA1) was obtained from Biolegend (San Diego, CA). Antibodies to EEA1, Rab7, and TAP were from Cell Signaling Technology (Beverly, MA, USA). RPMI-1640 medium and fetal bovine serum (FBS) were purchased from HyClone (Logan, UT, USA). BD Phosflow antibodies to phospho-p38 (p-T180/pY182) (Clone 36/p38), phospho-Erk1/2 (p-T202/pY204) (Clone 20A), phospho-Akt (pS473) (Clone M89-61), phospho-S6 (pS235/pS236) (Clone N7-548), and human IL-12 ELISA Kit were from BD Biosciences (San Jose, CA, USA). BrdU Cell Proliferation Kit was obtained from Roche (Roche Diagnostics GmbH, Germany). Fluorescence conjugated antibodies to human CD80, CD86, 4-1BBL, CD8, IFN-γ, MHC class I, and MHC class II molecules were obtained from eBioscience (San Diego, USA). Mounting medium for fluorescence with DAPI was obtained from Vector Laboratories, Inc. (Burlingame, CA, USA). Human PBMC isolation reagent was from Haoyang Biological Manufacture Co., Ltd. (Tianjin, China). Rab5, goat anti-mouse IgG and donkey anti-goat IgG secondary antibodies were from Abcam (New Territories, HK).

2.2. Generation of Human PBMC-Derived imDCs. Briefly, human PBMC was prepared from the donor's blood by gradient density centrifugation using PBMC isolation reagents and cultured at a density of 1×10^6 cells/mL in RPMI 1640 medium in the presence of 100 ng/mL recombinant human GM-CSF and 100 ng/mL IL-4. Nonadherent cells were gently washed out with PBS on day 4; the remaining loosely adherent clusters were used as hu-imDCs. Cells were synchronized by serum starvation (in RPMI 1640 with 0.5% FBS) for 4~6 h before the further treatment. This study was conducted with the understanding and the consent of all the blood donors and was approved by the Institutional Review Board for Human Subjects at the Medical College of Xiamen University.

2.3. Human imDCs Treatment. To determine the effect of *ex vivo* nicotine stimulation on surface molecules expression, hu-imDCs were exposed to nicotine (10^{-7} mol/L) for 12 to 15 h after cell synchronization by 0.5% serum starvation. The pretreatment with 2 μg/mL α-bungarotoxin or (4×10^{-5} mol/L) tubocurarine chloride 2 h prior to nicotine stimulation was conducted to investigate the role of α7 nAchR in nicotine-increased DCs' function. To elucidate the mechanism of nicotine-increased surface molecules expression, hu-imDCs were conferred with LY294002 (10 μmol/L) or Wortmannin (10 μmol/L) 2 h prior to nicotine (10^{-7} mol/L) exposure.

2.4. Flow Cytometric Measurement for Surface Molecules. The expression of surface molecules in hu-imDCs was determined by flow cytometry. Briefly, hu-imDCs were preincubated with 0.5 μg CD16/CD32 antibodies for 10 min. Then, aliquot cell suspension was stained with combined primary antibody at a concentration of 1 μg per 1×10^6 cells. Staining was performed on ice for 30 min and cells were washed with ice-cold PBS, containing 0.1% NaN3 and 0.5% BSA. Flow cytometry was done with FACSCalibur and data were analyzed with CellQuest software.

2.5. Flow Cytometric Measurement for Intracellular Signaling Molecules. To determine the effect of nicotine on kinases phosphorylation, hu-imDCs were collected by trypsination and treated with nicotine (10^{-7} mol/L) for 15 min. The phosphorylation of related kinase was determined by BD Phosflow. Briefly, at the end of nicotine treatment, the cells were immediately mixed with warmed BD Phosflow Fix Buffer I and incubated at 37°C for 10 min. Then, the cells were washed with BD Pharmingen Stain Buffer and permeabilized by incubation with cold BD Phosflow Perm Buffer III for 30 min on ice. After complete washes, the cells were stained with BD Phosflow antibodies and flow cytometry was done with FACSCalibur and data were analyzed with CellQuest software.

2.6. Confocal Microscope Analyses. The effect of nicotine on the endosomal translocation of antigen and the complex formation of ovalbumin-derived peptide-MHC class I and II molecules were investigated by confocal microscope analyses. Briefly, hu-imDCs were exposed to nicotine (10^{-7} mol/L) for 12~15 h. Then, the cells were conferred with endotoxin-free EndoGrade-ovalbumin (50 μg/mL) 60 min pulse with or without short period (20 min) LPS (1 ng/mL) stimulation. After that, the DCs were fixed and permeabilized in 100% methanol for 15 min, washed with PBS, and blocked with 10% nonfat milk for 3 h. Primary antibodies were incubated in a humid chamber overnight at 4°C. Finally, fluorescence-conjugated secondary antibodies were incubated for 1 h at 37°C. DAPI counterstaining was performed to visualize cell nuclei. The cell was washed three times in each step to remove nonbinding substance and images were recorded by a confocal fluorescence microscope at the wavelength of 488 nm.

2.7. Ag-Specific PBMC Proliferation and CTL Priming Assay. Briefly, hu-imDCs (cultured for 4 d) were pretreated with α-bungarotoxin (2 μg/mL) or tubocurarine chloride (4×10^{-5} mol/L) 2 h prior to nicotine treatment. Then, the DCs were conferred with 3 h endotoxin-free EndoGrade-ovalbumin (50 μg/mL) pulse with 60 min LPS (1 ng/mL) stimulation. Responder cells were prepared from PBMC of the same donor. Stimulator cells were mixed with responders at a ratio of 1 : 1. After 5 d of coculture, Ag-specific PBMC proliferation was determined by BrdU cell proliferation assay. To determine CTL priming, the proliferated PBMC cells were performed intracellular IFN-gamma and CD8 positive flow cytometric analyses.

2.8. Quantification of IL-12 Production. The release of IL-12 in the supernatant of MLR was determined by ELISA according to the standard procedure. Briefly, plates were treated with coating antibody at 4°C overnight, washed with PBS, and blocked with assay buffer at room temperature for 2 h. The blocked plates were washed twice with thorough aspiration of microwell contents between washes. After the last wash step, empty wells and tap microwell strip to remove excess wash buffer. Samples of assay buffer, biotin-conjugated detector antibodies were added to microwells and the plates were incubated at room temperature for 2 h. After incubation, plates were washed 5 times and added with streptavidin-HRP. After 1 h of incubation at room temperature, plates were washed and TMB substrate solution was added to all wells for color formation. Plates were incubated at room temperature and stop solution was added to stop the enzyme reaction at appropriate time. Absorbance of each microwell was read using 450 nm as primary wave length and 620 nm as reference wavelength, respectively.

2.9. Western Blot. For analysis of Akt and S6 phosphorylation regulated by nicotine on hu-imDCs, proteins were obtained in lysis buffer. Protein lysates (30 μg/mL) were electrophoresed on 10% SDS-PAGE gels, transferred to PVDF membranes, and blotted with phospho-Akt and phospho-S6 antibodies, followed by anti-mouse horseradish peroxidase and detection by chemiluminescence ECL. As loading controls, antibody against β-actin was used.

2.10. Statistical Analysis. All data were expressed as mean and standard error means. Statistical significance was tested using the Student t-test or one-way ANOVA with post-Newman-Keuls test. Statistical differences were considered to be significant if $P < 0.05$.

3. Results

3.1. Nicotine Upregulates Surface Molecules Expression in Human Semimature DCs. Human immature monocyte-derived DCs are commonly generated by culturing adherent peripheral monocytes with GM-CSF and IL-4 for up to 6 days [15–17]. Meanwhile, in a 4-day culture system, murine semimature DCs could differentiate into a regulatory DCs subset by splenic stromal cells [18] and have potential anti-tumor effects [3–6]. To explore the effect of nicotine on DCs' maturation and viability, hu-imDCs (cultured 4 days) were conferred with *ex vivo* nicotine stimulation. Consistent with murine semimature DCs' results [19, 20], 10^{-7} mol/L nicotine has no effect on cell viability of hu-imDCs (see Supplementary Figure 1 in Supplementary Material available online at http://dx.doi.org/10.1155/2015/741487). While 83.43% vehicle-treated hu-imDCs expressed human DCs specific marker CD1a, the treatment with nicotine increased the level of CD1a to about 150% (Supplementary Figure 2a). The analyses of CD11c expression also achieved the similar results (Supplementary Figure 2b). Considering *ex vivo* lower dose nicotine stimulation promotes the development of mouse semimature DCs [20, 21], the 4-day culture system might be a specific condition for the effect of lower dose nicotine stimulation on hu-imDCs.

MHC class I and II molecules are the components of antigenic peptide-MHC complex for antigen presentation [10–14]. While CD80/CD86 are important costimulatory molecules in T-cell-APC interaction [2, 22], 4-1BBL, which sends signals to 4-1BB-expressing cells [23, 24], was found to play critical roles in preventing activation-induced cell death [25, 26]. To explore the exact effect of nicotine stimulation on the expression of surface molecules, hu-imDCs were conferred with nicotine exposure and the expression of CD80, 4-1BBL, and MHC class I and II molecules was determined by flow cytometry. Compared with vehicle-treated cells, the treatment with nicotine obviously increased the expression of CD80, 4-1BBL, revealing about 177% and 131% upregulation, respectively (Figures 1(a) and 1(b)). The determination of MHC class I and II molecules also achieved similar results (Figures 1(c) and 1(d)). Interestingly, when dot plot of flow cytometry was used to investigate the effect of nicotine on DCs maturation, the treatment with nicotine not

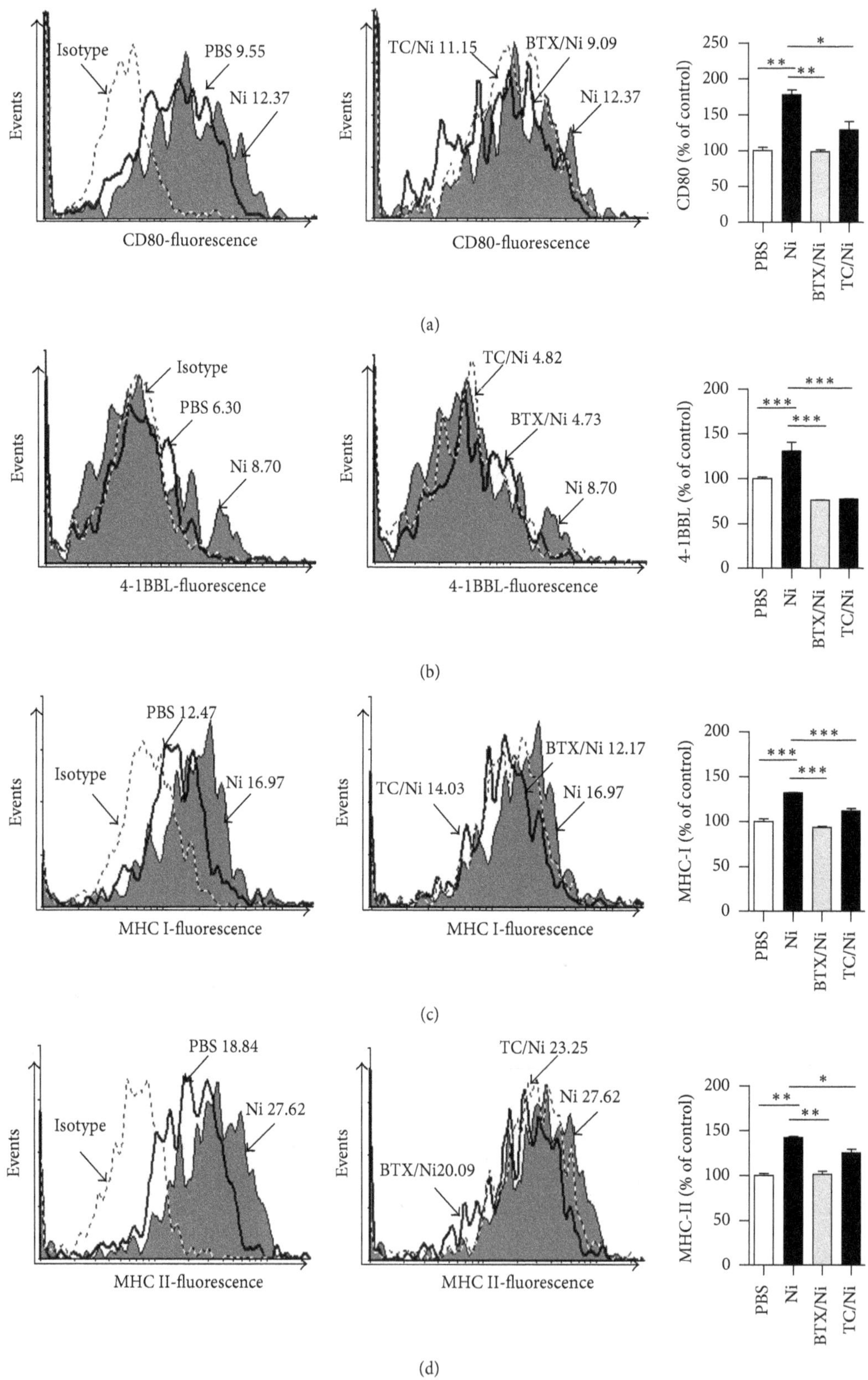

FIGURE 1: Nicotine upregulates surface molecules expression in human semimature DCs. (a–d) DCs derived from human PBMC with 100 ng/mL recombinant human GM-CSF and IL-4 were conferred with α-bungarotoxin (2 μg/mL) or tubocurarine chloride (4×10^{-5} mol/L) 2 h prior to nicotine (10^{-7} mol/L) 12~15 h stimulation. The effect of nicotine on the expression of CD80 (a), 4-1BBL (b), MHC class I (c), and MHC class II (d) molecules was determined by flow cytometry. Numbers in histogram indicated mean fluorescence intensity (MFI) of test samples. Data were given as mean ± SEM, one-way ANOVA with post-Newman-Keuls test. $^{*}P < 0.05$, $^{**}P < 0.01$, and $^{***}P < 0.001$. One representative from 3 independent experiments is shown. Ni: nicotine; BTX: α-bungarotoxin; and TC: tubocurarine chloride.

only increased CD1a-CD11c double positive DCs' percentage (Supplementary Figure 3a) but also augmented MHC class II-CD86 double positive cell population (Supplementary Figure 3b). These data indicate that *ex vivo* nicotine stimulation not only increases the expression of CD80 and 4-1BBL but also upregulates the expression of MHC class I and II molecules in hu-imDCs.

α7 nAchR, which is mainly expressed in DCs, is involved in nicotine-augmented expression of surface molecules in murine semimature DCs [19]. To investigate the potential roles of α7 nAchR in nicotine-increased surface molecules expression, hu-imDCs were treated with α7 nAchR specific α-bungarotoxin or nonspecific antagonist tubocurarine chloride prior to nicotine stimulation. Despite the expression of CD80, 4-1BBL, and MHC class I and II molecules obviously upregulated by the treatment with nicotine, the usage of α-bungarotoxin and tubocurarine chloride efficiently abrogated nicotine's effect on surface molecules expression (Figure 1), indicating that nicotine increasing surface molecules expression is α7 nAchR-dependent.

3.2. Ex Vivo Nicotine Stimulation Augments Semimature DCs-Mediated PBMC Proliferation and Promotes the Release of IL-12 in the Supernatant of Cocultured DCs-PBMC. Our previous studies showed that the treatment with lower dose nicotine promotes mouse semimature DCs-mediated cross priming [3–6]. Since *ex vivo* nicotine stimulation increases the expression of surface molecules in hu-imDCs (Figure 1, Supplementary Figure 3), we accessed the exact effect of nicotine stimulation on hu-imDCs-mediated PBMC proliferation and Th1 polarization by cocultured *ex vivo* nicotine-stimulated, ovalbumin-loaded hu imDCs with PBMC. As endotoxins increase antigen processing in both MHC class II–restricted antigen presentation and intracellular mechanisms of cross-presentation [27, 28], we mimic the ordinary antigen by giving traces of LPS (1 ng/mL) to endotoxin-free EndoGrade-ovalbumin. Compared with controls, while the loading with endotoxin-free ovalbumin and LPS promotes hu-imDCs-mediated PBMC proliferation, *ex vivo* nicotine stimulation efficiently augmented the ability of hu-imDCs-dependent PBMC proliferation ($P < 0.001$). The pretreatment with α-bungarotoxin or tubocurarine chloride dramatically abolished nicotine-increased hu-imDCs mediated PBMC proliferation, which revealed about 26.65% and 43.26% inhibitory rates, respectively, (Figure 2(a)), indicating that nicotine exposure-increased hu-imDCs-mediated PBMC proliferation is α7 nAchR-dependent.

IL-12, an indicator of antigen-specific CTL priming, can polarize Th0 to Th1 transition and subsequently induce antivirus and antitumor immune responses [29]. Since the treatment with nicotine increased hu-imDCs-mediated PBMC proliferation, we further explored if such stimulation could polarize Th0 to Th1 transition by the IL-12 determination in the supernatant of cocultured DCs-PBMC. Compared with controls, the pulse of endotoxin-free ovalbumin with traces of LPS obviously augmented IL-12 release in the supernatant. *Ex vivo* nicotine stimulation efficiently increased IL-12 release to about 167%. The pretreatment with α-bungarotoxin or tubocurarine chloride obviously abolished nicotine-increased IL-12 secretion with 58%~70% inhibitory rate (Figure 2(b)). Flow cytometric measurement of intracellular IFN-gamma showed that the percentage of double positive cell of IFN-gamma and CD8 was also increased by the treatment with *ex vivo* nicotine stimulation (Figure 2(c)). These data indicate that the treatment with nicotine facilitates Th1 polarization and CTL priming in DCs-mediated PBMC proliferation.

3.3. The Exposure of Traces of LPS Increases the Endosomal Translocation of Antigen and TAP-OVA-MHC Class I Molecules Complex Formation in Human Semimature DCs. Mannose receptor, which is expressed in human DCs, uptakes antigen and determines subcellular antigen localization [31]. The localization of model antigen ovalbumin in early endosomal compartment [13] did not further mature early endosome into lysosomes but promote antigen for cross-presentation [12]. Meanwhile, microbial products such as LPS were demonstrated to trigger a program of DCs maturation which enables DCs to activate T cells [14]. To elucidate the role of LPS in nicotine-increased antigen early endosomal translocation, we pulsed hu-imDCs briefly (60 min) with endotoxin-free EndoGrade-ovalbumin, concurrently either with short period (20 min) LPS (1 ng/mL) stimulation or for the same length of time but without LPS exposure (Figure 3). We assessed endosomal translocation of antigen by ovalbumin and EEA1/Rab7 antibodies staining. Coadministration of endotoxin-free EndoGrade-ovalbumin with short period LPS exposure resulted in significantly enhanced translocation of ovalbumin to endosomal compartment (Figure 3). As efficient cross-presentation requires the entrance of antigen into a specific intracellular pathway [12], the increased endosomal translocation of ovalbumin by lower dose LPS indicates that nicotine-increased cross-presentation needs mannose receptor-mediated endosomal translocation of internalized antigen.

While antigens internalization via mannose receptor-mediated endocytosis was routed into a distinct murine endosomal subset [10, 11], these endosomal subsets could reimport proteasome-derived peptides into the same endosomal compartment by LPS-inducing endosomal translocation of TAP, thereafter loading these peptides onto MHC I molecules [12]. To explore the role of LPS-inducing signaling in TAP-mediated antigenic transport, we assessed the translocation of antigen, TAP, and MHC class I and II molecules in lower dose LPS (1 ng/mL) presenting condition with related antibodies staining. Compared with nicotine-treated hu-imDCs, the signaling induced by LPS administration resulted in significantly enhanced translocation of OVA-TAP and OVA-MHC class I molecules (Figure 4). The colocalization of TAP-MHC class I molecules was also augmented by the treatment with LPS, whereas TAP-MHC class II molecules colocalization was not affected anymore (Figure 4). These results indicate that nicotine-increased cross-presentation needs LPS-induced endosomal recruitment of TAP.

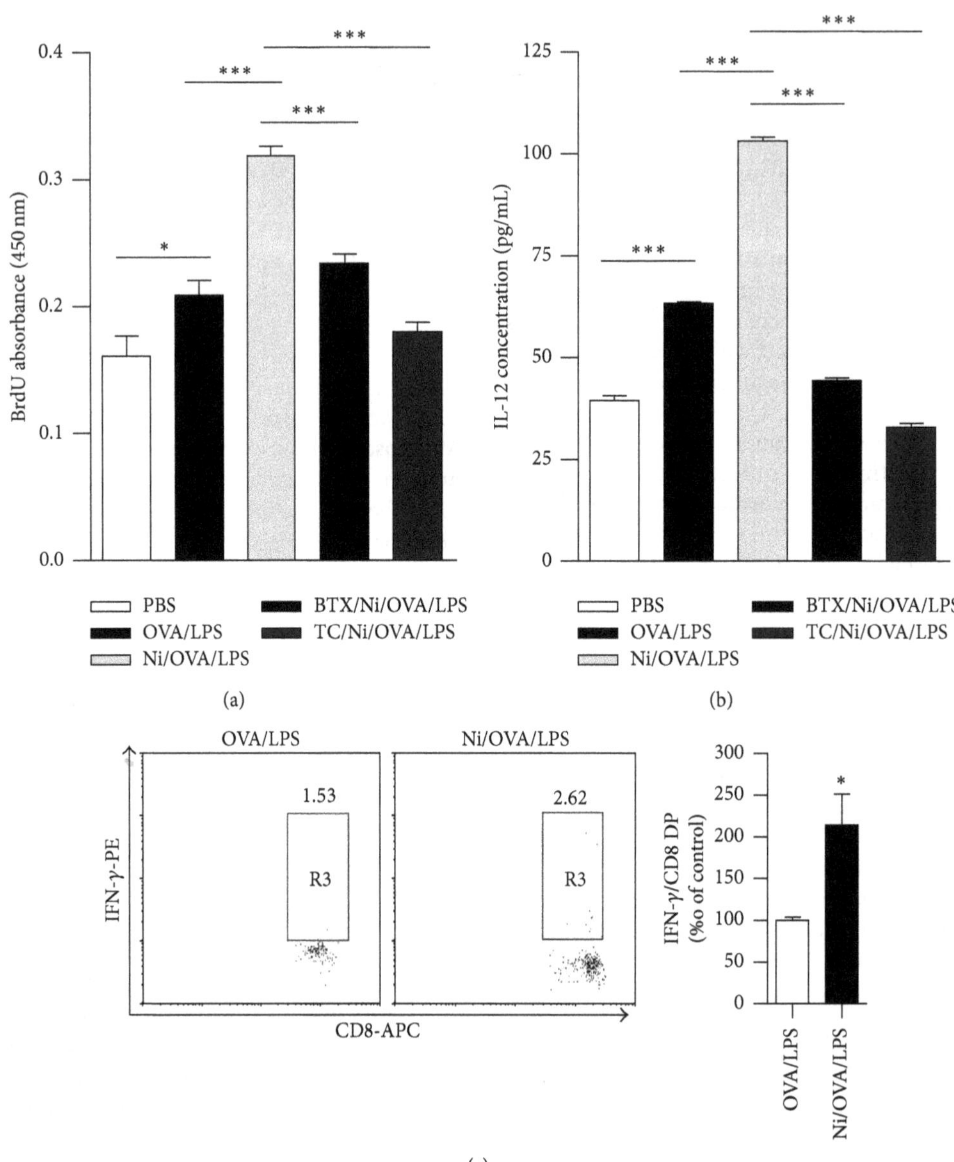

FIGURE 2: *Ex vivo* nicotine stimulation augments semimature DCs-mediated PBMC proliferation, promotes the release of IL-12, and increases the percentage of IFN-gamma/CD8 cells in the supernatant of cocultured DCs-PBMC. DCs derived from human PBMC with 100 ng/mL recombinant human GM-CSF and IL-4 were conferred with α-bungarotoxin (2 μg/mL) or tubocurarine chloride (4×10^{-5} mol/L) 2 h prior to nicotine (10^{-7} mol/L) 12~15 h stimulation. Then, the DCs were pulsed with endotoxin-free EndoGrade-ovalbumin (50 μg/mL) for 3 h, followed by 1 h LPS (1 ng/mL) stimulation. After that, the DCs were coincubated with PBMC of the same donor at a ratio of 1 : 1 for 5 d and the effect of nicotine on DCs-mediated PBMC proliferation, the IL-12 release in the supernatant, and IFN-gamma/CD8 cell percentage of cocultured DCs-PBMC were determined by BrdU cell proliferation assay (a), ELISA (b), and flow cytometry (c), respectively. Data were given as mean ± SEM, $n = 2$, one-way ANOVA with post-Newman-Keuls test. $^{*}P < 0.05$, and $^{***}P < 0.001$. One representative from 3 independent experiments is shown. Ni: nicotine; BTX: α-bungarotoxin; and TC: tubocurarine chloride.

3.4. The Treatment with Nicotine Induces Akt-S6 Pathway Activation in Human Semimature DCs. It was reported that the Erkl/2-p38-JNK MAPK and PI3K-Akt pathways could be activated by the treatment with nicotine and play important roles in nicotine-augmented surface molecules expression in murine DCs [5, 6, 19]. Meanwhile, the activation of Akt-mTORC1 induced by nicotine promotes structural plasticity in mesencephalic dopaminergic neurons was also documented [32]. To explore the role of Akt-mTOR in nicotine-increased DCs surface molecules expression, we thereafter tested the effect of nicotine on Erkl/2-p38 MAPK and Akt-S6 pathway activation. Unlike traditional methods such as Western blotting, intracellular phosphoprofiling could examine cellular subpopulations in complex samples and

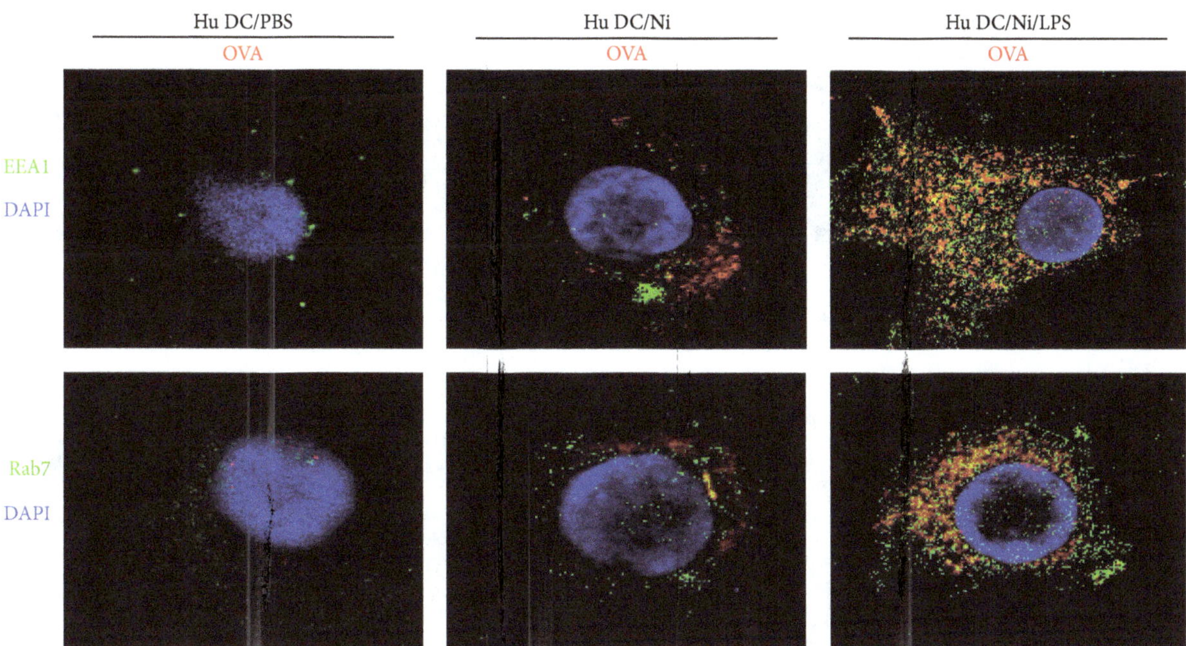

FIGURE 3: The exposure of traces of LPS increases the endosomal translocation of antigen in human semimature DCs. DCs derived from human PBMC with recombinant human GM-CSF and IL-4 were conferred with nicotine (10^{-7} mol/L) 12~15 h stimulation. Then, the DCs were exposed to 60 min endotoxin-free EndoGrade-ovalbumin (50 μg/mL) pulse and 20 min LPS (1 ng/mL) stimulation. The effect of nicotine and LPS on endosomal translocation of antigen was observed by confocal microscope analyses. One representative from 3 independent experiments is shown. Ni: nicotine.

analyze phosphoprotein signaling in rare cell subtypes [33, 34]. While the phosphorylation of Erk1/2 and p38 could be obviously augmented by nicotine stimulation (Supplementary Figure 4), the treatment with nicotine rapidly increased the phosphorylation status of Akt and S6 in the early 15 minutes, which revealed 163.5% and 191.8% increase, respectively, by flow cytometry assay (Figure 5(a)). Western blotting (Figure 5(b)) and confocal microscope analyses (Figure 5(c)) also showed that Akt-S6 pathway could be activated by the treatment with nicotine, indicating that Erk1/2-p38 and Akt-S6 pathways might be play potential roles in nicotine-increased surface molecules expression.

3.5. Nicotine Increases Surface Molecule Expression in Human Semimature DCs by Activating Akt-S6 Pathway. Despite the treatment with nicotine activates Akt-S6 pathway, the exact role of Akt-S6 in nicotine-increased surface molecule expression in hu-imDCs is still uncertain. We accessed the expression of surface molecules in human DCs by inhibition relevant kinases. Compared with vehicle-treated cells, the treatment with nicotine increased about 162.94%, 216.4%, 322.4%, 149%, and 126% expression of CD80, MHC class I, MHC class II, CD86, and 4-1BBL, respectively (Figure 6). Importantly, in contrast to the treatment with nicotine, the pretreatment with both Akt inhibitor LY294002 and Wortmannin obviously abolished nicotine's effect on these surface molecules upregulation (Figure 6). All these results indicate that the activation of Akt-S6 is involved in nicotine-increased surface molecules expression in hu-imDCs.

4. Discussion

In the present study, we investigated the effect of nicotine on surface molecules expression, the ability of cross-presentation, DCs-mediated PBMC priming, and activated signaling pathways by exposing hu-imDCs to nicotine stimulation. We demonstrate that the upregulation of surface molecules, the enhancement of hu-imDCs-mediated PBMC proliferation, and increased release of IL-12 in the supernatant of cocultured DCs-PBMC are α7 nAchR-dependent. Importantly, the percentage of CD8/IFN-gamma double positive cell was increased by the treatment with *ex vivo* nicotine stimulation. Moreover, the phosphorylation of Akt and ribosomal protein S6 induced by nicotine stimulation play vital roles in nicotine-increased surface molecules expression. Interestingly, the endosomal translocation of internalized ovalbumin and increased TAP-OVA colocalization are also augmented by the treatment with traces of LPS.

Nicotine, a major component of cigarette smoke which promotes established tumor metastasis and increases overall mortality in cancer patients [7], is widely accepted as a risk factor for atherosclerosis [19]. Since the nAchR is mainly expressed in neuron and affects neurodegenerative disease progression [35], the effects of nicotine on promoting lung cancer development, reducing the efficacy of chemotherapeutic agents [8], and activating hypoxia-inducible factor-1 α expression [9] can not exclude the potential roles of nAchR in regulating the function of DCs and neuron. Recently, α7 nAchR has been documented to exist in murine DCs and play pivotal roles in regulating DCs' function [3–6,

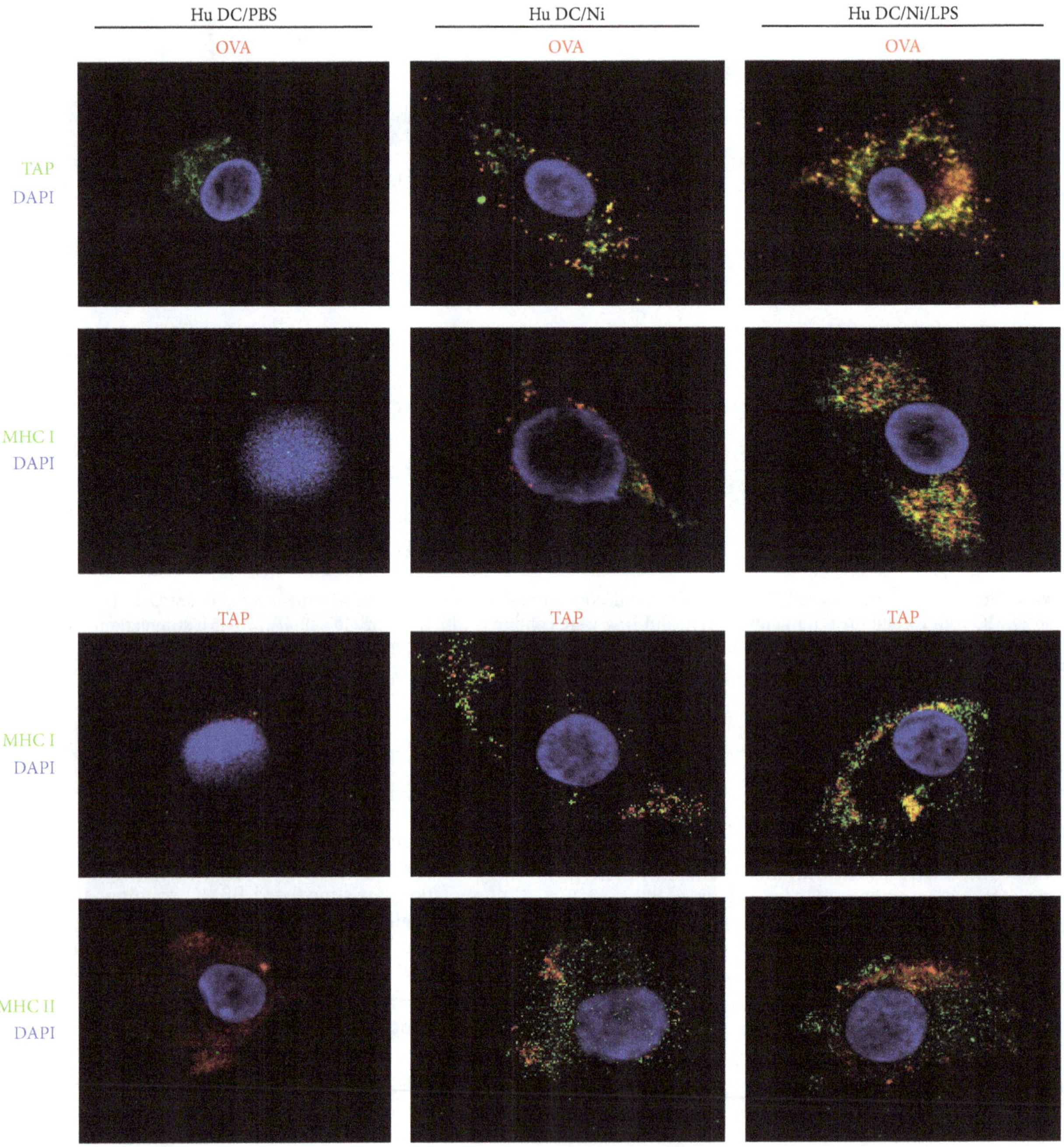

FIGURE 4: The exposure of traces of LPS increases TAP-OVA-MHC class I molecules complex formation in human semimature DCs. DCs derived from human PBMC with recombinant human GM-CSF and IL-4 were conferred with nicotine (10^{-7} mol/L) 12~15 h stimulation. Then, the DCs were exposed to 60 min endotoxin-free EndoGrade-ovalbumin (50 μg/mL) pulse and 20 min LPS (1 ng/mL) stimulation. The effect of nicotine and LPS on the complex formation of TAP, OVA, and MHC class I molecules was observed by confocal microscope analyses. One representative from 3 independent experiments is shown. Ni: nicotine.

22]. In response to Th2-promoting stimuli, both mouse and human DCs generated to 6-7 days in the presence of the immune modulator nicotine (nicDCs) preferentially support the differentiation of antigen-specific IL-4-producing Th2 effector cells [15]. Furthermore, NicDCs could produce lower levels of proinflammatory cytokines when compared with DCs differentiated in the absence of nicotine [16, 17], indicating the modulating role of nicotine in DCs' development. Hence, the exact effect of nicotine on DCs' function is currently contradictory. Using splenic stromal cells to mimic the immune microenvironment, murine immature DCs (cultured 4 days) could induce their differentiation into a new regulatory DC subset by both stromal cell contact and stromal cell-derived transforming growth factor-beta [18].

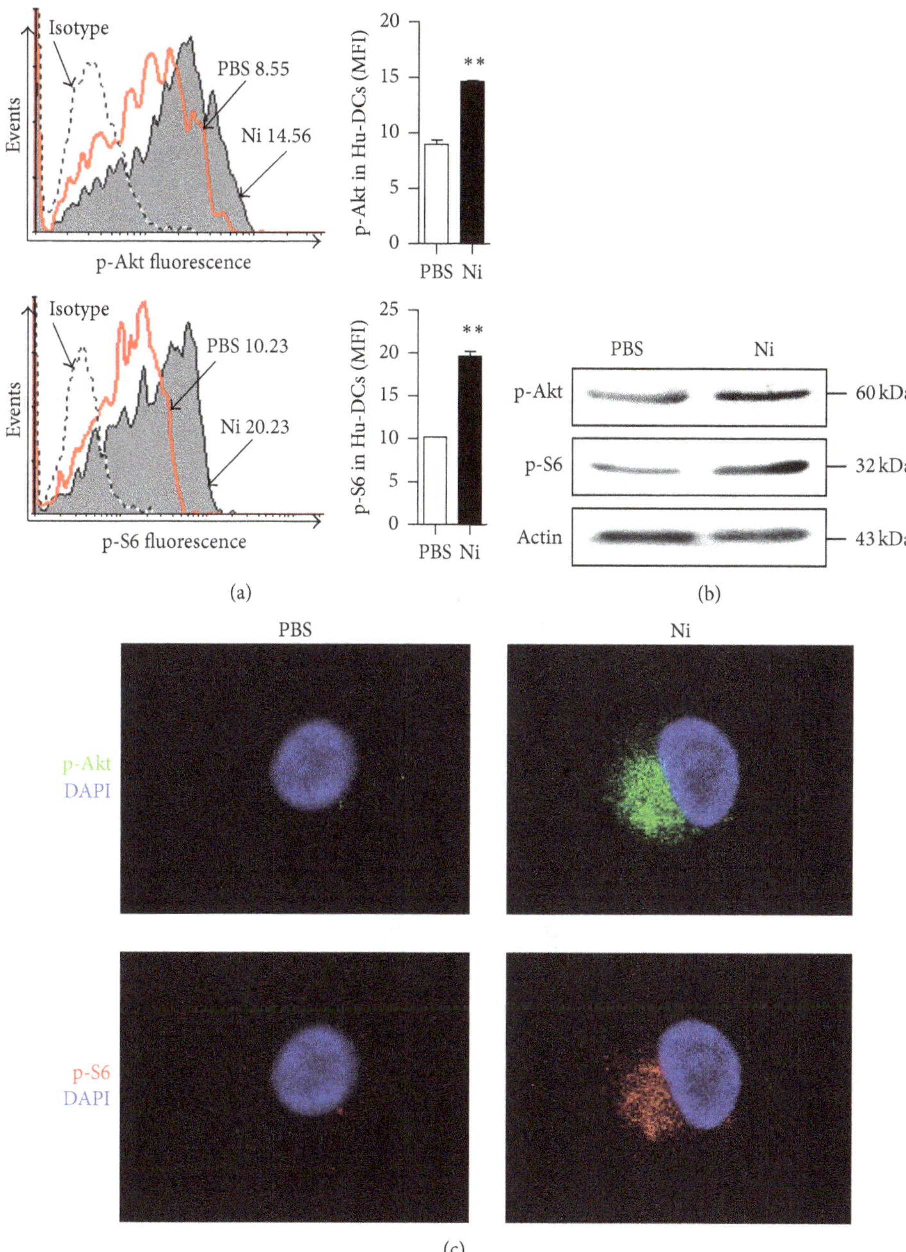

FIGURE 5: The treatment with nicotine induces Akt-S6 pathway activation in human semimature DCs. (a–c) Human PBMC-derived semimature DCs were stimulated with nicotine (10^{-7} mol/L) for 15 min and the phosphorylation of Akt and ribosomal protein S6 was determined by flow cytometry (a), Western blotting (b), and confocal microscope analyses (c), respectively. One representative from 3 independent experiments is shown. Numbers in histogram indicated mean fluorescence intensity (MFI) of test samples. Data were given as mean ± SEM, Student t-test, $^{**}P < 0.01$. Ni: nicotine.

In our previous studies, murine immature DCs (cultured 4 days) have been demonstrated to reveal potential antitumor effects by *ex vivo* nicotine stimulation [3–6]. Further studies reveal that although the treatment with nicotine and LPS upregulates surface molecules expression [20] and enables DCs to present Ags in the context of MHC I molecules, the $CD8^+$ T-cell priming is refractory [36]. As the biological effect of nicotine on lymphocyte is dependent on dose of nicotine, the duration of exposure[37], and the LPS existence in experiment system [20], the controversy of nicotine's effect on DCs might be attributed to the differences of experimental design, species, duration of exposure, and especially the nicotine concentration used in these experiments. With the treatment of 200 mg/mL nicotine, Nouri-Shirazi and Guinet found that the exposure to nicotine adversely affects the dendritic cell system and compromises host response to vaccination [38]. On the other hand, the presence of nicotine (0–200 μg/mL) promotes the development of mouse DC precursors into a semimature phenotype and supports the differentiation of ovalbumin- (OVA-) specific naïve T cells

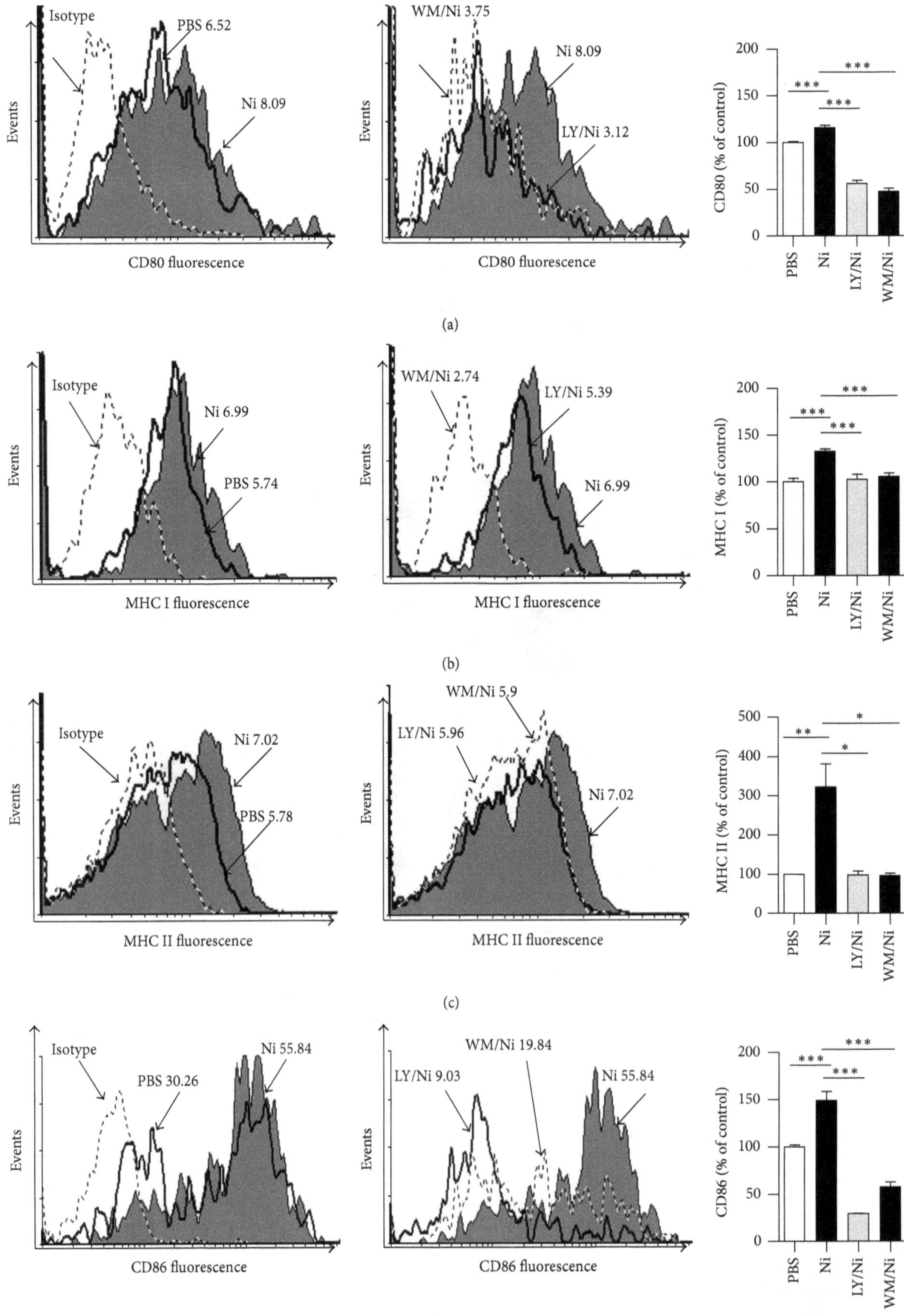

Figure 6: Continued.

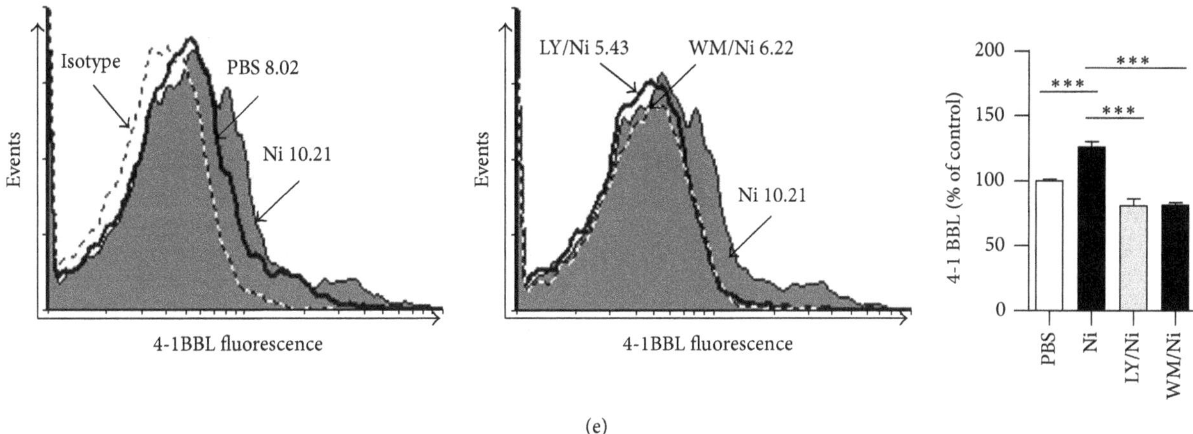

(e)

Figure 6: Nicotine increases surface molecule expression in human semimature DCs by activating Akt-S6 pathway. (a–e) DCs derived from human PBMC with human GM-CSF and IL-4 were conferred with LY294002 (10 μmol/L) or Wortmannin (10 μmol/L) 2 h prior to 12~15 h nicotine (10^{-7} mol/L) stimulation. The effect of Akt inhibition on nicotine-increased expression of CD80 (a), MHC class I (b), MHC class II (c), CD86 (d), and 4-1BBL (e) was determined by flow cytometry. Numbers in histogram indicated mean fluorescence intensity (MFI) of test samples. Data were given as mean ± SEM, one-way ANOVA with post Newman-Keuls test. $^{*}P < 0.05$, $^{**}P < 0.01$, and $^{***}P < 0.001$. One representative from 3 independent experiments is shown. Ni: nicotine; LY: LY294002; WM (Wort): Wortmannin.

into effector memory cells [21]. In our systematic studies, 10^{-7} mol/L nicotine (16.5 ng/mL) was used as α7 nAchR agonist to stimulate human or murine semimature DCs (cultured 4 days). Hence, lower dose nicotine stimulation (16.5 ng/mL) and DCs with a semimature phenotype were the specific conditions for achieving increased DCs vaccination. It does not implicate that nicotine itself has the similar biological effect on cancer growth.

Nicotine increasing mouse immature DCs-mediated cross priming could be abolished by α7 nAchR specific antagonist α-bungarotoxin and nonspecific antagonist tubocurarine chloride [3–6], indicating the vital role of α7 nAchR in nicotine-augmented murine DCs' function. In the present study, hu-imDCs were pretreated with α-bungarotoxin or tubocurarine chloride prior to *ex vivo* nicotine stimulation to investigate the role of α7 nAchR in nicotine-augmented hu-imDCs' function. Consistent with the finding of murine DCs, not only the upregulation of surface molecules (Figure 1) but also DCs-mediated PBMC priming (Figure 2) was abrogated by the blockage of α7 nAchR. These data indicate that nicotine-increased DCs-dependent PBMC proliferation and surface molecules upregulation are also α7 nAchR-dependent.

Antigens internalized by DCs via fluid phage pinocytosis or scavenger receptor-mediated endocytosis are rapidly targeted toward lysosomal structures, where they are degraded instantly and processed for presentation on MHC II molecules [39]. Meanwhile, antigens, which are internalized by the mannose receptor, are routed into endosome subpopulation. Antigens of endosome compartment are protected from lysosomal degradation and are processed exlusively for cross-presentation [12]. Recently, endotoxin was found to increase recruitment of TAP toward antigen-containing endosomes and enable the retranslocation of proteasome-derived peptides into the same endosome subset [12, 27, 28]. In this study, compared with endotoxin-free ovalbumin loading, the pulse of endotoxin-free ovalbumin with traces of LPS not only increased the endosomal translocation of antigen (Figure 3) but also augmented the formation of OVA-TAP-MHC class I complex (Figure 4), indicating that nicotine-enhanced hu-imDCs cross-presentation might also attribute to LPS-increased endosomal protection from lysosomal degradation and the endosomal recruitment of TAP.

Akt, which could be phosphorylated within the activation loop at threonine 308 and the C-terminus at serine 473, promotes cell survival by inhibiting proapoptotic function of Bad [40]. We have demonstrated that nicotine activates PI3K-Akt pathway and upregulates CD80 molecules expression in murine DCs [5, 6]. Jossin and Goffinet's study also showed that PI3K-Akt signal controls cortical development and regulates dendritic growth [41]. In the present study, Akt pathway was found to play vital role in nicotine-increased surface molecules expression in hu-imDCs (Figure 6). Ribosomal protein S6, which plays a role in regulating the translation of RNAs and thus controlling the growth and proliferation of cells [42], was efficient phosphorylated by the treatment with nicotine (Figure 5). Although mTORC1 was involved in nicotine-induced structural plasticity in mesencephalic dopaminergic neurons [32], the phosphorylation of S6 ribosomal protein was reported to upregulate ribosomal translocation of RNA species coding for other ribosomal proteins, peptide elongation factors [43]. Hence, the exact role of S6 ribosomal protein in nicotine-regulated surface molecules expression in human DCs still needs further investigation.

In conclusion, all the data presented here indicate that nicotine upregulating surface molecules and enhancing DCs-mediated PBMC proliferation and the release of IL-12 are α7 nAchR-dependent. Nicotine-enhanced hu-imDCs cross-presentation attributes to LPS-increased endosomal translocation of internalized ovalbumin and the endosomal recruitment of TAP.

Abbreviations

DCs: Dendritic cells
nAChR: Nicotinic acetylcholine receptor
S6: Ribosomal protein S6
PI3K: Phosphatidylinositol-3-kinase
Ni: Nicotine
MLRs: Mixed lymphocyte reactions
LPS: Lipopolysaccharide
PBMC: Peripheral blood monouclear cells
EEA1: Early endosome antigen 1
TAP: Transporter associated with antigen processing
Rab1: Ras-Related superfamily of guanine nucleotide binding proteins 1.

Conflict of Interests

The authors declare that they have no conflict of interests.

Authors' Contribution

Yan Yan Wang, Yi Wen Yang, and Xiang You contributed equally to this paper. Feng Guang Gao designed the research and copyedited the paper. Yan Yan Wang and Xiang You contributed to FACS, MLR, ELISA, and confocal microscope observation. Chun Fang Hu contributed to Western blot. Xiao Qian Deng and Yi Nan Wang contributed to MLR and ELISA. Cong Zhu, Jun Yao Wang, and Jiao Jiao Gu contributed to human DCs induction. Yi Wen Yang contributed to flow cytometry and confocal microscope observation. Qing Li wrote the paper.

Acknowledgments

This work was supported by Grants from the State Key Laboratory of Oncogenes and Related Genes (no. 90-14-05), Grants from the National Natural Science Foundation of China (no. 81273203; no. 81201275), and Grants from Natural Science Foundation of Fujian Province of China (nos. 2015J01353, 2013J05124).

References

[1] J. D. Bassett, T. C. Yang, D. Bernard et al., "CD8+ T-cell expansion and maintenance after recombinant adenovirus immunization rely upon cooperation between hematopoietic and nonhematopoietic antigen-presenting cells," *Blood*, vol. 117, no. 4, pp. 1146–1155, 2011.

[2] N.-L. L. Pham, L. L. Pewe, C. J. Fleenor et al., "Exploiting cross-priming to generate protective CD8 T-cell immunity rapidly," *Proceedings of the National Academy of Sciences of the United States of America*, vol. 107, no. 27, pp. 12198–12203, 2010.

[3] G. G. Feng, F. W. Da, and R. G. Jian, "Ex vivo nicotine stimulation augments the efficacy of therapeutic bone marrow-derived dendritic cell vaccination," *Clinical Cancer Research*, vol. 13, no. 12, pp. 3706–3712, 2007.

[4] F. G. Gao, H. T. Li, Z. J. Li, and J. R. Gu, "Nicotine stimulated dendritic cells could achieve anti-tumor effects in mouse lung and liver cancer," *Journal of Clinical Immunology*, vol. 31, no. 1, pp. 80–88, 2011.

[5] H. J. Jin, H. T. Li, H. X. Sui et al., "Nicotine stimulated bone marrow-derived dendritic cells could augment HBV specific CTL priming by activating PI3K-Akt pathway," *Immunology Letters*, vol. 146, no. 1-2, pp. 40–49, 2012.

[6] H. J. Jin, H. X. Sui, Y. N. Wang, and F. G. Gao, "Nicotine up-regulated 4-1BBL expression by activating Mek PI3K pathway augments the efficacy of bone marrow-derived dendritic cell vaccination," *Journal of Clinical Immunology*, vol. 33, no. 1, pp. 246–254, 2013.

[7] R. J. Rangani, M. A. Upadhya, K. T. Nakhate, D. M. Kokare, and N. K. Subhedar, "Nicotine evoked improvement in learning and memory is mediated through NPY Y1 receptors in rat model of Alzheimer's disease," *Peptides*, vol. 33, no. 2, pp. 317–328, 2012.

[8] S. Nikfar, S. Ehteshami-Ashar, R. Rahimi, and M. Abdollahi, "Systematic review and meta-analysis of the efficacy and tolerability of nicotine preparations in active ulcerative colitis," *Clinical Therapeutics*, vol. 32, no. 14, pp. 2304–2315, 2010.

[9] M. Orth, B. Amann, M. M. Robertson, and J. C. Rothwell, "Excitability of motor cortex inhibitory circuits in Tourette syndrome before and after single dose nicotine," *Brain*, vol. 128, no. 6, pp. 1292–1300, 2005.

[10] C. Kreer, J. Rauen, M. Zehner, and S. Burgdorf, "Cross-presentation: how to get there—or how to get the ER," *Frontiers in Immunology*, vol. 2, article 87, 2012.

[11] S. Burgdorf, V. Schuette, V. Semmling et al., "Steady-state cross-presentation of OVA is mannose receptor-dependent but inhibitable by collagen fragments," *Proceedings of the National Academy of Sciences of the United States of America*, vol. 107, no. 13, pp. E48–E49, 2010.

[12] S. Burgdorf, C. Schölz, A. Kautz, R. Tampé, and C. Kurts, "Spatial and mechanistic separation of cross-presentation and endogenous antigen presentation," *Nature Immunology*, vol. 9, no. 5, pp. 558–566, 2008.

[13] M. Zehner, A. I. Chasan, V. Schuette et al., "Mannose receptor polyubiquitination regulates endosomal recruitment of p97 and cytosolic antigen translocation for cross-presentation," *Proceedings of the National Academy of Sciences of the United States of America*, vol. 108, no. 24, pp. 9933–9938, 2011.

[14] M. Zehner and S. Burgdorf, "Regulation of antigen transport into the cytosol for cross-presentation by ubiquitination of the mannose receptor," *Molecular Immunology*, vol. 55, no. 2, pp. 146–148, 2013.

[15] M. Nouri-Shirazi, C. Kahlden, P. Nishino, and E. Guinet, "Nicotine exposure alters the mRNA expression of Notch ligands in dendritic cells and their response to Th1-/Th2-promoting stimuli," *Scandinavian Journal of Immunology*, vol. 81, no. 2, pp. 110–120, 2015.

[16] M. Yanagita, K. Mori, R. Kobayashi et al., "Immunomodulation of dendritic cells differentiated in the presence of nicotine with lipopolysaccharide from *Porphyromonas gingivalis*," *European Journal of Oral Sciences*, vol. 120, no. 5, pp. 408–414, 2012.

[17] M. Yanagita, R. Kobayashi, Y. Kojima, K. Mori, and S. Murakami, "Nicotine modulates the immunological function of dendritic cells through peroxisome proliferator-activated receptor-γ upregulation," *Cellular Immunology*, vol. 274, no. 1-2, pp. 26–33, 2012.

[18] M. Zhang, H. Tang, Z. Guo et al., "Splenic stroma drives mature dendritic cells to differentiate into regulatory dendritic cells," *Nature Immunology*, vol. 5, no. 11, pp. 1124–1133, 2004.

[19] A. Aicher, C. Heeschen, M. Mohaupt, J. P. Cooke, A. M. Zeiher, and S. Dimmeler, "Nicotine strongly activates dendritic cell-mediated adaptive immunity: potential role for progression of atherosclerotic lesions," *Circulation*, vol. 107, no. 4, pp. 604–611, 2003.

[20] S. X. Hu, H. X. Sui, H. J. Jin et al., "Lipopolysaccharide and dose of nicotine determine the effects of nicotine on murine bone marrow-derived dendritic cells," *Molecular Medicine Reports*, vol. 5, no. 4, pp. 1005–1010, 2012.

[21] M. Nouri-Shirazi, R. Tinajero, and E. Guinet, "Nicotine alters the biological activities of developing mouse bone marrow-derived dendritic cells (DCs)," *Immunology Letters*, vol. 109, no. 2, pp. 155–164, 2007.

[22] M. Grujic, C. Bartholdy, M. Remy, D. D. Pinschewer, J. P. Christensen, and A. R. Thomsen, "The role of CD80/CD86 in generation and maintenance of functional virus-specific CD8$^+$ T cells in mice infected with lymphocytic choriomeningitis virus," *Journal of Immunology*, vol. 185, no. 3, pp. 1730–1743, 2010.

[23] Z.-Y. Lu, M. Condomines, K. Tarte et al., "B7-1 and 4-1BB ligand expression on a myeloma cell line makes it possible to expand autologous tumor-specific cytotoxic T cells in vitro," *Experimental Hematology*, vol. 35, no. 3, pp. 443–453, 2007.

[24] C. Wu, H. Guo, Y. Wang, Y. Gao, Z. Zhu, and Z. Du, "Extracellular domain of human 4-1BBL enhanced the function of cytotoxic T-lymphocyte induced by dendritic cell," *Cellular Immunology*, vol. 271, no. 1, pp. 118–123, 2011.

[25] S. Kanagavelu, J. M. Termini, S. Gupta et al., "HIV-1 adenoviral vector vaccines expressing multi-trimeric BAFF and 4-1BBL enhance T cell mediated anti-viral immunity," *PLoS ONE*, vol. 9, no. 2, Article ID e90100, 2014.

[26] C. Wang, T. Wen, J.-P. Routy, N. F. Bernard, R. P. Sekaly, and T. H. Watts, "4-1BBL induces TNF receptor-associated factor 1-dependent Bim modulation in human T cells and is a critical component in the costimulation-dependent rescue of functionally impaired HIV-specific CD8 T cells," *Journal of Immunology*, vol. 179, no. 12, pp. 8252–8263, 2007.

[27] J. M. Blander and R. Medzhitov, "Toll-dependent selection of microbial antigens for presentation by dendritic cells," *Nature*, vol. 440, no. 7085, pp. 808–812, 2006.

[28] B. C. Gil-Torregrosa, A. M. Lennon-Duménil, B. Kessler et al., "Control of cross-presentation during dendritic cell maturation," *European Journal of Immunology*, vol. 34, no. 2, pp. 398–407, 2004.

[29] S. Gupta, R. Boppana, G. C. Mishra, B. Saha, and D. Mitra, "Interleukin-12 is necessary for the priming of CD4$^+$ T cells required during the elicitation of HIV-1 gp120-specific cytotoxic T-lymphocyte function," *Immunology*, vol. 124, no. 4, pp. 553–561, 2008.

[30] T. Hilmenyuk, I. Bellinghausen, B. Heydenreich et al., "Effects of glycation of the model food allergen ovalbumin on antigen uptake and presentation by human dendritic cells," *Immunology*, vol. 129, no. 3, pp. 437–445, 2010.

[31] S. B. Bazan, G. Geginat, T. Breinig, M. J. Schmitt, and F. Breinig, "Uptake of various yeast genera by antigen-presenting cells and influence of subcellular antigen localization on the activation of ovalbumin-specific CD8 T lymphocytes," *Vaccine*, vol. 29, no. 45, pp. 8165–8173, 2011.

[32] G. Collo, F. Bono, L. Cavalleri et al., "Nicotine-induced structural plasticity in mesencephalic dopaminergic neurons is mediated by dopamine D3 receptors and Akt-mTORC1 signaling," *Molecular Pharmacology*, vol. 83, no. 6, pp. 1176–1189, 2013.

[33] K. Blatt, H. Herrmann, I. Mirkina et al., "The PI3-kinase/mTOR-targeting drug NVP-BEZ235 inhibits growth and IgE-dependent activation of human mast cells and basophils," *PLoS ONE*, vol. 7, no. 1, Article ID e29925, 2012.

[34] L. van de Laar, A. van den Bosch, A. Boonstra et al., "PI3K-PKB hyperactivation augments human plasmacytoid dendritic cell development and function," *Blood*, vol. 120, no. 25, pp. 4982–4991, 2012.

[35] M. Q. Xue, X. X. Liu, Y. L. Zhang, and F. G. Gao, "Nicotine exerts neuroprotective effects against β-amyloid-induced neurotoxicity in SH-SY5Y cells through the Erk1/2-p38-JNK-dependent signaling pathway," *International Journal of Molecular Medicine*, vol. 33, no. 4, pp. 925–933, 2014.

[36] J. T. Tan, J. K. Whitmire, R. Ahmed, T. C. Pearson, and C. P. Larsen, "4-1BB ligand, a member of the TNF family, is important for the generation of antiviral CD8 T cell responses," *The Journal of Immunology*, vol. 163, no. 9, pp. 4859–4868, 1999.

[37] S. T. Hanna, "Nicotine effect on cardiovascular system and ion channels," *Journal of Cardiovascular Pharmacology*, vol. 47, no. 3, pp. 348–358, 2006.

[38] M. Nouri-Shirazi and E. Guinet, "Exposure to nicotine adversely affects the dendritic cell system and compromises host response to vaccination," *The Journal of Immunology*, vol. 188, no. 5, pp. 2359–2370, 2012.

[39] S. Burgdorf, A. Kautz, V. Böhnert, P. A. Knolle, and C. Kurts, "Distinct pathways of antigen uptake and intracellular routing in CD4 and CD8 T cell activation," *Science*, vol. 316, no. 5824, pp. 612–616, 2007.

[40] Y. Li, M. Zeng, W. Chen et al., "Dexmedetomidine reduces isoflurane-induced neuroapoptosis partly by preserving PI3K/Akt pathway in the hippocampus of neonatal rats," *PLoS ONE*, vol. 9, no. 4, Article ID e93639, 2014.

[41] Y. Jossin and A. M. Goffinet, "Reelin signals through phosphatidylinositol 3-kinase and Akt to control cortical development and through mTor to regulate dendritic growth," *Molecular and Cellular Biology*, vol. 27, no. 20, pp. 7113–7124, 2007.

[42] K. Höland, D. Boller, C. Hagel et al., "Targeting class Ia PI3K isoforms selectively impairs cell growth, survival, and migration in glioblastoma," *PLoS ONE*, vol. 9, no. 4, Article ID e94132, 2014.

[43] T. Wang, T. Kusudo, T. Takeuchi et al., "Evodiamine inhibits insulin-stimulated mTOR-S6K activation and IRS1 serine phosphorylation in adipocytes and improves glucose tolerance in obese/diabetic mice," *PLoS ONE*, vol. 8, no. 12, Article ID e83264, 2013.

20

The Role of "Bone Immunological Niche" for a New Pathogenetic Paradigm of Osteoporosis

Danilo Pagliari,[1] Francesco Ciro Tamburrelli,[2] Gianfranco Zirio,[2] Estelle E. Newton,[3] and Rossella Cianci[1]

[1] *Institute of Internal Medicine, Catholic University of the Sacred Heart, Largo A. Gemelli 8, 00168 Rome, Italy*
[2] *Institute of Orthopedics, Catholic University of the Sacred Heart, Largo A. Gemelli 8, 00168 Rome, Italy*
[3] *CytoCure LLC, 100 Cummings Center, Suite 430C, Beverly, MA 01915, USA*

Correspondence should be addressed to Rossella Cianci; rossellacianci@gmail.com

Academic Editor: Maryou Lambros

Osteoporosis is characterized by low bone mass and microarchitectural deterioration of bone tissue. The etiology and pathogenetic mechanisms of osteoporosis have not been clearly elucidated. Osteoporosis is linked to bone resorption by the activation of the osteoclastogenic process. The breakdown of homeostasis among pro- and antiosteoclastogenic cells causes unbalanced bone remodeling. The complex interactions among these cells in the bone microenvironment involve several mediators and proinflammatory pathways. Thus, we may consider the bone microenvironment as a complex system in which local and systemic immunity are regulated and we propose to consider it as an "immunological niche." The study of the "bone immunological niche" will permit a better understanding of the complex cell trafficking which regulates bone resorption and disease. The goal of a perfect therapy for osteoporosis would be to potentiate good cells and block the bad ones. In this scenario, additional factors may take part in helping or hindering the proosteoblastogenic factors. Several proosteoblastogenic and antiosteoclastogenic agents have already been identified and some have been developed and commercialized as biological therapies for osteoporosis. Targeting the cellular network of the "bone immunological niche" may represent a successful strategy to better understand and treat osteoporosis and its complications.

1. Osteoporosis: The Involvement of the Immune System in Osteoclastogenesis and Bone Resorption

Osteoporosis is a systemic skeletal disease, largely characterized by low bone mass and microarchitectural deterioration of bone tissue, leading to increased bone fragility and consequent increase in fracture risk. The etiology and pathogenetic mechanisms of osteoporosis have not been clearly elucidated [1].

Osteoporosis is a major health risk in people over 50. However, to date it is not completely clear whether osteoporosis is a separate bone disease or if it is secondary to the physiological bone aging process.

Osteoporosis is linked to bone tissue loss due to an activation of osteoclastogenic process. Osteoclastogenesis involves several cell subsets, in particular osteoblasts and osteoclasts. The final effector cells that determine bone matrix rearrangement and tissue loss are osteoclasts. Other cell types, such as macrophages and innate adaptive immune cells, also contribute to the tissue microenvironment that orchestrates osteoclastogenic process. In the ideal physiological condition all these cells subsets and their local related mediators are in perfect balance in the bone microenvironment. The result is balanced osteoclast and osteoblast activity and normal bone homeostasis. On the contrary, during osteoporosis and other bone pathological conditions, the harmony between cell subsets and their related mediators in the bone microenvironment breaks down and osteoclast activity increases relative to osteoblast activity. In such a case, activation of bone resorption occurs, resulting in bone tissue loss [2].

Proinflammatory cytokines, especially IL-1, IL-6, IFN-gamma, and TNF-alpha, have been shown to be involved in the pathogenesis of bone resorption in several bone diseases [3]. Proinflammatory T helper cells are now considered potent modulators of bone turnover and are important sources of osteoclastogenic cytokines under inflammatory conditions. It is well known that osteoclasts play a crucial role in osteoporosis [4]. Osteoclasts are specialized bone-resorbing cells regulated by RANKL and macrophage colony-stimulating factor (M-CSF) [5]; these cells are mainly implicated in the development of bone resorption. M-CSF is released by osteoblasts as a result of endocrine stimulation by parathormone and it acts on osteoclasts. M-CSF exerts its function on osteoclasts where it induces differentiation and activates bone resorption with consequent increase of serum calcium levels.

Bone resorption can be caused by three major mechanisms [6]:

(1) increasing osteoclast differentiation, activation, and survival;

(2) enhancing expression of receptor activator of NF-kappa B ligand (RANKL);

(3) inhibiting the bone-forming osteoblast, whilst stimulating osteoclast formation and function.

Functions and differentiation of both osteoblasts and osteoclasts, the principal cells involved in bone metabolism, are regulated by systemic hormones, such as estrogens and parathormone, and Vitamin D, cytokines, and other local tissue factors. Estrogen deficiency is the principal cause of accelerated bone loss in perimenopause and it is linked to the serum levels of particular cytokines, such as IL-1, TNF-alpha, M-CSF, IL-6, and IL-17 [7]. The levels of these cytokine are elevated during perimenopausal estrogen loss and they may potentiate bone resorption through osteoclast recruitment, differentiation, and activation. Several evidences reported the presence of lower calcitonin levels in women compared with men; however, calcitonin deficiency does not seem to be important in age-related osteoporosis [7].

2. Bone Destruction: The RANK/RANKL/OPG Pathway and Others

The principal cytokine involved in the osteoclastogenic process is the receptor activator of NF-kB ligand (RANKL). RANKL binding to its receptor RANK expressed on osteoclast precursors is able to activate NF-kB signaling, leading to the transcription of key osteoclastogenic factors [8]. RANKL activity is balanced in normal bone homeostasis by osteoprotegerin (OPG), a decoy receptor for RANKL secreted by osteoblasts and other cells. Experimental introduction of OPG results in a pronounced decrease in bone disruption [9].

The discovery of the receptor activator of nuclear factor-kB (RANK)/RANK ligand (RANKL)/osteoprotegerin (OPG) signaling pathway has permitted a better understanding of bone metabolism and remodeling. This system represents the major regulatory system for osteoclast formation and action, and it is a principal biological regulatory agent of the Tumor Necrosis Factor (TNF) superfamily in bone metabolism [10, 11].

In the late 1990s, the first component identified for a novel pathway regulating bone remodeling was osteoprotegerin (OPG). OPG was shown to encode a novel member of the TNF-receptor family. Overexpression of the OPG gene resulted in high bone mass and marked reduction in osteoclast number and activity [12]. Before that time, in 1980, it was suggested that osteoblasts might be involved in osteoclastogenesis. The nature of this hypothesized "osteoclast activating factor" remained elusive until 1998, when several laboratories independently identified RANKL as a new member of the TNF family of transmembrane and soluble ligands that could bind to OPG. RANK/RANKL/OPG are closely linked with each other in a single biological pathway [13].

RANKL is secreted by activated T cells and represents a crucial link between bone metabolism and the immune system, directly regulating osteoclastogenesis and bone remodeling [14]. Literature data have demonstrated that activated T and B cells can be the cellular source of RANKL for bone resorption in several bone diseases [15]. In most instances, RANKL relies on M-CSF as a cofactor for osteoclast differentiation, but RANKL can stimulate osteoclastogenesis and bone resorption in mice lacking functional M-CSF. Furthermore, no factor or combination of factors have been shown to be capable of restoring bone resorption when RANKL is absent, indicating the dominant role of RANKL in the regulation of bone resorption [16]. Recent experimental data have demonstrated that M-CSF loses its osteoclastogenic potential if it is present alone in osteoclast cultures [17]. On the other hand, when a fragment of bone is added to these cultures, the osteoclastogenic process is activated, thus demonstrating that the presence M-CSF is not sufficient to activate osteoclasts. The addition of the bone to the osteoclast culture provides other proosteogenic factors, such as RANKL, which are required for bone resorption.

Osteoclast precursors, called preosteoclasts, express the surface receptors RANK. Activation of RANK by RANKL promotes the maturation of preosteoclasts into osteoclasts. The activation of RANK in preosteoclasts results in the initiation of several intracellular signal transduction pathways involving NF-kB. After ubiquitination of the signal, NF-kB is released and it can translocate to the nucleus, where it upregulates cofactors that induce osteoclastogenic and proinflammatory transcription factors. Several growth factors, hormones, cytokines, and drugs that influence bone turnover have been shown to influence the expression of RANKL and OPG [16].

On the other hand, OPG protects the skeleton from excessive bone resorption by binding to RANKL and preventing it from binding to its receptor, RANK [18]. OPG expression is regulated by most of the factors that induce RANKL expression by osteoblasts. Although there are contradictory data, in general, upregulation of RANKL is associated with downregulation of OPG, or at least with lower induction of OPG; in this way, the ratio of RANKL to OPG changes in favor of osteoclastogenesis. Many reports have supported the fact that the RANKL/OPG ratio is an important determinant of bone mass and skeletal integrity [19].

Several cytokines can modulate the RANK/RANKL ratio by stimulating the expression of RANKL by immune cells. In particular, TNF-alpha, IL-1, and IL-18 can boost the activating effect of T cells on osteoclasts, because they upregulate RANKL expression on T cells [14].

Moreover, there are controversial data about the role of the well-known proinflammatory cytokine IFN-gamma in modulating bone resorption and homeostasis. In fact, in an *in vitro* model, IFN-gamma was shown to block RANKL signaling and the consequent osteoclastogenesis process; however, in an *in vivo* animal model, the same cytokine was shown to promote osteoclastogenesis process and the consequent bone resorption; thus, IFN-gamma may have, respectively, both destructing and protecting action on the bone [20]. These data lead to the hypothesis that the effect of IFN-gamma on bone homeostasis depends on the local microenvironment in which it is produced.

Another mode of interaction between immune cells and osteoclasts is via the surface receptor CD137, which is capable of antiosteoclastogenic activity. In fact, T cells may communicate with osteoclasts not only through RANK/RANKL interactions but also through CD137/CD137L ones. CD137 is a costimulatory member of the TNF receptor family induced by T-cell receptor activation and it is capable of transducing signals in both directions, through the receptor and into the cell that expresses the ligand. CD137L is expressed on dendritic cells and osteoclast precursors and it has been demonstrated *in vitro* that CD137L ligation suppresses osteoclastogenesis by inhibiting the multinucleation process [21]. Thus, the activation of the CD137/CD137L axis is a way in which T cells may block osteoclastogenesis process.

Considering bone resorption process, we have examined the role of osteoclastogenesis induction that involves osteoclasts activation. However, the same results in bone damage may be occur through the inhibition of osteoblasts activation. In fact, recent *in vivo* experimental data has demonstrated that at the bone level in human osteoporosis fracture there is an increase of osteoblasts inhibitors, such as the Wnt protein family molecules DKK-1 and sclerostin (SOST), and of osteoclastogenesis activators, such as RANKL, M-CSF and TGF-beta; moreover, this study demonstrated that an increase of RANKL/OPG ratio is present, further confirming the association of the RANK/RANKL/OPG axis in the pathogenesis of bone disruption in osteoporosis fractures [22].

3. The Breakdown of Cellular Network in the "Bone Immunological Niche": A Battle among Several Armies

Both Th1 and Th2 cytokine pattern producing cells are linked with bone resorption. In fact, both Th1 and Th2 cells may inhibit osteoclast differentiation by releasing IFN-gamma and IL-4, respectively [2]. The cytokines produced by Th1/Th2 cells mediate osteoclast formation and function and this cellular axis has been shown to be dysregulated in several bone pathologies [2]. Hence, literature data suggest that impairment of T-cell subpopulations and their related cytokine patterns is present in several bone pathologies.

The classic paradigm of Th1/Th2 axis was maintained until 2005, when a distinct lineage of proinflammatory T helper cells, named Th17 cells, was identified [23]. Indeed, it became evident that the T-cell subsets involved in regulation of osteoclasts differentiation are not limited to Th1 and Th2 cells. Th17 cells are characterized by proinflammatory action, the expression of the transcriptional factors STAT-3 and ROR gammaT, and the production of IL-17. IL-17 is an important proinflammatory factor that is mainly produced by Th17 cells and plays an important role in osteoclast differentiation [24]. Several studies have shown that Th17 cells are increased in many bone diseases and in osteoporosis in particular. Various cytokines, such as IL-6, TGF-beta, IL-23, and IL-1beta contribute to the differentiation and/or amplification of Th17 cells [25–27]. Indeed, it is certain that Th17 cells and IL-17 significantly contribute to the development of bone resorption [2, 28].

In addition, it has been demonstrated that T-cell subpopulations show a functional plasticity determined by the local microenvironment. Thus, microenvironment may modify T-cell function determining a shift from proinflammatory cytokine pattern producing cells to other proinflammatory ones, such as from Th1/Th2 to Th17 cells, or from proinflammatory cytokine producing cells to anti-inflammatory ones, such as from Th1/Th2/Th17 cells to T regulatory cells (Tregs). For example, IL-23 may induce the differentiation of naive T cells into highly pathogenic Th17 cells. Th17 cells produce IL-17 that induces osteoclast function supporting cells, such as synovial fibroblast and osteoblasts, and induces them to express RANKL. IL-17 strongly induces the secretion of TNF-alpha and IL-1 by synovial macrophages and induces osteoclast formation [29]. On the other hand, Th17 cells may directly contribute to bone loss by producing RANKL. In fact, IL-17 stimulates fibroblasts and osteoblasts to produce RANKL [30]. This cytokine is critical for the development of osteoclasts, the major cells responsible for bone erosion. The role of Th17 cells in inducing bone resorption has recently been recognized as mediating systemic bone loss in several inflammatory bowel diseases, such as Crohn's disease [5, 31]. It has been shown that IL-17 not only stimulates RANKL expression in cultures of osteoblasts but also induces osteoclast differentiation. IL-17 directly stimulates human osteoclastogenesis from peripheral blood mononuclear cells (PBMCs) and it also promotes the formation of actin rings in mature osteoclasts [32]. Moreover, Th17 cells play a critical role in the pathogenesis of several bone diseases, such as rheumatoid arthritis, but the mechanisms by which these cells regulate the development of these diseases are not yet fully understood [33].

Additionally, Th17 cells may be a potent osteoclastogenic mediator in estrogen-deficient osteoporosis. In fact, estrogen deficiency promotes osteoclastogenesis by upregulating Th17 cell populations in bone marrow and IL-17 levels in peripheral blood [34]. In postmenopausal women, the production of proinflammatory cytokines is greater than that in premenopausal subjects and it is related to estrogen deficiency [14, 35].

Functions and development of proinflammatory cells are regulated by the activity of several transcriptional factors.

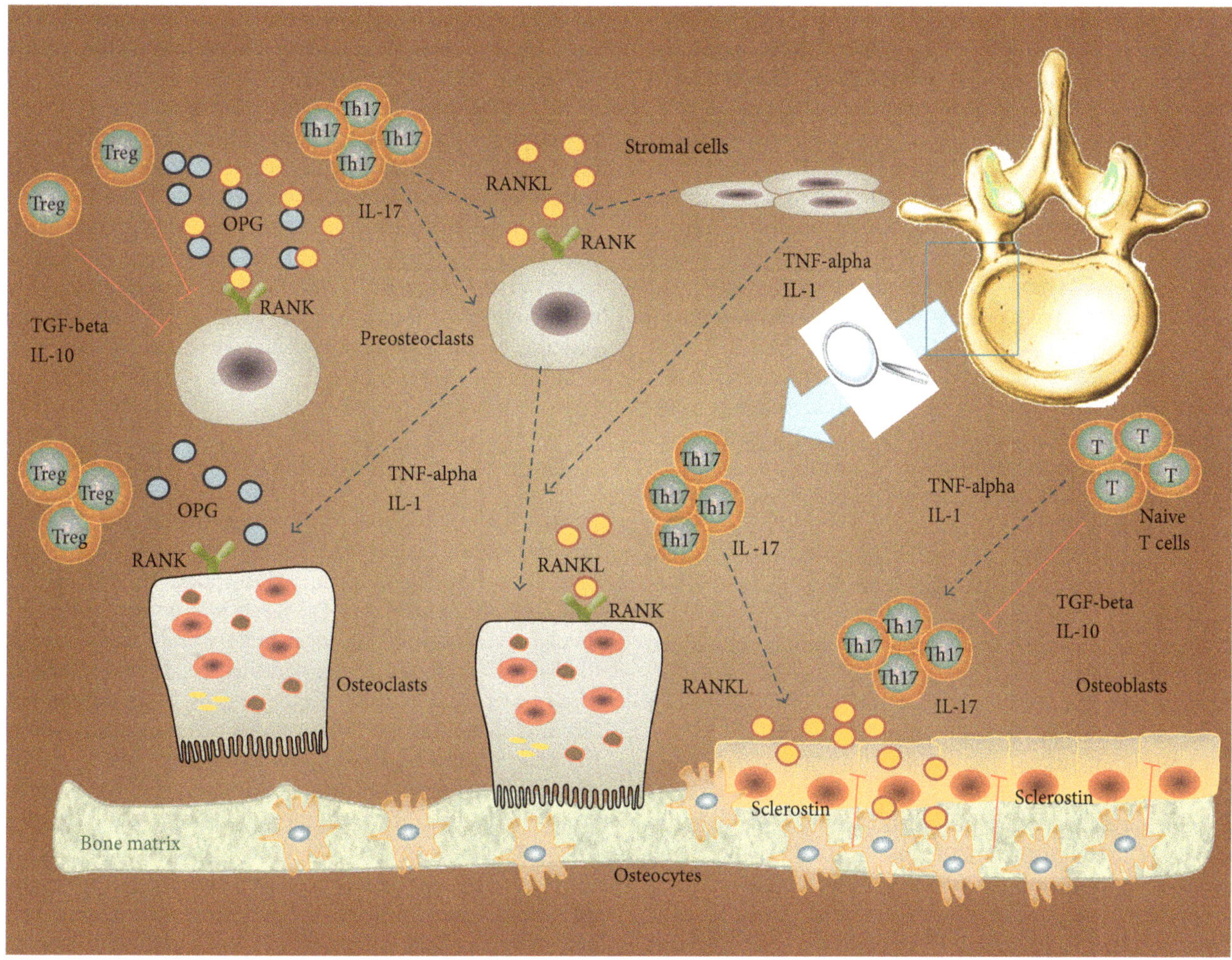

FIGURE 1: The complex cellular network of the "bone immunological niche." OPG: osteoprotegerin.

STAT-3 is the major transcription factor that is critical for Th17 cell differentiation [36]. STAT-3 protein exists in a latent form in the cytoplasm. STAT-3 becomes phosphorylated on tyrosine residues upon receptor activation by cytokines, such as IL-6, and forms homo- or heterodimers that translocate to the cell nucleus, where they act as transcription activators. Activated STAT-3 translocated into the nucleus promotes the transcription of ROR-gammaT, the essential transcription factor of Th17 cells [37]. STAT-3 also regulates the expression of IL-17, IL-21, and IL-23R, which are all of the utmost importance in the effector function of Th17 cells [28]. STAT-3 is activated in inflamed synovium [38]: in fact, it has been demonstrated that STAT-3 plays essential roles in inflammatory arthritis. STAT-3 is critical in the growth, differentiation, and survival of cells, and it was reported that STAT-3 activation in stromal/osteoblastic cells is required for the induction of RANKL and osteoclast formation [28].

On the other hand, STA-21 is a small molecule with potent STAT-3 inhibiting activity [39]. It impedes STAT-3 DNA binding activity, STAT-3 dimerization, and STAT-3 dependent luciferase activity. It has been demonstrated in a knock-out animal model that STA-21 acts in decreasing the proportion of Th17 cells and of their related proinflammatory cytokines and in increasing the proportion of the anti-inflammatory Tregs [28]. Thus, the activation of STA-21 may reduce tissue inflammation pathways and may further reduce osteoclastic activity and the related bone resorption. Hence, STA-21 could be a promising biological therapeutic agent for several bone diseases.

We have extensively examined the potential bone destructing role of several T-cell subpopulations, such as Th1, Th2, and Th17 cells (Figure 1). However, not all T cells promote bone destruction. In fact, T-cell subpopulations can also inhibit osteoclast resorption interacting within the bone microenvironment by the release of cytokines that inhibit osteoclastogenesis, including IFN-gamma, TGF-beta, GM-CSF, IL-4, IL-10, IL-18, and IL-23 [4]. Among these cytokines, as described above in this review, we have to remember that TGF-beta and IFN-gamma may function in a dichotomic way on bone homeostasis. Hence, further *in vivo* studies are needed to better understand the effective role of these cytokines in human bone pathology. Moreover, a new antiosteoclastogenic factor produced by osteoblast lineage has been identified. It is IL-33, a cytokine that influences osteoclast formation. IL-33 is produced by osteoblasts and sporadically by osteocytes. In osteoblasts, it was strongly stimulated by parathormone (PTH) and oncostatin M, two agents that promote bone formation. IL-33 inhibits osteoclast formation *in vitro*, through the induction of other osteoclast inhibitors: GM-CSF, IL-14, IL-13, and IL-10 [40].

Furthermore, literature data have revealed that the newly discovered T regulatory cells (Tregs) [23], a T-cell subpopulation recognized for its anti-inflammatory activity, its role in immune tolerance, the capacity to suppress immune responses, and the expression of the transcription factor FoxP3, take part in bone homeostasis inhibiting osteoclast differentiation by their release of the antiosteoclastogenic cytokines TGF-beta, GM-CSF, IFN-gamma, IL-5, and IL-10 [41, 42]. The potential role of Tregs in modulating bone homeostasis in a FoxP3-overexpressing mouse model characterized by increased numbers of Tregs has been demonstrated; these mice showed high bone volume and low osteoclast numbers, with no change in bone formation showing partial attenuation of bone loss [43].

Nevertheless although there is extensive experimental evidence about the role of Tregs in limiting bone resorption, to date there are no data that describe the impact of these cells in human osteoporosis. So, further studies are needed to better understand the involvement of Tregs in the pathogenesis of disease and their potential role in the developing of osteoporosis biological based therapies.

Some recent studies have demonstrated that cross-talk within the bone microenvironment is not limited to bone cell lineages; in fact, other cells of the immune system may be involved in the regulation of bone homeostasis, such as a particular population of resident tissue macrophages.

Resident tissue macrophages (osteomacs) are a recently identified distinct population of bone resident macrophage cells that function in the bridge between innate and adaptive immune responses. These cells are defined by their expression of the cell surface antigen F4/80 and are usually located close to bone surfaces where they form a canopy over bone-forming osteoblasts. Osteomacs have been found to be associated with bone surfaces but their frequency, distribution, and tissue-specific functional contributions have not been explored. Osteomacs are involved in regulating osteoblast maturation and function and they are important in bone homeostasis and repair [44].

Normally, in a bone microenvironment characterized by chronic inflammation, macrophages are closely related to bone-resorbing osteoclasts and share a dependence on the lineage-specific growth factor CSF-1. They function as proinflammatory cells producing proinflammatory mediators and cytokines that induce the differentiation of osteoclast from preosteoclasts and the osteoclasts function [45]. This active presence of macrophages in bone tissue raises the question of whether they may be considered a third player in bone homeostasis and turnover. Thus, in such a proinflammatory tissue microenvironment, bone resorption is activated with consequent bone loss. Indeed, the bone microenvironment is characterized for the simultaneous presence of proinflammatory and anti-inflammatory mediators and cells. So, as described above in this review, at bone level, on one hand there are the proinflammatory Thl, Th2, and Th17 cells and other immune cells such as proinflammatory macrophages, and on the other hand there are the anti-inflammatory Tregs and other immune cells with regulatory functions, such as osteomacs. In this manner, the bone microenvironment functions as a dynamic model in which a continuous balancing between proinflammatory and anti-inflammatory mediators is performed. When the side of the scale leans in the proinflammatory sense, bone resorption and remodeling develop; on the contrary, when the side of the scale leans in the anti-inflammatory sense, bone homeostasis is conserved (Figure 2). Thus, we may consider the bone microenvironment as a complex system in which local and systemic immunity is regulated and we propose to consider it as an "immunological niche."

4. Bone Homing Pathways

Rather than hypothesizing a stochastic model in which immunological cells are recruited into bone tissue, we think that bone homing is regulated through several systemic and local mechanisms in the bone microenvironment that involve cytokines, tissue local factors, Toll Like Receptors (TLRs), adhesion molecules and their related receptors, and other innate and adaptive immune cells. Studying the bone "immunological niche" will permit a better understanding of the complex cell trafficking regulating bone resorption and disease. The concept of "immunological niche" has been previously introduced by our group with the aim of explaining the pathogenesis of other inflammatory diseases [27, 46].

Furthermore, as it has been well established for different diseases, a crucial role in the pathogenetic mechanisms is played by Toll Like Receptors (TLRs). TLRs are transmembrane proteins that are typically expressed either on the cell surface or in endosomes. They act as pathogen recognition receptors (PRRs), identifying microbe-associated molecular patterns (MAMPs), that are specific for microbes and essential for their survival. TLR signaling is involved in epithelial cell proliferation, immunoglobulin production, and antimicrobial peptide expression; TLRs are also expressed by other immune cells and can activate an inflammatory response involving both innate and adaptive components [47]. TLRs mediate the interconnection between pathogens and innate immunity [48]. When activated by a pathogen or other specific signals, TLRs determine the initiation of immune response. Dysregulation of TLRs expression is linked to several pathologies, such as bone disease. TLRs are also expressed in osteoclasts and in other cells present at bone tissue, such as macrophages, dendritic cells, and T cells, and their activation affects these cells' differentiation and activity. TLR3, TLR4, and TLR9 have been connected to bone physiology and pathology [49]. Several potential mechanisms have been proposed to explain how bacteria might cause bone destruction. In addition to release of inflammatory cytokines from the immune system, these mechanisms include the release of substances acting directly on the bone matrix, the release of factors capable of directly or indirectly stimulating bone-resorbing cells, and the release of factors capable of inhibiting bone-forming cells, causing apoptosis or other effects. The expression of functional TLRs by osteoclasts

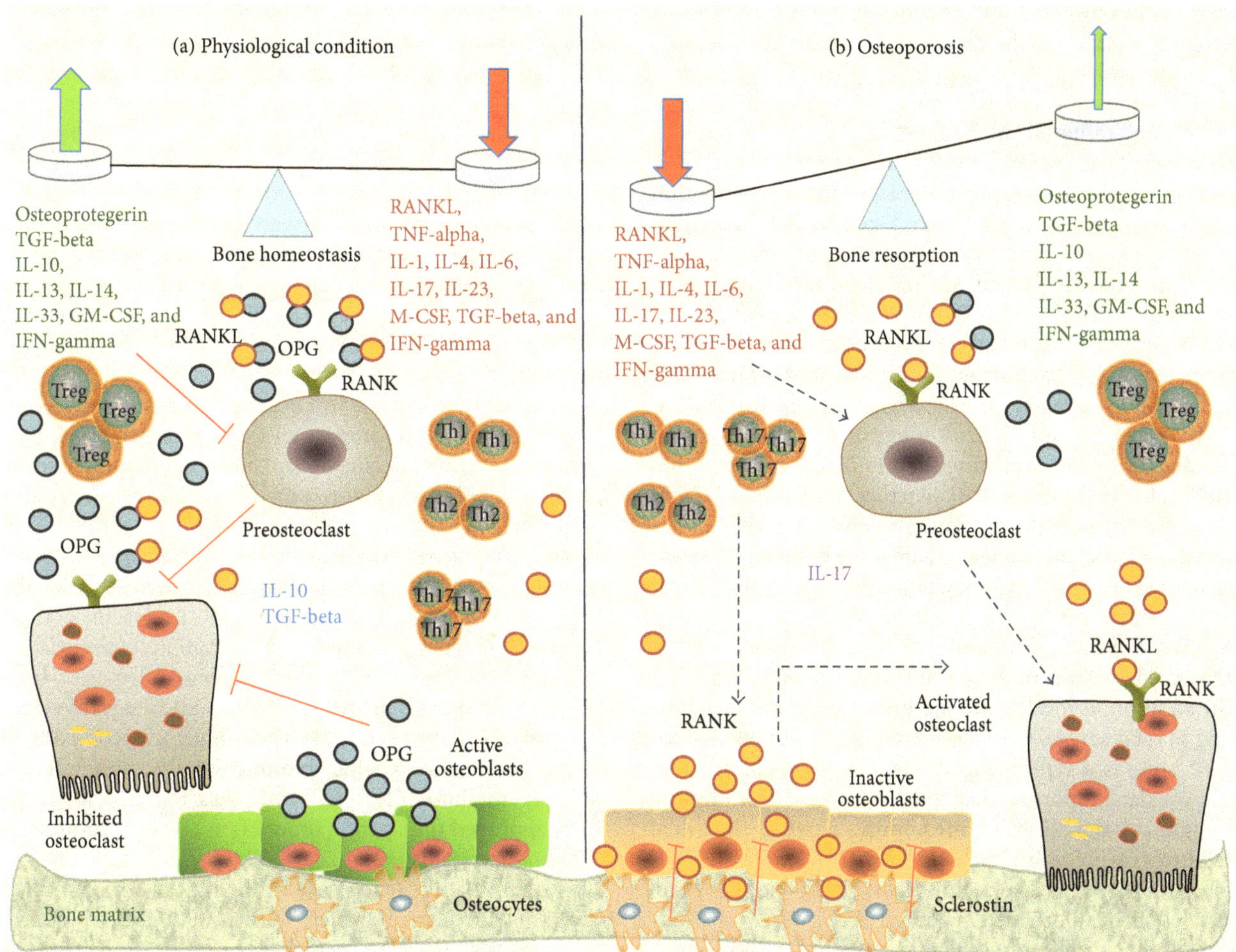

FIGURE 2: Osteoclastogenic pathways in "bone immunological niche." At bone tissue level, on one hand, there are the proinflammatory Th1, Th2, and Th17 cells with related proosteoclastogenic cytokines (RANKL, TNF-alpha, IL-1, IL-4, IL-6, IL-17, IL-23, M-CSF, TGF-beta, and IFN-gamma) and other immune cells such as proinflammatory macrophages; on the other hand, there are the anti-inflammatory Tregs with related antiosteoclastogenic cytokines (OPG, TGF-beta, IL-10, IL-13, IL-14, IL-33, GM-CSF, and IFN-gamma) and other immune cells with regulatory functions, such as osteomacs. The bone microenvironment functions as a dynamic model in which a continuous balancing between proosteoclastogenic and antiosteoclastogenic mediators is performed. (a) In physiological condition anti- and proosteoclastogenic factors are in *equilibrium* and bone homeostasis is conserved. (b) In osteoporosis condition, proosteoclastogenic factors prevail and bone resorption and remodeling develop. OPG: osteoprotegerin, GM-CSF: granulocyte-macrophage colony stimulating factor, and M-CSF: macrophage colony stimulating factor.

raises the possibility of direct modulation of these cells' differentiation and resorptive activity by pathogen-derived TLR ligands [49]. Several studies in animal models have taken in consideration the role of infections in causing bone resorption; hence, it has been shown that bacterial infections are linked to bone loss due to an increase of osteoclastogenesis activity. Nevertheless, these studies do not consider the direct effect of TLRs on osteoclasts activity [50]. Other animal models confirm the role of *bacteria* in bone resorption; in fact, the injection of LPS into mice induces osteoclast differentiation. On the other hand, the activation of TLRs may mediate both activation and inhibition of osteoclastic differentiation and related bone resorption. For example, the activation of TLR9 results in inhibition of RANKL-induced osteoclastogenesis [51], while the activation of TLRs in committed osteoclasts results in increased osteoclastogenesis and is probably the mechanism by which pathogen-induced bone loss occurs. The inhibition of osteoclastogenesis by TLRs activation may play a role in reducing the excessive bone loss caused by pathogenic infection and shifting the balance between the bone and immune systems during infection to recruit immune cells [49].

Moreover, chemokines and other proinflammatory mediators may regulate cellular homing to bone tissue. Multiple cytokines are responsible for increased chemotaxis and homing to the bone marrow.

The interactions between integrins and extracellular matrix (ECM) may modulate bone development and growth as these are strictly regulated by bone microenvironment mediators. The Beta1 subfamily of integrins is the largest integrin subfamily and constitutes the main integrin binding partners of collagen I, the major ECM component of bone [52]. In particular, the interaction of Alpa2/Beta1 integrin with collagen I is a crucial signal for osteoblastic differentiation and mineralization. Emerging evidence suggests that Alpha2/Beta1 integrin can be a major regulator of T-cell activation. In fact, Alpha2/Beta1 integrin may function as receptor for collagen type I on T cells and is expressed only on effector T cells associated with inflammation in extravascular tissues. Hence, Alpha2/Beta1 integrin protects human effector T cells from Fas-mediated apoptosis [53]. In addition, Alpha2/Beta1 integrin is the major collagen-binding integrin expressed by human Th17 cells. It mediates Th17 cell adhesion to collagen, which costimulates the production of IL-17; for this, Alpha2/Beta1 integrin may constitute an important factor for regulating the migration and retention of Th17 cells to the bone [54]. Furthermore, Alpha2/Beta1 integrin can regulate the migration of effector T cells to the tissues that are rich in collagen, such as the bone marrow and the synovium [55]. All these data confirm that Alpha2/Beta1 integrin is a major mediator of cellular bone homing. Finally, integrins are broadly implicated in bone metastasis due to their ability to induce mitogenic intracellular signaling.

In addition, a model of bone homing and cellular trafficking is represented by bone metastasis in human cancer. In fact, bone is a typical metastatic site of several tumors. Literature data reported that integrins mediate mitogenic and migratory signaling of bone homing, whereas the initial attachment of metastatic cells to bone endothelial cells is largely attributed to the lectin class of protein adhesion molecules. It has been demonstrated that cancer cells may modify their surface molecules in order to permit them to achieve bone metastatic tissue targets. Several molecular mechanisms have been elucidated endowing bone metastatic circulating tumor cells with the ability to attach and invade bone tissue. Broad classes of stromal interactions, such as integrin- and lectin-mediated attachment or protease-dependent invasion have been characterized [9]. It has been established that bone metastatic cells can express chemokine receptor 4 (CXCR4) that provokes actin polymerization and pseudopodia formation resulting in migration upon exposure to bone endothelial cell secretions; thus, CXCR-4 enables circulating cancer cells to migrate into bone tissue to form the pre-metastatic niche [56].

Three major integrins are linked to bone seeding of metastatic cells: integrins AlphaV/Beta3, Alpha2/Beta1, and Alpha4/Beta1. AlphaV/Beta3 integrin functions in bone metastasis through binding either osteopontin (OPN), bone sialoprotein (BSP), or CD44. OPN is a major extracellular component of multiple bone tissue cells, and engagement by AlphaV/Beta3 integrin results in MEK induced upregulation of matrix metalloproteinase 9 (MMP9). BSP is a distinct AlphaV/Beta3 ligand expressed in normal bone tissue that is upregulated in bone metastatic lesions compared to metastases in other organs [57]. Then, Alpha2/Beta1 and Alpha4/Beta1 integrins bind collagen I (COL1) and VCAM1 in bone metastasis. COL1 is the major structural component of the bone matrix whereas VCAM1 is constitutively expressed by bone endothelial cells; when bound by Alpha2/Beta1, subsequent RhoC activation primes cell morphology for invasion [58, 59]. Multiple *in vitro* studies have demonstrated that Beta1 integrins are crucial regulators of osteogenesis and mineralization, whereas *in vivo* studies have revealed only mild and sometimes contradictory results on the use of Beta1 integrins in bone repair [52].

Moreover, the initial attachment of metastatic cells to bone endothelial cells is largely attributed to the lectin class of protein adhesion molecules. Glycosylated ligands present on circulating tumor cells, such as PSGL1 and CD44, engage endothelial selectin (SELE) and mediate initial cell attachment and subsequent rolling along bone endothelial cells [60].

The study of cellular trafficking and bone homing may help to identify additional potential pathways to develop new biological therapeutical strategies for osteoporosis. For example, in the field of regenerative medicine, the knowledge about bone homing has been utilized to develop drugs directly able to arrive on their targets in the bone. Hence, regenerative medicine strategies include the use of vehicles for drug delivery to the bone in order to permit the specific action of these drugs on target tissue sites. For example, hydrogels, such as polyethylene glycol (PEG), are water-swollen cross-linked polymer networks that offer significant advantages as vehicles for protein delivery due to their high cytocompatibility, low inflammatory profile, biofunctionality, and injectable delivery method [61]. PEG hydrogels are widely used in FDA approved therapeutic products as covalent modifiers of proteins and lipids [62].

Moreover, a potential use of biological vehicles may be driving bone morphogenetic protein (BMP) therapies to bone targets. BMP therapy has emerged as a promising alternative to autografts and allografts. In fact, BMP therapy has been shown to be successful in stimulating bone repair. It has recently been demonstrated in a mouse model that an Alpha2/Beta1 integrin-specific PEG hydrogel BMP-2 carrier may allow better clinical results in inducing bone repair than traditional therapies [61].

5. Traditional Therapies and New Osteoporosis Therapeutical Approach Based on Biological Agents

At present, the main aim of osteoporosis treatment is to preserve bone mass and prevent fractures. Despite this, exploration into the disease mechanisms might lead to the development of discoveries of new or improved therapies.

As explained in this review, there is a close cross-communicatio among osteoblasts, osteoclasts, macrophages, and innate and adaptive immune cells; this cellular network is essential for bone homeostasis. Hence, studying this cellular cross-communication and its interference with the "bone immunological niche" may help to introduce new biologically based therapies for bone diseases.

To date, the more common therapies for osteoporosis are those that act to reduce bone resorption. This goal can be achieved both by osteoclast inhibition therapy and by osteoblast stimulation therapy. Among osteoclast inhibition

TABLE 1: Traditional and potential therapies for osteoporosis.

Molecular target	Mechanism of action	Approved agent
Prenylation	Osteolysis inhibitor	*Zoledronic acid and other bisphosphonates*
RANK/RANKL/OPG axis	Osteoclastogenesis inhibitor	*Denosumab*
Recombinant osteoprotegerin (OPG)	Osteoclastogenesis inhibitor	
STA-21 (STAT-3 inhibitor)	Osteoclastogenesis inhibitor	
TGF-beta	Osteoclastogenesis inhibitor	
Alpha2/Beta1 integrin	Bone homing and drug vehicles	

therapies, two drugs have shown efficacy; these are bisphosphonates and the monoclonal antibody Denosumab (anti-RANKL antibody). Additional pharmacological agents have demonstrated promise in preclinical experiments but have to be tested in clinical trials [9].

Bisphosphonates act in diminishing bone resorption; they became a standard of care in the treatment of osteoporosis. Bisphosphonates, such as zoledronic acid, pamidronate, or ibandronate, specifically bind to the bone matrix and are internalized by osteoclasts upon resorption. Once internalized, these drugs inhibit various metabolic processes such as prenylation and lead to apoptosis [63].

Denosumab is a fully human monoclonal antibody inhibiting RANKL; it is recommended for the treatment of osteoporosis, bone metastases, multiple myeloma, and giant cell tumor of bone. Denosumab inhibits the maturation of preosteoclast into osteoclasts by binding and inhibiting RANKL. This mimics the natural action of the endogenous RANKL inhibitor osteoprotegerin that results decreased in osteoporotic patients. This protects bone from degradation and helps to stabilize the progression of the disease [13, 64].

Compared to bisphosphonates, Denosumab and recombinant OPG demonstrate higher clinical efficacy by targeting RANKL (Table 1). Both have shown similar promise in clinical trials [9].

In this review we have already examined the role of Th17 cells in inducing osteolysis and bone resorption. The molecule STA-21 is able to block the principal Th17 cell transcription factor STAT-3 that activates the transcription of proinflammatory cytokines genes. Thus, the activation of STA-21 may reduce tissue inflammatory patterns, osteoclastic activity, and the consequent bone resorption. Hence, STA-21 could be a promising biological therapeutical agent for several bone diseases. In fact, recent experimental data performed in an *in vivo* mouse model and in an *ex vivo* human model have demonstrated the potential therapeutic role of STA-21; treatment with STA-21 induced the increase of bone protective T regulatory cells (Tregs) and reduced the number of bone destructive Th17 cells and their related production of proinflammatory IL-17 [28]. Considering that Th17 cell maturation, growth, and proliferation are dependent on a various number of cytokines as described in this review will help to introduce new biological therapies for bone remodeling which utilize these cytokine patterns.

It has been shown that Alpha2/Beta1 integrin is the major collagen-binding integrin expressed by human synovial proinflammatory and proosteoclastogenic Th17 cells and it is the pivotal mediator of lymphocytes bone homing. An *in vivo* mouse model has recently demonstrated that blocking Alpha2/Beta1 integrin with a specific monoclonal antibody led to a decrease in the number of Th17 cells in the joint and to a reduction of IL-17 levels in mice; this was associated with a reduction of bone loss due to an inhibition of RANKL levels and osteoclast numbers and activity [3]. Thus, Alpha2/Beta1 integrin may be a promising mediator to develop new drugs for biological therapies of human osteoporosis.

In conclusion, studying the complex cellular network engaging bone and immune cells responsible of the pathogenesis of osteoporosis has permitted the individuation of new pathological mediators, mechanisms and pathways. This cellular interplay involves both circulating and tissue cells, and it is strictly regulated by the complex microworld of the "bone immunological niche." However, further data are needed to better explain some other pathogenetic disease mechanisms. There are several potential warriors in this disease battle, such as osteoblasts, osteoclasts, macrophages, and innate and adaptive immune cells. The breakdown of the homeostasis among these warriors causes unbalanced bone remodeling. The goal of a perfect therapy may potentiate good warriors and block bad ones. In this scenario, additional factors may take part in helping or hindering the warriors. Hence, several proosteoblastogenic and antiosteoclastogenic agents have been individuated and some of them have been developed and commercialized as biological therapies for osteoporosis. Many others are currently under investigation. Thus, targeting the cellular network of the "bone immunological niche" may represent a successful strategy to better understand and treat osteoporosis and its complications.

Conflict of Interests

The authors declare that they have no conflict of interests.

References

[1] E. Canalis, "Update in new anabolic therapies for osteoporosis," *Journal of Clinical Endocrinology and Metabolism*, vol. 95, no. 4, pp. 1496–1504, 2010.

[2] F. Yuan, X. Li, W. Lu et al., "Type 17 T-helper cells might be a promising therapeutic target for osteoporosis," *Molecular Biology Reports*, vol. 39, no. 1, pp. 771–774, 2012.

[3] M.-A. El Azreq, M. Boisvert, A. Cesaro et al., "$\alpha 2\beta 1$ integrin regulates Th17 cell activity and its neutralization decreases the

severity of collagen-induced arthritis," *Journal of Immunology*, vol. 191, no. 12, pp. 5941–5950, 2013.

[4] N. A. Sims and N. C. Walsh, "Intercellular cross-talk among bone cells: new factors and pathways," *Current Osteoporosis Reports*, vol. 10, no. 2, pp. 109–117, 2012.

[5] U. Syrbe and B. Siegmund, "Bone marrow Th17 TNFalpha cells induce osteoclast differentiation and link bone destruction to IBD," *Gut*, vol. 64, no. 7, pp. 1011–1012, 2015.

[6] R. R. McLean, "Proinflammatory cytokines and osteoporosis," *Current Osteoporosis Reports*, vol. 7, no. 4, pp. 134–139, 2009.

[7] S. H. Tella and J. C. Gallagher, "Prevention and treatment of postmenopausal osteoporosis," *Journal of Steroid Biochemistry and Molecular Biology*, vol. 142, pp. 155–170, 2014.

[8] B. K. Park, H. Zhang, Q. Zeng et al., "NF-κB in breast cancer cells promotes osteolytic bone metastasis by inducing osteoclastogenesis via GM-CSF," *Nature Medicine*, vol. 13, no. 1, pp. 62–69, 2007.

[9] M. Esposito and Y. Kang, "Targeting tumor-stromal interactions in bone metastasis," *Pharmacology and Therapeutics*, vol. 141, no. 2, pp. 222–223, 2014.

[10] D. L. Lacey, W. J. Boyle, W. S. Simonet et al., "Bench to bedside: elucidation of the OPG-RANK-RANKL pathway and the development of denosumab," *Nature Reviews Drug Discovery*, vol. 11, no. 5, pp. 401–419, 2012.

[11] D. Vega, N. M. Maalouf, and K. Sakhaee, "CLINICAL review #: the role of receptor activator of nuclear factor-kappaB (RANK)/RANK ligand/osteoprotegerin: clinical implications," *The Journal of Clinical Endocrinology & Metabolism*, vol. 92, no. 12, pp. 4514–4521, 2007.

[12] W. S. Simonet, D. L. Lacey, C. R. Dunstan et al., "Osteoprotegerin: a novel secreted protein involved in the regulation of bone density," *Cell*, vol. 89, no. 2, pp. 309–319, 1997.

[13] P. Geusens, "Emerging treatments for postmenopausal osteoporosis—focus on denosumab," *Clinical Interventions in Aging*, vol. 4, pp. 241–250, 2009.

[14] L. D'Amico and I. Roato, "Cross-talk between T cells and osteoclasts in bone resorption," *BoneKEy Reports*, vol. 1, no. 6, article 82, 2012.

[15] T. Kawai, T. Matsuyama, Y. Hosokawa et al., "B and T lymphocytes are the primary sources of RANKL in the bone resorptive lesion of periodontal disease," *The American Journal of Pathology*, vol. 169, no. 3, pp. 987–998, 2006.

[16] A. E. Kearns, S. Khosla, and P. J. Kostenuik, "Receptor activator of nuclear factor κB ligand and osteoprotegerin regulation of bone remodeling in health and disease," *Endocrine Reviews*, vol. 29, no. 2, pp. 155–192, 2008.

[17] T. J. De Vries, T. Schoenmaker, D. Aerts et al., "M-CSF priming of osteoclast precursors can cause osteoclastogenesis-insensitivity, which can be prevented and overcome on bone," *Journal of Cellular Physiology*, vol. 230, no. 1, pp. 210–225, 2015.

[18] B. F. Boyce and L. Xing, "Biology of RANK, RANKL, and osteoprotegerin," *Arthritis Research & Therapy*, vol. 9, no. 1, article S1, 2007.

[19] L. C. Hofbauer and M. Schoppet, "Clinical implications of the osteoprotegerin/RANKL/RANK system for bone and vascular diseases," *Journal of the American Medical Association*, vol. 292, no. 4, pp. 490–495, 2004.

[20] Y. Gao, F. Grassi, M. R. Ryan et al., "IFN-γ stimulates osteoclast formation and bone loss in vivo via antigen-driven T cell activation," *Journal of Clinical Investigation*, vol. 117, no. 1, pp. 122–132, 2007.

[21] R. Senthilkumar and H.-W. Lee, "CD137L- and RANKL-mediated reverse signals inhibit osteoclastogenesis and T lymphocyte proliferation," *Immunobiology*, vol. 214, no. 2, pp. 153–161, 2009.

[22] P. DAmelio, I. Roato, L. Damico et al., "Bone and bone marrow pro-osteoclastogenic cytokines are up-regulated in osteoporosis fragility fractures," *Osteoporosis International*, vol. 22, no. 11, pp. 2869–2877, 2011.

[23] F. Pandolfi, R. Cianci, D. Pagliari, R. Landolfi, S. Kunkel, and G. Cammarota, "Cellular mediators of inflammation: tregs and T H 17 cells in gastrointestinal diseases," *Mediators of Inflammation*, vol. 2009, Article ID 132028, 11 pages, 2009.

[24] X. Li, F. L. Yuan, W. G. Lu et al., "The role of interleukin-17 in mediating joint destruction in rheumatoid arthritis," *Biochemical and Biophysical Research Communications*, vol. 397, no. 2, pp. 131–135, 2010.

[25] C. Dong, "Differentiation and function of pro-inflammatory Th17 cells," *Microbes and Infection*, vol. 11, no. 5, pp. 584–588, 2009.

[26] D. Pagliari, R. Cianci, S. Frosali et al., "The role of IL-15 in gastrointestinal diseases: a bridge between innate and adaptive immune response," *Cytokine & Growth Factor Reviews*, vol. 24, no. 5, pp. 455–466, 2013.

[27] R. Cianci, G. Cammarota, G. Frisullo et al., "Tissue-infiltrating lymphocytes analysis reveals large modifications of the duodenal 'immunological niche' in coeliac disease after gluten-free diet," *Clinical and Translational Gastroenterology*, vol. 3, article e28, 2012.

[28] J.-S. Park, S.-K. Kwok, M.-A. Lim et al., "STA-21, a promising STAT-3 inhibitor that reciprocally regulates Th17 and Treg cells, inhibits osteoclastogenesis in mice and humans and alleviates autoimmune inflammation in an experimental model of rheumatoid arthritis," *Arthritis and Rheumatology*, vol. 66, no. 4, pp. 918–929, 2014.

[29] K. Sato, A. Suematsu, K. Okamoto et al., "Th17 functions as an osteoclastogenic helper T cell subset that links T cell activation and bone destruction," *Journal of Experimental Medicine*, vol. 203, no. 12, pp. 2673–2682, 2006.

[30] L. Rifas and M. N. Weitzmann, "A novel T cell cytokine, secreted osteoclastogenic factor of activated T cells, induces osteoclast formation in a RANKL-independent manner," *Arthritis & Rheumatism*, vol. 60, no. 11, pp. 3324–3335, 2009.

[31] A. E. Oostlander, V. Everts, T. Schoenmaker et al., "T cell-mediated increased osteoclast formation from peripheral blood as a mechanism for crohn's disease-associated bone loss," *Journal of Cellular Biochemistry*, vol. 113, no. 1, pp. 260–268, 2012.

[32] T. Korn, M. Oukka, V. Kuchroo, and E. Bettelli, "Th17 cells: effector T cells with inflammatory properties," *Seminars in Immunology*, vol. 19, no. 6, pp. 362–371, 2007.

[33] K. Okamoto and H. Takayanagi, "Regulation of bone by the adaptive immune system in arthritis," *Arthritis Research & Therapy*, vol. 13, no. 3, article 219, 2011.

[34] R. Zhao, "Immune regulation of bone loss by Th17 cells in oestrogen-deficient osteoporosis," *European Journal of Clinical Investigation*, vol. 43, no. 11, pp. 1195–1202, 2013.

[35] M. F. Faienza, A. Ventura, F. Marzano, and L. Cavallo, "Postmenopausal osteoporosis: the role of immune system cells," *Clinical and Developmental Immunology*, vol. 2013, Article ID 575936, 6 pages, 2013.

[36] T. Mori, T. Miyamoto, H. Yoshida et al., "IL-1β and TNFα-initiated IL-6-STAT3 pathway is critical in mediating inflammatory cytokines and RANKL expression in inflammatory arthritis," *International Immunology*, vol. 23, no. 11, pp. 701–712, 2011.

[37] T. J. Harris, J. F. Grosso, H.-R. Yen et al., "An in vivo requirement for STAT3 signaling in TH17 development and TH17-dependent autoimmunity," *Journal of Immunology*, vol. 179, no. 7, pp. 4313–4317, 2007.

[38] A. S. K. de Hooge, F. A. J. van de Loo, M. I. Koenders et al., "Local activation of STAT-1 and STAT-3 in the inflamed synovium during zymosan-induced arthritis: exacerbation of joint inflammation in STAT-1 gene-knockout mice," *Arthritis and Rheumatism*, vol. 50, no. 6, pp. 2014–2023, 2004.

[39] H. Song, R. Wang, S. Wang, and J. Lin, "A low-molecular-weight compound discovered through virtual database screening inhibits Stat3 function in breast cancer cells," *Proceedings of the National Academy of Sciences of the United States of America*, vol. 102, no. 13, pp. 4700–4705, 2005.

[40] H. Saleh, D. Eeles, J. M. Hodge et al., "Interleukin-33, a target of parathyroid hormone and oncostatin m, increases osteoblastic matrix mineral deposition and inhibits osteoclast formation *in vitro*," *Endocrinology*, vol. 152, no. 5, pp. 1911–1922, 2011.

[41] M. M. Zaiss, R. Axmann, J. Zwerina et al., "Treg cells suppress osteoclast formation: a new link between the immune system and bone," *Arthritis & Rheumatism*, vol. 56, no. 12, pp. 4104–4112, 2007.

[42] M. M. Zaiss, B. Frey, A. Hess et al., "Regulatory T cells protect from local and systemic bone destruction in arthritis," *Journal of Immunology*, vol. 184, no. 12, pp. 7238–7246, 2010.

[43] M. M. Zaiss, K. Sarter, A. Hess et al., "Increased bone density and resistance to ovariectomy-induced bone loss in FoxP3-transgenic mice based on impaired osteoclast differentiation," *Arthritis and Rheumatism*, vol. 62, no. 8, pp. 2328–2338, 2010.

[44] A. R. Pettit, M. K. Chang, D. A. Hume, and L.-J. Raggatt, "Osteal macrophages: a new twist on coupling during bone dynamics," *Bone*, vol. 43, no. 6, pp. 976–982, 2008.

[45] M. K. Chang, L.-J. Raggatt, K. A. Alexander et al., "Osteal tissue macrophages are intercalated throughout human and mouse bone lining tissues and regulate osteoblast function in vitro and in vivo," *Journal of Immunology*, vol. 181, no. 2, pp. 1232–1244, 2008.

[46] R. Cianci, D. Pagliari, R. Landolfi et al., "New insights on the role of T cells in the pathogenesis of celiac disease," *Journal of Biological Regulators and Homeostatic Agents*, vol. 26, no. 2, pp. 171–179, 2012.

[47] L. Shang, M. Fukata, N. Thirunarayanan et al., "Toll-like receptor signaling in small intestinal epithelium promotes B-cell recruitment and IgA production in lamina propria," *Gastroenterology*, vol. 135, no. 2, pp. 529.e1–538.e1, 2008.

[48] R. Cianci, S. Frosali, D. Pagliari et al., "Uncomplicated diverticular disease: innate and adaptive immunity in human gut mucosa before and after rifaximin," *Journal of Immunology Research*, vol. 2014, Article ID 696812, 11 pages, 2014.

[49] T. Krisher and Z. Bar-Shavit, "Regulation of osteoclastogenesis by integrated signals from toll-like receptors," *Journal of Cellular Biochemistry*, vol. 115, no. 12, pp. 2146–2154, 2014.

[50] B. Henderson and S. P. Nair, "Hard labour: bacterial infection of the skeleton," *Trends in Microbiology*, vol. 11, no. 12, pp. 570–577, 2003.

[51] A. Amcheslavsky and Z. Bar-Shavit, "Toll-like receptor 9 ligand blocks osteoclast differentiation through induction of phosphatase," *Journal of Bone and Mineral Research*, vol. 22, no. 8, pp. 1301–1310, 2007.

[52] A. Shekaran, J. T. Shoemaker, T. E. Kavanaugh et al., "The effect of conditional inactivation of beta 1 integrins using twist 2 Cre, Osterix Cre and osteocalcin Cre lines on skeletal phenotype," *Bone*, vol. 68, pp. 131–141, 2014.

[53] Y.-P. Lin, C.-C. Su, J.-Y. Huang et al., "Aberrant integrin activation induces p38 MAPK phosphorylation resulting in suppressed Fas-mediated apoptosis in T cells: implications for rheumatoid arthritis," *Molecular Immunology*, vol. 46, no. 16, pp. 3328–3335, 2009.

[54] M. Boisvert, N. Chetoui, S. Gendron, and F. Aoudjit, "Alpha2beta1 integrin is the major collagen-binding integrin expressed on human Th17 cells," *European Journal of Immunology*, vol. 40, no. 10, pp. 2710–2719, 2010.

[55] K. Tokoyoda, S. Zehentmeier, A. N. Hegazy et al., "Professional Memory $CD4^+$ T Lymphocytes Preferentially Reside and Rest in the Bone Marrow," *Immunity*, vol. 30, no. 5, pp. 721–730, 2009.

[56] S. Brenner, N. Whiting-Theobald, T. Kawai et al., "CXCR4-transgene expression significantly improves marrow engraftment of cultured hematopoietic stem cells," *Stem Cells*, vol. 22, no. 7, pp. 1128–1133, 2004.

[57] C. Hayashi, S. Rittling, T. Hayata et al., "Serum osteopontin, an enhancer of tumor metastasis to bone, promotes B16 melanoma cell migration," *Journal of Cellular Biochemistry*, vol. 101, no. 4, pp. 979–986, 2007.

[58] C. L. Hall, C. W. Dubyk, T. A. Riesenberger, D. Shein, E. T. Keller, and K. L. Van Golen, "Type I collagen receptor ($\alpha_2\beta_1$) signaling promotes prostate cancer invasion through RhoC GTPase," *Neoplasia*, vol. 10, no. 8, pp. 797–803, 2008.

[59] Y.-S. Guo, R. Zhao, J. Ma et al., "βig-h3 promotes human osteosarcoma cells metastasis by interacting with integrin $\alpha2\beta1$ and activating PI3K signaling pathway," *PLoS ONE*, vol. 9, no. 3, Article ID e90220, 2014.

[60] S. R. Barthel, D. L. Hays, E. M. Yazawa et al., "Definition of molecular determinants of prostate cancer cell bone extravasation," *Cancer Research*, vol. 73, no. 2, pp. 942–952, 2013.

[61] A. Shekaran, J. R. García, A. Y. Clark et al., "Bone regeneration using an alpha 2 beta 1 integrin-specific hydrogel as a BMP-2 delivery vehicle," *Biomaterials*, vol. 35, no. 21, pp. 5453–5461, 2014.

[62] P. Bailon and C.-Y. Won, "PEG-modified biopharmaceuticals," *Expert Opinion on Drug Delivery*, vol. 6, no. 1, pp. 1–16, 2009.

[63] G. R. Mundy, "Metastasis to bone: causes, consequences and therapeutic opportunities," *Nature Reviews Cancer*, vol. 2, no. 8, pp. 584–593, 2002.

[64] M. R. McClung, E. Michael Lewiecki, S. B. Cohen et al., "Denosumab in postmenopausal women with low bone mineral density," *The New England Journal of Medicine*, vol. 354, no. 8, pp. 821–831, 2006.

Permissions

All chapters in this book were first published in ACP, by Hindawi Publishing Corporation; hereby published with permission under the Creative Commons Attribution License or equivalent. Every chapter published in this book has been scrutinized by our experts. Their significance has been extensively debated. The topics covered herein carry significant findings which will fuel the growth of the discipline. They may even be implemented as practical applications or may be referred to as a beginning point for another development.

The contributors of this book come from diverse backgrounds, making this book a truly international effort. This book will bring forth new frontiers with its revolutionizing research information and detailed analysis of the nascent developments around the world.

We would like to thank all the contributing authors for lending their expertise to make the book truly unique. They have played a crucial role in the development of this book. Without their invaluable contributions this book wouldn't have been possible. They have made vital efforts to compile up to date information on the varied aspects of this subject to make this book a valuable addition to the collection of many professionals and students.

This book was conceptualized with the vision of imparting up-to-date information and advanced data in this field. To ensure the same, a matchless editorial board was set up. Every individual on the board went through rigorous rounds of assessment to prove their worth. After which they invested a large part of their time researching and compiling the most relevant data for our readers.

The editorial board has been involved in producing this book since its inception. They have spent rigorous hours researching and exploring the diverse topics which have resulted in the successful publishing of this book. They have passed on their knowledge of decades through this book. To expedite this challenging task, the publisher supported the team at every step. A small team of assistant editors was also appointed to further simplify the editing procedure and attain best results for the readers.

Apart from the editorial board, the designing team has also invested a significant amount of their time in understanding the subject and creating the most relevant covers. They scrutinized every image to scout for the most suitable representation of the subject and create an appropriate cover for the book.

The publishing team has been an ardent support to the editorial, designing and production team. Their endless efforts to recruit the best for this project, has resulted in the accomplishment of this book. They are a veteran in the field of academics and their pool of knowledge is as vast as their experience in printing. Their expertise and guidance has proved useful at every step. Their uncompromising quality standards have made this book an exceptional effort. Their encouragement from time to time has been an inspiration for everyone.

The publisher and the editorial board hope that this book will prove to be a valuable piece of knowledge for researchers, students, practitioners and scholars across the globe.

List of Contributors

Sugapriya Dhanasekaran
Stem Cell and Molecular Biology Lab, Department of Biotechnology, Bhupat and Jyoti Mehta School of Biosciences, Indian Institute of Technology Madras, Chennai, Tamil Nadu 600036, India
Department of Medical Laboratory Sciences (Haematology), College of Applied Medical Sciences, Prince Sattam Bin Abdul-Aziz University, Wadi Ad Dawaser Campus, P.O. Box 54, Riyadh, Saudi Arabia

Devilakshmi Sithambaram, Kavitha Govarthanan, Bijesh Kumar Biswal and Rama S. Verma
Stem Cell and Molecular Biology Lab, Department of Biotechnology, Bhupat and Jyoti Mehta School of Biosciences, Indian Institute of Technology Madras, Chennai, Tamil Nadu 600036, India

Ewa PocheT, Marta Zdbczy Nska and Anna Lity Nska
Department of Glycoconjugate Biochemistry, Institute of Zoology, Faculty of Biology and Earth Science, Jagiellonian University, Gronostajowa 9, 30-387 Krakow, Poland

Katarzyna Bocian
Department of Immunology, Institute of Zoology, Faculty of Biology, University of Warsaw, Miecznikowa 1, 02-096Warsaw, Poland

Grahyna Korczak-Kowalska
Department of Immunology, Institute of Zoology, Faculty of Biology, University of Warsaw, Miecznikowa 1, 02-096Warsaw, Poland
Department of Clinical Immunology, Transplantation Institute, Medical University of Warsaw, Nowogrodzka 59, 02-006Warsaw, Poland

Chi-Hsuan Tsou and Chung-Ming Chen
Institute of Biomedical Engineering, College of Medicine and College of Engineering, National Taiwan University, No. 1, Section 1, Jen-Ai Road, Taipei 100, Taiwan

Yi-Chien Lu and Yeun-Chung Chang
Department of Radiology, National Taiwan University College of Medicine and Department of Medical Imaging, National Taiwan University Hospital, No. 7, Chung-Shan South Road, Taipei 100, Taiwan

Ang Yuan
Department of Internal Medicine, National Taiwan University College of Medicine, No. 7, Chung-Shan South Road, Taipei 100, Taiwan

Cassia Calixto-Campos, Mab P. Corrêa, Thacyana T. Carvalho, Ana C. Zarpelon, Miriam S. N. Hohmann, Ana C. Rossaneis, Leticia Coelho-Silva, Wander R. Pavanelli, Phileno Pinge-Filho, Jefferson Crespigio and Jr. Waldiceu A. Verri
Department of Pathology, Biological Sciences Centre, Londrina State University, Rodovia Celso Garcia Cid KM480 PR445, Caixa Postal 10.011, 86057-970 Londrina, PR, Brazil

Catia C. F. Bernardy
Department of Nursing, Health Science Centre, Londrina State University, Avenue Robert Koch 60, 86038-350 Londrina, PR, Brazil

Rubia Casagrande
Department of Pharmaceutical Sciences, Health Science Centre, Londrina State University, Avenue Robert Koch 60, 86038-350 Londrina, PR, Brazil

Yi-Cheng Chang
Graduate Institute of Medical Genomics and Proteomics, National Taiwan University, Taipei 100, Taiwan
Department of Internal Medicine and Center for Obesity, Lifestyle and Metabolic Surgery, National Taiwan University Hospital, Taipei 100, Taiwan
Institute of Biomedical Science, Academia Sinica, Taipei 100, Taiwan

Siow-Wey Hee
Department of Internal Medicine and Center for Obesity, Lifestyle and Metabolic Surgery, National Taiwan University Hospital, Taipei 100, Taiwan

Meng-Lun Hsieh
Graduate Institute of Medical Genomics and Proteomics, National Taiwan University, Taipei 100, Taiwan

Yung-Ming Jeng
Graduate Institute of Pathology, National Taiwan University, Taipei 100, Taiwan
Department of Pathology, National Taiwan University Hospital, Taipei 100, Taiwan

Lee-Ming Chuang
Department of Internal Medicine and Center for Obesity, Lifestyle and Metabolic Surgery, National Taiwan University Hospital, Taipei 100, Taiwan
College of Medicine, National Taiwan University, Taipei 100, Taiwan
Institute of Preventive Medicine, College of Public Health, National Taiwan University, Taipei 100, Taiwan

Sônia Cristina Almeida da Luz
Departamento de Patologia, Universidade Federal de Santa Maria (UFSM), Campus Universitário, Camobi, 97105-900 Santa Maria, RS, Brazil

Melissa Falster Daubermann
Serviço de Patologia, Hospital Universitário de Santa Maria (UFSM), Campus Universitário, Camobi, 97105-900 Santa Maria, RS, Brazil

Gustavo Roberto Thomé, Matheus Mülling dos Santos, Angelica Ramos, Gerson Torres Salazar, João Batista Teixeira da Rocha and Nilda Vargas Barbosa
Departamento de Bioquímica e Biologia Molecular, Universidade Federal de Santa Maria (UFSM), Campus Universitário, Camobi, 97105-900 Santa Maria, RS, Brazil

Kaouther Hadj Ayed Tka, Asma Mahfoudh Boussaid, Mohamed Amine Zaouali and Hassen Ben Abdennebi
Unit of Molecular Biology and Anthropology Applied to Development and Health (UR12ES11), Faculty of Pharmacy, University of Monastir, rue Avicenne, 5000 Monastir, Tunisia

Rym Kammoun and Sonia Ghoul Mazgar
Laboratory of Histology and Embryology, Faculty of Dental Medicine, University of Monastir, rue Avicenne, 5000 Monastir, Tunisia

Joan Rosello Catafau and Mohamed Bejaoui
Unit of Experimental Hepatic Ischemia-Reperfusion, Institute of Biomedical Investigations, Higher Council of Scientific Investigations, 08036 Barcelona, Spain

Yicheng Chen, Yanlan Yu, Liwei Xu, Youyun Zhang, Shicheng Yu, Gonghui Li and Zhigeng Zhang
Department of Urology, Sir Run-Run Shaw Hospital, College of Medicine, Zhejiang University, Hangzhou 310016, China

Yueping Wang
Department of Urology, Wuyi First People's Hospital, Zhejiang 321200, China

Rehab M. Samaka, Hayam A. Aiad, Mona A. Kandil, Nancy Y. Asaad and Nanes S. Holah
Pathology Department, Faculty of Medicine, Menoufia University, Shebin El-Kom, Egypt

Kenneth Maiese
Cellular and Molecular Signaling, Newark, NJ 07101, USA

Arif Malik, Misbah Sultana, Gulshan Parveen and Sulayman Waquar
Institute of Molecular Biology and Biotechnology (IMBB), The University of Lahore, Pakistan

Aamer Qazi and Mahmood Husain Qazi
Center for Research in Molecular Medicine (CRiMM), The University of Lahore, Pakistan

Abdul Basit Ashraf
University College of Medicine and Dentistry, The University of Lahore, Pakistan

Mahmood Rasool
Center of Excellence in Genomic Medicine Research (CEGMR), King Abdulaziz University, Jeddah, Saudi Arabia

Mei Lin
Clinical Medical Institute, Taizhou People's Hospital Affiliated to Nantong University, Taizhou, Jiangsu 225300, China
Medical School, Southeast University, Nanjing, Jiangsu 210009, China

Junxing Huang, Hong Yu, Yanhong Xiao, Yujuan Shi and Ting Guo
Clinical Medical Institute, Taizhou People's Hospital Affiliated to Nantong University, Taizhou, Jiangsu 225300, China

Dongsheng Zhang
Medical School, Southeast University, Nanjing, Jiangsu 210009, China
Jiangsu Key Laboratory for Biomaterials and Devices, Nanjing, Jiangsu 210009, China

Xingmao Jiang
Key Laboratory of Advanced Catalytic Material and Technology, Changzhou University, Changzhou, Jiangsu 213000, China

Jia Zhang
Medical School, Southeast University, Nanjing, Jiangsu 210009, China

Rene Franzen
Department of Conservative Dentistry, Periodontology and Preventive Dentistry, RWTHAachen University Hospital, Pauwelsstrasse 30, 52074 Aachen, Germany
AALZ Aachen Dental Laser Center, Center for Biomedical Technology, RWTH Aachen Campus, Pauwelsstrasse 17, 52074 Aachen, Germany

Nasrin Kianimanesh and Asma Ahmed
AALZ Aachen Dental Laser Center, Center for Biomedical Technology, RWTH Aachen Campus, Pauwelsstrasse 17, 52074 Aachen, Germany

Rudolf Marx
Medical Material Science, RWTH Aachen University Hospital, Pauwelsstrasse 30, 52074 Aachen, Germany

Norbert Gutknecht
Department of Conservative Dentistry, Periodontology and Preventive Dentistry, RWTHAachen University Hospital, Pauwelsstrasse 30, 52074 Aachen, Germany

Kallirroi Voudouri, Aikaterini Berdiaki, George N. Tzanakakis and Dragana Nikitovic
Laboratory of Anatomy-Histology-Embryology, School of Medicine, University of Crete, 71003 Heraklion, Greece

Maria Tzardi
Laboratory of Pathology, School of Medicine, University of Crete, 71003 Heraklion, Greece

Alex Stepan, Cristiana Simionescu, Raluca Ciurea and Claudiu Margaritescu
Department of Pathology, University of Medicine and Pharmacy of Craiova, Petru Rares Street 2, Dolj, 200349 Craiova, Romania

Daniel Pirici
Department of Pathology, University of Medicine and Pharmacy of Craiova, Petru Rares Street 2, Dolj, 200349 Craiova, Romania
Department of Research Methodology, University of Medicine and Pharmacy of Craiova, Petru Rares Street 2, Dolj, 200349 Craiova, Romania

Matthias Bartneck, Klaudia Theresa Warzecha, Felix Heymann, Christian Trautwein and Frank Tacke
Department of Medicine III, RWTH University Hospital Aachen, Pauwelsstrasse 30, 52074 Aachen, Germany

Ralf Weiskirchen
Institute of Molecular Pathobiochemistry, Experimental GeneTherapy and Clinical Chemistry, RWTH University Hospital Aachen, Pauwelsstrasse 30, 52074 Aachen, Germany

Carmen Gabriele Tag and Sibille Sauer-Lehnen
Department of Medicine III, RWTH University Hospital Aachen, Pauwelsstrasse 30, 52074 Aachen, Germany
Institute of Molecular Pathobiochemistry, Experimental GeneTherapy and Clinical Chemistry, RWTH University Hospital Aachen, Pauwelsstrasse 30, 52074 Aachen, Germany

Zaneta Swiderska
Warsaw University of Technology, Pl. Politechniki 1, 00-661Warsaw, Poland

Anna Korzynska, Anna Wesolowska and Lukasz Roszkowiak
Nalecz Institute of Biocybernetics and Biomedical Engineering PAS, Trojdena 4, 02-109Warsaw, Poland

Tomasz Markiewicz
Warsaw University of Technology, Pl. Politechniki 1, 00-661Warsaw, Poland
Military Institute of Medicine, Szaserow 128, 04-141Warsaw, Poland

Malgorzata Lorent, Janina Slodkowska and Bartlomiej Grala
Military Institute of Medicine, Szaserow 128, 04-141Warsaw, Poland

Jakub Zak
Warsaw University of Technology, Pl. Politechniki 1, 00-661Warsaw, Poland
Nalecz Institute of Biocybernetics and Biomedical Engineering PAS, Trojdena 4, 02-109Warsaw, Poland

Yan Yan Wang, Yi Wen Yang, Xiang You, Xiao Qian Deng, Chun Fang Hu, Cong Zhu, Jun Yao Wang, Jiao Jiao Gu, Yi Nan Wang and Qing Li
Department of Immunology, Basic Medicine Science, Medical College, Xiamen University, Xiamen 361102, China

Feng Guang Gao
Department of Immunology, Basic Medicine Science, Medical College, Xiamen University, Xiamen 361102, China
The State Key Laboratory for Oncogenes and Related Genes, Shanghai Jiao Tong University, Shanghai 200032, China

Danilo Pagliari and Rossella Cianci
Institute of Internal Medicine, Catholic University of the Sacred Heart, Largo A. Gemelli 8, 00168 Rome, Italy

Francesco Ciro Tamburrelli and Gianfranco Zirio
Institute of Orthopedics, Catholic University of the Sacred Heart, Largo A. Gemelli 8, 00168 Rome, Italy

Estelle E. Newton
CytoCure LLC, 100 Cummings Center, Suite 430C, Beverly, MA 01915, USA

www.ingramcontent.com/pod-product-compliance
Lightning Source LLC
Chambersburg PA
CBHW080250230326
41458CB00097B/4241

9781632424556